PROGRESS IN BRAIN RESEARCH

VOLUME 67

VISCERAL SENSATION

Recent volumes in PROGRESS IN BRAIN RESEARCH

Volume 46: Membrane Morphology of the Vertebrate Nervous System. A Study with Freeze-etch Technique, by C. Sandri, J. M. Van Buren and K. Akert — *revised edition* — 1982

Volume 53: Adaptive Capabilities of the Nervous System, by P. S. McConnell, G. J. Boer, H. J. Romijn, N. E. Van de Poll and M. A. Corner (Eds.) — 1980

Volume 54: Motivation, Motor and Sensory Processes of the Brain: Electrical Potentials, Behaviour and Clinical Use, by H. H. Kornhuber and L. Deecke (Eds.) — 1980

Volume 55: Chemical Transmission in the Brain. The Role of Amines, Amino Acids and Peptides, by R. M. Buijs, P. Pévet and D. F. Swaab (Eds.) — 1982

Volume 56: Brain Phosphoproteins, Characterization and Function, by W. H. Gispen and A. Routtenberg (Eds.) — 1982

Volume 57: Descending Pathways to the Spinal Cord, by H. G. J. M. Kuypers and G. F. Martin (Eds.) — 1982

Volume 58: Molecular and Cellular Interactions Underlying Higher Brain Functions, by J.-P. Changeux, J. Glowinksi, M. Imbert and F. E. Bloom (Eds.) — 1983

Volume 59: Immunology of Nervous System Infections, by P. O. Behan, V. Ter Meulen and F. Clifford Rose (Eds.) — 1983

Volume 60: The Neurohypophysis: Structure, Function and Control, by B. A. Cross and G. Leng (Eds.) — 1983

Volume 61: Sex Differences in the Brain: The Relation Between Structure and Function, by G. J. De Vries, J. P. C. De Bruin, H. B. M. Uylings and M. A. Corner (Eds.) — 1984

Volume 62: Brain Ischemia: Quantitative EEG and Imaging Techniques, by G. Pfurtscheller, E. J. Jonkman and F. H. Lopes da Silva — 1984

Volume 63: Molecular Mechanisms of Ischemic Brain Damage, by K. Kogure, K.-A. Hossmann, B. K. Siesjö and F. A. Welsh (Eds.) — 1985

Volume 64: The Oculomotor and Skeletal Motor Systems: Differences and Similarities, by H.-J. Freund, U. Büttner, B. Cohen and J. Noth (Eds.) — 1986

Volume 65: Psychiatric Disorders: Neurotransmitters and Neuropeptides, by J. M. Van Ree and S. Matthysse (Eds.) — 1986

Volume 66: Peptides and Neurological Disease, by P. C. Emson, M. N. Rossor and M. Tohyama (Eds.) — 1986

Volume 67: Visceral Sensation, by F. Cervero and J. F. B. Morrison (Eds.) — 1986

Volume 68: Coexistence of Neuronal Messengers — A New Principle in Chemical Transmission, by T. G. M. Hökfelt, K. Fuxe and B. Pernow (Eds.) — 1986

PROGRESS IN BRAIN RESEARCH

VOLUME 67

VISCERAL SENSATION

F. CERVERO

Department of Physiology, University of Bristol Medical School, University Walk, Bristol BS8 1TD, U.K.

and

J. F. B. MORRISON

Department of Physiology, University of Leeds Medical School, Leeds LS2 9TJ, U.K.

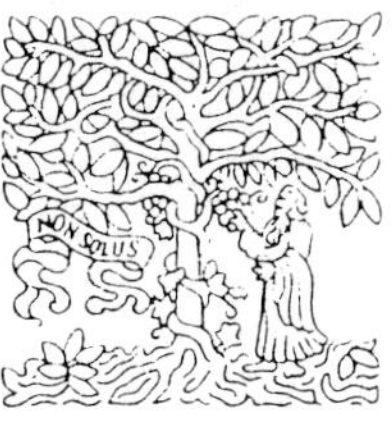

ELSEVIER
AMSTERDAM – NEW YORK – OXFORD
1986

ISBN 0-444-80757-8 (volume)
ISBN 0-444-80104-9 (series)

Published by:
Elsevier Science Publishers B.V. (Biomedical Division)
P.O. Box 211
1000 AE Amsterdam
The Netherlands

Sole distributors for the USA and Canada:
Elsevier Science Publishing Company, Inc.
52 Vanderbilt Avenue
New York, NY 10017
USA

Library of Congress Cataloging in Publication Data

Visceral sensation.

(Progress in brain research; v. 67)
"Originates from a Symposium on "Visceral Sensation" that took place in Bristol in February 1985 ... organized by the Physiological Society" — Pref.
Includes bibliographies and index.
1. Senses and sensation — Congresses. 2. Viscera — Innervation — Congresses. 3. Afferent pathways — Congresses. 4. Sensory-motor integration — Congresses. I. Cervero, Fernando. II. Morrison, J. F. B. (John Finlay Benzie). III. Physiological Society (Great Britain). IV. Symposium on "Visceral Sensation" (1985: Bristol, Avon). V. Series. [DNLM: 1. Afferent Pathways — congresses. 2. Central Nervous System — congresses. 3. Sensation — physiology — congresses. W1 PR667J v.67 / WL 702 V822 1985]
QP376.P7 vol. 67 612′.82 s [612′.8] 86-2160
[QP435]
ISBN 0-444-80757-8 (U.S.)

Printed in The Netherlands

List of Contributors

W. S. Ammons, Department of Physiology and Biophysics, University of Oklahoma Health Sciences Centre, P.O. Box 26901, Oklahoma City, OK 73190, U.S.A.

P. L. R. Andrews, Department of Physiology, St. George's Hospital Medical School, Cranmer Terrace, London SW17 0RE, U.K.

R. W. Blair, Department of Physiology and Biophysics, University of Oklahoma Health Sciences Centre, P.O. Box 26901, Oklahoma City, OK 73190, U.S.A.

F. Cervero, Department of Physiology, University of Bristol Medical School, University Walk, Bristol BS8 1TD, U.K.

W. C. De Groat, Department of Pharmacology, University of Pittsburgh, School of Medicine, 518 Scaife Hall, Pittsburgh, PA 15261, U.S.A.

G. J. Dockray, M.R.C. Secretory Control Research Group, Physiological Laboratory, University of Liverpool, Brownlow Hill, P.O. Box 147, Liverpool L69 3BX, U.K.

R. D. Foreman, Department of Physiology and Biophysics, University of Oklahoma Health Sciences Centre, P.O. Box 26901, Oklahoma City, OK 73190, U.S.A.

H. Higashi, Department of Physiology, Kurume University School of Medicine, Kurume 830, Japan.

A. Iggo, Department of Veterinary Physiology, Royal (Dick) School of Veterinary Studies, University of Edinburgh, Summerhall, Edinburgh EH9 1QH, U.K.

W. Jänig, Physiological Institute, Christian-Albrechts University, Olshausenstrasse 40, D-2300 Kiel, F.R.G.

D. Jordan, Department of Physiology, Royal Free Hospital School of Medicine, Rowland Hill Street, London NW3 2PF, U.K.

T. Kumazawa, Department of Nervous and Sensory Functions, The Research Institute of Environmental Medicine, Nagoya University, Furo-cho, Chikusa-ku, Nagoya 464, Japan.

F. Lombardi, Institute of Cardiovascular Research, C.N.R., Pathological Medicine, "Fidia" Centre, "L. Sacco" Hospital, University of Milan, Milan, Italy.

B. M. Lumb, Department of Physiology, University of Leeds Medical School, Leeds LS2 9TJ, U.K.

A. Malliani, Institute of Cardiovascular Research, C.N.R., Pathological Medicine, "Fidia" Centre, "L. Sacco" Hospital, University of Milan, Milan, Italy.

M. Maresca, Institute of Clinical Medicine I, University of Florence, Viale G. B. Morgagni 85, 50134 Florence, Italy.

S. B. McMahon, Sherrington School of Physiology, St. Thomas's Hospital Medical School, London SE1 7EH, U.K.

J. F. B. Morrison, Department of Physiology, University of Leeds Medical School, Leeds LS2 9TJ, U.K.

M. Pagani, Institute of Cardiovascular Research, C.N.R., Pathological Medicine, "Fidia" Centre, "L. Sacco" Hospital, University of Milan, Milan, Italy.

A. S. Paintal, D.S.T. Centre for Visceral Mechanisms, Vallabhbhai Patel Chest Institute, University of Delhi, Delhi 110007, India.

P. Procacci, Institute of Clinical Medicine I, University of Florence, Viale G. B. Morgagni 85, 50134 Florence, Italy.

K. A. Sharkey, Department of Physiology, University of Bristol Medical School, University Walk, Bristol BS8 1TD, U.K.

K. M. Spyer, Department of Physiology, Royal Free Hospital School of Medicine, Rowland Hill Street, London NW3 2PF, U.K.

J. E. H. Tattersall, Department of Physiology, University of Bristol Medical School, University Walk, Bristol BS8 1TD, U.K.

J. G. Widdicombe, Department of Physiology, St. George's Hospital Medical School, Cranmer Terrace, London SW17 0RE, U.K.

W. D. Willis Jr., Marine Biomedical Institute and Departments of Anatomy and of Physiology and Biophysics, University of Texas Medical Branch, 200 University Boulevard, Galveston, TX 77550-2772, U.S.A.

M. Zoppi, Institute of Clinical Medicine I, University of Florence, Viale G. B. Morgagni 85, 50134 Florence, Italy.

Preface

The last few years have witnessed a considerable surge of scientific interest in the neural mechanisms of visceral sensation, reflected in the fact that many laboratories throughout the world are now actively studying various aspects of visceral sensory systems. New and detailed information has been obtained on the types of sensory receptor activated by natural forms of visceral stimulation, which has helped in assessing whether or not visceral sensory receptors encode information by an "intensity" mechanism. The mode of termination of visceral afferent fibres within the central nervous system has been studied in considerable detail using neuroanatomical tracing techniques, and the functional organisation of viscero-somatic convergence in the spinal cord and brain stem has also been the object of extensive investigations. In addition, research on the pharmacology and neurochemistry of visceral afferent fibres and on the functional role of putative neurotransmitters used by visceral sensory pathways has thrown new light on the involvement of gut peptides in the regulation of visceral function.

The time has now come to take stock of all these recent advances and to extract from the mass of accumulated data the experimental findings that have changed the direction of research in this field. This reappraisal will also help in assessing what progress has been made in our knowledge of the neurophysiological mechanisms of visceral sensation.

This book originates from a symposium on "Visceral sensation" that took place in Bristol in February, 1985. The symposium was organised by The Physiological Society and attracted some 120 members of the Society and guests, who listened to and actively discussed with the eight main speakers. In addition, some of the participants in the symposium presented poster communications with their more recent data. Because of the lack of comprehensive publications on the topic of visceral sensation, we felt that rather than editing a simple proceedings account of the symposium, it would be more helpful to produce a multi-author book that included contributions not only by those who attended the symposium but also by active researchers in this field who had not been present at the meeting.

The intention of this book is to review those aspects of the neural mechanisms of visceral sensation which have been the subject of recent experimental studies. We realise that this approach will exclude some important facets of this area of knowledge, most notably those related to the psychological and perceptual components of visceral sensory experiences. This is only a reflection of the state of physiological knowledge on visceral sensory mechanisms and we hope that these gaps will be adequately filled in the not very distant future.

The contributions to this book have been divided into those that discuss visceral afferent systems and those that deal with CNS organisation of visceral sensory pathways. In addition, three introductory chapters have been grouped in a section where the reader will find reviews of basic ideas and concepts about visceral sensation. This introductory section includes chapters by A. S. Paintal and A. Iggo, to whom we owe much of our physiological knowledge on visceral sensory receptors, and a contribution by P. Procacci and his colleagues, who discuss normal and abnormal sensory perceptions from viscera in the context of their vast clinical experience.

The section on visceral afferent systems includes several chapters that survey the innervation of most internal organs, and two contributions that deal with the neurochemical and pharmacological approaches to the study of visceral afferent fibres. A central element of discussion in many of the chapters that review CNS mechanisms of visceral sensation is whether the reflex and unconscious control of internal organs shares a common organisation with the systems that mediate the perception of visceral sensation. This is still an unresolved question that perhaps can be best analysed by the study of viscera whose reflex activity is under substantial central control and from which a variety of sensory experiences can be evoked. The urinary bladder, the heart and the respiratory system come to mind as potential candidates for such studies.

Like most active and developing fields of science, ours is not free from conflictive interpretations of the experimental data or from controversial hypotheses and disputed functional models. We firmly believe that rational arguments based on sound and carefully made experimental observations will always stand the test of time. Therefore, we have not imposed an editorial line on our contributors nor have we chosen to ignore the views of those who disagree with ours. All authors have freely expressed their ideas, so that the reader will be able to judge the coherence of the arguments and the strength of the experimental observations that back every hypothesis.

The symposium from which this book originated was made possible thanks to the generosity of some medical charities and of members of the pharmaceutical industry. It is a pleasure to acknowledge the financial support given by the Physiological Society, the Wellcome Trust, Merck Sharp and Dohme, Smith Kline and French, Glaxo group, Beecham Pharmaceuticals and Parke-Davis. We also thank Elsevier Publications for offering the vehicle of this series for our book and, in particular, the editorial help of Dr. N. J. Spiteri.

Ten years ago, Elsevier published a volume in the series Progress in Brain Research, entitled "Somato-sensory and visceral receptor mechanisms", which covered some of the aspects of visceral sensation dealt with in the present volume. It is interesting to compare some of the observations reported then with the updates of the present book in order to realise how much this field has advanced in 10 years. We are quite sure that a substantial number of the new observations reported in this volume will still form the core of a future publication in 10 years time.

F. Cervero
J. F. B. Morrison

Contents

Section III — Central Nervous System Mechanisms of Visceral Sensation

SECTION I

Basic Ideas on Visceral Sensation

F. Cervero and J. F.B. Morrison
Progress in Brain Research, Vol. 67

CHAPTER 1

The visceral sensations — some basic mechanisms

A. S. Paintal

D.S.T. Centre for Visceral Mechanisms, Vallabhbhai Patel Chest Institute, University of Delhi, Delhi 110007, India

Introduction

Compared to the considerable amount of information on the special and cutaneous senses, the amount of information available about the sensations from the viscera, i.e., breathlessness, satiation of hunger and thirst, bladder and rectal fullness, is very small. Perhaps the reason for this is that man could go through life without noticing any visceral sensations. Thus, this field held little excitement for physiologists as well as clinicians, except when it came to determining the mechanisms underlying the origin of pain in various visceral diseases. Moreover, ever since the early observations on the genesis of pain reviewed in the classical monograph on pain by Lewis (1942), the view that has been held is that the viscera are remarkably insensitive.

Interest in the visceral sensations has lagged behind the interest in the detailed study and analysis of the pattern of flow of sensory impulses in the nerve fibres of sensory receptors, beginning with the classical paper on pulmonary stretch receptors by Adrian (1933) and the papers on arterial baroreceptors (Bronk and Stella, 1932, 1935) and chemoreceptors (Euler et al., 1939, 1941). A wealth of information on the sensory systems of lungs, heart and the gastrointestinal tract accumulated in the fifties and sixties, following the introduction of greatly simplified techniques for dissecting single units and determining the conduction velocities of individual fibres. However, all this information did not stimulate enquiries into the sensations produced by these receptors in a manner comparable to the interest in the somato-sensory system.

It was only in 1980 that a short symposium on "Visceral Sensory Mechanisms and Sensations" was held during the International Physiological Congress at Budapest, and the present symposium volume is actually the first serious attempt to take stock of what is known about the subject.

The visceral sensations experienced normally are breathlessness during exercise, the immediate satiation of hunger and thirst, bladder fullness and rectal fullness. These sensations are experienced apparently also by animals, as shown by their behaviour. In addition, man experiences the sensations associated with hunger pangs, for which the sensory mechanism has yet to be determined. Another sensation whose peripheral mechanism has yet to be determined is nausea, which although not a normal sensation, occurs in man and apparently must occur in animals, who also vomit. Cough is the result of sensation of irritation in the throat. This sensation can also be regarded as a normal sensation as it constitutes the afferent limb of a protective reflex and is experienced fairly frequently by both man and animals during imperfect deglutition. The other sensations, such as choking, anginal pain, biliary, gastric, intestinal and renal colics and pleural pain, are nociceptive and occur under pathological conditions.

Value of chemical stimulation of receptors for studying visceral sensations

The great usefulness of chemical substances for locating and studying visceral sensory receptors is now well known (see Paintal, 1973, 1981a). However, it is not generally known that chemical stimulation of receptors can also be of great value for studying visceral sensations. This fact has been brought to light in connection with a recent investigation on various sensations produced by J receptors (Paintal, 1983a,b) and will be elaborated below as the approach may be of value in future investigations.

Use of lobeline

In the past, lobeline injected intravenously has been used as a method for determining the circulation time (Lilienfeld and Berliner, 1942). With the advent of cardiac catheterization for evaluating cardiovascular performance, the determination of circulation time with chemical indicator substances such as lobeline fell into disuse. Before this finally occurred, Hillis and Kelly (1951) tried to determine the origin of cough following lobeline injections, by applying local anaesthesia on the pharynx and larynx, injection of various drugs, and general anaesthesia. In the same year Eckenhoff and Comroe (1951) reported that the substernal burning pain following intravenous injections of lobeline was probably due to stimulation of pain endings in the pleura. Subsequently, Beven and Murray (1963) and Stern et al. (1966) concluded that cough and other effects were due to the stimulation of certain mechanoreceptors, then thought to be located in the wall of the pulmonary artery (see Paintal, 1972). Subsequently, after it became known that lobeline stimulated the J receptors of cats (Paintal, 1971b), Jain et al. (1972) used it for studying the reflex effects of J receptors in man. They rightly attributed the apnoea following injection of lobeline, into the pulmonary artery of their subjects, as being due to the stimulation of J receptors. However, they were reluctant to attribute the cough and the accompanying sensations that followed injections of lobeline to impulses from J receptors because stimulation of these receptors had not been known to produce cough in anaesthetized animals (see Paintal, 1973). This was a powerful argument, which misled several investigators. However, there could be no doubt that the observations of Jain et al. (1972) and Stern et al. (1966) showed clearly that only receptors upstream from the left ventricle were involved in producing cough, leading to the inevitable conclusion that the J receptors must be responsible for the cough after injection of lobeline into the pulmonary artery (or intravenously) of man. This conclusion was presented at a symposium held in Philadelphia in 1976 (Paintal, 1977b) but it did not arouse sufficient interest and was largely ignored, perhaps because lobeline was an unnatural stimulus and it could not be linked with normal sensations as it had not been established at that time that J receptors could be stimulated in normal men at sea level. That this must be so became clear later on when it was found that in cats, at sea level, doubling pulmonary blood flow, as would be expected to occur in moderate exercise, clearly stimulates J receptors to levels of activity (Fig. 1A) that produce marked reflex effects, e.g., inhibition of somatic muscles (Fig. 1B) (Anand and Paintal, 1980).

Correlation of effects of chemical stimulation with effects of natural stimulation

The J receptors are intensely stimulated during pulmonary oedema (Fig. 1C) (Paintal, 1969, 1970), which also occurs not infrequently in man at high altitude. Therefore, the possibility that cough could be a consequence of natural stimulation of J receptors was considered and the available data on the effects of lobeline (Hillis and Kelly, 1951; Eckenhoff and Comroe, 1951; Bevan and Murray, 1963; Jain et al., 1972) compared with the available data on the effects of high-altitude pulmonary oedema (HAPO) (Hultgren et al., 1961; Menon, 1965). From this it became evident that the effects of lobeline were in some ways similar to the effects of HAPO, not only with regard to cough but also with regard to the sensation of substernal pain. Unfortunately, the earlier data relating to HAPO were complicated by the fact that the HAPO patients had fever and infection, i.e., the patients could have had

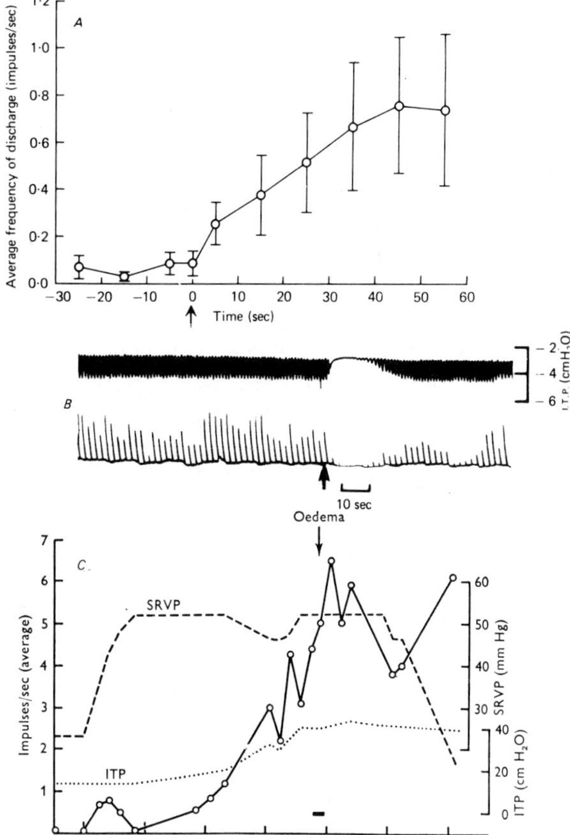

Fig. 1. Two levels of activity, generated by natural stimulation in J receptors of cats and their reflex effects. A shows the development of average activity in ten J receptors in the right lung (of five cats) following increase in pulmonary blood flow, in the right lung, by 133%, by occluding the left pulmonary artery at the arrow. Vertical bars represent standard errors. Note that the activity plateaued at 0.75 impulses/second. Activity of this intensity generated by injecting 18 μg/kg phenyl diguanide into the right atrium at arrow in B resulted in the marked respiratory reflex effects (upper trace = intrathoracic pressure) and also marked inhibition of the knee jerk elicited every 2 seconds (lower trace). Note the prolonged depression of the knee jerk after the injection (from Anand and Paintal, 1980). C shows the intense activity in another J receptor following pulmonary oedema produced by injecting alloxan at arrow. Note that the ordinate in C is ten times greater than in A. Also note the gradual reduction in pulmonary compliance, as shown by the rise in the intrathoracic pressure curve (ITP). The curve with dashed lines represents systolic right ventricular pressure (SRVP) (from Paintal, 1969).

upper respiratory tract infection and the cough could have been due to this. In order to exclude this possibility, the symptoms accompanying HAPO in apparently normal individuals were studied on the one hand and, on the other, the sensations produced by lobeline were re-examined. The data relating to HAPO, reported briefly earlier (Paintal, 1983a), are given in Table I.

The 36 subjects of Table I were selected from a group of 72 young males, mostly between the ages of 18 and 30, who had developed HAPO within 12–96 hours of arrival by air at a height of 3,200 m and were kept under close observation. 36 of the 72 subjects were excluded from further study as they showed evidence of some infection, i.e., raised body temperature (37.5–38°C) or body ache. The remaining 36 subjects (Table I) had no fever, bodyache, rhinitis or pharyngitis but they had HAPO, as established by physical signs, radiographs of the chest and the fact that all of them improved or were cured within a few hours or a day following standard treatment for HAPO, which consisted of rest, intravenous injections of furosemide, oxygen and morphine.

As shown in Table I, most of these 36 otherwise normal subjects complained of dry cough, dyspnoea, and pain in the chest, and since upper respiratory tract infection had been excluded in all of them, it followed that the dry cough and pain in the chest must have been due to impulses from J recep-

TABLE I

Frequency of complaints of cough, pain in the chest and breathlessness in 36 otherwise normal subjects with HAPO

Symptom	Frequency	
	Number	% of total (36)
Cough	35	97
Dry cough[a]	27	75
Pain in the chest	26	72
Breathlessness	31	86

[a] 10 out of these 27 cases (37%) did not complain of cough at the first clinical examination that took place, 1 or 2 hours before the second examination.

tors, which are known to be intensely stimulated during pulmonary oedema (Paintal, 1969, 1970; Coleridge, H. M. and Coleridge, 1977; Coleridge, J. C. G. and Coleridge, 1984). Impulses in pulmonary stretch receptors (as the cause of cough) can be excluded as they are not obviously stimulated during pulmonary oedema (Paintal, 1969) and because deep inspiration which stimulates them intensely never gives rise to cough. Similarly, as pointed out earlier (Paintal, 1977a), marked stimulation of the rapidly adapting receptors does not produce any unpleasant sensations. In fact, it can be readily demonstrated by repeated forced expiration at a frequency of 120/minute from functional residual capacity level, so as to generate a high-frequency discharge greater than 200/second in the rapidly adapting receptors (see Fig. 14 in Widdicombe, 1954), that no feeling of irritation in the throat or a desire to cough develops. Finally, the C-fibre bronchial receptors are little, if at all, stimulated during pulmonary oedema (Coleridge and Coleridge, 1977).

An interesting feature of Table I is that 37% of the subjects did not complain of cough at the first clinical examination, which shows that the cough and the sensations associated with it (attributable to impulses in J receptors) did not constitute an unusual feature prominent enough to complain of. From this it can be concluded that the sensations (and cough) produced by impulses in J receptors are similar to that produced by irritation of the upper airways, e.g., in upper respiratory tract infections. Thus, a dry cough in the absence of upper respiratory airways inflammation must be regarded with suspicion as it may originate at the alveolar level.

Is the cough of J receptor origin a reflex?

The cough following lobeline injection (i.e., sudden burst of impulses in J receptors) is preceded by sensations in the throat and upper chest (Paintal, 1983b). This was confirmed by injecting small doses (<1 mg) of lobeline intravenously, when it was found that sensations in the throat and upper chest appeared without any cough in one subject (A. Anand, A. S. Paintal and A. Guz, unpublished observations), and subsequently confirmed by Raj (1984) in many more subjects studied systematically with various doses of lobeline injected intravenously. The sensations, depending on the dose and the sensitivity of the individuals, are variously described as a feeling of itching, tickling, irritation, choking, suffocation, fumes, smoke or cold air in the throat. Several individuals have likened the sensation to that which they perceive during exercise (Raj, 1984). The threshold dose for producing cough is about 1 mg in most individuals. In two schizophrenic patients the dose was found to be more than 4 times greater in repeated trials (S. Haq, A. S. Paintal and S. Sharma, unpublished observations). This is to be expected as even the threshold for pain is raised in such patients, as indicated by the reduced affective responses in them. Thus, it is certain that the primary effect of impulses from J receptors is to produce irritating sensations in the throat and that man tries to remove them by coughing or clearing his throat. Therefore, the cough is not a reflex act following J receptor stimulation and so it is understandable why no cough is produced in cats, rabbits and dogs, even following intense inputs from J receptors. The sensations are not secondary to constriction of the larynx produced by J receptors (Stransky et al., 1973; Rex and Paintal, 1983) as the sensations are present in laryngectomized patients following lobeline injections (Jain, 1980).

Pain through J receptor inputs

It is known that impulses from J receptors produce pain referred to the chest (Paintal, 1983a). This information has been brought into the limelight through the use of a chemical substance, notably lobeline, and it was first reported by Eckenhoff and Comroe (1951), who used large doses of lobeline (5.0–7.5 mg) and concluded that the pain originated in the pleura. Their observations relating to pain

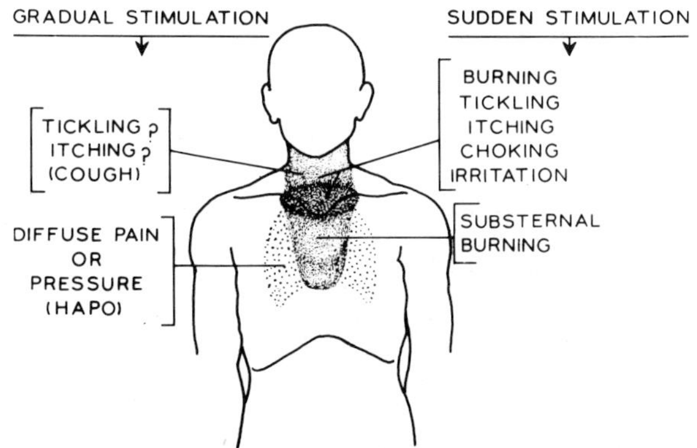

Fig. 2. The kinds of sensations produced by J receptors and the regions to which they are referred. Note the qualitative difference between the sensations produced by sudden stimulation by lobeline on the right and by gradual stimulation during HAPO on the left. See text for source of data.

were subsequently confirmed by Bevan and Murray (1963) and Jain et al. (1972). The pain was described as substernal burning, and its approximate location is shown in Fig. 2. The fact that this is not merely a physiological curiosity but is an important feature is indicated by the fact that it occurs in HAPO in otherwise normal individuals (Table I). As shown in Table I, about 72% of otherwise normal individuals complained of pain, which was felt as a dull ache substernally and on either side of the sternum. It is important to note that the level of activity in J receptors at which pain was produced following injections of lobeline must have been small because apnoea (index of J receptor stimulation, see Anand and Paintal, 1980) was either absent or was of short duration (Bevan and Murray, 1963; Jain et al., 1972). It follows that activity in J receptors does not necessarily have to be intense in order to produce pain.

Location of sensations

The locations of various sensations produced by J receptors are summarized in Fig. 2, which also shows the qualitative differences in the sensations resulting from sudden or gradual stimulation by lobeline and HAPO, respectively. Following sudden and intense stimulation by injecting 5–7.5 mg lobeline, 86% of the subjects (seven) of Eckenhoff and Comroe reported substernal burning and discomfort. On the other hand, because they used much smaller doses, only 16% of the subjects (18) of Jain et al. (1972) reported this sensation. Fig. 2 shows that gradual stimulation by HAPO produces diffuse pain or pressure in the chest substernally or on either side of the chest. It also shows that the HAPO subjects (Table I) obviously must have had the sensations of throat irritation, as indicated by (?) in Fig. 2, before developing the urge to cough, but they did not complain of them, just as several of them did not even complain of cough itself, as they apparently did not regard it as a significant feature.

Other possible uses of chemical substances

The approach involving the use of a chemical substance in evaluating the sensations of J receptors described above can also be of value in the case of other receptors. For example, in the case of gastric or intestinal receptors it should be possible to stimulate them selectively with chemical substances (e.g., phenyl diguanide, capsaicin) with the help of balloon-tipped catheters.

Another use is in studying in more detail the sensations generated during hyperventilation resulting from sudden stimulation of carotid and aortic chemoreceptors. In this connection, using lobeline and phenyl diguanide, Stern et al. (1966) and Jain et al. (1972) noted that impulses from the chemoreceptors did not produce any primary sensations, even though they had been stimulated sufficiently to give rise to marked hyperpnoea. All that the subjects of Jain et al. (1972) reported after injection of phenyl diguanide was that the only sensation felt was that of being forced to breathe deeply. They denied breathlessness. Although this is consistent with the fact that hypoxia does not produce any unpleasant sensations, even though ventilation may be increased considerably (Guz et al., 1966), there is sufficient justification to repeat the observations because it is most interesting that the respiratory

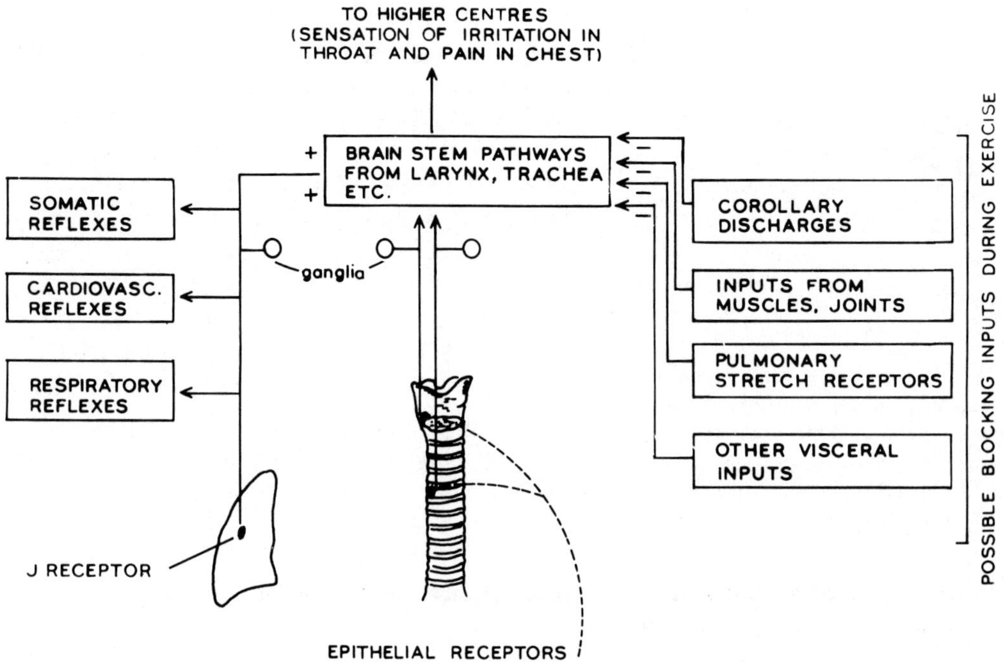

Fig. 3. Possible mechanism that could operate normally during exercise for blocking the referred sensations of throat irritation and pain in chest produced by J receptors at rest (by lobeline or HAPO). Note that intense activity is not an essential requirement for producing pain. See text for details.

stimulation produced by chemoreceptor inputs lacks the unpleasant features of the respiratory drive produced by J receptor inputs during HAPO, such as breathlessness, sensations of irritation in the throat and pain in the upper chest (see above).

Mechanisms that block sensations

An important point that has emerged is that all the referred sensations produced by sudden or gradual stimulation of J receptors (Fig. 2) are not experienced by most people when their J receptors are considerably stimulated, such as during moderate or severe exercise (see Anand and Paintal, 1980), when pulmonary blood flow increases several-fold. The conclusion follows that at some point(s) in the central pathways a block occurs (Paintal, 1983a). Although the precise mechanisms of the block are not known, certain possible mechanisms are suggested in Fig. 3. It is possible that the extensive flow of impulses from pulmonary stretch receptors resulting from the greatly increased ventilation could inhibit the inputs from the J receptors, as has been observed in the case of phrenic activity (unpublished observations). Inputs from muscles and joints could constitute the basic blocking mechanism and other visceral inputs may also be involved. Finally, corollary discharges may play an important part in producing the block. On the other hand, it is also possible that since the general pain threshold is raised during exercise (Clark et al., 1983) the block of J receptor-produced sensation is part of the generalized rise in threshold for nociception.

J receptors are not nociceptors

It must be noted that because the J receptors can produce pain under abnormal conditions in the absence of normally active blocking mechanisms, it

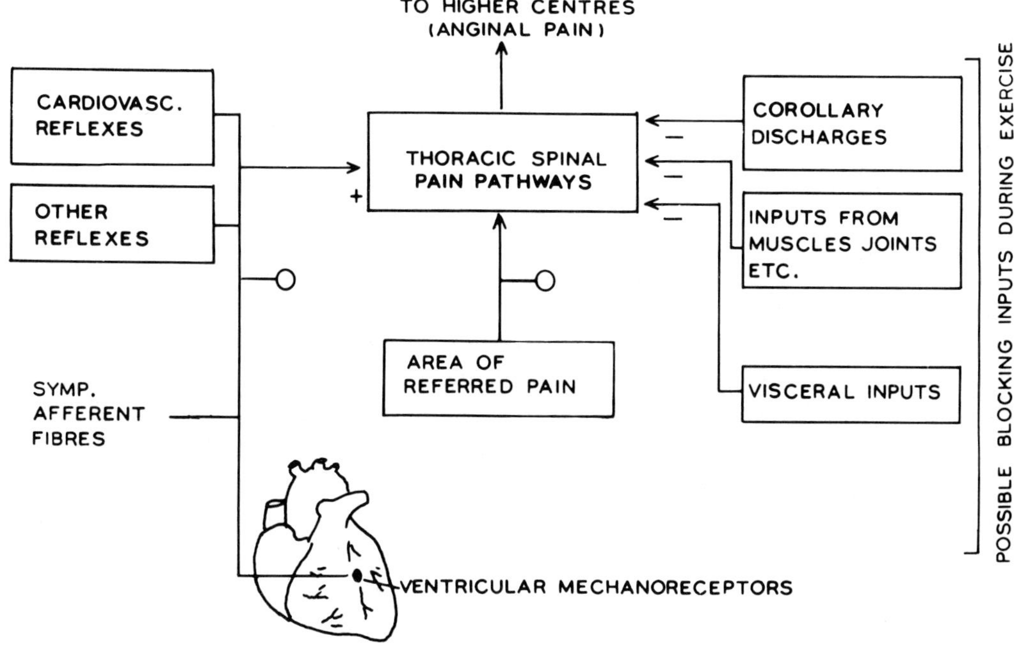

Fig. 4. Suggested mechanism that could operate normally during exercise for blocking the referred sensations of anginal pain by ventricular receptors when stimulated at rest during cardiac ischaemia.

does not follow that they are part of a nociceptive system. From what is known so far they are mechanoreceptors whose natural stimulus is increase in interstitial volume following increasing in pulmonary capillary pressure (Fig. 1A,C).

Possible mechanisms of anginal pain

The clear evidence showing that normally non-nociceptive impulses from J receptors can produce pain in the absence of blocking inputs generated during exercise ("exercise inputs") raises important questions regarding the occurrence of pain through non-nociceptive inputs under abnormal conditions from other viscera, notably the heart. It is possible that here also inputs from ventricular receptors normally are prevented from activating the thoracic segmental pain pathways by "exercise inputs". On the other hand, when the same pain pathways are activated, at rest during cardiac ischaemia by the ventricular receptors in the absence of "exercise inputs", the well-known pain of cardiac ischaemia results. A scheme showing how this could happen is shown in Fig. 4. It is known that activity in the ventricular mechanoreceptors with sympathetic medullated and non-medullated fibres is increased following coronary occlusion (Brown, 1967; Malliani et al., 1973; Uchida and Murao, 1974; and see Malliani, 1982). It is also known that the activity in these receptors also increases when intraventricular pressure is increased (see Malliani, 1982). Thus, there must be greatly increased input from various ventricular receptors during exercise, when the force of contraction and heart rate increases greatly. (Increase in heart rate alone can double or triple the input from ventricular receptors.) This level of activity would be expected to be far greater than that during coronary occlusion, which appears to be only twice the resting activity (see Malliani, 1982). As in the case of J receptor inputs, it is possible that the increased inputs from the ventricular receptors during exercise are prevented from activating the pain-producing pathways in the thoracic region of the spinal cord by the greatly increased impulse traffic from other sources, such as muscles and joints, other visceral inputs (e.g., pulmonary stretch receptors and J receptors) and possibly from corollary discharges coming down from the brain (Fig. 4). However, if the same ventricular receptors are activated at rest during cardiac ischaemia then the inputs from them, apparently well within normal limits (see Malliani, 1982), succeed in activating the pain-producing pathways in the absence of the inhibitory "exercise inputs", and this leads to the appearance of anginal pain. Presumably, such pain when it occurs could be blocked by engaging in muscular exercise. Perhaps, in the absence of increased coronary flow, this could be one mechanism used by patients for "running out their angina", with of course disastrous results. Indeed, as stated by De Bono and Julian (1984), some patients find that the pain comes when they start walking and that later it does not return despite greater effort. Others can "walk it off". It would be worthwhile to investigate further the nature of the blocking inputs, their sources and their relative effectiveness. In particular, it would be worth knowing whether the impulses from J receptors can block anginal pathways in the spinal cord.

Another point that merits consideration is that, as in the case of J receptor-produced sensations, it is possible that weak inputs from the ventricular receptors (in the absence of blocking inputs) may produce non-painful sensations (corresponding to J receptor-produced irritations in the throat), the nature of which have yet to be elucidated. Re-evaluation of carefully documented description of symptoms in patients with angina available on this subject in older literature may prove fruitful.

In contrast to the above, there is the alternative hypothesis that there are specific pain receptors that are activated only under pathophysiological conditions. If this is so, then it follows that such a pain-producing system may never be activated in numerous people during their entire lifetime. Nevertheless, it is necessary to consider the view that pain is due to the activation of such pathways, e.g., through specific chemosensitive endings.

Chemosensitive endings

According to Coleridge and co-workers, there exist in the heart, lungs and vessels endings with both vagal and sympathetic afferent fibres that are specifically stimulated by certain locally released chemical substances (autocoids), such as bradykinin and prostaglandins and histamine (Coleridge, J. C. G. and Coleridge, 1979a; Coleridge, H. M. and Coleridge, 1980, 1981; Baker et al., 1980; Kaufman et al., 1980). According to them, there is no other natural stimulus for these receptors, such as mechanical events in the heart, blood vessels or lungs. In the case of pulmonary endings, Coleridge and Coleridge (1981) believe that these endings form part of a defence system against noxious external agents and internal noxious substances travelling in the bloodstream. In fact, they even regard the J receptors (their pulmonary C-fibres) as chemosensitive endings forming part of this system. They apparently do not attach much significance to the many observations, including their own (Coleridge and Coleridge, 1977), showing that the natural stimulus of the J receptors is an increase in interstitial volume and that this occurs normally due to the increase in pulmonary blood flow during exercise, which the receptors reflexly inhibit (Paintal, 1969, 1970; Anand and Paintal, 1980). Coleridge and Coleridge (1984) regard the muscle inhibition by the J receptors as a kind of sham death response, presumably as part of a defensive mechanism.

With regard to anginal pain which originates from impulses in sympathetic afferent fibres, Coleridge and Coleridge (1980) state "It seems reasonable to suggest that the pain of angina, for example, results mainly from stimulation of chemosensitive nerve endings by substances released in the ischaemic myocardium rather than from stimulation of sympathetic mechanoreceptors by purely mechanical events". They do not believe that the increase in activity of ventricular mechanoreceptors with medullated fibres following coronary arterial occlusion reported by Uchida and Murao (1974) could be mainly responsible for the pain of angina. On the other hand, they believe that it is the sympathetic afferent C-fibres, that were previously silent but which yield an irregular discharge and are sensitive to lactic acid, that are responsible for cardiac pain (Coleridge and Coleridge, 1980) (see Malliani, 1982, for detailed references).

It should be noted that Coleridge and Coleridge (1980) have mentioned that many receptors stimulated by mechanical events in the heart (i.e., cardiac contraction and pressure and volume changes in the heart) were stimulated much more after applying bradykinin to the epicardial surface. In fact, they fired at high frequency continuously or in bursts for 2–3 minutes. Coleridge and Coleridge (1980) do not think that such receptors could be responsible for cardiac pain since mechanoreceptors are also stimulated by mechanical changes, which according to them are unlikely to be perceived as painful.

The view that the chemosensitive endings respond to purely local chemical changes (Coleridge and Coleridge, 1980) is based on the assumption that bradykinin and prostaglandins are involved in the transduction mechanisms at afferent nerve terminals in both physiological and pathological circumstances (Coleridge, J. C. G. and Coleridge, 1979). However, for this there is no evidence. Kaufman et al. (1980) have stated that "the chemosensitive endings, first identified in the ventricles (Coleridge, H. M. et al., 1964; Sleight and Widdicombe, 1965) and later in the atria, aorta and pulmonary artery (Coleridge, H. M. et al., 1973), are stimulated by a number of chemicals, including capsaicin, phenyl diguanide, nicotine and the veratrum alkaloids, and also by naturally occurring substances, bradykinin (present results) and PGE_2 (Baker et al., 1980)" (see Kaufman et al. (1980) for references in above quotation). The above statement excludes specificity, which is a required essential feature if a chemical substance is to be involved in any transduction process at sensory nerve endings. Secondly, the above view (i.e., that the cardiac chemosensitive endings respond to purely locally released chemical substances) is further weakened by the inclusion of the J receptors in the group of chemosensitive endings (Coleridge and Coleridge, 1980), because in the case of these receptors it is almost certain that their natural stimulus is an increase in interstitial volume (Paintal, 1969, 1970, 1973; 1977a), i.e., they are mechanoreceptors. Therefore, as in the case of many other mechanoreceptors, their stimulation by chemical substances, such as phenyl diguanide, capsaicin, etc., is merely the result of non-specific action by these substances on the regenerative region, which is far more sensitive to chemical substances than the generator region (Paintal, 1964, 1971a, 1976, 1977c). Thus far, there is no concrete evidence indicating, in the case of any receptor, that transduction involves a specific transmitter, although hopes that this may be so are entertained from time to time (e.g., Iggo and Findlater, 1984). So far it is possible to reconcile all the known facts relating to sensory transduction with the hypothesis that the generator membrane of sensory receptors produces a generator potential when it is mechanically deformed by an external stimulus either directly or indirectly, without the involvement of any chemical transmitter (Paintal, 1976).

There are several other investigators who are also not convinced about the existence of specific chemosensitive endings, particularly since the effects of chemical substances appear to be highly unspecific and various kinds of receptors (e.g., mechanoreceptors) are stimulated by bradykinin (see Paintal, 1981b). Moreover, specific chemosensitive endings have not been encountered by others. For example, Morrison has stated that in spite of a deliberate search for specific chemosensitive endings he and his co-workers found that all the receptors that were stimulated by bradykinin in their search were also stimulated by bladder contractions (see Paintal, 1981b).

Pain due to increase in non-nociceptive inputs

It has been believed that inputs from non-nociceptive receptors can cause pain through impulses in the smallest medullated and non-medullated fibres (Brindley, 1977). Evidence is now available in favour of this view. As mentioned above in the case of J receptors, if the input from them is small then subjects experience a mild itch in the throat but when the dose of lobeline is larger they experience a painful type of sensation (substernal burning, Fig. 2). However, this pain (produced artificially by lobeline or naturally by HAPO) is experienced, as mentioned above, under abnormal conditions, when other blocking inputs generated during muscular exercise are absent. However, it does show that non-nociceptive J receptor inputs, not necessarily large, can produce pain, and therefore this evidence provides a clear exception to the Muller-Volkmann hypothesis (see Brindley, 1977). This also supports Morrison's view that there are no specific pain endings that signal pain when the bladder is greatly distended. Morrison admits that his view was at variance with the accepted concept that each type of sensory receptor was responsible for signalling a specific type of sensation (see Paintal, 1981b) (see also Leek, 1972; Morrison, 1977; and Jänig and Morrison in this volume).

Sensations produced by pulmonary receptors

Pulmonary stretch receptors

The slowly and rapidly adapting receptors can be regarded as one group as they have in common many properties, such as the natural stimulus (lung inflation), relative accessibility to the pulmonary and bronchial circulations and the other stimuli that excite them (Paintal, 1983c). It well known that stimulation of these receptors by large inflations of the lungs produces relief from unpleasant sensa-

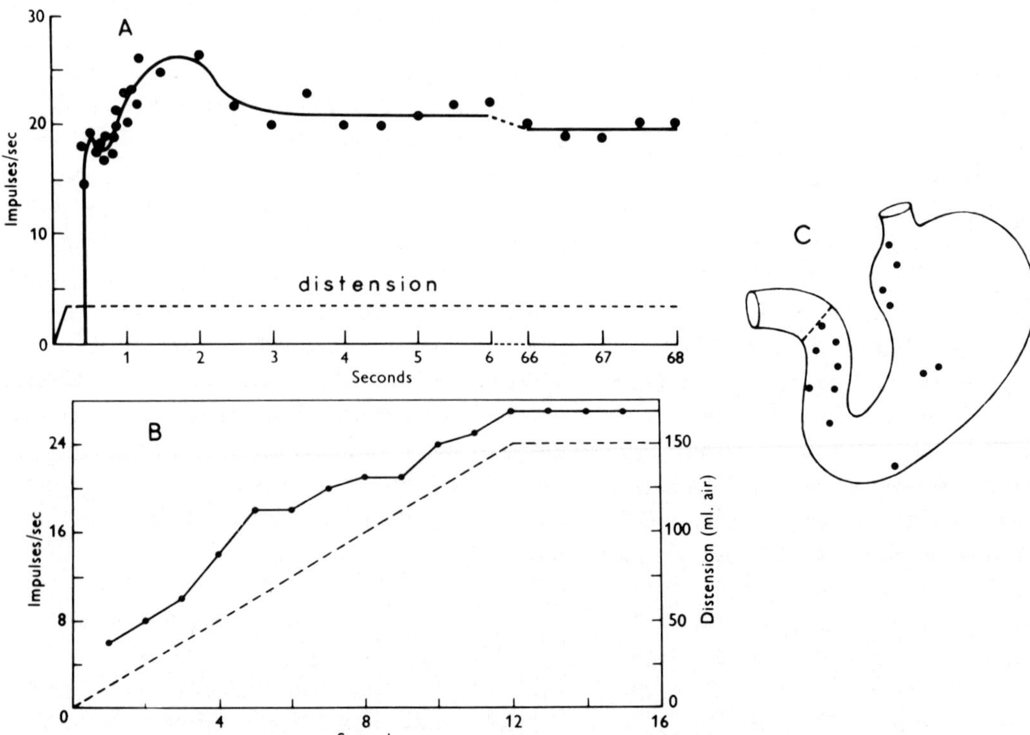

Fig. 5. Location and responses of gastric stretch receptors to distension of the stomach. A shows the response to distension, of the stomach, maintained for over a minute; note the slow adaptation. B shows the response of another slowly adapting receptor to gradual distension of the stomach. In the latter case, a gastric balloon was distended with 150 ml air in 12 seconds, as shown by the interrupted line. C shows the location of gastric stretch receptors in the stomach. From Paintal (1954).

tions of breath-holding (Fowler, 1954; Mithoefer, 1959). On the other hand, when these receptors are blocked by surface local anaesthesia the unpleasant sensations of dyspnoea that appear on breathing CO_2-enriched mixtures are increased (Cross et al., 1976). To what extent the feeling of relief of unpleasantness is a primary sensation is unknown. It appears that the reflex inhibition of contractions of the diaphragm following deep inspiration could play an important role in the genesis of relief (see Campbell and Guz, 1981; Killian and Campbell, 1983).

Bronchial C-fibre receptors

It has been suggested that broncial C-fibre receptors may produce a sensation of sub-sternal rawness or burning and irritation and an urge to cough (Coleridge and Coleridge, 1981). Evidence in support of this suggestion is needed.

J receptors

Evidence obtained with lobeline and during HAPO has already been presented above, showing that impulses from J receptors produce referred sensations in the throat and chest (Fig. 2). These are produced under abnormal conditions, when blocking "exercise inputs" are absent, i.e., at rest. However, the most important sensation produced by J receptors normally is breathlessness.

Sensations of breathlessness

Sensations of breathlessness during exercise are the most important visceral sensations which are experienced normally. They could be largely due to the stimulation of J receptors (see Paintal, 1977a), a conclusion that is fairly convincing in otherwise normal people with HAPO at high altitude. Guz et al. (1970) have observed that vagotomy (or vagal block) abolished the sensation of dyspnoea in certain patients in whom the J receptors would be expected to be stimulated owing to the existing pathophysiological condition of their lungs. Man complains of these sensations when they are expected to be absent. Breathlessness is the most prominent and frequent complaint of otherwise normal people with HAPO (Table I), and it can be attributed to the likely intense stimulation of J receptors that must occur during pulmonary oedema (Paintal, 1969, 1970) (Fig. 1C). Severe dyspnoea is also a common clinical feature of left heart failure. The sensations of breathlessness are complex and are linked with the increased respiratory drive that can be produced by J receptors (Anand et al., 1982), a conclusion for which, using phosgene gas, further evidence has been obtained recently (Anand et al., 1985). The sensations which are essentially vague and unlocalized can be experienced by men with spinal transection at C3 without any involvement of the diaphragm (Prys-Roberts, 1970). However, in normal man the available evidence indicates that the sensation is the result of a complex series of events requiring the involvement of diaphragmatic contractions (see Campbell and Guz, 1981; Killian and Campbell, 1983). On the other hand, it has recently been observed by Raj (personal communication) that the sensations referred to in the throat by individuals during exercise are similar to those experienced after lobeline.

Feeling of muscle weakness

Although not produced immediately, it seems that a feeling of generalized muscle weakness is experienced by certain individuals in whom the J receptors have been stimulated for a sufficient period, as in HAPO. The muscle weakness is apparently a manifestation of the J reflex, i.e., the inhibition of muscles by J receptor inputs so as to terminate exercise (Paintal, 1970). Evidence for the existence of this reflex in man has been obtained in patients with sustained ankle clonus. In these patients the clonus was abolished for a while following injection of lobeline (i.e., presumably by stimulating their J receptors (A. S. Paintal, V. Virmani and E. G. Walsh, unpublished observations)). The J reflex is not only a life-saving mechanism at high altitude (Ginzel and Eldred, 1977; Coleridge, H. M. and Coleridge, 1979) but it also operates physiologically at sea level. In fact, it has been shown that brief levels of activity equivalent to that generated by doubling pulmonary blood flow can produce marked inhibition of somatic muscles (Fig. 1B) (Anand and Paintal, 1980), and therefore it is to be expected that more prolonged stimulation, as in HAPO, will produce greater inhibition of muscles. In man the inhibition of muscles seems to manifest itself as a feeling of muscle weakness, because of the need for greater voluntary effort for the performance of motor tasks (see McCloskey, 1982). Thus, it is easy to understand why patients with left ventricular failure accompanied with pulmonary oedema complain of muscle weakness. It would be expected that this would be a major complaint of patients with HAPO. In fact, it was reported in 42% of the patients of Hultgren et al. (1961). Unfortunately, this was not examined in the recent study on otherwise normal individuals. (Table I).

Epithelial receptors signalling irritation in upper airways

There must exist receptors in the airways that are specifically stimulated by mechanical stimuli and/or chemical irritants and which produce the sensations of irritation in the throat leading to the production of cough. Although there have been some studies on the receptors of the larynx and trachea (see Korpas and Tomori, 1979; Saint'Ambrogio, 1982), it appears that detailed reports on receptors stimulated solely by mechanical and/or chemical irritants are not available. It is important to note that the receptors that would be expected to signal irritation of the upper airways should not be stimulated by airflow even during high flow rates as no noteworthy sensations (or cough) are produced during forced expiration (or inspiration), as pointed out in the earlier part of this review.

Receptors with sympathetic fibres

Receptors in the lungs and mediastinum with sympathetic afferent fibres have been described (Holmes and Torrance, 1959), but so far no sensations have been associated with them. Perhaps there are none, because blocking the vagus and glossopharyngeal nerves in man seems to abolish all noteworthy sensations (Guz et al., 1970).

Sensations produced by cardiovascular receptors

So far none of the cardiovascular receptors with vagal afferent fibres are associated with any visceral sensation (Paintal, 1977a). The same is true of the various receptors with sympathetic fibres (i.e., atrial and vascular), except for the ventricular receptors with sympathetic medullated and non-medullated fibres, which must be responsible for the pain following cardiac ischaemia. This has been discussed above in detail (Fig. 4). However, as has already been mentioned, this field should be re-explored through the use of chemical excitants for the production of non-painful sensations that have so far been overlooked.

Sensations produced by oesophageal receptors

It is possible that the oesophageal receptors described by Andrew (1956a,b), especially those located in the mucosa (Andrew, 1957), and others described by Iggo (1957a) and Mei (1970, 1983) in the cat may produce some sensations during the passage of food or fluids but they do not enter consciousness normally — perhaps because they are overshadowed by the far more overpowering sensations generated by the various receptors in the oropharynx before the oesophageal receptors are stimulated. Heartburn is apparently due to certain receptors at the cardiac end of the oesophagus (see Wolf and Wolff, 1947), but their precise nature is not known.

Sensations produced by gastrointestinal receptors

The responses of the gastrointestinal receptors have been described by Andrews and Jänig and Morrison in this volume and reviewed previously by Mei

(1983) (see also Morrison, 1977). Here, mainly receptors that produce the sensations will be dealt with briefly.

Gastric stretch receptors

The gastric stretch receptors mostly consist of slowly adapting receptors that seem to be suited for signalling the degree of distension of the stomach and the slow arrival of food or fluid into the stomach (Fig. 5). Such receptors have also been described by Iggo (1955) and Mei (1970) in the cat and by Iggo (1955) and Leek (see Leek, 1972, 1977) in the goat and sheep (see also review by Mei, 1983). It is now generally accepted (e.g., see Davson and Segal, 1976) that, as suggested earlier (Paintal, 1954), these receptors are ideally suited for generating the sensations of the immediate satiation of hunger and thirst. From Fig. 5B one can see what would happen while drinking fluid (or during a meal on a longer time scale). With gradual entry of food or fluids there would be a gradually increasing activity in the gastric stretch receptors, which would continue to increase in proportion to the amount of food or fluid ingested. This would be associated with a gradual increase in the sensation of satiation (developing within seconds or minutes), which would build up to a maximum when food or fluid intake would be terminated. This is what one generally experiences, and experimentally the mechanism has been shown to operate in dogs by Share et al. (1952) and by Towbin (1955), who showed that inhibition of fluid intake (presumably due to immediate satiation of thirst) is abolished by vagotomy.

It is possible that great stimulation of the gastric stretch receptors by producing intense sensations of satiety may also lead to feeling of nausea, although evidence for this is lacking (but see Wolf and Wolff, 1947). The sensation of fullness may, as suggested by Leek (1977), be the result of complex inputs from the stomach and mesenteric attachments.

Gastric mucosal receptors

In view of the fact that the gastric mucosal "chemoreceptors" described by Iggo (1957b) can no longer be regarded as pH receptors (Leek, 1977) and because it seems that these endings signal the passage or presence of gastric contents (Paintal, 1973), they might be involved in the sensations arising from the stomach following a meal and they also could be involved in some way with the sensations of immediate satiation following distension of the stomach with food.

Intestinal receptors

There can be no doubt that one or more of various intestinal receptors, e.g., distension-sensitive (Iggo, 1957a), distension-insensitive mucosal mechanoreceptors (Paintal, 1957) or those with sympathetic fibres (see Morrison, 1977), should be responsible for the sensations and/or reflex effects that result in the anorexia following distension of an isolated loop of the intestines as the anorexia is abolished by denervating the isolated loop (Herrin and Meek, 1933). However, at this stage one cannot enter into any justifiable speculations regarding which receptor could be involved in the anorexia as one does not even know whether the anorexia is mediated through vagal or sympathetic afferent fibres.

Sympathetic innervation of the viscera

Because of the relatively greater difficulties encountered in recording impulses in sympathetic afferent fibres quantitative studies on the responses of their sensory receptors have lagged behind those relating to vagal afferent fibres. They have been reviewed recently by Mei (1983), and discussed previously by Morrison (1977). There can be no doubt that many receptors signal mechanical events in the gastrointestinal and urinary tracts (Niijima, 1962; Morrison, 1973, 1977; Floyd and Morrison, 1974; Floyd et al., 1976). They may also produce some nonpainful sensations of which there is no knowledge at present.

Origin of visceral referred pain

Pain from the abdominal and pelvic viscera seems to be mediated almost entirely through sympathetic afferent fibres (see Lewis, 1942). On the one hand, pain could originate from specific nociceptors, as would be indicated by the observations of Cervero (1982) on the responses of the high-threshold receptors in the biliary system. On the other hand, it now looks more likely that it is not necessary to postulate the existence of specific nociceptors in view of the fact that it is almost certain that pain can be produced through non-nociceptive inputs provided that (1) the intensity of the sensory input is adequate (intense activity not being an essential requirement) and (2) the normal pain-blocking inputs are absent, as in the case of J receptors (see Fig. 3 and related text). A similar mechanism probably also exists in the case of the ventricular mechanoreceptors responsible for producing anginal pain (see Fig. 4 and related text). In this connection it will therefore be useful to obtain information about the following aspects in the case of each viscus: (1) Which of the various types of mechanoreceptors in the viscus could be responsible for the pain characteristic of that viscus. (2) The natural stimulus of these receptors. (3) The threshold level of activity in these receptors for pain. (4) The qualitative nature of the sensations (and their localization) felt when the level of activity is below that for producing pain (e.g., equivalent to itching in the throat in the case of J receptors (Fig. 2)). (5) The nature and intensity of the normal pain-blocking inputs (equivalent to exercise inputs in the case of J receptors (Fig. 3) and possibly also ventricular mechanoreceptors (Fig. 4)).

Summary

The main normal visceral sensations are (1) breathlessness during exercise, (2) sensations of irritation in the upper airways, (3) satiation of hunger and thirst, (4) bladder fullness and (5) rectal fullness. These sensations are produced respectively by (1) J receptors, (2) so far unidentified epithelial receptors in the upper airways, (3) gastric stretch receptors, (4) bladder mechanoreceptors and (5) mechanoreceptors in the rectum and colon. To these may be added the sensation of relief of breathlessness by pulmonary stretch receptors.

In addition to the above normal sensations, visceral receptors produce certain other sensations under pathophysiological conditions. For example, the J receptors produce sensations of irritation in the throat and pain in the upper chest; these sensations are normally blocked during exercise, which would be expected to produce much more intense activity than that necessary for producing pain. Certain ventricular mechanoreceptors with sympathetic afferent fibres are activated (activity doubled) during cardiac ischaemia and these produce anginal pain. It is suggested that as in the case of J receptors this anginal pain results from the absence of normal pain-blocking mechanisms operative during exercise.

Thus, it is not necessary to postulate the existence of specific nociceptors to account for visceral pain which results from adequate (but not necessarily intense) activity in non-nociceptive receptors, as shown in the case of J receptors by the effects of lobeline and HAPO, provided the normal pain-blocking mechanisms are absent (e.g., those generated during exercise).

Acknowledgements

I am grateful to the Scientific Advisor, Ministry of Defence, and the Director General, Armed Forces Medical Services, for their help in connection with the observations on HAPO reported in this paper.

References

Adrian, E. D. (1933) Afferent impulses in the vagus and their effect on respiration. J. Physiol., 79: 332–358.

Anand, A. and Paintal, A. S. (1980) Reflex effects following selective stimulation of J receptors in the cat. J. Physiol., 299: 553–572.

Anand, A., Loeschcke, H. H., Marek, W. and Paintal, A. S. (1982) Significance of the respiratory drive by impulses from J receptors. J. Physiol., 325: 14P.

Anand, A., Paintal, A. S. and Whitteridge, D. (1986) Phosgene stimulates J receptors and produces increased respiratory drive in cats. J. Physiol., 325: 14P.

Andrew, B. L. (1956a) A functional analysis of the myelinated fibres of the superior laryngeal nerve of the rat. J. Physiol., 133: 420–432.

Andrew, B. L. (1956b) The nervous control of the cervical oesophagus of the rat during swallowing. J. Physiol., 134: 729–740.

Andrew, B. L. (1957) Activity in afferent nerve fibres from the cervical oesophagus. J. Physiol., 135: 54–55.

Baker, D. G., Coleridge, H. M., Coleridge, J. C. G. and Nerdrum, T. (1980) Search for a cardiac nociceptor: stimulation by bradykinin of sympathetic afferent nerve endings in the heart of the cat. J. Physiol., 306: 519–536.

Bevan, J. A. and Murray, J. F. (1963) Evidence for a ventilation modifying reflex from the pulmonary circulation in man. Proc. Soc. Exp. Biol. Med., 114: 393–396.

Brindley, G. S. (1977) Somatic and visceral sensory mechanisms: Introduction. Br. Med. Bull., 33: 89–90.

Bronk, D. W. and Stella, G. (1932) Afferent impulses in the carotid sinus nerve. I. The relation of the discharge from single end organs to arterial blood pressure. J. Cell. Comp. Physiol., 1: 113–130.

Bronk, D. W. and Stella, G. (1935) The response to steady pressures of single end organs in the isolated carotid sinus. Am. J. Physiol., 110: 708–714.

Brown, A. M. (1967) Excitation of afferent cardiac sympathetic nerve fibres during myocardial ischaemia. J. Physiol., 190: 35–53.

Campbell, E. J. M. and Guz, A. (1981) Breathlessness. In T. F. Hornbein (Ed.), Regulation of Breathing, Part II, Marcel Dekker, New York, pp. 1181–1195.

Cervero, F. (1982) Afferent activity evoked by natural stimulation of biliary system in the ferret. Pain, 13: 137–151.

Clark, W. C., Janal, M. L., Colt, E. W. D. and Glusman, M. (1983) The effects of long distance running on pain sensitivity, mood and endocrine levels: reversal by nalaxone. Proc. Int. Union Physiol. Sci., 15: 105.

Colerdige, H. M. and Coleridge, J. C. G. (1977) Afferent vagal C-fibers in the dog lung: their discharge during spontaneous breathing, and their stimulation by alloxan and pulmonary congestion. In A. S. Paintal and P. Gill-Kumar (Eds.), Respiratory Adaptations, Carpillary Exchange and Reflex Mechanisms, Vallabhbhai Patel Chest Institute, Delhi, pp. 396–405.

Coleridge, H. M. and Coleridge, J. C. G. (1979) Afferents of the pulmonary vascular bed and their role. In McC. C. Brooks, K. Koizumi and A. Sato (Eds.), Integrative Function of the Autonomic Nervous System, University of Tokyo Press, Tokyo, pp. 98–110.

Coleridge, H. M. and Coleridge, J. C. G. (1980) Cardiovascular afferents involved in regulation of peripheral vessels. Annu. Rev. Physiol., 42: 413–427.

Coleridge, H. M. and Coleridge, J. C. G. (1981) Afferent fibres involved in defence reflexes from the respiratory tract. In I. Hutas and L. A. Debreczeni (Eds.), Advances in Physiological Sciences, Vol. 10, Pergamon Press, Budapest, pp. 467–477.

Coleridge, H. M., Coleridge, J. C. G. and Kidd, C. (1964) Cardiac receptors in the dog, with particular reference to two types of afferent ending in the ventricular wall. J. Physiol., 174: 323–339.

Coleridge, H. M., Coleridge, J. C. G., Dangel, A., Kidd, C., Luck, J. C. and Sleight, P. (1973) Impulses in slowly conducting vagal fibers from afferent endings in veins, atria and arteries of dogs and cats. Circ. Res., 33: 87–97.

Coleridge, J. C. G. and Coleridge, H. M. (1979) Chemoreflex regulation of the heart. In R. M. Berne (Ed.), Handbook of Physiology, Section 2, Cardiovascular System, The Heart, American Physiological Society, Bethesda, pp. 653–676.

Coleridge, J. C. G. and Coleridge, H. M. (1984) Afferent vagal C fibre innervation of the lungs and airways and its functional significance. Rev. Physiol. Biochem. Pharmacol., 99: 1–110.

Cross, B. A., Guz, A., Jain, S. K., Archer, S., Stevens, J. and Reynolds, F. (1976) The effect of anaesthesia of the airway in dog and man: a study of respiratory reflexes, sensations and lung mechanics. Clin. Sci., 50: 439–454.

Davson, H. and Segal, M. B. (1976) Introduction to Physiology, Vol. 3, Academic Press, London, p. 305.

De Bono, D. P. and Julian, D. G. (1984) Diseases of the cardiovascular system. In J. Macleod (Ed.), Davidson's Principles and Practice of Medicine, Churchill Livingstone, Hong Kong, pp. 122–201.

Eckenhoff, J. E. and Comroe, J. H. Jr. (1951) Blocking action of tetraethylammonium on lobeline-induced thoracic pain. Proc. Soc. Exp. Biol. Med., 76: 725–726.

Euler, U. S. V., Liljestrand, G. and Zotterman, Y. (1939) The excitation mechanism of chemoreceptors of the carotid body. Scand. Arch. Physiol., 83: 132–152.

Euler, U. S. V., Liljestrand, G. and Zotterman, Y. (1941) Über den Reizmechanismus der Chemorezeptoren im Glomus caroticum. Acta Physiol. Scand., 1: 383–385.

Floyd, K. and Morrison, J. F. B. (1974) Splanchnic mechanoreceptors in the dog. Q. J. Exp. Physiol., 59: 359–364.

Floyd, K., Hick, V. E. and Morrison, J. F. B. (1976) Mechanosensitive afferent units in the hypogastric nerve of the cat. J. Physiol., 259: 457–471.

Fowler, W. S. (1954) Breaking point of breath-holding. J. Appl. Physiol., 6: 539–545.

Ginzel, K. H. and Eldred, E. (1977) Reflex depression of somatic motor activity from heart, lungs and carotid sinus. In A. S. Paintal and P. Gill-Kumar (Eds.), Respiratory Adaptations, Capillary Exchange and Reflex Mechanisms, Vallabhbhai Patel Chest Institute, Delhi, pp. 358–394.

Guz, A., Noble, M. I. M., Widdicombe, J. G., Trenchard, D. and Mushin, W. W. (1966) Peripheral chemoreceptor block in man. Resp. Physiol., 1: 38–40.

Guz, A., Noble, M. I. M., Eisele, J. H. and Trenchard, D. (1970) Experimental results of vagal block in cardiopulmonary disease. In R. Porter (Ed.), Breathing: Hering-Breuer Centenary Symposium, Churchill, London, pp. 315–329.

Herrin, R. C. and Meek, W. J. (1933) Distension as a factor in intestinal obstruction. Arch. Intern. Med., 51: 152–168.

Hillis, B. R. and Kelly, J. C. C. (1951) Effect of hexamathonium iodide on lobeline-stimulated coughing. Glasgow Med. J., 32: 72–76.

Holmes, R. and Torrance, R. W. (1959) Afferent fibres of the stellate ganglion. Q. J. Exp. Physiol., 44: 271–281.

Hultgren, H. N., Spickard, W. B., Hellriegel, K. and Houston, C. S. (1961) High altitude pulmonary edema. Medicine, 40: 289–313.

Iggo, A. (1955) Tension receptors in the stomach and the urinary bladder. J. Physiol., 128: 593–607.

Iggo, A. (1957a) Gastro-intestinal tension receptors with unmyelinated afferent fibres in the vagus of the cat. Q. J. Exp. Physiol., 42: 130–143.

Iggo, A. (1957b) Gastric mucosal chemoreceptors with vagal afferent fibres in the cat. Q. J. Exp. Physiol., 42: 389–409.

Iggo, A. and Findlater, C. S. (1984) A review of Merkel cell mechanisms. In W. Hamann and A. Iggo (Eds.), Sensory Receptor Mechanisms, World Scientific Publ. Co., Singapore, pp. 117–131.

Jain, S. K. (1980) Pulmonary vagal receptors and respiratory sensations. In E. Grastyán and P. Molnár (Eds.), Advances in Physiological Sciences, Vol. 16, Sensory Functions, Akademiai Kiado, Budapest, pp. 315–323.

Jain, S. K., Subramanian, S., Julka, D. B. and Guz, A. (1972) Search for evidence of lung chemoreflexes in man: study of respiratory and circulatory effects of phenyldiguanide and lobeline. Clin. Sci., 42: 163–177.

Kaufman, M. P., Baker, D. G., Coleridge, H. M. and Coleridge, J. C. G. (1980) Stimulation by bradykinin of afferent vagal C-fibers with chemosensitive endings in the heart and aorta of the dog. Circ. Res., 46: 476–484.

Killian, K. J. and Campbell, E. J. M. (1983) Dyspnea and exercise. Annu. Rev. Physiol., 45: 465–479.

Korpás, J. and Tomori, Z. (1979) Cough and other respiratory reflexes. Prog. Resp. Res., 12: 1–356.

Leek, B. R. (1972) Abdominal visceral receptors. In E. Neil (Ed.), Handbook of Sensory Physiology, Vol. III/I: Enteroceptors, Springer-Verlag, Berlin, pp. 113–160.

Leek, B. R. (1977) Abdominal and pelvic visceral receptors. Br. Med. Bull., 33: 163–168.

Lewis, T. (1942) Pain, The Macmillan Company, New York.

Lilienfeld, A. and Berliner, K. (1942) Duplicate measurements of circulation time made with the alpha lobeline method. Arch. Int. Med., 69: 739–745.

Malliani, A. (1982) Cardiovascular sympathetic afferent fibers. Rev. Physiol. Biochem. Pharmacol., 94: 11–74.

Malliani, A., Recordarti, G. and Schwartz, P. J. (1973) Nervous activity of afferent cardiac sympathetic fibres with atrial and ventricular endings. J. Physiol., 229: 457–469.

McCloskey, D. I. (1982) Corollary discharges: motor commands and perception. In J. M. Brookhart and V. B. Mountcastle (Eds.), Handbook of Physiology. The Nervous System: Motor Control, Vol II, Part II, American Physiological Society, Bethesda, pp. 1415–1447.

Mei, N. (1970) Mécanorécepteurs vagaux digestifs chez le chat. Exp. Brain Res., 11: 502–514.

Mei, N. (1983) Sensory structures in the viscera. Prog. Sensory Physiology, 4: 1–42.

Menon, N. D. (1965) High-altitude pulmonary edema. N. Engl. J. Med., 273: 66–73.

Mithoefer, J. C. (1959) Lung volume restriction as a ventilatory stimulus during breath holding. J. Appl. Physiol., 14: 701–705.

Morrison, J. F. B. (1973) Splanchnic slowly adapting mechanoreceptors with punctate receptive fields in the mesentery and gastrointestinal tract of the cat. J. Physiol., 233: 349–361.

Morrison, J. F. B. (1977) The afferent innervation of the gastrointestinal tract. In F. P. Brooks and P. W. Evers (Eds.), Nerves and the Gut, Charles B. Slack Inc., Thorofare, NJ, pp. 297–322.

Niijima, A. (1962) Afferent impulses in the vagal and splanchnic nerves of toad's stomach, and their rôle in sensory mechanism. Jpn. J. Physiol., 12: 25–44.

Paintal, A. S. (1954) A study of gastric stretch receptors. Their role in the peripheral mechanism of satiation of hunger and thirst. J. Physiol., 126: 255–270.

Paintal, A. S. (1957) Responses from mucosal mechanoreceptors in the small intestine of the cat. J. Physiol., 139: 353–368.

Paintal, A. S. (1964) Effects of drugs on vertebrate mechanoreceptors. Pharmacol. Rev., 16: 341–380.

Paintal, A. S. (1969) Mechanism of stimulation of type J pulmonary receptors. J. Physiol., 203: 511–532.

Paintal, A. S. (1970) The mechanism of excitation of type J receptors, and the J reflex. In R. Porter (Ed.), Breathing: Hering-Breuer Centenary Symposium, Churchill, London, pp. 59–71.

Paintal, A. S. (1971a) Action of drugs on sensory nerve endings. Annu. Rev. Pharmacol., 11: 231–240.

Paintal, A. S. (1971b) The J reflex. Proc. Int. Union Physiol. Sci., 8: 79–80.

Paintal, A. S. (1972) Cardiovascular receptors. In E. Neil (Ed.), Handbook of Sensory Physiology, Vol. III/I: Enteroceptors, Springer-Verlag, Berlin, pp. 1–45.

Paintal, A. S. (1973) Vagal sensory receptors and their reflex effects. Physiol. Rev., 53: 159–227.

Paintal, A. S. (1976) Natural and paranatural stimulation of sensory receptors. In Y. Zotterman (Ed.), Sensory Functions of the Skin, Pergamon Press, Oxford, pp. 3–12.

Paintal, A. S. (1977a) Thoracic receptors connected with sensation. Br. Med. Bull., 33: 169–174.

Paintal, A. S. (1977b) The nature and effects of sensory inputs into the respiratory centres. Fed. Proc., 30: 2428–2432.

Paintal, A. S. (1977c) Effects of drugs on chemoreceptors, pulmonary and cardiovascular receptors. Pharmac. Ther. B., 3: 41–63.

Paintal, A. S. (1981a) Vagal sensory mechanisms and sensations. In E. Grastyán and P. Molnár (Eds.), Advances in Physiological Sciences, Vol. 16, Akademiai Kiado, Budapest, pp. 309–313.

Paintal, A. S. (1981b) Concluding remarks on visceral sensory mechanisms and sensations. In E. Grastyán and P. Molnár (Eds.) Advances in Physiological Sciences, Vol. 16, Akademiai Kiado, Budapest, pp. 335–337.

Paintal, A. S. (1983a) Localization of the sensations produced by J receptors (J area). Proc. Int. Union Physiol. Sci., 15: 245.

Paintal, A. S. (1983b) The central effects of J receptors. Proc. Int. Union Physiol. Sci., 15: 290.

Paintal, A. S. (1983c) Lung and airway receptors. In D. J. Pallot (Ed.), Control of Respiration, Croom Helm, London, pp. 78–107.

Prys-Roberts, C. (1970) In R. Porter (Ed.), Breathing: Hering-Breuer Centenary Symposium, Churchill, London, p. 249.

Raj, H. (1984) Sensations and reflex effects produced by J receptors in man. M.D. Thesis, Delhi University.

Rex, M. A. E. and Paintal, A. S. (1983) Stimulation of laryngeal constrictor muscles by J receptors and cardiac receptors. Proc. Int. Union Physiol. Sci., 15: 245.

Sant'Ambrogio, G. (1982) Information arising from the tracheobronchial tree of mammals. Physiol. Rev., 62: 531–569.

Share, I., Martyniuk, E. and Grossman, M. I. (1952) Effect of prolonged intragastric feeding on oral food intake in dogs. Am. J. Physiol., 169: 229–235.

Sleight, P. and Widdicombe, J. G. (1965) Action potentials in fibres from receptors in the epicardium and mycardium of the dog's left ventricle. J. Physiol., 181: 235–258.

Stern, S., Bruderman, I. and Braun, K. (1966) Localization of lobeline-sensitive receptors in the pulmonary circulation in man. Am. Heart J., 71: 651–655.

Stransky, A., Szeredaprzestaszewska, M. and Widdicombe, J. G. (1973) The effects of lung reflexes on laryngeal resistance and motoneurone discharge. J. Physiol., 231: 417–438.

Towbin, E. J. (1955) Thirst and hunger behavior in normal dogs and the effects of vagotomy and sympathectomy. Am. J. Physiol., 182: 377–382.

Uchida, Y. and Murao, S. (1974) Excitation of afferent cardiac sympathetic nerve fibers during coronary occlusion. Am. J. Physiol., 226: 1094–1099.

Widdicombe, J. G. (1954) Respiratory reflexes from the trachea and bronchi of the cat. J. Physiol., 123: 55–70.

Wolf, S. and Wolff, H. G. (1947) Human Gastric Function, Oxford University Press, London.

F. Cervero and J. F.B. Morrison
Progress in Brain Research, Vol. 67

CHAPTER 2

Clinical approach to visceral sensation

Paolo Procacci, Massimo Zoppi and Marco Maresca

Istituto di Clinica Medica I, Servizio di Algologia, Università di Firenze, Viale G.B. Morgagni 85, 50134 Firenze, Italy

Introduction

Normal visceral sensations are generally known as "common sensations" or "coenaesthesia" (from the Greek κοινή (koiné) = common, and αἴσθησις (aìsthesis) = sensation). This term corresponds to the German *Gemeingefühl.* These sensations are many and are not as well defined as somatic sensations. Typical examples are the feeling of appetite in the stomach, and the feeling of fullness in the rectum and in the bladder. It is a matter of discussion whether sensations that originate in the sexual organs during coitus could be considered as visceral; in our opinion they have particular characters and we prefer to consider them under the separate heading of "sexual sensations".

The concept of common sensations derives from the Aristotelian ancient idea of *sensorium commune.* Aristotle considered pain as an increased sensitivity to every sensation, especially to touch (Procacci and Maresca, 1984). This "intensity theory" is still an open question in visceral pain mechanisms.

A common sensation can become clearly unpleasant but not necessarily painful, as in motion sickness or in the sensation of "air hunger". The term that defines this kind of unpleasant sensation is "coenaesthesiopathia". Visceral pain can arise from a visceral common sensation, i.e., sensations from the bladder. The common sensation is the feeling of fullness, accompanied by a desire to micturate. If it is inconvenient to micturate, the desire to do so becomes stronger and unpleasant, but it is still not painful. During severe urinary retention, as occurs in acute urinary bladder obstruction, this unpleasant feeling becomes increasingly painful. The transitional and often unpleasant feeling which when it rises to a certain level becomes painful was termed "metaesthesia" by Keele (1962) in his studies of sensations induced by chemicals on the skin. This term seems very appropriate for many visceral sensations that are unpleasant but below the level of pain, such as a feeling of disagreeable fullness or acidity of the stomach or undefined and unpleasant thoracic or abdominal sensations. These metaesthesic sensations generally remain under the level of pain, but can also precede the onset of visceral pain, such as a typical attack of angina pectoris or a renal or biliary colic.

The most important visceral sensation is visceral pain. The stimuli that induce pain in viscera are different from those which induce pain in somatic structures. This explains why in the past the viscera were considered to be insensitive to pain (see Bonica, 1953). In fact, it was observed that viscera could be exposed to such stimuli as burning or cutting without evoking pain. This apparent insensitivity of viscera was due to failure to apply adequate stimuli.

The main factors capable of inducing pain in visceral structures are the following (Ayala, 1937; Lunedei and Galletti, 1953; Procacci et al., 1978): (1) Abnormal distension and contraction of the muscle walls of hollow viscera. (2) Rapid stretching of the capsule of such solid visceral organs as the liver, spleen, and pancreas. (3) Abrupt anoxemia of visceral muscle. (4) Formation and accumulation of pain-producing substances. (5) Direct action of chemical stimuli (especially important in the oesophagus and stomach). (6) Traction or compression of ligaments and vessels. (7) Inflammatory states. (8) Necrosis of some structures (myocardium, pancreas). Some of these factors may be concomitant, and interact in many clinical conditions.

As regards the contraction of hollow viscera, it must be noted that a strong contraction in approximately isometric conditions provokes a more severe pain than in approximately isotonic conditions. This may explain the strong pain of some diseases, such as acute intestinal obstruction and biliary or ureteral colics.

The different visceral structures show different pain sensitivity. Serosal membranes have the lowest pain threshold and are followed, in order of ascending threshold, by the wall of hollow viscera and the parenchymatous organs.

Experimental investigations have been carried out in man on algogenic visceral conditions. Oesophageal pain has been induced by many authors, using mechanical, electrical and chemical stimuli. Gastric algogenic conditions were studied by Wolf and Wolff (1947) on a patient with a large gastric stoma. Different kinds of stimuli were applied. No pain could be induced when the healthy mucosa of the fundus of the stomach was squeezed between the blades of a forceps. Electrical stimuli, intense enough to cause pain in the tongue, and chemical stimuli, such as 50 or 90% alcohol, 1.0 N HCl, 0.1 N NaOH and 1:30 suspension of mustard, were also ineffective in evoking pain when applied to healthy gastric mucosa. However, if the mucosa was inflamed, all the above-mentioned procedures induced a strong pain. Kinsella (1948) observed that squeezing the inflamed appendix provoked pain.

The sensibility of pleura was investigated by means of electrical, thermal and mechanical stimuli during a Jacobaeus operation (section of pleural synechiae) (Teodori and Galletti, 1962). Pain was induced by stimulation of areas of normal and inflamed pleura. When the stimuli were applied to the inflamed serosa, pain was more intense, sharp and localized than when the stimuli were applied to the normal pleura. Similar phenomena were observed in cases of electrical, mechanical and chemical endobronchial stimulation.

All these findings suggest that inflammation plays an important role in the genesis of pain in many viscera, inducing a sensitization to normally non-painful stimuli. Many pain-producing substances have been identified, such as kinins, 5-hydroxytriptamine, histamine, prostaglandins and K^+, which could be active in visceral painful diseases. The algogenic activity of some substances has been demonstrated in experiments in which the substances were introduced in the arteries or in the peritoneum (Lim, 1966, 1967). However, it must be noted that when an algogenic substance is released in pathologic conditions, several factors may be present, such as activating or inhibiting agents, changes of pH and of capillary permeability, which may modify the effect of the substance. This complex biochemical and biophysical situation cannot be reproduced in experiments.

Visceral pain has different characteristics in different patients, or in the same patient at different times. The clinical classification of visceral pain used in this chapter is derived from the classical studies of Lewis (1942), Bonica (1953), Lunedei and Galletti (1953), Hansen and Schliack (1962) and Wolff (1963) (Table I).

True visceral pain

This pain is deep, dull, not well defined, but described by the patient with especial terms. It is difficult to locate this type of pain, which tends to ra-

TABLE I

Classification of visceral pain

A. True visceral pain
B. Referred pain
  i: with superficial and/or deep hyperalgesia
  ii: without superficial and/or deep hyperalgesia

diate and frequently reaches parts of the body that are far from the affected organ. It is often accompanied by a sense of malaise. It induces strong autonomic reflex phenomena, including diffuse sweating, vasomotor responses, changes of arterial pressure and heart rate, and an intense psychic alarm reaction.

An example of true visceral pain is the pain which is observed as the earliest manifestation in most cases of myocardial infarction and, less frequently, in cases of angina pectoris. This pain is deep and poorly localized. It is always midline, usually substernal or epigastric, and sometimes interscapular as well. Instead of pain, some patients experience unpleasant common sensations, described as heaviness, pressure, smothering, tightness, choking, squeezing, or as a sense of gastric fullness. Pain or the other unpleasant common sensations are frequently accompanied by nausea, vomiting and profuse sweating. In many cases, there is an intense alarm reaction. No cutaneous or deep hyperalgesia can be detected.

Referred pain

When an algogenic process affecting a viscus recurs frequently or becomes more intense and prolonged, the location becomes more exact and the painful sensation is progressively felt in more superficial structures, sometimes far from the site of origin. This phenomenon is usually called in English "referred pain", whereas German authors use the less well known but, in our opinion, more appropriate term of "transferred pain" *(übertragener Schmerz)* (Hansen and Schliack, 1962).

Referred pain with superficial and/or deep hyperalgesia

This type of referred pain is generally felt within the metamere or metameres that include the viscus giving rise to pain. The sensation is often limited to a part of the metamere. Such pain is accompanied by an increased pain sensitivity of the skin and/or of the muscles. The cutaneous pain threshold is lowered and non-noxious stimuli applied to the skin induce pain (allodynia). An abnormal dermographic response (white dermographism) is sometimes present. Acute muscle pain is evoked even when only light pressure is applied, and in many cases a sustained muscular contraction occurs. A characteristic property of cutaneous and deep hyperalgesia is that they often subside after an injection of local anaesthetic.

Muscular pain and tenderness are often restricted to small areas of the abdominal wall, from where pain radiates. These algogenic points, named after different authors, were considered in the past as points of true visceral pain. It is now evident that the cholecystic, appendicular and ureteral points of tenderness are generally due to pain arising from the musculo-cutaneous structures of the abdominal wall. Knowledge of these points and of the radiation pattern of pain as a consequence of diseases of visceral organs is of great importance for a correct diagnosis.

Another example of referred pain is often observed during myocardial infarction or angina pectoris. This pain, constrictive and well localized, is reported by the patients as originating in the thoracic wall and/or in the upper limbs. It is felt in various sites: in the chest, in the precordial, sternal or left interscapulo-vertebral areas, in the upper limbs, more often the left, diffusely in the whole limb or only in the forearm, with a sense of numbness and constriction at the elbow and wrist. Pain is accompanied by sweating but not by nausea and vomiting; muscular tenderness is often present, with well-defined myalgic spots or trigger points and cutaneous hyperalgesia. In infarction, this type of pain often follows the deep visceral pain after an interval varying from 10 minutes to some hours; in angina pectoris, and sometimes in infarction, it is the first type of pain perceived. In many cases, this referred pain with hyperalgesia does not replace but only inhibits the perception of true visceral pain. As an example, we shall report some of our observations on patients suffering from angina of effort (Procacci and Zoppi, 1983, 1984). Pain during stress testing was referred to the anterior chest wall. These patients had typical myalgic spots on the chest wall, which were blocked with a local anaesthetic. After the block, stress testing caused a different type of pain or of general discomfort, which appeared at the time of the S-T segment displacement in the electrocardiogram and in most cases had never been felt before. Pain was substernal or epigastric, with the characteristics of true visceral pain.

Referred pain without superficial and/or deep hyperalgesia

This form of pain is felt in large sections of the metamere or metameres that include the viscus of origin of an algogenic process. It may also extend to adjacent metameres, far from the site of origin. Cutaneous hyperalgesia is never observed. Injection of a local anaesthetic into superficial or deeper regions of the area where this referred pain is experienced will not reduce the intensity of the sensation. Deep palpation of the abdomen, which would produce a tolerable painful sensation under normal conditions, causes intense pain and defensive reactions in the patients. The clinical interpretation of this type of pain is rather difficult. It often occurs in extensive but not very intense pathological processes, but it can also be an indication of the onset of serious diseases that develop slowly, for example, tumours of the digestive system or of the lungs.

Mechanisms of referred pain

Mackenzie (1909), on the basis of previous observations by Sturge (1883) and Ross (1887), offered a classical interpretation of referred pain which, though modified by many authors, has remained unaltered in its fundamental concept. According to this interpretation, sensory impulses from the viscera create an "irritable focus" in the segment at which they enter into the spinal cord. Afferent impulses from the skin are thereby facilitated, giving rise to true cutaneous pain: hyperalgesia and referred pain are the consequence of this "irritable focus". This interpretation is called the "convergence-facilitation theory".

Ruch (1960) proposed a somewhat different thesis: some visceral afferents subserving pain sensation converge with cutaneous afferents, to end on the same neuron at some point in the sensory pathway. The resulting impulses, on reaching the brain, are interpreted as having come from the skin, an interpretation that has been learned from previous experiences in which the same tract fibre was stimulated by cutaneous afferents. This "convergence-projection theory" can explain the references of pain but not the hyperalgesia of dermatomal distribution.

Many experimental findings support the above theories by showing that nociceptive impulses from visceral and cutaneous areas converge at the level of the spinal cord, brainstem, thalamus and cortex (Hugon, 1971; Mountcastle, 1974; Wall, 1974; Nathan, 1977; Willis and Coggeshall, 1978; Cervero, 1980). The convergence of pain impulses in the central nervous system can explain some of the clinical phenomena observed, i.e., referred pain without hyperalgesia. However, the presence of hyperalgesia is more difficult to explain, and according to Wolff (1963) it is characteristic of an initial local alteration of tissues.

The suggestion can be advanced that, in the referred pain areas in which hyperalgesia is present, algogenic conditions develop in the cutaneous and muscular structures through a reflex mechanism and provoke the onset of a true parietal pain. This explanation is widely accepted for muscle structures which become the site of referred pain as a consequence of sustained contractions. A classic experiment was performed by MacLellan and Goodell (1943), who observed that, following stimulation of the ureter or of the pelvis of the kidney, the muscles of the abdominal wall on the stimulated side remained contracted and, after about half an hour, this side of the body began to ache. The ache became quite severe and lasted for 6 hours, with the side still tender the following day. Therefore, it is clear that painful stimulation of visceral structures evokes a visceromuscular reflex, so that some muscles contract and become a new source of pain. As regards cutaneous structures, Wolff (1963) has suggested that pain can be induced through impulses that pass antidromically in afferent peripheral nerves and provoke the formation and release of pain-producing substances of the kinin type (neurokinin). Wolff reached this conclusion through experiments in which dorsal roots were stimulated and cutaneous perfusate was subsequently collected.

According to Procacci (1969), algogenic conditions in the skin and some related phenomena are induced through a reflex arc whose efferent limb is sympathetic. This hypothesis had previously been proposed by Penfield (1925) and by Davis and Pollock (1930). Some studies were carried out in patients suffering from myofascial pain originating in tender muscle spots (trigger points) and with referred pain with hyperalgesia in areas of the metamere or metameres that included the painful muscle. Local anaesthetic block of the muscle spots (i.e., the source of pain) caused both deep and referred pain to subside, as had previously been observed by Lewis (1942). Local anaesthetic block of the sympathetic ganglia led to the disappearance, or at least to a marked decrease, of referred pain, hyperalgesia, and alterations of dermographia and of cutaneous impedance (Galletti et al., 1963; Galletti and Procacci, 1966, 1968). Moreover, local anaesthetic block of sympathetic ganglia produced long-lasting changes in the cutaneous pain threshold, measured with a thermal algometer (Procacci et al., 1975) or by means of electrical stimuli (Procacci et al., 1979a), as well as changes in the skin potential responses (Procacci et al., 1979a).

In conclusion, referred pain seems to be caused by two different mechanisms which, at least in part, overlap. A central convergence of visceral and cutaneous impulses is certainly present and can explain the referred pain without hyperalgesia irradiated to large segmental areas. The same mechanism is presumably present in referred pain with hyperalgesia, but, in addition, a group of visceromuscular and viscerocutaneous reflexes gives rise to algogenic conditions in the periphery, with subsequent excitation of the pain receptors. In some conditions, this parietal pain is long lasting, increases progressively, even if the affected organ is removed, and is accompanied by obvious dystrophy of somatic structures, as in the shoulder-hand syndrome that may follow a myocardial infarction. This is probably the result of a vicious circle of impulses (periphery–CNS–periphery), as suggested by Livingston (1943) and Bonica (1953) for causalgia and other reflex dystrophies.

Intricate conditions

In clinical practice the distinction between visceral pain, referred pain and somatic pain is often difficult: these are the so-called "intricate conditions". The concept was firstly proposed by Froment and Gonin (1956), who observed that angina pectoris can be related to cervical osteoarthritis, oesophageal hernia or cholecystitis. It is difficult to ascertain whether these "intricate conditions" are due to a simple addition of impulses from different sources in the CNS, or to somatovisceral and viscerosomatic mechanisms, which may induce a classical "vicious circle" between different structures. The pathogenesis of pain is probably different in different subjects. It is beyond the scope of this chapter to consider every "intricate condition", but a typical example is that of painful scars (Leriche, 1949; Bonica, 1953). These scars are painful per se, although algogenic conditions in viscera metamerically related to the scar may often be observed. In this case, associated reflex phenomena are probably responsible for the painful scar.

Mnemonic traces

Every level of the central nervous system can hold learned experiences and give them back when necessary. It has been demonstrated that the mnemonic process is facilitated if the experience to be retained is repeated many times or is accompanied by pleasant or unpleasant emotions (Benedetti, 1969). It has also been demonstrated that pain, like other sensory modalities, is, at least in part, a learned experience (Melzack, 1973). Pain experience develops not only in learning avoidance reflexes but also as memory. This is not a memory in the sense that it can be called to the conscious mind by action of the will. Therefore, the processes of retained painful experience were appropriately termed memory-like processes by Melzack (1973). Nathan (1962) observed that in some subjects different kinds of stimuli could call to mind forgotten painful experiences.

A very interesting method of sensory stimulation is the ischaemia of the limbs experimentally provoked with a pneumatic cuff. The limbs may be maintained at rest, according to some techniques (Weddell and Sinclair, 1947; Merrington and Nathan, 1949; Galletti and Procacci, 1958), or may be tested during a muscular contraction (Smith et al., 1966). In the technique of Galletti and Procacci, ischaemia is induced at the same time in both upper or lower limbs kept at rest. Ischaemia is maintained for 10 minutes and the induced sensations are recorded. With this method it is possible to obtain a comparative evaluation of the sensory changes in both limbs. In normal subjects ischaemia induces paraesthesic sensations (tingling, "pins and needles", numbness), but never pain.

We performed experiments in patients with previous myocardial infarction, but with normal sensibility as judged by accurate examination. Ischaemia of the upper limbs was induced according to our technique. In most patients ischaemia caused pain with characteristics similar to those of the pain felt during the episode of infarction. Thus, in the patients in whom the pain of the infarction had radiated to the left limb the pain induced by the ischaemia was felt in the same limb, whereas in the patients in whom the pain of the infarction had radiated to both limbs the pain induced by the ischaemia was felt in both limbs. During the ischaemia, some patients of this group felt common sensations accompanied by alarm reaction, with sweating, nausea, tachycardia, and tachypnea (Procacci et al., 1968). The test was promptly interrupted at the onset of these symptoms. In all patients electrocardiogram and arterial pressure were accurately monitored as the test was performed in an intensive care unit. We also examined patients with previous painless myocardial infarction. First of all, it must be noted that most of these patients remembered an episode variously defined as fullness of the stomach, nausea or indigestion, whereas in other patients the history was completely silent. In most of the patients the ischaemia of the upper limbs provoked the onset of diffuse common sensations, often accompanied by autonomic and emotional reactions. In a few of the patients, these reactions called to mind a similar but long-forgotten episode of diffuse sensation (Procacci et al., 1976, 1979b).

Ischaemia of the upper limbs was also induced in patients suffering from angina pectoris (Procacci et al., 1972). Most patients whose anginal pain radiated to the left arm reported pain in the same limb and with the same radiation as their spontaneous pain. Most of the patients whose anginal pain was felt only in the chest or radiated to both upper limbs reported pain in both limbs.

These results suggest that ischaemic pain can evoke mnemonic traces of previous painful experiences. Some patients did not remember the painful episode but later experienced similar sensations. The formation of mnemonic traces in patients suffering from angina is probably due to the repetition of painful attacks whereas in patients with previous painful or painless infarction it is probably due to the strong aversive emotions with feeling of impending death that accompanied the single episode.

Similar mechanisms may also be active in painful diseases of the abdominal organs. We observed that during the first episode of colicky biliary or ureteral pain, true parietal pain followed true visceral pain after a variable interval. In subsequent episodes, parietal pain developed promptly and was not preceded by true visceral pain. This phenomenon was probably due to the activation of mnemonic traces (Procacci and Zoppi, 1983).

Conclusions

We have seen that in experiments on man and in clinical practice different types of sensations arise from viscera, ranging from unpleasant sensations of fullness of the stomach to the excruciating pain of myocardial infarction.

As regards pain, a clear-cut distinction between visceral and somatic pain can be made only in some cases, most commonly in the early stages of the disease. Otherwise, we observe a mixture of visceral and somatic pain, both in the phenomenon of referred pain and in the "intricate conditions" in which pain arises from viscera and from somatic tissues. This is an important point, because pain can only be useful for an accurate diagnosis if correctly interpreted.

References

Ayala, M. (1937) Douleur sympathique et douleur viscérale. Rev. Neurol., 68: 222–242.

Benedetti, G, (1969) Neuropsicologia, Feltrinelli, Milano, pp. 45–81.

Bonica, J. J. (1953) The Management of Pain, Lea and Febiger, Philadelphia.

Cervero, F. (1980) Deep and visceral pain. In H. W. Kosterlitz and L. Y. Terenius (Eds.), Pain and Society, Verlag Chemie, Weinheim, pp. 263–282.

Davis, L. and Pollock, L. J. (1930) The peripheral pathway for painful sensations. Arch. Neurol. Psychiat., 24: 883–898.

Froment, R. and Gonin, A. (1956) Les Angors Coronariens Intriqués, Expansion Scientifique Française, Paris.

Galletti, R. and Procacci, P. (1958) Su l'esplorazione funzionale delle vie sensitive degli arti per mezzo dell'ischemia da compressione. Norme tecniche per l'esecuzione della prova e risultati nei soggetti normali. Rass. Neurol. Veg., 13: 143–150.

Galletti, R. and Procacci, P. (1966) The role of the sympathetic system in the control of somatic pain and of some associated phenomena. Acta Neuroveg., 28: 495–500.

Galletti, R. and Procacci, P. (1968) Basi fisiopatologiche per una razionale terapia antalgica delle affezioni viscerali. Rass. Neurol. Veg., 23, Suppl. 1: 1–204.

Galletti, R., Procacci, P., Marchetti, P. G., Rocchi, P. and Buzzelli, G. (1963) Esplorazione della funzione sensitiva dell'arto superiore e dei fenomeni cutanei correlati nelle fibromialgie. Effetti del blocco delle vie sensitive e del ganglio stellato. Arch. Fisiol., 62: 313–331.

Hansen, K. and Schliack, H. (1962) Segmentale Innervation: Ihre Bedeutung fur Klinik und Praxis, Thieme, Stuttgart, pp. 166–325.

Hugon, M. (1971) Transfer of somatosensory information in the spinal cord. In W. A. Cobb (Ed.), Handbook of Electroencephalography and Clinical Neurophysiology, Vol. 9: Somatic Sensation, Elsevier, Amsterdam, pp. 33–44.

Keele, C. A. (1962) Sensations aroused by chemical stimulation of the skin. In C. A. Keele and R. Smith (Eds.), The Assessment of Pain in Man and Animals, Livingstone, Edinburgh, pp. 28–31.

Kinsella, V. J. (1948) The Mechanism of Abdominal Pain, Australasian Medical Publishing Company, Sidney.

Leriche, R. (1949) La Chirurgie de la Douleur, Masson, Paris.

Lewis, T. (1942) Pain, Macmillan, New York, pp. 118–172.

Lim, R. K. S. (1966) A revised concept of the mechanism of analgesia and pain. In R. S. Knighton and P. R. Dumke (Eds.), Henry Ford International Symposium, Pain, Churchill, London, pp. 117–154.

Lim, R. K. S. (1967) Pharmacologic viewpoint of pain and analgesia. In E. L. Way (Ed.), New Concepts in Pain and its Clinical Management, Davis, Philadelphia, pp. 33–47.

Livingston, W. K. (1943) Pain Mechanisms, Macmillan, New York, pp. 224–235.

Lunedei, A. and Galletti, R. (1953) Il meccanismo di insorgenza del dolore dei visceri nei suoi recenti sviluppi. Rass. Neurol. Veg., 10: 3–22.

Mackenzie, J. (1909) Symptoms and their Interpretation, Shaw and Sons, London.

MacLellan, A. M. and Goodell, H. (1943) Pain from the bladder, ureter and kidney pelvis. Proc. Ass. Res. Nerv. Ment. Dis., 23: 252–262.

Melzack, R. (1973) The Puzzle of Pain, Penguin Books, Harmondsworth.

Merrington, W. R. and Nathan, P. W. (1949) A study of postischaemic paraesthesiae. J. Neurol. Neurosurg. Psychiat., 12: 1–18.

Mountcastle, V. B. (1974) Pain and temperature sensibilities. In V. B. Mountcastle (Ed.), Medical Physiology, 12th edn., Mosby, St. Louis, pp. 348–381.

Nathan, P. W. (1962) Pain traces left in the central nervous system. In C. A. Keele and R. Smith (Eds.), The Assessment of Pain in Man and Animals, Livingstone, Edinburgh, pp. 129–134.

Nathan, P. W. (1977) Pain. Br. Med. Bull., 33: 149–156.

Penfield, W. (1925) Neurological mechanism of angina pectoris and its relation to surgical therapy. Am. J. Med. Sci., 170: 864–873.

Procacci, P. (1969) A survey of modern concepts of pain. In P. J. Vinken and G. W. Bruyn (Eds.), Handbook of Clinical Neurology, Vol. 1, North-Holland Publishing Company, Amsterdam, pp. 114–146.

Procacci, P. and Maresca, M. (1984) Pain concept in Western civilization: a historical review. In C. Benedetti, C. R. Chapman and G. Moricca (Eds.), Advances in Pain Research and Therapy, Vol. 7, Raven Press, New York, pp. 1–11.

Procacci, P. and Zoppi, M. (1983) Pathophysiology and clinical aspects of visceral and referred pain. In J. J. Bonica, U. Lindblom and A. Iggo (Eds.), Advances in Pain Research and Therapy, Vol. 5, Raven Press, New York, pp. 643–658.

Procacci, P. and Zoppi, M. (1984) Heart pain. In P. D. Wall and R. Melzack (Eds.), Textbook of Pain, Churchill Livingstone, Edinburgh, pp. 309–318.

Procacci, P., Buzzelli, G., Voegelin, M. R. and Bozza, G. (1968) Esplorazione della funzione sensitiva degli arti superiori in soggetti con pregresso infarto miocardico. Rass. Neurol. Veg., 22: 403–418.

Procacci, P., Passeri, I., Zoppi, M., Burzagli, L., Voegelin, M. R. and Maresca, M. (1972) Esplorazione della funzione sensitiva degli arti superiori in soggetti con angina pectoris. Giorn. Ital. Cardiol., 2: 978–984.

Procacci, P., Francini, F., Zoppi, M. and Maresca, M. (1975) Cutaneous pain threshold changes after sympathetic block in reflex dystrophies. Pain, 1: 167–175.

Procacci, P., Zoppi, M., Padeletti, L. and Maresca, M. (1976) Myocardial infarction without pain. A study of the sensory function of the upper limbs. Pain, 2: 309–313.

Procacci, P., Maresca, M. and Zoppi, M. (1978) Visceral and deep somatic pain. Acupuncture Electrother. Res., 3: 135–160.

Procacci, P., Francini, F., Maresca, M. and Zoppi, M. (1979a) Skin potential and EMG changes induced by cutaneous electrical stimulation. II. Subjects with reflex sympathetic dystrophies. Appl. Neurophysiol., 42: 125–134.

Procacci, P., Zoppi, M. and Maresca, M. (1979b) Tracce mnemoniche nel dolore cardiaco. Dolore, 1: 17–20.

Ross, J. (1887) On the segmental distribution of sensory disorders. Brain, 10: 333–361.

Ruch, T.C. (1960) Pathophysiology of pain. In T. C. Ruch and J. F. Fulton (Eds.), Medical Physiology and Biophysics, Saunders, Philadelphia, pp. 350–368.

Smith, G. M., Egbert, L. D., Markowitz, R. A., Mosteller, F. and Beecher, H. K. (1966) An experimental pain method sensitive to morphine in man: the submaximum effort tourniquet technique. J. Pharmacol. Exp. Ther., 154: 324–332.

Sturge, W. A. (1883) The phenomena of angina pectoris, and their bearing upon the theory of counter-irritation. Brain, 5: 492–510.

Teodori, U. and Galletti, R. (1962) Il Dolore nelle Affezioni degli Organi Interni del Torace, Pozzi, Roma.

Wall, P. D. (1974) Physiological mechanisms involved in the production of pain. In J. J. Bonica, P. Procacci and C. A. Pagni (Eds.), Recent Advances on Pain, Thomas, Springfield, pp. 36–63.

Weddell, G. and Sinclair, D. C. (1947) "Pins and needles": observations on some of the sensations aroused in a limb by the application of pressure. J. Neurol. Neurosurg. Psychiat., 10: 26–46.

Willis, W. D. and Coggeshall, R. E. (1978) Sensory Mechanisms of the Spinal Cord, Plenum Press, New York.

Wolf, S. and Wolff, H. G. (1947) Human Gastric Function. An Experimental Study of a Man and his Stomach, Oxford University Press, New York.

Wolff, H. G. (1963) Headache and Other Head Pain, Oxford University Press, New York, pp. 28–46.

F. Cervero and J. F.B. Morrison
Progress in Brain Research, Vol. 67

CHAPTER 3

Afferent C-fibres and visceral sensation

A. Iggo

Department of Veterinary Physiology, University of Edinburgh, Summerhall, Edinburgh EH9 1QH, U.K.

Introduction

The existence of sensations elicited from the viscera is not in question, although the qualities or modalities evocable are very limited. In 1911, Hurst published a monograph in which he argued, on the basis of clinical observations, for a primitive form of muscle sense. About the same time, Head et al. (1905) were attributing a capacity for "protopathic" sensitivity to viscera partly on the grounds of their innervation by thin, in his view primitive, nerves. Sherrington also made a contribution, although in terms of reflexes, with the demonstration of potent effects of gallbladder distension on systemic blood pressure (Sherrington and Sowton, 1915). The existence of an afferent innervation of the viscera is thus attested by these classical contributions. Two other "classical" papers are relevant to the topic — the first by Payne and Poulton (1927), who, in an investigation of the sensations associated with swallowing, reported that the normal propulsive contractions of the oesophagus are unfelt; in contrast, if the subject attempted to swallow an incompressible balloon, lodged in the oesophagus, an extremely painful sensation was aroused, associated with a strong contraction of the oesophagus. The other paper is by Denny-Brown and Robertson (1933), who measured the intravesical pressure and reported the sensation experienced when the urinary bladder was filled to different volumes. The pressure showed sudden increments with successive increments in volume, followed by a slow fall as the muscle relaxed, until large volumes of fluid were present, when the pressure tended to remain high and reflex contractions and emptying were elicited. A range of sensations from a sense of distension, through fullness to discomfort, and varying degrees of pain were reported.

The viscera, therefore, can be the source of sensations but also of reflexes, and varying degrees of the same stimulus appear to be capable of evoking a variety of responses. Questions prompted by these results are: what kinds of visceral sensory receptors are there? Does a single receptor have multiple sensory functions? Are there specific nociceptors?

An answer can be sought by electrophysiological analysis. One of the earliest attempts was by Adrian (1933) who showed that the cervical vagus contained afferent units excited by pulmonary inflation — these form the afferent limb of the Hering-Breuer inflation reflex, and normally do not enter consciousness. They are proprioceptors. The thoracic viscera have yielded many other afferents with cardiovascular and respiratory functions. In contrast, the abdominal and pelvic viscera were in the 1940s a terra incognita. Germandt and Zotterman in 1946 recorded from mesenteric nerves and reported activity evoked by mechanical stimuli, and of course the Pacinian corpuscles, especially of the cat, were investigated by Gray and Sato (1953), among others.

Visceral nerves, however, contain a preponderance of non-myelinated fibres. Agostoni et al. (1957), at University College, London, found those in the vagus to be afferent, with cell bodies in the nodose ganglion. At the same time I was attempting

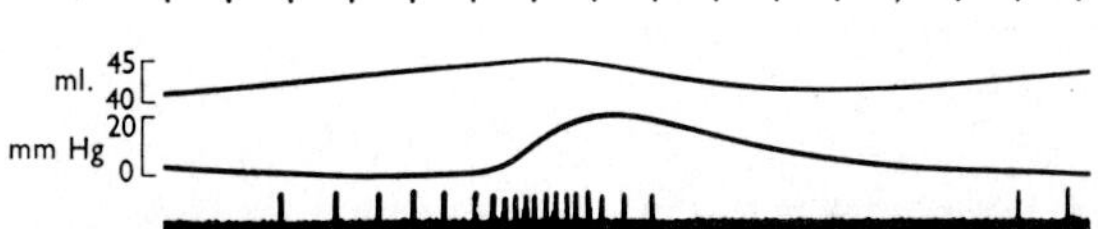

Fig. 1. "In series" tension receptor in urinary bladder of the cat. A single unit recording showing the relatively weak effect of distension, during filling of the bladder, and strong effect of a bladder contraction. The upper trace records bladder volume, middle trace shows the intravesicle pressure and lower trace the afferent discharge in a single fibre. From Iggo (1955).

to analyse the mechanisms underlying the well-organised contractions of the ruminant stomach and, in order to develop suitable techniques, was working on the afferent innervation of the bladder. The experiments, using single unit dissection of the pelvic nerves, established what has turned out to be a characteristic property of many visceral mechanoreceptors — excitation during distension, and a further enhancement of the discharge during muscular contraction of the viscus, as is clearly illustrated in Fig. 1. The receptors are seen to be excited as the bladder distends, during the increase in volume of its contents, with only a small rise in intravesicular pressure. Then, during a reflexly elicited contraction, the bladder pressure increases sharply, while volume also increases and there is a substantial acceleration of the afferent discharge. What is particularly notable is that the discharge of impulses continues as the volume of the bladder is decreasing, and the contraction continues until, with progressive emptying and as the intravesicle pressure is falling, the afferent unit falls silent, to begin again only after filling of the bladder has started again. The receptor is responding not just to distension, but to contraction as well — it is an "in series" tension receptor (Iggo, 1955). A complication is introduced when more than one receptor is examined, in that different receptors do not necessarily respond in concert. These differences are attributed to the independent action smooth muscle of the bladder wall, with asynchronous contractions of various parts. The urinary bladder can be persuaded to make sustained contractions, for example, by suddenly switching from isotonic to isometric re-

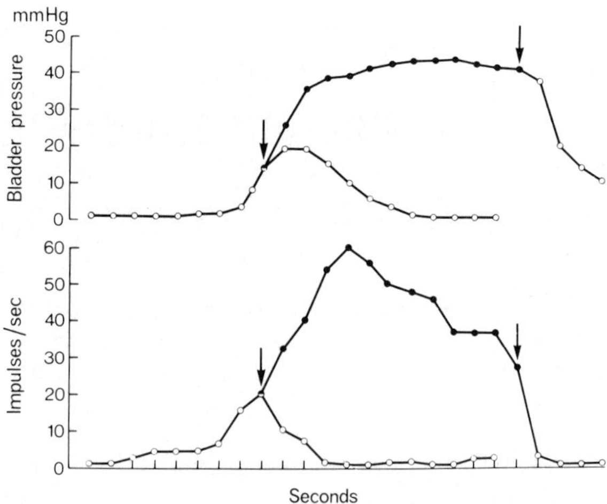

Fig. 2. An "in series" tension receptor in urinary bladder during an isotonic contraction (open circles) as in Fig. 1, and the response during a sustained isometric contraction (closed circles). From Iggo (1966).

cording conditions during a contraction. Fig. 2 illustrates the effect of such a manoeuvre. The small pressure rise seen during isotonic distension in Fig. 1 is now transformed to a vigorous 3-fold rise in pressure which is sustained for more than 10 seconds, until the isotonic conditions are restored by allowing fluid to leave the bladder. Here we see the same receptor responding in a stimulus-related manner, over a wide range of pressures. The sensory analogy is from unawareness to intense pain — to be tested quite simply by suddenly interrupting the free flow of urine during micturition. Are the sensory consequences to be attributed to the same receptor, firing at different rates?

One unsettled question in the bladder afferent study was the size of the afferent fibres. The pelvic nerves contain small myelinated axons, and it was more or less tacitly assumed at the time that the afferent fibres were myelinated. Indeed, it was generally assumed that non-myelinated axons, if they carried impulses at all, were inaccessible to single unit recording. This view was reinforced by Gasser's (1955) electron microscope analysis of cutaneous nerves, which showed the non-myelinated fibres as small clusters of up to 10–15 axons, each cluster in association with a Schwann cell (Fig. 3).

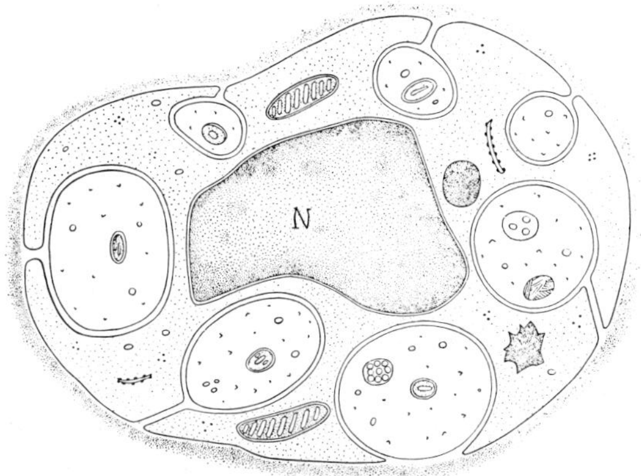

Fig. 3. Diagrammatic representation of non-myelinated axons and the associated Schwann cell, with its nucleus (N). From Elfvin (1958).

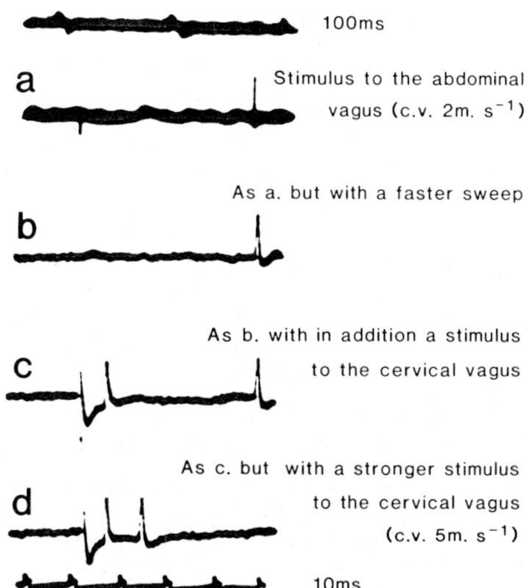

Fig. 4. Conduction velocity measurements in an abdominal vagal afferent unit, illustrating the collision method for the identification of an afferent fibre for conduction velocity (c.v.) measurement. From Iggo (1958).

His own further analysis however, did establish that individual axons, in the whole nerve, were capable of independent conduction. Nevertheless, the morphology of the nerve did raise serious doubts about the possibility of a unitary analysis of afferent C-fibres by electrophysiological methods. Indeed, the first reports to the Physiological Society of single-unit C-fibre afferent activity in mammals (Iggo, 1957a) were greeted with scepticism by scientists more familiar with giant non-myelinated axons of invertebrates.

TABLE I

A comparison of three estimates of the conduction velocity in ten single vagal fibres

Fibre No.	Receptor	Conduction velocity (m/second)		
		I, Short distance S1–R (19–25 mm)	II, Long distance S2–R (47–55 mm)	III, by difference
44	Pulmonary inflation	34	33.5	32.5
43	Pulmonary inflation	19.6	19.2	18.5
54	Pulmonary inflation	17.6	16.9	16.5
53	Gastric mucosal	2.8	2.6	2.4
50	Unidentified	2.0	1.5	1.2
55	Gastric mucosal	1.8	1.5	1.3
45	Oesophageal tension	1.4	1.1	1.0
47	Gastric tension	1.3	1.2	1.1
52	Gastric mucosal	1.2	1.1	1.0
51	Gastric tension	1.1	1.05	1.0

The velocities were computed from $v = d/t$; in columns I and II, d is the distance from S to R, and t is the time interval between the stimulus artifact and the arrival of the impulse at R; in column III, d is the distance between S1 and S2 and t is the difference between the conduction times in columns I and II. From Iggo (1958).

The original single C-fibre methods, based on microdissection of small strands dissected from the vagus (Iggo, 1957a), depended on conduction velocity measurements for identification. Fig. 4 illustrates an example, where conduction velocities were measured over two lengths of the nerve, in which, although one velocity corresponds to a non-myelinated axon, the other over a shorter distance adjacent to the proximally placed recording electrode was that expected for a thin myelinated axon. This possibility that apparent C-fibre units were actually thinly myelinated at the recording electrodes was tackled systematically (Iggo, 1958), with results as in Table I that established uniformity of conduction velocity, at values well within the C range. Confirmation of the conclusion that unit spikes could be recorded from mammalian non-myelinated axons was provided by Bower (1966), working with abdominal visceral nerves that did not contain any myelinated axons.

A further technical development, the use of the collision technique (Iggo, 1958), greatly eased the task of obtaining verifiable single C-units, and such analyses are now generally available.

What of the results?

Single-unit analyses of abdominal afferent systems are directed at either the vagal or the splanchnic nerves. My own studies were directed principally at the vagus, because of an interest in the reflex regulation of gastric activity, and because the vagus was often considered, in clinical situations, to be a motor nerve. It is, in fact, as Agostoni et al. (1957) first established, at least 80% afferent.

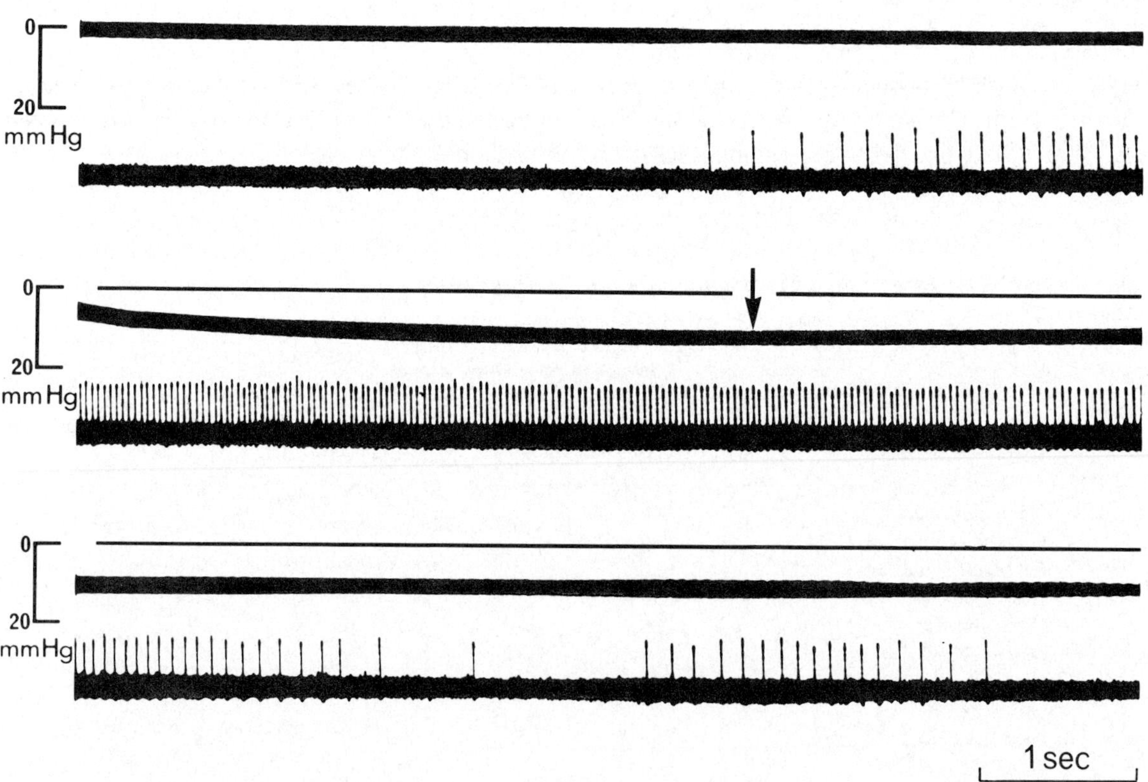

Fig. 5. Gastric "in series" tension receptor with a non-myelinated (C) afferent fibre during distension of the stomach. Inflow of fluid began at start of upper record and stopped at the arrow. Upper trace is intraluminal pressure and lower trace is afferent discharge in a single C-fibre. From Iggo (1957a).

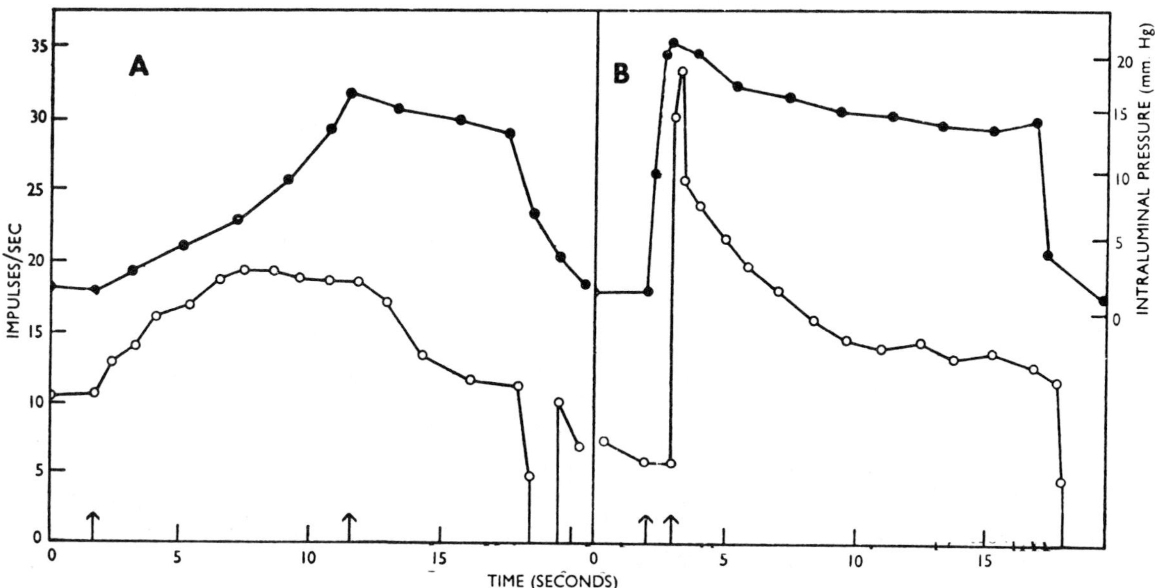

Fig. 6. Jejunal "in series" tension receptor with C afferent fibre in an isolated segment of the intestine during distension with the same volume of fluid, during slow inflow in A, and during rapid inflow in B. From Iggo (1957a).

The first clearly established category of alimentary C-fibres were the "in series" tension receptors (Iggo, 1955), originally reported in ruminants, with small myelinated axons in the cervical vagus and excited by distension, compression and contraction. The C-fibre "in series" tension receptors in the cat stomach had similar properties (Fig. 5) and similar units were present in the intestines (Fig. 6), where it was also easier to establish the importance of smooth muscle in affecting the dynamic aspects of distension. The evidence pointed to a location of the "in series" receptors in the muscularis externa, a location since confirmed in a detailed analysis by Cottrell and Iggo (1984a) (Fig. 7).

Another category of C-mechanoreceptor is the distension-sensitive unit, lying beneath the serosa (or in the omentum) but unaffected by contraction. This kind of unit, with afferent fibres in the vagus, is relatively uncommon, and it is probable that most of the vagal C-units in the outer coats of the alimentary canal are "in series" tension receptors. Other muscular viscera, such as the gallbladder and its ducts, presumably have similar receptors (see Paintal, this volume).

The other major source of afferent input from the alimentary canal is the mucosa. The early single unit studies indicated that their properties were different from the "in series" tension receptors and also that more of the axons were myelinated, at least in their more rostral parts. They are mechanically sensitive, but do not give sustained discharges to distension or contraction; instead, they can be excited by stroking or dragging a probe across the mucosal surface. Some of them are excited by either acid (Fig. 8) or alkali placed on the mucosa, and, in the cat stomach, may give a sustained and repeatable response to such a stimulus (Iggo, 1966). In the non-glandular forestomach and the glandular abomasum (Harding and Leek, 1972) and in the duodenum (Cottrell and Iggo, 1984c) of the sheep the response characteristics are incompatible with the [H^+] being the only or major factor determining the response of the units, in contrast to the older report for cat gastric units (Iggo, 1957b). Instead, they appear to have sensitivity correlated with the titratable acidity and molality of short-chain aliphatic organic acids (such as acetic) rather than pH. The recent detailed analysis by Cottrell and Iggo

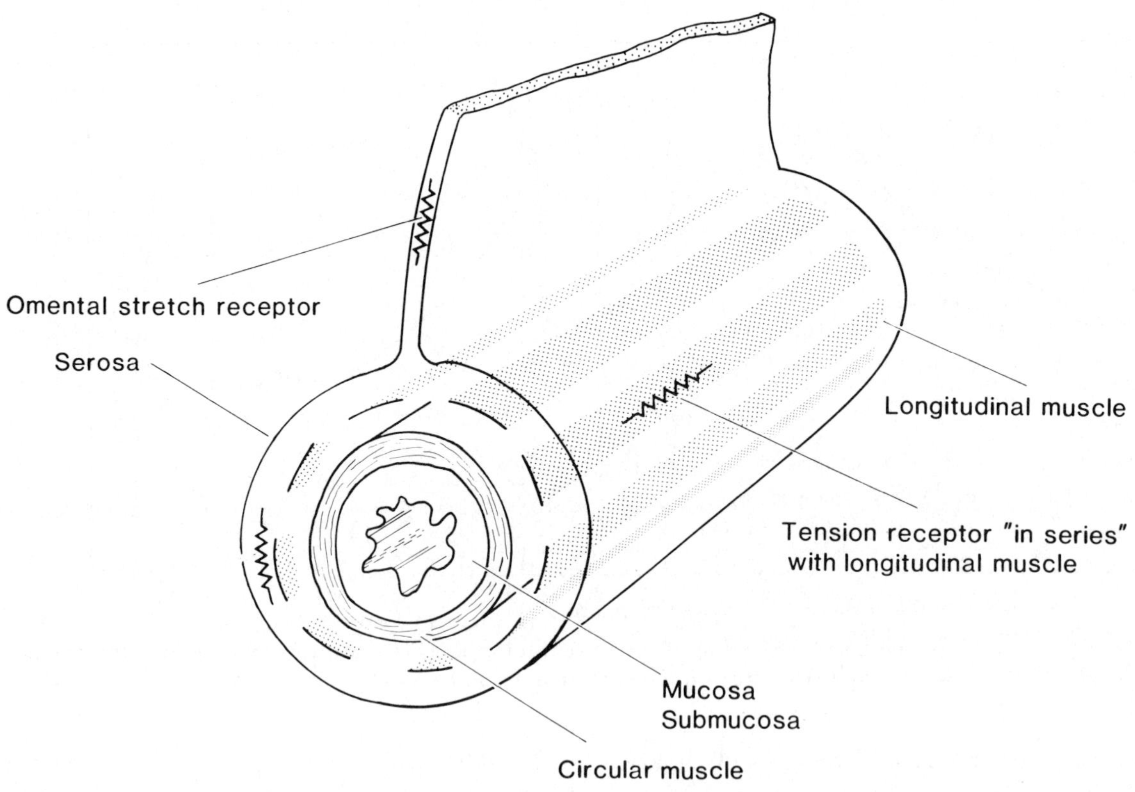

Fig. 7. Diagram to illustrate the postulated organisation of sensory receptors with vagal afferent fibres in the muscularis externa of the duodenum of the sheep. From Cottrell and Iggo (1984b).

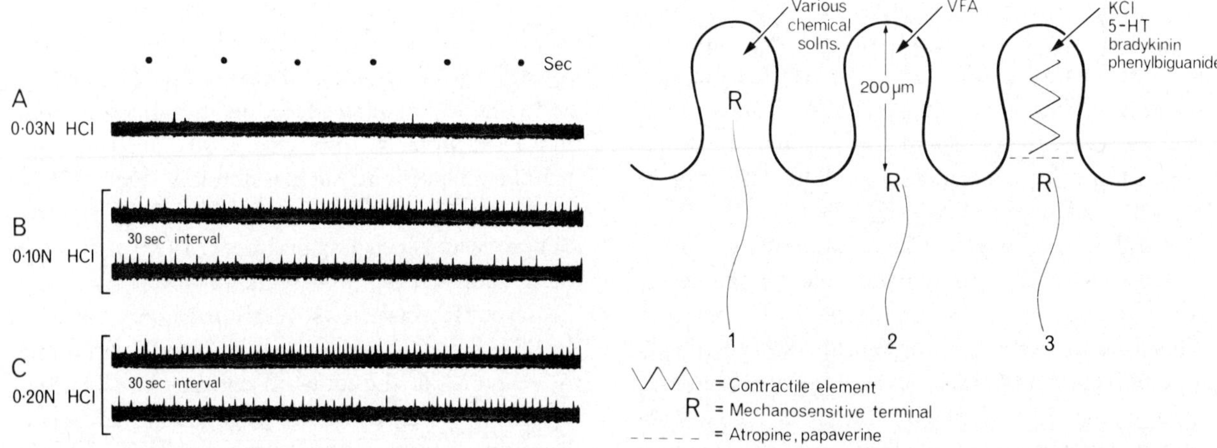

Fig. 8. Mucosal receptors with vagal afferent fibres in the cat, responding to acid solution (1 N HCl) on the mucosal surface. In B and C, the lower record is a continuation, after 30 seconds, of the upper record. From Iggo (1957b).

Fig. 9. Diagram to illustrate the postulated organisation of sensory receptors in the duodenal mucosa and muscularis mucosa of the sheep. 5-HT, 5-hydroxytryptamine; VFA, vagal fibre afferent. From Cottrell and Iggo (1984c).

(1984a,b,c) brings up-to-date knowledge of the duodenal sensory receptors (Fig. 9), with the suggestion of several categories of unit according to the responses to mechanical and chemical stimuli.

New varieties of chemical agents now available include the neuropeptides, some of which were first studied in the gastrointestinal tract, such as gastrin and cholecystokinin. Because they have, or may have, a role in neurally mediated responses of the alimentary canal in digestion they have recently been examined in single-unit C-fibre preparations of the duodenum (Cottrell and Iggo, 1984b). There were often clear excitatory effects on "in series" tension receptors, but these were blocked by atropine or hexamethanium, and could usually be correlated with changes in muscular activity. The conclusion reached was that although clear excitatory effects were seen, the responses were secondary to an action of the peptides either directly or indirectly evoking contractions.

This brief survey establishes the viscera as the source of a diversity of afferent inputs to the central nervous system. The inputs go centrally along visceral nerves, such as the vagus, splanchnic and pelvic nerves, that are also the routes by which the autonomic system exerts its controlling influence on the viscera. It is now well established that the afferent inflow is important, among other things, in regulating through reflex actions the activity of viscera, as for example the cyclical contractile activity of the ruminant stomach (e.g., Iggo and Leek, 1967). It is also clear that the afferent inflow can reach consciousness and result in a variety of sensations, from comfortable repletion after a meal, to hunger pangs and even completely disabling pain from gallstones.

What is still not completely resolved is whether the same afferent unit provides the only sensory inflow that, depending on circumstances, results in these different sensations. Or are there several kinds of afferent unit, as is now so clearly established for the cutaneous senses? Are there visceral nociceptors, distinct from other mechanoreceptors? The answers to these questions will surely come from the detailed analysis of spinal and cerebral mechanisms of the kind now under way, and reported in other chapters of the present volume.

References

Adrian, E. D. (1933) Afferent impulses in the vagus and their effect on respiration. J. Physiol., 79: 332–358.

Agostoni, E., Chinnock, J. E., Daly, M. De B. and Murray, J. G. (1957) Functional and histological studies of the vagus nerve and its branches to the heart, lungs and abdominal viscera. J. Physiol., 135: 182–205.

Bower, E. A. (1966) The activity of post-ganglionic sympathetic nerves to the uterus of the rabbit. J. Physiol., 183: 748–767.

Cottrell, D. F. and Iggo, A. (1984a) Tension receptors with vagal afferent fibres in the proximal duodenum and pyloric sphincter of sheep. J. Physiol., 345: 457–475.

Cottrell, D. F. and Iggo, A. (1984b) The responses of duodenal tension receptors in sheep to pentagastrin, cholecystokinin and some other drugs. J. Physiol., 354: 477–495.

Cottrell, D. F. and Iggo, A. (1984c) Mucosal enteroceptors with vagal afferent fibres in the proximal duodenum of sheep. J. Physiol., 354: 497–522.

Denny-Brown, D. and Robertson, E. G. (1933) The physiology of micturition. Brain, 56: 149–190.

Elfvin, L.-G. (1958) The ultrastructure of unmyelinated fibres in the splenic nerve of the cat. J. Ultrastruct. Res., 1: 428–454.

Gasser, H.S. (1955) Properties of dorsal root unmedullated fibers on the two sides of the ganglion. J. Gen. Physiol., 38: 709–728.

Gray, J. A. B. and Sato, M. (1953) Properties of the receptor potential in Pacinian corpuscles. J. Physiol., 122: 610–636.

Germandt, B. and Zotterman, Y. (1946) Intestinal pain: An electrophysiological investigation on mesenteric nerves. Acta Physiol. Scand., 12: 56–72.

Harding, R. and Leek, B. F. (1972) Rapidly adapting mechanoreceptors in the reticulo-rumen which also respond to chemicals. J. Physiol., 223: 32–33P.

Head, H., Rivers, W. H. R. and Sherren, J. (1905) The afferent nervous system from a new aspect. Brain, 28: 99–115.

Hurst, A. F. (1911) The Sensibility of the Alimentary Canal, Oxford University Press, London.

Iggo, A. (1955) Tension receptors in the stomach and the urinary bladder. J. Physiol., 128: 593–607.

Iggo, A. (1957a) Conduction velocity in vagal afferent fibres. J. Physiol., 138: 21P.

Iggo, A. (1957b) Gastric mucosal chemoreceptors with vagal afferent fibres in the cat. Q. J. Exp. Physiol., 42: 398–409.

Iggo, A. (1958) The electrophysiological identification of single nerve fibres, with particular reference to the slowest conducting vagal afferent fibres in the cat. J. Physiol., 142: 110–126.

Iggo, A. (1966) Physiology of visceral afferent systems. Acta Neuroveg., 28: 121–134.

Iggo, A. and Leek, B. F. (1967) An electrophysiological study of some reticulo-ruminal and abomasal reflexes in sheep. J. Physiol., 193: 95–119.

Payne, W. W. and Poulton, E. P. (1927) Experiments on visceral sensation. Part I: The relation of pain to activity of the human oesophagus. J. Physiol., 63: 217–241.

Sherrington, C. S. and Sowton, S. C. M. (1915) Observations on reflex responses to single break shocks. J. Physiol. (Lond.), 49: 331–348.

SECTION II

Visceral Afferent Systems

F. Cervero and J. F.B. Morrison
Progress in Brain Research, Vol. 67

CHAPTER 4

Sensory innervation of the heart

Alberto Malliani, Federico Lombardi and Massimo Pagani

Istituto Ricerche Cardiovascolari, CNR; Patologia Medica, Centro "Fidia", Ospedale "L. Sacco"; Università di Milano, Milano, Italy

Introduction

From a pathophysiological point of view, derived more from a clinical oversimplification than from adequate observations, there is a tendency to consider cardiac pain as the most alarming message from the jeopardised heart.

This is not to deny the general validity of the biological principle that pain has a protective, or self-preserving, value to the organism (Adams, 1980), but rather to anticipate that, where the heart is concerned, "noxious" does not necessarily mean pain and that non-painful sensations can sometimes represent a more ominous clinical message than pain per se.

A few and very elementary notes on the anatomy and physiology of the sensory substratum of the heart, although they may sound obvious and too schematised to the experts, will have to be included for those readers who, interested in visceral sensation, are not acquainted with the complexity of cardiac innervation.

The dual afferent pathway

The heart possesses a double sensory innervation made up of afferent nerve fibres coursing into the vagal and sympathetic nerves to, respectively, the medulla and the spinal cord.

As a consequence of this double sensory innervation, selective degeneration studies have been necessary in order to discriminate from an anatomical point of view between vagal and sympathetic sensory endings, and the ensuing scanty evidence is what has been so far obtained and will probably last as such until selective labelling techniques are also used in this field.

The existence of sensory endings in the heart was first suggested by Berkley (1894), Smirnov (1895) and Dogiel (1898). As to the contribution of vagal or sympathetic fibres to these endings, Woollard (1926) concluded that a large proportion of cardiac sensory terminals were of vagal origin, as he observed that experimental bilateral stellectomy did not markedly modify what he considered to be the normal aspect of the sensory apparatus of the heart. The conclusions reached by Nettleship (1936) were somewhat different: the removal of the dorsal root ganglia produced a degeneration of fibres in the endocardial net at the apex of the ventricles and from the walls of the coronary vessels, thus proving that a portion of sensory afferents from the heart were projecting to the spinal cord through the sympathetic nerves. In favour of a more substantial balance between the dual input seems the opinion of Khabarova (1963), when she writes that sympathetic endings "frequently lie side by side with ... endings of the vagus nerves", a statement that seems to reflect the electrophysiological findings which, so far, have suggested that vagal and sympathetic receptors are intermingled in all regions of the heart.

Vagal afferent fibres

Afferent vagal fibres innervating the heart (Hainsworth et al., 1979; Bishop et al., 1983) can be divided, on the basis of the location of their receptors and of the characteristics of the fibres, into: (a) atrial myelinated fibres, (b) ventricular myelinated fibres and (c) cardiac receptors with unmyelinated fibres.

Atrial receptors with myelinated fibres, since the first analytical study by Paintal (1953), have been divided, according to the patterns of their impulse activity, into type A and type B (Paintal, 1973).

Type A receptors, which yield a burst of impulses during atrial systole, have been suggested to respond to atrial systolic pressure (Dickinson, 1950), active wall tension (Struppler and Struppler, 1955; Recordati et al., 1976), and heart rate (Arndt et al., 1971), while the pattern of discharge during the cardiac cycle might depend on both the degree of atrial distension and the contractile state of the atrial muscle (Recordati et al., 1976).

Conversely, type B atrial receptors, which generate impulses during atrial filling, have been shown to be slowly adapting stretch sensors that respond to pulsatile changes in atrial filling (Paintal, 1953, 1973) and, in more detail, to both static and dynamic changes in atrial wall tension (Recordati et al., 1975).

These vagal atrial receptors have a reflex regulatory role of probable paramount importance, including reflex tachycardia or alterations in renal function, which has been extensively reviewed recently (Hainsworth et al., 1979; Bishop et al., 1983).

Ventricular vagal receptors with myelinated fibres discharge in phase with the rise of the intraventricular pressure (Paintal, 1955).

Thus, vagal afferent myelinated fibres innervate all chambers of the heart and, in addition, the coronary tree (Brown, 1965). Their responsiveness to mechanical stimuli indicates their prevalent mechanosensitive nature, although they can also be excited by various drugs (Paintal, 1964; Coleridge, J. G. G. and Coleridge, 1979; Bishop et al., 1983).

Cardiac receptors with unmyelinated fibres innervating the atria and the ventricles have recently been submitted to numerous investigations and reviews (Oberg and Thorén, 1972; Thames et al., 1977; Thorén, 1979; Bishop et al., 1983).

In general, atrial and ventricular unmyelinated afferents display a lower frequency impulse activity, when compared to their myelinated counterpart.

Atrial endings seem to respond to both atrial filling and contraction, while in the case of ventricular receptors the end-diastolic pressure seems to represent a more important determinant than do systolic events (Thames et al., 1977; Thorén, 1979; Bishop et al., 1983). All of these unmyelinated afferents can also be markedly excited by chemical substances (Coleridge and Coleridge, 1979).

It is interesting that the afferent unmyelinated cardiac vagal fibres seem to mediate cardiovascular reflexes of a solely inhibitory nature (Thorén, 1979; Bishop et al., 1983).

Sympathetic afferent fibres

Afferent sympathetic fibres can also be divided, on the basis of the distribution of their receptors, into atrial and ventricular afferents, both of which can be either myelinated or unmyelinated (Malliani, 1982). In this context, we shall simply outline their general functional characteristics.

Afferent sympathetic nerve fibres with cardiac receptors, in the anaesthetised animal under apparently normal resting conditions, display a tonic impulse activity in relation to normal and specific haemodynamic events (Malliani, 1982; Bishop et al., 1983). The peculiarity of this spontaneous activity is that it usually consists of, at most, one action potential per cardiac cycle. Their mechanosensitivity to natural stimuli can be extreme, while no truly major differences seem to characterise, from this point of view, myelinated from unmyelinated afferents (Ueda et al., 1969; Malliani et al., 1973; Hess et al., 1974; Uchida, 1975; Casati et al., 1979).

Afferent sympathetic cardiac fibres are also extremely sensitive to chemicals (Uchida and Murao, 1974; Nishi et al., 1977; Coleridge and Coleridge, 1979; Coleridge, H. M. and Coleridge, 1980; Baker et al., 1980; Lombardi et al., 1981; Malliani, 1982), a property which has been used in order to investigate whether cardiac nociception was more likely to be based on "specificity" (Baker et al., 1980) or "intensity" (Malliani and Lombardi, 1982) mechanisms. Suffice it to say, in this context, that as ventricular sympathetic receptors always displayed, in our hands, a spontaneous impulse activity if the haemodynamic conditions were within the normal range and as bradykinin or coronary occlusion increased this ongoing impulse activity without recruiting silent afferents, the conclusion was reached that the "intensity" theory appeared the most likely candidate to account for the properties of the neural substrate subserving cardiac nociception (Malliani and Lombardi, 1982). In short, in our experiments we never found sensory units fitting the fundamental criterion for a specific nociceptor, i.e., of being deprived of a spontaneous background activity (Burgess and Perl, 1973) and of being recruited exclusively by stimuli considered to be "noxious".

The role of vagal and sympathetic afferent nerve fibres in transmitting nociceptive information

The concept that the afferent fibres running in the cardiac sympathetic nerves were the only essential pathway for the transmission of cardiac pain arose from observations on both humans and experimental animals.

In man, thoracic sympathectomy or section of the higher thoracic dorsal roots was found to be a manoeuvre capable of relieving anginal pain (Jonnesco, 1921; Leriche and Fontaine, 1927; Lindgren and Olivecrona, 1947; White, 1957), while stellate ganglionectomy could abolish behavioural reactions accompanying coronary occlusion in acute experiments (Sutton and Lueth, 1930; Brown, 1967). Observations which were consistent with Langley's statement (1903) that "most of the afferent fibres, which on electrical stimulation give rise to pain, pass by the sympathetic strands and not by the vagus". This view is still tenable nowadays, although some contribution by vagal afferent fibres in the mediation of cardiac nociception cannot be dismissed too hastily. Indeed, the anginal pain referred to the jaw, head and neck, more frequent after sympathectomy (the phenonemon of "migration of pain" (Lindgren and Olivecrona, 1947), may indicate an additional central site, besides the spinal cord, where the mechanisms for referred pain may be activated: in this case by cardiac vagal afferent fibres. Moreover, even when nociception would be transmitted through afferent sympathetic fibres, an important modulatory role might be exerted by vagal afferents (Ammons et al., 1983).

Yet, in the present context, aware of possible over-simplifications, we can affirm that afferent sympathetic cardiac fibres do mediate cardiac nociception.

The adequate stimuli for cardiac pain and the importance of the experimental model

When Harvey and Charles I, an unusual team, touched the beating heart of the son of the Earl of Montgomery, incredibly exposed through a large thoracic wound, they had to acknowledge "that the heart was without the sense of touch" (Willis, 1847). That was the dawn of a future certitude: for the viscera as much as for the soma, touch and pain cannot be equated. Or, from another perspective, that was the beginning of searching for the adequate stimulus eliciting cardiac pain. When Sherrington (1906) focused attention on the "nocuous" event, which threatened the integrity of a tissue — the stimulus capable, by definition, of triggering nociception — he furnished more a piece of understanding of some sensory systems rather than a universal key to all sensory mechanisms.

As to the heart, it has long been known that, for instance, "in acute endocarditis, pain is rarely present, and ulceration of valves or of the wall may proceed to a most extreme degree without any sensory disturbance" (Osler, 1910).

In experimental terms, pain being a conscious experience that can be explored only indirectly with experimental models, the crucial problems presented by specific models will now be briefly reviewed (Malliani and Lombardi, 1982; Malliani et al., 1984).

In animals recovering from anaesthesia or in decerebrate acute preparations, it is quite easy to obtain "pseudoaffective reflexes" (Woodworth and Sherrington, 1904) by applying "noxious" stimuli to the heart. Thus, Sutton and Lueth (1930) observed that traction on a ligature placed around a coronary artery could elicit "evidence of severe pain".

Leaving unsolved whether the possible adequate stimulus for cardiac pain is mainly mechanical (Martin and Gorham, 1938), chemical (Lewis, 1932; Baker et al., 1980) or a mixture of both, a question that we have recently discussed in detail (Malliani and Lombardi, 1982; Malliani et al., 1984), we would rather like to focus, on this occasion, on the fundamental fact that a similar stimulus appears algogenic or not, depending only on the specific experimental set.

The nonapeptide bradykinin was likely to furnish a remarkable tool for the experimental analysis of this subject, as it was considered the most powerful of natural algogenic substances, and hence able to be quantified when used as a stimulus (Lombardi et al., 1981).

Indeed, the initial observations by Guzman et al. (1962) appeared extremely sound and easy to interpret when they reported that intracoronary injections of bradykinin produced overt pain reactions very effectively in dogs recovering from recent surgery.

However, we have recently analysed the reflex haemodynamic effects of the chemical stimulation with bradykinin of the cardiac sensory innervation

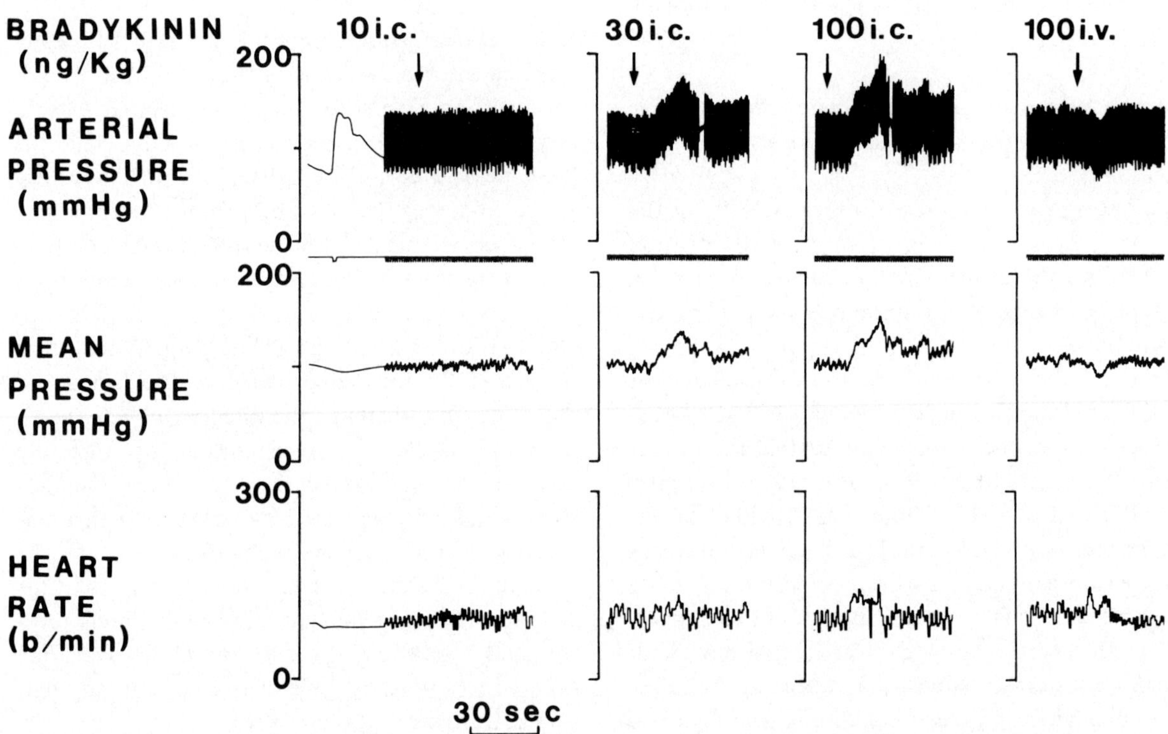

Fig. 1. Progressive pressor responses to graded injections of bradykinin into the cannulated circumflex coronary artery of a conscious dog. Note that hypotension and tachycardia are produced by intravenous injections (100 ng/kg, right panel). From Pagani et al. (1985).

in conscious dogs after full recovery from the operation necessary for their instrumentation (Pagani et al., 1985).

In these animals the injections of bradykinin in either the left anterior descending or the circumflex coronary artery consistently produced a marked gradual increase in systemic arterial pressure and heart rate (Fig. 1) as well as left ventricle pressure and d*P*/d*t* (Fig. 2, right panel).

It is important to point out that these changes were never accompanied by any pain reaction, as expressed by agitation and vocalisation of the animals. In this study the amounts of bradykinin injected into the cannulated coronary artery ranged

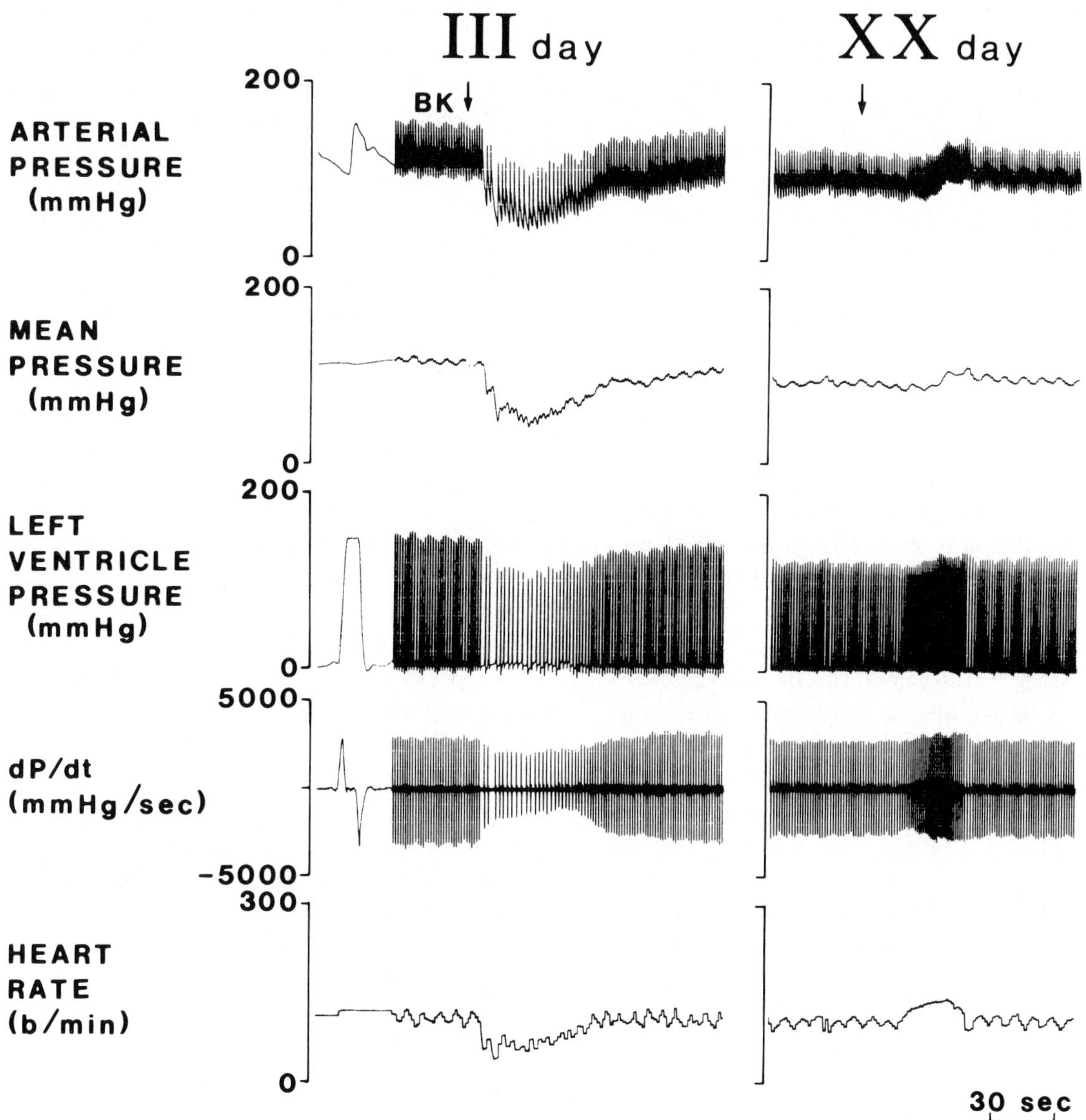

Fig. 2. Contrasting effects of intracoronary bradykinin (100 ng/kg) in a conscious dog when examined early (left panel) and late (right panel) after surgery. Note that while a depressor response was obtained on the third day post-operatively, it reverted to a pressor response at a time of complete recovery from surgery (20th day post-operatively).

from 10 ng/kg (the threshold dose for the response) to 3 μg/kg. When this latter, very large dose was used, however, the direct vasodilatory effects of the drug prevailed and hypotension and tachycardia were observed, again in absence of any pain reactions (see figure in Malliani et al., 1984). A similar pressor response, in the absence of pain reactions, was also seen when bradykinin was injected into the pericardial sac (Pagani et al., 1985).

The importance of recovery from anaesthesia and recent surgery, in explaining the apparent discrepancy with the finding by Guzman et al. (1962), was demonstrated by experiments performed soon after surgery, when recovery of the animals was still incomplete. Injections of bradykinin into the coronary bed of nine animals during the first week after surgery provoked either an early depressor (Fig. 2, left panel) or pressor response which became the usual constant pressor response at a time of complete recovery from surgery (Fig. 2, XX day). Moreover, out of the nine dogs, three animals exhibited vocalisation and agitation, suggesting a pain reaction, in response to the bradykinin injections performed during the first week after surgery. Such a reaction was no longer present when the animals were tested later on, at a time of complete recovery from surgery (Pagani et al., 1985).

An absence of pain was also reported (Barron and Bishop, 1982) in relation to intracoronary injections of veratridine, a non-physiological compound likely to stimulate directly (Paintal, 1971) the nerve fibres, and surely capable of activating both vagal (Von Bezold and Hirt, 1867, Thorén, 1979) and sympathetic afferent fibres (Malliani et al., 1972).

The observation that, under appropriate experimental conditions, an excitation of the cardiac sensory supply, likely to be massive, did not elicit pain appears as a total defeat for the "specificity" theory, at least if nociceptors were postulated to be exquisitely sensitive to bradykinin (Baker et al., 1980). On the other hand, the "intensity" theory also does not explain in simple terms the lack of induction of pain.

As a working hypothesis we propose a modified version of the intensity mechanism. Cardiac pain would result from the extreme excitation of a spatially restricted population of afferent sympathetic fibres (Malliani, 1982, 1986; Malliani et al., 1984). The result shown in Fig. 3 could be interpreted in this sense: indeed, a peculiar position maintained in this experiment by the coronary cannula, lying just outside the wall of the vessel and below the adventitia, determined that each minute injection distended a very limited portion of the adventitia. It should be noted that a similarly marked pressor, inotropic and heart rate reponse was observed with injections of either bradykinin or saline. The animal displayed overt pain reactions to every trial, independent of the pressor effect, as they persisted when the hypertensive responses were blunted by alpha adrenergic receptor blockade with phentolamine (Fig. 3, panels B and C). The pain reaction was similarly induced by both bradykinin and saline; hence, the effective stimulus was likely to be the mechanical distension of the adventitia.

One experiment should not be the basis for a theory, but it is well known that experimental casuality has often offered new perspectives on a problem. The implications of this hypothesis could be relevant. A spatially restricted mechanical abnormality localized in the myocardium or in the abundantly innervated coronary arteries could lead to pain more efficiently than a more widely distributed myocardial ischaemia with its chemical components. Thus, coronary spasm could be a highly effective stimulus, while a restricted coronary denervation accompanying by-pass interventions could produce a strategic interruption of afferent fibres. Obviously, we are not equating anginal pain for which mechanical factors could be prevalent and pain in the course of myocardial infarction, when the interaction between accumulation of chemicals and mechanical factors is likely to be maximal.

To summarize, it is our current hypothesis that when the activation of the sympathetic afferent fibres is widely distributed, as in the case of intracoronary injections of bradykinin, some central in-

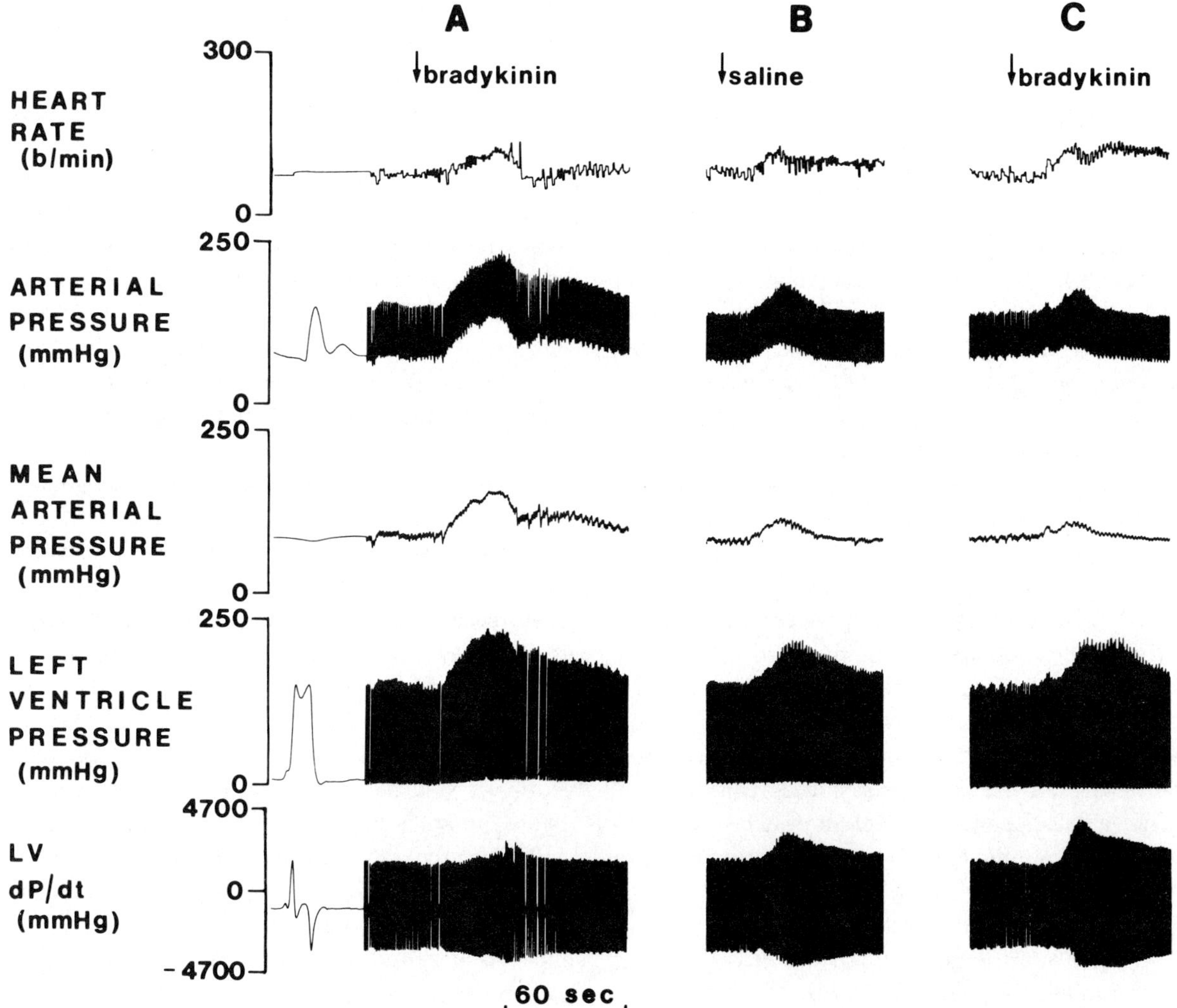

Fig. 3. Effects of mechanical distensions of the adventitia of the left circumflex coronary artery produced in a conscious dog by sub-adventitial injections of either bradykinin or saline. Similar pain reactions (vocalisation and agitation) were observed even if the pressor response was blunted by alpha adrenergic receptor blockade with phentolamine (1 mg/kg between A and B and again between B and C). LV, left ventricle.

hibitory modulation (Melzack and Wall, 1965; Besson et al., 1979; Wall and Melzack, 1984) would be more effective in preventing pain mechanisms.

Non-painful sensations from the heart

It is largely extra-medical knowledge that the consciousness of heartbeat can be increased by proper training. Yet almost every person has experienced, in addition to the normal tachycardia sensation, the ill-definable perception of premature beats or, more in general, of arrhythmias.

It is obvious that it has not been proved at all that the receptors initiating these various perceptions are located in the heart. For instance, tachycardia may stimulate parietal receptors belonging to the chest wall and, similarly, so can arrhythmias, especially when some of the beats are accompanied by abnormal mechanics.

However, the fact that the conscious sensations are more likely to arise from small and healthy hearts rather than from chronically enlarged ones suggests that the sensors are within the heart and signal unusual events.

Were this to be true, vagal afferent fibres with their mechanosensitive endings might well provide a fast information pathway on abnormal cardiac motion. On the other hand, it is remarkable how many devastating events, from inflammatory ones such as myocarditis to traumatic ones such as valve rupture, can be signalled only by the extra-cardiac consequences of congestion or low output.

Pathophysiological considerations

In a general conception which has often considered health and disease as two qualitatively different processes, the afferent sympathetic path has been historically assigned to the kingdom of abnormality and, more specifically, has been linked with the transmission of cardiac pain. In fact, this represents perhaps the most committed conceptualisation of a specific nociceptive channel, not only in terms of a peculiar contingent of small diameter afferent nerve fibres but as the whole sensory input contained in an ensemble of nerves.

On the other hand, multifarious reasons, from the abundance of information obtainable from the highly sophisticated afferent impulse traffic coursing from the heart to the medulla to the relative lack of reflexes elicitable from acutely vagotomised hearts, have surely contributed to the conviction that only cardiac vagal afferent fibres were involved in regulatory mechanisms. Current medical opinion has been furnishing the best proof of this: thus, when atrial or ventricular receptors were alluded to as reflexogenic sources, they were intended to be, by definition, sensory endings of afferent vagal fibres.

It is now known that the afferent sympathetic fibres with cardiovascular endings can mediate powerful cardiovascular reflexes, mainly characterised by their positive-feedback sign (Pagani et al., 1982): a finding which suggests that the neural control of circulation might well operate, for each specific performance, through an integration of opposite mechanisms possessing either negative or positive feedback properties (Malliani, 1982; Bishop et al., 1983).

If it is realised how oversimplified the traditional view on cardiac afferent sympathetic fibres was, it is reasonable that in the future a similar oversimplification will be revealed in the exclusion of afferent vagal fibres from the mechanisms of cardiac nociception. Indeed, the fact that they are not essential does not rule out that they might play an important part.

A call for caution in respect to what we know, at the moment, about the pathophysiology of this double afferent input emerges very clearly from the following clinical considerations.

In recent years, it has been amply documented that in patients exhibiting spontaneous and reversible electrocardiographic changes typical of ischaemic episodes of the myocardium, the haemodynamic profile of the episodes can appear substantially similar whether or not accompanied by pain (Guazzi et al., 1971, 1975, 1976; Maseri et al., 1978; Chierchia et al., 1980). The lack of pain has been attributed to a "defective warning system" (Cohn, 1980). Instead, we think that the fact that in some or many cases the alarm system appropriately signals myocardial ischaemia, does not mean at all that the afferent sympathetic cardiac fibres have been conceived or, if one prefers, have developed with the purpose of constituting a "warning system". Indeed, the porosity of this system would be too high, letting too many dangers filter through.

For instance, there is little question that malignant arrhythmias are among the most important risk factors for sudden death (Lown, 1979): the severity of arrhythmias can often be appreciated by a patient, such an appraisal being totally independent of pain but rather dependent on the degree of awareness and culture.

In conclusion, the local damage in the heart, symbolised by ischaemia, is not always accompanied by pain, while even greater dangers may jeopardise the heart and yet activate sensations that only a high degree of consciousness transforms into alarm.

Hence, damage leading to pain, proportionate to risk, is only one of the possibilities. Moreover, around it there is probably a much larger halo, including multifarious cardiac dysfunctions which can lead silently to death, if we call silence the absence of pain.

References

Adams, R. D. (1980) Pain. General considerations. In K. I. Isselbaker, R. D. Adams, E. Braunwald, R. G. Petersdorf and J. D. Wilson (Eds.), Harrison's Principles of Internal Medicine, McGraw-Hill Inc., New York.

Ammons, S. N., Blair, R. W., Hindorf, K. and Foreman, R. D. (1983) Vagal afferent inhibition of spinothalamic cell responses to sympathetic afferents and bradykinin in the monkey. Circ. Res., 53: 603–612.

Arndt, J. O., Brambring, P., Hindorf, K. and Rohnelt, M. (1971) The afferent impulse traffic from atrial A type receptors in cats. Pfluegers Arch., 326: 300–315.

Baker, D. G., Coleridge, H. M., Coleridge, J. C. G. and Nerdrum, T. (1980) Search for a cardiac nociceptor: stimulation by bradykinin of sympathetic afferent nerve endings in the heart of the cat. J. Physiol., 306: 519–536.

Barron, K. W. and Bishop, V. S. (1982) Reflex cardiovascular changes with veratridine in the conscious dog. Am. J. Physiol., 242: H810–H817.

Berkley, H. J. (1894) The intrinsic nerve supply of cardiac ventricles in certain vertebrates. Johns Hopkins Hosp. Rep., 4: 248–255.

Besson, J. M., Dickenson, A. H. and Le Bars, D. (1979) Plurisegmental noxious inhibitory controls on rat dorsal horn convergent neurones. J. Physiol., 292: 41P–42P.

Bishop, V. S., Malliani, A. and Thorén, P. (1983) Cardiac mechanoreceptors. In J. T. Shepherd, F. M. Abbond and S. R. Geiger (Eds.), Handbook of Physiology. Section 2, The Cardiovascular System. Vol. III, Peripheral Circulation and Organ Blood Flow. American Physiological Society, Washington, DC, pp. 497–555.

Brown, A. M. (1965) Mechanoreceptors in or near the coronary arteries. J. Physiol., 177: 203–214.

Brown, A. M. (1967) Excitation of afferent cardiac sympathetic nerve fibres during myocardial ischaemia. J. Physiol., 190: 35–53.

Burgess, P. R. and Perl, E. R. (1973) Cutaneous mechanoreceptors and nociceptors. In A. Iggo (Ed.), Handbook of Sensory Physiology, Somatosensory System, Vol. 2, Springer-Verlag, Berlin, pp. 29–78.

Casati, R., Lombardi, F. and Malliani, A. (1979) Afferent sympathetic unmyelinated fibres with left ventricular endings in cats. J. Physiol., 292: 135–148.

Chierchia, S., Brunelli, C., Simonetti, I., Lazzari, M. and Maseri, A. (1980) Sequence of events in angina at rest: primary reduction in coronary flow. Circulation, 61: 759–768.

Cohn, P. F. (1980) Silent myocardial ischemia in patients with a defective anginal warning system. Am. J. Cardiol. 45: 697–702.

Coleridge, H. M. and Coleridge, J. C. G. (1980) Cardiovascular afferents involved in regulation of peripheral vessels. Am. Rev. Physiol., 42: 413–427.

Coleridge, J. C. G. and Coleridge, H. M. (1979) Chemoreflex regulation of the heart. In R. M. Berne, N. Sperlakis and S. R. Geiger (Eds.), Handbook of Physiology, Section 2, The Cardiovascular System. Vol. 1, The Heart, American Physiological Society, Washington, DC, pp. 653–676.

Dickinson, C. J. (1950) Afferent nerves from the heart region. J. Physiol., 111: 399–407.

Dogiel, A. S. (1898) Die sensiblen nervenendigungen in Herzen und in den Blutgefässen der Säugethiere. Arch. Mikrosk. Anat. 52: 44–70.

Guazzi, M., Polese, A., Fiorentini, C., Magrini, F. and Bartorelli, C. (1971) Left ventricular performance and related haemodynamic changes in Prinzmetal's variant angina pectoris. Br. Heart J., 33: 84–94.

Guazzi, M., Polese, A., Fiorentini, C., Magrini, F., Olivari, M. T. and Bartorelli, C. (1975) Left and right heart haemodynamics during spontaneous angina pectoris. Comparison between angina with ST segment depression and angina with ST segment elevation. Br. Heart J., 37: 401–413.

Guazzi, M., Olivari, M. T., Polese, A., Fiorentini, C. and Magrini, F. (1976) Repetitive myocardial ischemia of Prinzmetal type without angina pectoris. Am. J. Cardiol., 37: 923–927.

Guzman, F., Braun, C. and Lim, R. K. S. (1962) Visceral pain and the pseudoaffective response to intra-arterial injection of bradykinin and other algesic agents. Arch. Intern. Pharmacol., 136: 353–384.

Hainsworth, R., Kidd, C. and Linden, R. J. (Eds.) (1979) Cardiac Receptors, Cambridge University Press, Cambridge.

Hess, G. L., Zuperku, E. J., Coon, R. L. and Kampine, J. P. (1974) Sympathetic afferent nerve activity of left ventricular origin. Am. J. Physiol., 227: 543–546.

Jonnesco, T. (1921) Traitement chirurgical de l'angine de poitrine par la résection du sympathique cervico-thoracique. La Presse Medicale, 29: 193–194.

Khabarova, A. Y. (1963) The Afferent Innervation of the Heart, Consultants Bureau, New York, pp. 1–175.

Langley, J. N. (1903) The autonomic nervous system. Brain, 26: 1–26.

Leriche, R. and Fontaine, R. (1927) The surgical treatment of angina pectoris. Am. Heart J., 3: 649–671.

Lewis, T. (1932) Pain in muscular ischemia — its relation to anginal pain. Arch. Int. Med., 49: 713–727.

Lindgren, I. and Olivecrona, H. (1947) Surgical treatment of angina pectoris. J. Neurosurg., 4: 19–39.

Lombardi, F., Della Bella, P., Casati, R. and Malliani, A. (1981) Effects of intracoronary administration of bradykinin on the impulse activity of afferent sympathetic unmyelinated fibers with left ventricular endings in the cat. Circ. Res., 48: 69–75.

Lown, B. (1979) Sudden cardiac death: the major challenge confronting contemporary cardiology. Am. J. Cardiol., 43: 313–328.

Malliani, A. (1982) Cardiovascular sympathetic afferent fibers. Rev. Physiol. Biochem. Pharmacol., 94: 11–74.

Malliani, A. (1986) The elusive link between transient myocardial ischemia and pain. Circulation, 73: 201–204.

Malliani, A. and Lombardi, F. (1982) Consideration of the fundamental mechanisms eliciting cardiac pain. Am. Heart J., 103: 575–578.

Malliani, A., Peterson, D. F., Bishop, V. S. and Brown, A. M. (1972) Spinal sympathetic cardiocardiac reflexes. Circ. Res. 30: 158–166.

Malliani, A., Recordati, G. and Schwartz, P. J. (1973) Nervous activity of afferent cardiac sympathetic fibres with atrial and ventricular endings. J. Physiol., 229: 457–469.

Malliani, A., Pagani, M. and Lombardi, F. (1984) Visceral versus somatic mechanisms. In P. D. Wall and R. Melzack (Eds.), Textbook of Pain, Churchill Livingstone, pp. 100–109.

Martin, S. J. and Gorham, L. W. (1938) Cardiac pain. An experimental study with reference to the tension factor. Arch. Int. Med., 62: 840–852.

Maseri, A., Severi, S., De Nes, M., L'Abbate, A., Chierchia, S., Marzilli, M., Ballestra, A. M., Parodi, O., Biagini, A. and Distante, A. (1978) "Variant" angina: one aspect of a continuous spectrum of vasospastic myocardial ischemia. Am. J. Cardiol., 42: 1019–1035.

Melzack, R. and Wall, P. D. (1965) Pain mechanisms: a new theory. Science, 150: 971–979.

Nettleship, W. A. (1936) Experimental studies on the afferent innervation of the cat's heart. J. Comp. Neurol., 64: 115–131.

Nishi, K., Sakanashi, M. and Takenaka, F. (1977) Activation of afferent cardiac sympathetic nerve fibers of the cat by pain producing substances and by noxious heat. Pflügers Arch., 372: 53–61.

Oberg, B. and Thorén P. (1972) Studies on left ventricular receptors, signalling in non-modulated vagal afferents. Acta Physiol. Scand., 85: 145–163.

Osler, W. (1910) The Lumleian lectures on "Angina pectoris" (lecture II). Lancet, 1: 839–844.

Pagani, M., Pizzinelli, P., Bergamaschi, M. and Malliani, A. (1982) A positive feedback sympathetic pressor reflex during stretch of the thoracic aorta in conscious dogs. Circ. Res. 50: 125–132.

Pagani, M., Pizzinelli, P., Furlan, R., Guzzetti, S., Rimoldi, O., Sandrone, G. and Malliani, A. (1985) Analysis of the pressor sympathetic reflex produced by intracoronary injections of bradykinin in conscious dogs. Circ. Res., 56: 175–183.

Paintal, A. S. (1953) A study of right and left atrial receptors. J. Physiol., 120: 596–610.

Paintal, A.S. (1955) A study of ventricular pressure receptors and their role in the Bezold reflex. Q. J. Exp. Physiol., 40: 348–368.

Paintal, A. S. (1964) Effects of drugs on vertebrate mechanoreceptors. Pharmacol. Rev., 16: 341–380.

Paintal, A. S. (1971) Action of drugs on sensory nerve endings. Am. Rev. Pharmacol., 11: 231–240.

Paintal, A. S. (1973) Vagal sensory receptors and their reflex effects. Physiol. Rev., 53: 159–227.

Recordati, G., Lombardi, F., Bishop, V. S. and Malliani, A. (1975) Response of type B atrial vagal receptors to changes in wall tension during atrial filling. Circ. Res., 36: 682–691.

Recordati, G., Lombardi, F., Bishop, V. S. and Malliani, A. (1976) Mechanical stimuli exciting type A atrial vagal receptors in the cat. Circ. Res., 38: 397–403.

Sherrington, C. S., (1906) The Integrative Action of the Nervous System, Yale University Press, New Haven, pp. 1–400.

Smirnov, A. (1895) Ueber die sensiblen nervenendigungen im herzen bei amphibien und säugetieren. Anat. Anz., 10: 737–749.

Struppler, A. and Struppler, E. (1955) Uber spezielle charakteristika afferennter vagaler herznerven impulse und ihre beziehungen zur herzdynamik. Acta. Physiol. Scand., 33: 219–231.

Sutton, D. C. and Lueth, H. C. (1930) Experimental production of pain on excitation of the heart and great vessels. Arch. Intern. Med., 45: 827–867.

Thames, M. D., Donald D. E. and Shepherd, J. T. (1977) Behaviour of cardiac receptors with nonmyelinated vagal afferents during spontaneous respiration in cats. Circ. Res., 41: 694–701.

Thorén, P. (1979) Role of cardiac vagal c-fibers in cardiovascular control. Rev. Physiol. Biochem. Pharmacol., 86: 1–94.

Uchida, Y. (1975) Afferent sympathetic nerve fibers with mechanoreceptors in the right heart. Am. J. Physiol., 228: 223–230.

Uchida, Y. and Murao, S. (1974) Bradykinin-induced excitation of afferent cardiac sympathetic nerve fibers. Jpn. Heart J., 15: 84–91.

Ueda, H., Uchida, Y. and Kamisaka, K. (1969) Distribution and responses of the cardiac sympathetic receptors to mechanically induced circulatory changes. Jpn. Heart J., 10: 70–81.

Von Bezold, A. and Hirt, L. (1867) Ueber die physiologischen Wirkungen des essigsauren Veratrins. Untersuch Physiol. Lab. Würzburg, 1: 73–156.

Wall, P. D. and Melzack, R. (Eds.) (1984) Textbook of Pain, Churchill Livingstone, Edinburgh.

White, J. C. (1957) Cardiac pain. Anatomic pathways and physiologic mechanisms. Circulation, 16: 644–655.

Willis, R. (1847) The Works of William Harvey, Sydenham Society, London.

Woodworth, R. S. and Sherrington, C. S. (1904) A pseudoaffective reflex and its spinal path. J. Physiol., 31: 234–243.

Woollard, H. H. (1926) The innervation of blood vessels. Heart, 13: 319–336.

F. Cervero and J. F.B. Morrison
Progress in Brain Research, Vol. 67

CHAPTER 5

Sensory innervation of the lungs and airways

J. G. Widdicombe

Department of Physiology, St. George's Hospital Medical School, Cranmer Terrace, London SW17 0RE, U.K.

Introduction

Extensive studies of reflexes from the lungs and airways have not been paralleled by investigations of sensation. Research on reflexes has usually been with experimental animals, and its counterpart in man, including sensation, is more difficult. Also, the stimulus/receptor interactions leading to reflexes and sensation have seldom been identified. To give a simple example: irritation of the larynx causes both cough and a sensation of rawness; we do not know whether the two responses have a common afferent pathway or even the histological appearance of the end-organs activated. When respiratory sensation has been reported, it has seldom been quantitated. Until recently, only respiratory proprioception had been accurately measured, although in the last few years psychometric tests have been applied to breathlessness; there has been virtually no quantitation of common respiratory sensations such as pain and irritation.

Proprioception

Most parts of the lungs and airways, but not the nose, are distensible and contain proprioceptors in their walls. However, distension and collapse will also affect afferent information from surrounding somatic muscles of breathing, and the volume change may be initiated by contraction of these muscles. Therefore, it is not always easy to determine the site of origin of proprioceptive sensation: most analytical studies have depended on nervous blockade by local anaesthesia or by disease (Guz et al., 1970; Guz, 1977; Campbell and Guz, 1981), and quantitative extrapolation to healthy man is difficult.

Respiratory proprioception can be of pressure, volume, flow, ventilation or loading, elastic or resistive loads frequently being studied (Zechman and Wiley, 1986). A mouthpiece or nose-clip is usually used, thus distorting an important part of the airway sensing system. Flow and pressure can certainly be detected in the nose and mouth, but there is little evidence for their detection more peripherally. Detection of volume changes and loading is thought to be confined to the respiratory muscles and possibly lungs (Campbell and Guz, 1981; Zechman and Wiley, 1985), although the latter may be less important since load detection is unaffected by bilateral vagal blockade (Guz, 1970) or by airway anaesthesia (Chaudhary and Burki, 1978).

Two studies are illustrative. Gandevia et al. (1981) showed that healthy subjects had a threshold for detecting negative pressure at the mouth during active inspiration of 0.5 cm H_2O, and that this was increased to 1–1.5 cm H_2O when the glottis was closed. This suggested that the mouth was 2–3 times less sensitive than the mouth plus lower respiratory tract for pressure detection. On the other hand, Noble et al. (1972) found that patients with tracheostomies could detect resistive loads less easily when breathing through the tracheostomy than through the upper airway, suggesting that the upper airway was the more important sensor of added load. Clearly, comparison of healthy subjects and patients, with different respiratory stimuli must be cautious.

Noxious and irritant stimuli

Sensation evoked by inhaled irritants varies greatly (Douglas, 1981). A gas like ammonia is odorous in concentrations (3500 $\mu g \cdot m^{-3}$) far lower than those that cause unpleasant sensation (20,000–40,000 $\mu g \cdot m^{-3}$); gases like hydrogen chloride "irritate" at the threshold detection level (7200 $\mu g \cdot m^{-3}$) (Henderson and Haggard, 1943). The distinction between smell and irritation may depend on interaction between olfactory (smell) and trigeminal (irritation) pathways (Beidler, 1961). In addition, the quality of unpleasant sensation varies widely in the same subject, different irritant gases giving rise to sensations such as burning, rawness, nausea, itching, tickling, pain, etc. The sensations may be felt in the nose, mouth, pharynx, throat and upper chest, but rarely deep in the chest (see later). The response has been called the "common chemical sense" by Parker (1922) to distinguish it from taste and smell, and may be distributed over the whole body surface in fish and lower animals. In man, mammals and birds, with horny, hairy or feathery skins, this chemical sensibility seems to be more concentrated in the respiratory mucosa than in the skin.

The sense of chemical irritation has been distinguished from pain on several counts, although if the concentration of an inhaled irritant is high enough, pain results and the same afferent pathways could be involved. Classical experiments by Sheldon (1909) and Parker (1922) showed that cocaine could block noxious responses to mechanical stimulation while those to chemical irritants persisted. More recently, Jansco et al. (1977) have shown that depletion of substance P from nociceptive afferent nerves, by use of capsaicin, blocks the chemical irritant responses while leaving those to mechanical stimuli intact. However, these types of experiment probably only show that more than one afferent pathway is involved in responses to noxious stimuli.

Many of the afferent mechanisms underlying sensation from inhaled irritants are also involved in sensation with respiratory disease. The latter sensation has the same range of qualities: e.g., in rhinitis — tickling, a desire to sneeze, rawness, finally pain; in asthma — tightness in the chest; in laryngitis and tracheitis — rawness, desire to cough, burning, and pain. Some irritants that cause these sensations may initially be restricted to the airway epithelium, since chemicals such as sulphur dioxide, hydrogen chloride and ammonia rapidly become part of the large body pools of sulphate, chloride and ammonium and only exert surface actions; however, disease processes may extend deeper into tissue. Both types of condition may involve release of mediators and cellular breakdown products that could diffuse into deeper tissues.

Temperature sensation

Although it is general experience that we can sense warmth and cold in the nose and mouth, these sensations have been little studied.

The nose

Olfaction is outside the scope of this chapter; it can interact with other nasal pathways to give quality to sensation, and there is reflex interaction between olfactory and trigeminal pathways.

Nervous receptors

There has been no definitive description of nervous end-organs in the nose, apart from the olfactory ones. Light and electron microscopies show non-myelinated fibres in and under the nasal epithelium (Cauna et al., 1969) (Fig. 1); their EM appearance suggests that they are afferent, and this is supported by degeneration studies (Grote et al., 1975). No specialised receptors have been described for the nasal mucosa. Recent studies have shown the presence of substance P in nerves in and under the nasal epithelium (Lundblad, 1984). These fibres are prob-

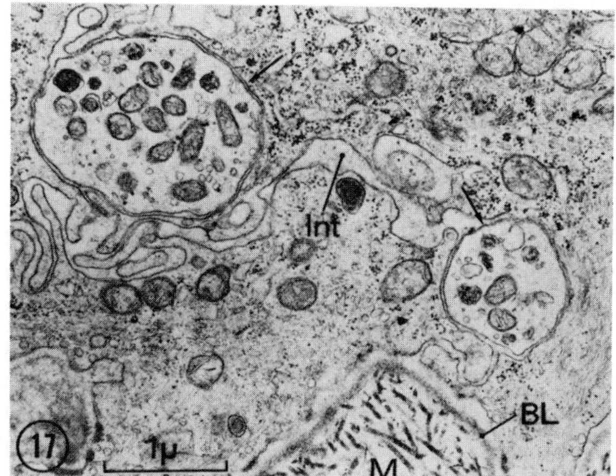

Fig. 1. Two intraepithelial nerve endings (arrows) from the respiratory mucosa of the nasal septum. The axon terminals are enwrapped by the cell membranes of the epithelial cells. The axoplasm of the endings contains accumulations of typical small mitochondria and some microvesicles. Int, intercellular space; BL, epithelial basal lamina; M, part of the basal or Bowman's membrane. Electron micrograph. Male, 11 years old. From Cauna et al. (1969).

ably the same as those that stain for acetylcholinesterase, and they can be destroyed by afferent denervation or by capsaicin (Uddman et al., 1983). As with other viscera, their appearance suggests that they may underlie axon and local reflexes, as well as set up central nervous reflexes.

Afferent nerves

These, for the nose, are complex and surgically somewhat inaccessible, which may explain the paucity of studies with single-fibre afferent recording; this is in striking contrast to the extensive studies for the lower respiratory tract and the larynx. The few records show that both myelinated and nonmyelinated fibres in the trigeminal nerve are activated by odours and irritants, and some receptors by temperature changes (Andersen, 1954; Beidler, 1961). The same stimuli may set up discharges in the olfactory nerve (Adrian, 1942). A few sensory fibres are found in the sympathetic nerves to the nose, but the predominant afferent pathway is parasympathetic.

Reflexes

These have been extensively studied for the nose, and are reviewed fully elsewhere (Angell-James and Daly, 1969; Korpas and Tomori, 1979; Widdicombe, 1981, 1986). They include:

Breathing

Nasal irritation more commonly causes apnoea than the sneeze under experimental conditions. The apnoeic reflex is part of the complex diving response (Elsner and Gooden, 1983; Daly, 1986). The physiological stimulus is water applied to the face or into the nose. Apnoea can be induced by odours or irritants, and by water (sensed as an irritant) in the nose (Allen, 1929). It occurs in all mammalian and terrestrial vertebrate species that have been studied, including birds and humans, and also in neonates and fetuses. Associated with the apnoea are conspicuous cardiovascular changes that "centralise" the circulation to brain and heart, with a greatly reduced cardiac output, and laryngeal closure that presumably helps to prevent water entering the lungs (Daly, 1986).

Mechanical and a wide variety of chemical stimuli applied to the nasal mucosa can cause sneezing, and it is not known why the same stimulus may cause apnoea or sneeze. Chemical mediators such as histamine can also cause sneezing, as can secretion of mucus in the nose (Mygind et al., 1983). Because local application of capsaicin, which depletes substance P-containing nerves of their neuropeptide, can prevent the sneeze due to inhaled irritants, the nonmyelinated nerves containing substance P may be the receptors for the sneeze (Lundblad, 1984).

Irritants and odours in the nose can cause sniffing, by a reflex (Allen, 1929; Korpas and Tomori, 1979). Because sniffing may direct airflow towards the olfactory mucosa, at least in humans, the physiology of sniffing may be related to detection of smells. This may be especially important for sexual odours.

Positive pressure in the nose and nasopharynx can stimulate breathing in man and experimental animals, and negative pressure has the opposite effect (Mathew et al., 1982a; Van Lunteren et al., 1984). Since most of the nose is not distensible, the receptors may be in the nasopharynx. The same stimuli affect the patency of the pharynx and the larynx, negative pressure in the nose tending to make the dilator muscles contract more strongly (Mathew, 1984; Roberts et al., 1984; Van Lunteren et al., 1984). The mechanism may be important in snoring and sleep apnoeas (Phillipson and Bowes, 1986). Nasal airflow, as distinct from pressure, can also set up respiratory and nasal muscular reflexes (Widdicombe, 1986).

Other reflexes

The cardiovascular reflex changes are generally similar to those for the diving response and include hypertension, bradycardia, release of adrenal hormones, and adjustment of circulation through various vascular beds (Elsner and Gooden, 1983; Daly, 1986).

Nasal irritation can cause bronchoconstriction or bronchodilatation reflexly, and probably at least two afferent pathways from the nose are present, with opposite effects on bronchomotor tone (Nadel, 1980; Widdicombe, 1985). In patients with asthma, nasal irritation enhances the bronchoconstriction by cholinergic reflexes (Nolte and Berger, 1933; Yan and Salome, 1983). Cold applied to the nose of sensitive subjects and patients may also cause reflex bronchoconstriction (Wells et al., 1960; Melville and Morris, 1972).

Nasal irritation constricts the larynx, both transiently during sneeze and also maintained during the apnoea of the diving response (Szereda-Przestaszewska and Widdicombe, 1973). The same stimuli cause reflex secretion of mucus in the lower respiratory tract as well as in the nose (Phipps, 1981). This presumably has a protective function.

Irritation of the nose can inhibit the tone of skeletal muscle at spinal level (Andersen, 1954). This response seems to contrast with the arousal responses that can be derived from the nose (Phillipson and Bowes, 1986), and presumably are the basis of the use of "smelling salts" and smoke to promote revival.

Naso-nasal and local reflexes

Irritation of one side of the nose causes mucus secretion and congestion on the opposite side, by a reflex cholinergic pathway (Borum et al., 1983; Mygind et al., 1983). Similarly, stimulation of receptors in the nasal mucosa may release substance P from local axon pathways, which will cause vascular dilatation and oedema (Lundblad, 1984). The same receptors are thought to be responsible for sneeze and, possibly, the sensation that goes with it.

Sensation

It is claimed that pain and touch are the only sensations that can be aroused from the nose (Cauna et al., 1969), but detailed descriptions include tickling, irritation, rawness and a desire to sneeze (Korpas and Tomori, 1979). Since the nervous receptors and afferent pathways for nasal reflexes have scarcely been analysed, it is impossible to link them to particular nasal sensations. In view of the frequency of rhinitis, nasal sensation and its quantitation are important subjects for study.

In summary, nasal end-organs have not been identified histologically, and afferent activities have not been defined, so it is impossible at present to link either with reflexes or sensation.

Pharynx and nasopharynx

Nervous receptors and afferent nerves

Nonmyelinated branches of nerve terminals occur under the squamous cell epithelium of the nasopharynx (Fillenz and Widdicombe, 1971) (Fig. 2). Single-fibre recordings show two types of receptor: rapidly-adapting (Nail et al., 1969) and slowly-adapting (Hwang et al., 1984b) endings that respond mainly to mechanical stimuli, especially distension and collapse. Although presumably the region contains nonmyelinated afferent receptors and nerves, these have not been studied by fibre recording. There is no evidence of sympathetic afferent nerves from the pharynx.

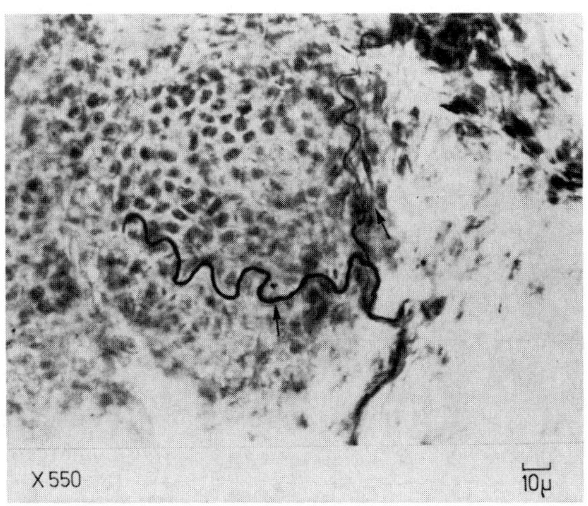

Fig. 2. Frozen section of cat epipharyngeal region showing nerve fibres ramifying among epithelial cells. Schofield's silver stain. Photograph by Mrs. A. M. S. White. From Fillenz and Widdicombe (1971).

Reflexes

Breathing

The aspiration reflex is the rapidly repeated powerful contractions of the diaphragm set up by mechanical stimulation of the nasopharynx and probably related to sniffing (Tomori and Widdicombe, 1969; Korpas and Tomori, 1979; Widdicombe, 1986). Presumably, the function of the reflex is to clear the nasopharynx of obstruction. It is probably mediated by the rapidly-adapting receptors.

Another important reflex is the stimulation of breathing due to distension of the upper airways. Collapse of the pharynx reflexly contracts the dilator muscles of the pharynx (Hwang et al., 1984a). The weakness of these reflexes may be associated with snoring and sleep apnoea, and distension of the upper airways may inhibit these undesirable effects (Phillipson and Bowes, 1986). The afferent pathway is probably the slowly-adapting receptors (Hwang et al., 1984b).

Swallowing

This can be elicited from the posterior pharyngeal wall and surrounding structures by mechanical and chemical stimuli (Miller, 1982). It is associated with inhibition of breathing and closure of the larynx.

Other reflexes

These include bronchodilatation, hypertension, tachycardia, closure of the larynx and secretion of mucus (Korpas and Tomori, 1979; Widdicombe, 1986).

Sensation

Apart from anecdotal evidence that one can have the sensations of pain, nausea, rawness and irritation from the pharyngeal region, studies on pharyngeal sensation have been neglected.

The larynx

Probably because of ease of access to the larynx and its nerve supply, the structure has been a playground for physiologists for many decades. Despite this, we still cannot identify any reflex with any receptor end-organ, and there are virtually no analytical studies of laryngeal sensation.

Nervous receptors

Various types of nerve ending have been identified in and under the laryngeal epithelium. Some are specialised structures, resembling taste buds or small encapsulated terminals (Koizumi, 1953; Feindel, 1956), but most descriptions are of free nerve endings in the mucosa and submucosa (Hatakeyama, 1969; Lewis and Prentice, 1980). Receptors are also seen around joints and in the laryngeal intrinsic muscles.

Afferent nerves

There have been many single-fibre recordings from laryngeal receptors (see Widdicombe, 1986). The fibres run mainly in the superior laryngeal nerves, although a few are in the recurrent laryngeal nerves.

There is no evidence of sympathetic afferent innervation. Different authors use different systems of classification of receptors. The following patterns of response are seen.

Pressure receptors

These are the commonest receptors studied. They respond with slowly-adapting discharges to distension and/or collapse of the larynx (Mathew et al., 1982b; Sant'Ambrogio et al., 1983; Hwang et al., 1984b). They have been studied for rat, lamb, dog, cat and rabbit, and there are clear species differences. They are inhibited by 5–10% CO_2 (Boushey et al., 1974), but otherwise are not very chemosensitive.

Drive receptors

These are characterised by depending on upper airway skeletal muscle contraction (Sant'Ambrogio et al., 1983). They comprise about 20% of the endings studied. They discharge phasically, usually in inspiration, following the activity of the posterior cricoarytenoid muscle. They may include the joint and muscle receptors seen by histologists.

Cold/flow receptors

These constitute 8–15% of receptors studied. They were initially thought to respond to flow, but have now been shown to respond to cold, since airflow at less than ambient temperature and humidity will cool the receptors (Sant'Ambrogio et al., 1983, 1985). They adapt rapidly to a maintained mechanical stimulus, and normally show inspiratory modulation, as would be expected.

Irritant-sensitive endings

A wide variety of irritant gases and aerosols can stimulate laryngeal receptors, the usual stimuli tested being ammonia, SO_2, cigarette smoke and 10–30% CO_2 (Andrew, 1956; Boushey et al., 1974). The receptors are also mechanically sensitive, with a rapidly-adapting irregular discharge and an off-response, in this respect resembling the pattern seen with lower airway receptors thought to be responsible for cough and irritant-induced reflexes.

Chemosensitive endings

Water in the larynx stimulates end-organs (Boggs and Bartlett, 1982) (Fig. 3). They respond primarily to a deficiency in permeant anions, chloride in particular, rather than to low osmolarity of water.

Nonmyelinated afferents

These have been established in the larynx by degeneration experiments (Agostoni et al., 1957) and recordings from the nodose ganglion (Mei and Nourigat, 1967), but have not been studied much by fibre recordings (Boushey et al., 1974).

Joint and muscle receptors

Discharges from these receptors have been studied (Andrew, 1956), but it has seldom been possible to identify the receptors and their distinction from other laryngeal mechanoreceptors has not always been clear (Wyke and Kirchner, 1979).

Reflexes

The list of reflexes from the larynx is even longer

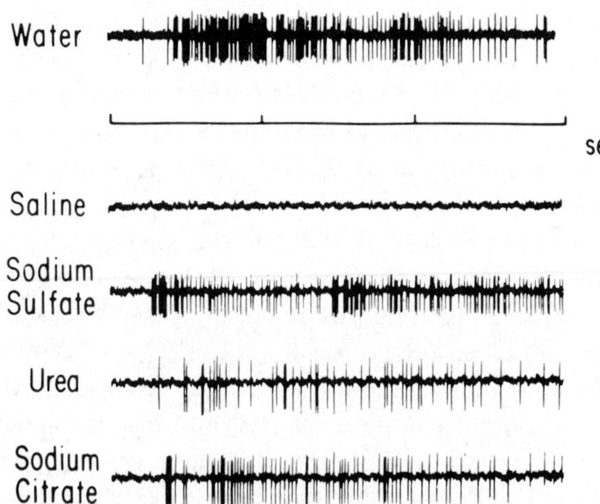

Fig. 3. Recordings from a single water-sensitive fibre in the superior laryngeal nerve of an adult dog. Onset of discharge coincided with arrival of fluids in the larynx with negligible latency. Time marks denote 1-second intervals. The four solutions applied in the lower records were isotonic (300 mmol · l^{-1}). Only saline did not stimulate the receptor. From Boggs and Bartlett (1982).

than that of receptors studied by fibre recording (Korpas and Tomori, 1979; Daly, 1985; Widdicombe, 1986). With a few exceptions, it is almost impossible to say which fibres may be responsible for which reflexes.

Breathing

Chemical and mechanical irritation of the larynx causes apnoea in anaesthetised animals with thresholds lower than those needed for cough or expiration (Boushey et al., 1972; Korpas and Tomori, 1979). Since the apnoea can be induced by hypotonic solutions, and is mediated at least in part by myelinated afferent fibres, it seems likely that the chemosensitive endings are involved (Boggs and Bartlett, 1982).

In unanaesthetised animals the apnoeic reflex is weak or replaced by coughing, so possibly the same afferent pathway may mediate both responses, anaesthesia being critical (Boggs and Bartlett, 1982). Coughing can be induced by mechanical, irritant and hypo-osmolar stimuli. There are large species differences in the sensitivity of the cough reflex (Bucher, 1958). Presumably, the irritant-sensitive and chemosensitive receptors are involved. There are recent reviews on the neural mechanisms of coughing (Korpas and Tomori, 1979; Widdicombe, 1981, 1986).

The expiration reflex has been extensively studied by Korpas and his colleagues (Korpas and Tomori, 1979), and consists of a sudden and brief expiratory effort when the vocal folds are touched mechanically. The reflex is more resistant to general anaesthesia than is the cough, and is present in newborn animals before the cough reflex develops.

Negative pressure in the entire upper airway, or in the pharynx and larynx, slows breathing, mainly by increasing inspiratory time. Positive pressure has the opposite effect (Mathew et al., 1982a; Hwang et al., 1984a; Van Lunteren et al., 1984). Since the response is greatly reduced by cutting the superior laryngeal nerves, it presumably comes mainly from laryngeal receptors. The response is slowly-adapting and the most likely afferent pathway is from the pressure receptors of the larynx.

Swallow

With hypo-osmolar liquids, this can be more readily elicited from the epiglottis and larynx than from other parts of the upper respiratory tract, at least in anaesthetised animals (Miller, 1982; Boggs and Bartlett, 1982). It is concurrent with a brief apnoea and, since the same stimuli cause the two, the same reflex pathway could be involved. The state of development and the condition of the animal may determine whether the response is apnoea or a swallow, or both.

Other reflexes

Hypertension and vagal bradycardia are the main primary cardiovascular reflexes when the laryngeal mucosa is stimulated (Tomori and Widdicombe, 1969; Daly, 1985; Widdicombe, 1986). Cardiac arrhythmias may occur. There is also bronchoconstriction by an atropine-sensitive vagal reflex (Nadel, 1980). Irritation of the larynx causes mucus secretion in the trachea, mainly by a vagal cholinergic reflex (Phipps, 1981). The receptors and afferent nerves for these reflexes are unknown.

Mechanical or chemical irritation of the laryngeal mucosa causes laryngeal adduction (Szereda-Przestaszewska and Widdicombe, 1971) even if the stimulus is too weak to cause coughing or apnoea. In man and dogs the reflex is absent at birth, and its absence may be inducive to the aspiration syndrome in the newborn.

Negative pressure in the entire upper airway, or in the orolarynx alone, causes reflex contraction of the dilator muscles of the pharynx, larynx and nose, especially genioglossus, posterior cricoarytenoid and alae nasi (Mathew et al., 1982b; Mathew, 1984; Roberts et al., 1984; Van Lunteren et al., 1984). This helps to maintain upper airway patency. Positive pressure has the opposite effect. The dominant afferent pathway is the superior laryngeal nerves. Since the response is slowly-adapting, it seems probable that the pressure receptors mentioned above are the main afferent pathway. The reflexes may be weak in obstructive sleep apnoea, when the pharyngeal airway may collapse.

Sensation

Inflammation and irritation of the larynx can cause sensations of rawness, irritation, tickling, desire to cough and pain. There are no indications as to which of the receptors listed above may be responsible for these sensations, nor have the sensations been analysed or quantified. There is no evidence that we can sense pressure, airflow or temperature from the larynx.

In summary, for the larynx, as for the nose and pharynx, we cannot relate receptor structure to afferent patterns of activity or the latter to sensation; however, there are a few indications as to which afferent fibres cause which reflex.

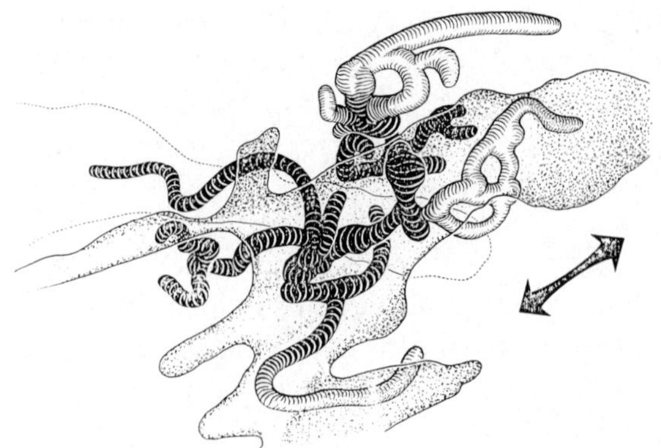

Fig. 4. Reconstruction from electron micrographs of a slowly-adapting stretch receptor from the trachea of a dog. The stippled areas represent smooth muscle and the tubular structure the receptor complex. The arrows show the longitudinal direction of contraction of the muscle. From Krauhs (1984).

Tracheobronchial tree and lungs

Probably because of the length and ease of access of the vagus nerves, afferents from the lungs have been more studied than those from the upper respiratory tract. The extensive literature has been reviewed (Sant'Ambrogio, 1982; Coleridge, J. C. G. and Coleridge, 1984; Coleridge, H. M. and Coleridge, 1986; Widdicombe, 1986).

There are three main groups of lung receptors, the slowly-adapting stretch receptors, the rapidly-adapting "irritant" stretch receptors, and the C-fibre receptors. Each group is distributed throughout the tracheobronchial tree, and the last is also in the alveolar walls. The same type of receptor may have different reflex actions, depending on its site. A fourth type of receptor, associated with neuroepithelial bodies, has less well-defined physiology (Pack and Widdicombe, 1984).

Nervous receptors

Recent studies by Krauhs (1984) have shown the structure of the pulmonary stretch receptor (Fig. 4) located in airway smooth muscle on anatomical and functional grounds. Its distribution is fairly compact. It has a close relation with surrounding collagen and smooth muscle fibres, but how these interact in terms of receptor stimulation is not very clear.

Much indirect evidence suggests that the rapidly-adapting "irritant" receptors have some branches close to the lumen of the airways, and are concentrated at points of airway branching (Widdicombe, 1954, 1986). Histologically, the only nerves seen that could correspond are the intra-epithelial free nerve fibres (Das et al., 1978) (Fig. 5) that connect to myelinated nerves higher up. Degeneration experiments show that they are sensory (Das et al., 1979). However, the histological pictures only show single nerves, and the whole nerve complex has not been unravelled. Physiological studies suggest that the single receptor may ramify not only in the epithelium but also deep into airway muscle (Fisher, 1964; Sant'Ambrogio et al., 1978).

C-fibre receptors have not been definitely identified, except possibly at the alveolar level (Coleridge and Coleridge, 1984). Here there are nonmyelinated fibres, presumed afferent, but they are rather rare (Meyrick and Reid, 1971). Similar nerves have not been identified in the tracheobronchial tree, although it is impossible to say whether any observed nonmyelinated fibre might be part of a C-fibre receptor complex.

Neuroepithelial bodies, the cells of which contain amine-rich granules and are secretory, are said to

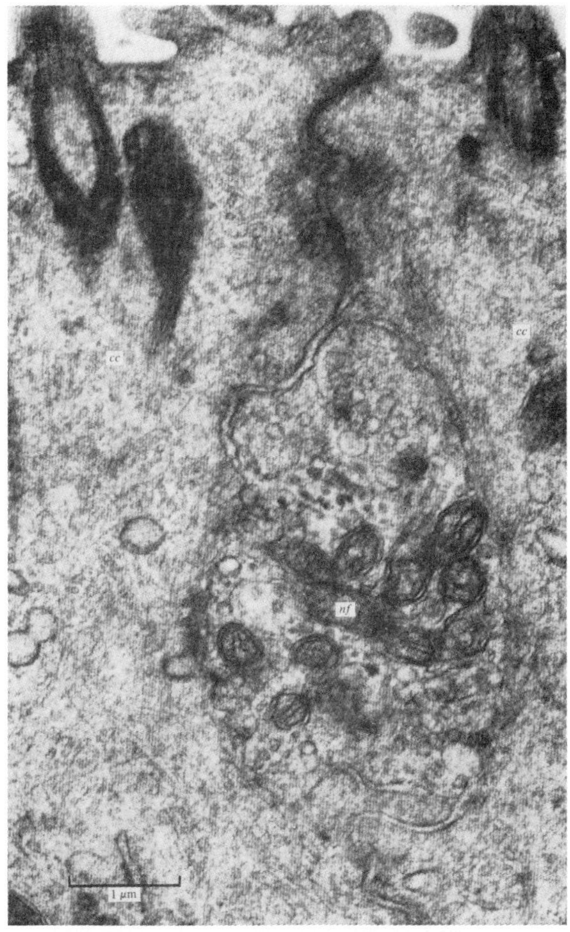

Fig. 5. Luminal edge of airway epithelium showing a nerve fibre (nf) containing numerous inclusions. The nerve lies between ciliated cells (cc) with a double cell membrane. Fixed with glutaraldehyde and osmium tetroxide, stained with uranyl acetate and lead citrate. From Widdicombe (1981).

have an afferent innervation. However, this sensory pathway has not been studied nor has its role been defined (Pack and Widdicombe, 1984).

Afferent nerves

There have been many studies of single-fibre vagal recording from the lung receptors. A few afferent fibres in sympathetic nerves have been studied, but the supply is predominantly vagal. A summary of their properties follows, and more detailed reviews can be consulted (Sant'Ambrogio, 1982; Coleridge, J. C. G. and Coleridge, 1984; Coleridge, H. M. and Coleridge, 1986).

Slowly-adapting stretch receptors

These are localised in airway smooth muscle, the greatest concentration being in the extrapulmonary and large intrapulmonary airways. They discharge during inflation (Fig. 6) and adapt slowly to main-

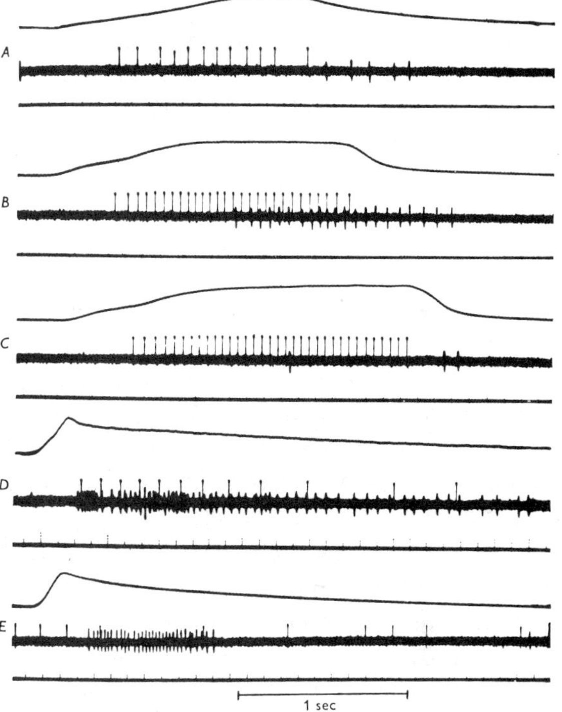

Fig. 6. Responses of J type receptor (small diphasic spike) to inflation of the lung (A, B, C) with open chest and insufflation of halothane (60 ml) at (D) and (E). The large monophasic spikes in A, B, C and D are those of a pulmonary stretch receptor fibre and these show the consistent response to inflation of the lung with 60 ml in A and about 150 ml in B and C, in contrast to the variable response in the J type fibre, which is excited during the deflation phase in A and during the inflation phase in B (but after a significant delay); there is comparatively little response in C (again about 150 ml inflation). Insufflation of halothane had an excitatory effect on the J type receptor, which is excited with a similar latency in E after cutting the great vessels and removing the ventricles. From above downward in each record: intratracheal pressure, impulses in filament and 0.1-second time marks. Gain of amplifier for intratracheal pressure in A, D and E is twice that in B and C. From Paintal (1969).

tained stretch of the airway wall, and collapse of the airway may either inhibit or stimulate them. They have low volume thresholds, many being tonically active at FRC. Their activity is enhanced by contraction of the surrounding smooth muscle, indicating the possibility of vago-vagal feedback control.

Although the receptors are primarily mechanosensitive, they have some response to endogenous chemicals. Bronchoconstrictor drugs such as histamine and acetylcholine increase their discharge, probably acting primarily via smooth muscle contraction. CO_2 can inhibit their discharge, but there is some dispute whether this has physiological importance.

Rapidly-adapting "irritant" stretch receptors

Since their first detailed description by Knowlton and Larrabee (1946), these receptors have been intensively studied. They respond to inflation and deflation of the airways and lungs with rapidly-adapting irregular discharges, often with a prominent off-response (Widdicombe, 1954). They occur throughout the trachea and larger bronchi, with concentrations at the carina and the points of bronchial branching. Those in the lungs are less rapidly-adapting than those in the trachea. They are distinct from slowly-adapting receptors, not only in their response to mechanical stimuli but in the fact that they are sensitive to many inhaled irritants. They are also sensitive to inhaled dusts and gentle touch with an intraluminal catheter, suggesting that they may be superficial in the mucosa. Ammonia, ether, SO_2 and cigarette smoke have been frequently tested and, although the sensitivity and uniformity of response varies, in general the receptors are excited, with maintained responses not showing much adaptation (Mills et al., 1969, 1970; Sellick and Widdicombe, 1971). The receptors are also stimulated by a number of chemical mediators such as histamine, 5-hydroxytryptamine, prostaglandin $F_{2\alpha}$ (Fig. 7) and acetylcholine; this applies whether the drugs are given by aerosol or intravenously (Sampson and Vidruk, 1978).

The discharge and sensitivity of the receptors are

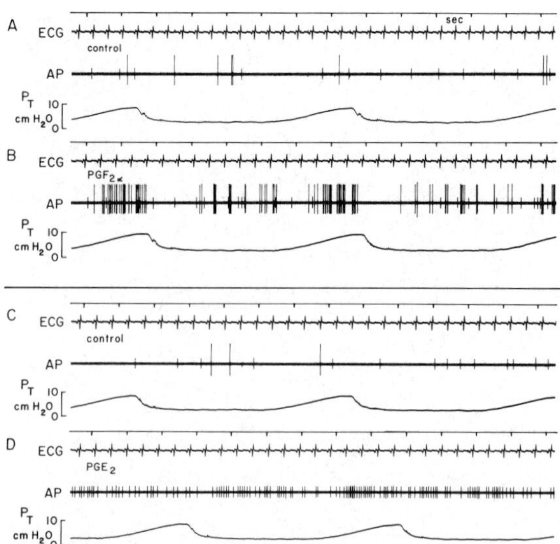

Fig. 7. Comparison of the effects of prostaglandin (PG) $F_{2\alpha}$ and PGE_2 on an "irritant" receptor (large spikes) and a pulmonary C-fibre (small spikes) in a dog with open chest and on positive-pressure ventilation. Both endings were located in the lower lobe of the left lung. A was taken before and B 16 seconds after injection of 4 μg $PGF_{2\alpha} \cdot kg^{-1}$ body weight in the right atrium. The interval between B and C was 6 minutes. C was taken before and D 42 seconds after injection of 20 $\mu g \cdot kg^{-1}$ PGE_2 into the right atrium. From above downward in each record: 1-second time trace, electrocardiogram (ECG), action potentials (AP) recorded from an afferent slip of the left vagus nerve, tracheal pressure (P_T). From Coleridge and Coleridge (1985).

increased in a number of pathological conditions, including congestion, microembolisation, anaphylaxis, pneumothorax and bronchoconstriction due to various drugs (Sellick and Widdicombe, 1969, 1970; Mills et al., 1970). In some instances the response can be related to a fall in compliance. The response to endogenous mediators may depend in part on airway smooth muscle contraction and changes in compliance, although some of the mediators also seem to have a direct action on the receptors (Sampson and Vidruk, 1978). In general, the irritant receptors are polymodal and respond to physiological and pathological changes.

C-fibre receptors

These were first studied by Paintal (1955), who investigated receptors at the alveolar level and subsequently called them J receptors (Paintal, 1969). There are two groups of similar receptors, now called pulmonary and bronchial C-fibre receptors, names which indicate their sites. They can be localised by mechanical stimulation or by sensitivity to drugs injected by various vascular routes (Coleridge and Coleridge, 1984).

The receptors normally have little tonic discharge, but are activated by large inflations in dogs, and by strong deflations in cats. However, the main stimulus to the receptors seems to be endogenous mediators such as bradykinin, PGE (Fig. 7), 5-hydroxytryptamine, acetylcholine and histamine. They are excited by some inhaled gases (Fig. 6). The C-fibre receptors are also stimulated or sensitised in a variety of lung conditions, in particular, congestion and lung oedema, pneumonia and microembolisation (Paintal, 1973).

Thus, both the irritant and C-fibre receptors have many properties in common, and it is likely that both groups of receptor are activated simultaneously in many conditions. However, there are some differences, for example, in sensitivities to prostaglandins and bradykinin, and to pneumothorax and lung volume changes.

Reflexes

Slowly-adapting stretch receptors

These receptors are responsible for the Hering-Breuer reflex, the inhibition of inspiratory activity in inflation (Bradley, 1977; Coleridge and Coleridge, 1986). They also prolong expiratory time (Knox, 1973). They control the pattern of breathing in experimental animals, although not in eupnoeic healthy man. Other reflex actions are relaxation of tracheobronchial muscle and cardio-acceleration (Daly, 1985). The major role of the receptors is mainly physiological, although in pathological conditions they may influence breathing pattern. There is no evidence that their activity reaches consciousness (see later).

Rapidly-adapting "irritant" stretch receptors

The epithelial site of these receptors and their responses to intraluminal stimuli indicate that reflexly they cause cough (from the carina and large bronchi) and hyperpnoea (from smaller bronchi) (Mills et al., 1970; Widdicombe, 1981). This conclusion is based mainly on a correlation between reflexes from the airways and receptor discharges recorded from the vagus. Species which lack intraepithelial nerves (mouse and ferret) have no cough reflex from the tracheobronchial tree (Korpas and Widdicombe, 1983; Pack et al., 1984). The irritant receptors are also thought to cause other reflex changes associated with coughing, namely bronchoconstriction, laryngoconstriction and mucus secretion (Coleridge and Coleridge, 1986). There is no evidence that they cause cardiovascular effects.

Pulsatile stimuli that excite irritant receptors, in the presence of block of slowly-adapting receptors, can cause tachypnoea by shortening expiratory time (Davies and Roumy, 1982); this is consistent with the view that the receptors deep in the lungs cause hyperpnoea rather than coughing (Davies et al., 1978). The same stimuli can cause augmented breaths, the occasional deep inspirations that reverse the tendency to collapse of the lung (Larrabee and Knowlton, 1946; Davies and Roumy, 1982). Thus, the irritant receptors play a role in physiological control of breathing as well as in pathological conditions.

C-fibre receptors

Reflexes from these receptors have been studied mainly with their excitation by exogenous chemicals. In most mammals these cause apnoea at FRC, followed by rapid shallow breathing (Paintal, 1973; Coleridge and Coleridge, 1984). The same patterns of breathing can be seen in the pathological conditions that stimulate C-fibre receptors (and often irritant receptors), e.g., in microembolism, lung congestion and oedema, and pneumonia.

C-fibre activation also causes reflex bronchoconstriction, laryngoconstriction, tracheal mucus secretion, hypotension, bradycardia and inhibition of spinal reflexes (Coleridge, J. C. G. and Coleridge, 1984; Coleridge, H. M. and Coleridge, 1986). These widespread responses, some of them long-lasting, indicate a profound defensive response by the animal.

Sensation

Proprioception

There is no evidence that slowly-adapting stretch receptors are involved in respiratory sensation, whether physiological or pathological (Zechman and Wiley, 1986). The awareness of lung volume changes and of resistive loads is normal in subjects whose vagi have been blocked by local anaesthesia (Guz et al., 1970). On the other hand, spinal block at T1 (denervating the abdomen and chest wall) makes no difference to detection of added loads (Newsom Davis, 1967). The diaphragm might provide the primary sensory input for load perception, but here the evidence is in conflict. For example, bilateral phrenic nerve block makes no difference to the detection of resistive loads (Noble et al., 1970, 1972). One subject, with spinal transection at C2–C3, could also detect loads normally, although his accessory muscles of breathing might have been involved in this (Noble et al., 1970). In general, the diaphragm and possibly the chest wall muscles seem important in volume and load detection, but a subsidiary role for lung receptors is possible if the other systems fail; if this is so, then the pulmonary stretch receptors seem the most likely mechanism.

"Unpleasant sensations"

There is much stronger evidence that unpleasant sensations can be derived from lung receptors. The burning sensation when an endotracheal/bronchial catheter is passed is abolished by vagal block (Klassen et al., 1951; Morton et al., 1951), and the rawness due to tracheitis is abolished by local anaesthesia of the airways. Inflation of collapsed lung gives rise to an unpleasant sensation of "tearing" (Burger and Macklem, 1968). The tightness in the chest felt by asthmatics during an attack is abolished by local anaesthesia to the airways or to the vagus nerves (Guz et al., 1970; Guz, 1977). Inhalation of irritant aerosols, as of citric acid or ammonia, causes rawness and irritation, which is blocked by local anaesthesia (Cross et al., 1976). These sensations must be derived from airway receptors. Cough accompanies many of the "irritations" and is undeniably reflex.

There are three possibilities for the afferent pathway of these unpleasant sensations — irritant receptors, C-fibre receptors, or both. The experimental problem is that there are few stimuli that act on only one of the two groups of receptor. Both $PGF_{2\alpha}$ and bradykinin aerosols cause coughing and rawness in man, and in animals stimulate irritant and C-fibre receptors, respectively (Coleridge and Coleridge, 1984). However, one cannot rule out an action of these aerosols on the larynx. Pneumothorax, which stimulates irritant receptors but has little action on C-fibre endings in animals, is a powerful cause of breathlessness but it is difficult to establish this as a vagal reflex in man. However, one of the most powerful excitants of pulmonary C-fibre activity, namely pulmonary congestion and oedema, is not associated with distressing lung sensation at rest, although exertion may lead to breathlessness. Gases such as phosgene cause pulmonary oedema before any unpleasant respiratory sensation (Henderson and Haggard, 1943). In man, drugs can be injected intravenously to stimulate lung C-fibre endings. With lobeline, when it reaches the lungs it sometimes causes cough and sensation near the larynx, but no sensation referred to the lungs (Jain et al., 1972); however, the specificity of lobeline has not been clarified in either animals or man. With intravenous capsaicin there is a raw sensation in the chest but no changes in breathing, heart rate or blood pressure (Winning et al., 1985). Capsaicin powerfully stimulates lung C-fibres in animals, but the differences in responses between humans and animals make interpretation very difficult. In unanaesthetised cats intravenous injections of drugs that stimulate lung C-fibres cause considerable cardiovascular and spinal reflex changes, but give rise to no apparent distress (Kalia et al., 1973; Ginzel and Eldridge, 1977).

It is clear that stimulation of lung receptors can cause a variety of unpleasant sensations in man, but which afferent pathways are involved is not certain.

As with other tissues, it is likely that more than one pathway may lead to unpleasant sensation, and that the intensity and quality of the sensation may depend on the interaction of these pathways.

Dyspnoea

Dyspnoea is one of the respiratory sensations which has been quantitated and is being studied with psychometric tests. However, dyspnoea in patients and breathlessness in conditions such as exercise in healthy subjects have their primary afferent input from respiratory muscles, especially the diaphragm (Campbell and Guz, 1981; Fishman and Ledlie, 1979). In this respect, if lung receptors are stimulated, their main effect on dyspnoea will not be a direct one on viscero-sensory areas of the brain, but a secondary one via imposed respiratory alterations of muscle activity. It is not possible to exercise subjects with bilateral vagal blockade, and studies on exercising subjects with complete anaesthetisation of the airways might provide valuable information as to the importance of lung sensory pathways. There are excellent reviews of dyspnoea (Guz, 1977; Fishman and Ledlie, 1979; Campbell and Guz, 1981).

Conclusions

There are glaring deficiencies in our knowledge of sensation from the lungs and airways. A few of the sensations have been quantitated, and those that have, such as dyspnoea and responses to loading, seem to come primarily from somatic structures. Qualities of sensation from the respiratory system have been described frequently, but it has seldom been possible to identify these with either a precise afferent pathway or a histological structure in the tissues. Nonetheless, the subject is an important one for research. Quite apart from breathlessness, respiratory distressful sensations in conditions such as rhinitis, asthma and respiratory infections must be one of the commonest unpleasant visceral sensations.

References

Adrian, E. D. (1942) Olfactory reactions in the brain of the hedgehog. J. Physiol., 100: 459–473.

Agostoni, E., Chinnock, J. E., Daly, M. De B. and Murray, J. G. (1957) Functional and histological studies of the vagus nerve and its branches to the heart, lungs and abdominal viscera in the cat. J. Physiol., 135: 182–205.

Allen, W. F. (1929) Effect on respiration, blood pressure and carotid pulse of various inhaled and insufflated vapours when stimulating one cranial nerve and various combinations of cranial nerve. III. Olfactory and trigeminals stimulated. Am. J. Physiol., 88: 117–129.

Andersen, P. (1954) Inhibitory reflexes elicited from the trigeminal and olfactory nerves in rabbits. Acta Physiol. Scand., 30: 137–148.

Andrew, B. L. A. (1956) A functional analysis of the myelinated fibres of the superior laryngeal nerve of the rat. J. Physiol., 133: 420–432.

Angell-James, J. E. and Daly, M. De B. (1969) Nasal reflexes. Proc. Roy. Soc. Med., 62: 1287–1293.

Beidler, L. M. (1961) The chemical senses. Annu. Rev. Psychol., 12: 363–388.

Boggs, D. F. and Bartlett, D. (1982) Chemical specificity of a laryngeal apneic reflex in puppies. J. Appl. Physiol., 53: 455–462.

Borum, P., Gronborg, H., Brofeld, S. and Mygind, N. (1983) Nasal reactivity in rhinitis. Eur. J. Resp. Dis. Suppl., 128: 65–71.

Boushey, H. A., Richardson, P. S. and Widdicombe, J. G. (1972) Reflex effects of laryngeal irritation on the pattern of breathing and total lung resistance. J. Physiol., 224: 501–513.

Boushey, H. A., Richardson, P. S., Widdicombe, J. G. and Wise, J. C. M. (1974) The response of laryngeal afferent fibres to mechanical and chemical stimuli. J. Physiol., 240: 153–175.

Bradley, G. W. (1977) Control of the breathing pattern. In J. G. Widdicombe (Ed.), Respiratory Physiology, II, Vol. 14, University Park Press, Baltimore, pp. 185–217.

Bucher, K. (1958) Pathophysiology and pharmacology of cough. Pharmacol. Rev., 10: 43–58.

Burger, E. J. and Macklem, P. (1968) Airway closure: demonstration by breathing 100% O_2 at low lung volume and N_2 washout. J. Appl. Physiol., 25: 139–148.

Campbell, E. J. M. and Guz, A. (1981) Breathlessness. In T. F. Hornbein (Ed.), Regulation of Breathing, Part II, Marcel Dekker, New York, pp. 1181–1195.

Cauna, N., Hinderer, K. H. and Wentges, R. T. (1969) Sensory receptor organs of the human nasal and respiratory mucosa. Am. J. Anat., 14: 295–300.

Chaudhary, B. A. and Burki, N. K. (1978) The effects of airway anaesthesia and the ability to detect added inspiratory resistive loads. Clin. Sci. Mol. Med., 54: 621–626.

Coleridge, H. M. and Coleridge, J. C. G. (1986) Reflexes evoked from tracheobronchial tree and lungs. In N. S. Cherniack and J. G. Widdicombe, (Eds.), Handbook of Physiology, The Respiratory System, II, American Physiological Society, Washington, DC, pp. 395–430.

Coleridge, J. C. G. and Coleridge, H. M. (1984) Afferent vagal C-fibre innervation of the lungs and airways and its functional significance. Rev. Physiol. Biochem. Pharmacol., 99: 1–110.

Cross, B. A., Guz, A., Jain, S. K., Archer, S., Stevens, J. and Reynolds, F. (1976) The effect of anaesthesia of the airways in dog and man: a study of respiratory reflexes, sensations and lung mechanics. Clin. Sci. Mol. Med., 50: 439–454.

Daly, M. De B. (1986) Interactions between respiration and circulation. In N. S. Cherniack and J. G. Widdicombe (Eds.), Handbook of Physiology, The Respiratory System, II, American Physiological Society, Washington, DC, pp. 529–594.

Das, R. M., Jeffery, P. J. and Widdicombe, J. G. (1978) The epithelial innervation of the lower respiratory tract of the cat. J. Anat., 126: 123–131.

Das, R. M., Jeffery, P. K. and Widdicombe, J. G. (1979) Experimental degeneration of intra-epithelial nerve fibres in cat airways. J. Anat., 128: 259–263.

Davies, A. and Roumy, M. (1982) The effect of transient stimulation of lung irritant receptors on the pattern of breathing in rabbits. J. Physiol., 324: 389–401.

Davies, A., Dixon, M., Callanan, D., Huszczuk, A., Widdicombe, J. G. and Wise, J. C. M. (1978) Lung reflexes in rabbits during pulmonary strech receptor block by sulphur dioxide. Respir. Physiol., 34: 83–101.

Douglas, R. (1981) Inhalation of irritant gases and aerosols. In J. G. Widdicombe (Ed.), Respiratory Pharmacology, Pergamon Press, Oxford, pp. 297–333.

Elsner, R. and Gooden, B. (1983) Diving and Asphyxia. Monographs of the Physiological Society, No. 40. Cambridge University Press, Cambridge.

Feindel, W. J. (1956) The neural pattern of the epiglottis. J. Comp. Neurol., 105: 269–280.

Fillenz, M. and Widdicombe, J. G. (1971) Receptors of the lungs and airways. In E. Neil (Ed.), Handbook of Sensory Physiology, Vol. III, Springer-Verlag, Berlin, pp. 81–112.

Fisher, A. W. F. (1964) The intrinsic innervation of the trachea. J. Anat., 98: 117–124.

Fishman, A. P. and Ledlie, J. F. (1979) Dyspnoea. Bull. Eur. Physiopath. Resp., 15: 789–804.

Gandevia, S. C., Killian, K. J. and Cambell, E. J. M. (1981) The contribution of upper airway and respiratory muscle mechanisms to the detection of pressure changes at the mouth in normal subjects. Clin. Sci., 60: 513–518.

Ginzel, K. H. and Eldred, E. (1977) Reflex depression of somatic motor activity from heart, lungs and carotid sinus. In A. S. Paintal and G. Gill-Kumar (Eds.), Krogh Centenary Symposium on Respiratory Adaptations, Capillary Exchange and Reflex Mechanisms, Vallabhbhai Chest Institute, Delhi, pp. 358–394.

Grote, J. J., Kuijpers, W. and Huygen, P. L. M. (1975) Selective denervation of the autonomic nerve supply of the nasal mucosa. Acta Otolaryngol., 79: 124–132.

Guz, A. (1977) Control of ventilation in man with special reference to abnormalities in asthma. In M. L. Lichtenstein and K. F. Austen (Eds.), Asthma, Physiology, Immunopharmacology and Treatment, Academic Press, New York, pp. 211–222.

Guz, A., Noble, M. I. M., Eisele, J. H. and Trenchard, D. (1970) Experimental results of vagal block in cardiopulmonary disease. In R. Porter (Ed.), Breathing: Hering-Breuer Centenary Symposium, Churchill, London, pp. 315–329.

Hatakeyama, S. (1969) Histological study of the nerve distribution in the larynx in the cat. Arch. Jpn. Histol., 19: 369–389.

Henderson, Y. and Haggard, H. W. (1943) Noxious Gases and the Principles of Respiration Influencing their Action, Reinhold, New York.

Hwang, J. C., St. John, W. M. and Bartlett, D. Jr. (1984a) Afferent pathways for hypoglossal and phrenic responses to changes in upper airway pressure. Respir. Physiol., 55: 341–354.

Hwang, J. C., St. John, W. M. and Bartlett, D. Jr. (1984b) Receptors corresponding to changes in upper airway pressure. Respir. Physiol., 55: 355–366.

Jain, S. K., Subramanian, S., Julka, D. B. and Guz, A. (1972) Search for evidence of lung chemoreflexes in man: study of respiratory and circulatory effects of phenyldiguanide and lobeline. Clin. Sci., 42: 163–177.

Jansco, G., Kiraly, E. and Jansco-Gabor, A. (1977) Pharmacologically induced selective degeneration of chemosensitive primary sensory neurones. Nature, 270: 741–743.

Kalia, M., Paintal, A. S. and Koepchen, H. P. (1973) Motor behavioural responses to J-receptor stimulation in an awake walking cat. Pflugers Arch., 339: Suppl., R80.

Klassen, K. P., Morton, D. R. and Curtis, G. M. (1951) The clinical physiology of the human bronchi. III. The effect of vagus section on the cough reflex, bronchial caliber and clearance of bronchial secretions. Surgery, 29: 483–490.

Knowlton, G. C. and Larrabee, M. G. (1946) A unitary analysis of pulmonary volume receptors. Am. J. Physiol., 147: 100–114.

Knox, C. K. (1973) Characteristics of inflation and deflation reflexes during expiration in the cat. J. Neurophysiol., 36: 284–295.

Koizumi, H. (1953) On sensory innervation of the larynx in dog. Tohoku J. Exp. Med., 58: 199–210.

Korpas, J. and Tomori, Z. (1979) Cough and Other Respiratory Reflexes, S. Karger, Basel.

Korpas, J. and Widdicombe, J. G. (1983) Defensive respiratory reflexes in ferrets. Respiration, 44: 128–135.

Krauhs, J. M. (1984) Morphology of presumptive slowly adapting receptors in dog trachea. Anat. Res., 210: 73–85.

Larrabee, M. J. and Knowlton, G. C. (1946) Excitation and inhibition of phrenic motoneurones by inflation of the lungs. Am. J. Physiol., 147: 90–99.

Lewis, D. J. and Prentice, D. E. (1980) The ultrastructure of rat laryngeal epithelia. J. Anat., 130: 617–632.

Lundblad, L. (1984) Protective reflexes and vascular effects in the nasal mucosa elicited by activation of capsaicin-sensitive substance P-immunoreactive trigeminal neurons. Acta Physiol. Scand. Suppl., 529: 1–42.

Mathew, O. P. (1984) Upper airway negative-pressure effects on respiratory activity in upper airway muscles. J. Appl. Physiol., 56: 500–505.

Mathew, O. P., Abu-Osba, Y. K. and Thach, B. T. (1982a) Influence of upper airway pressure changes on respiratory frequency. Respir. Physiol., 49: 223–233.

Mathew, O. P., Abu-Osba, Y. K. and Thach, B. T. (1982b) Genio-glossus muscle responses to upper airway pressure changes: afferent pathways. J. Appl. Physiol., 52: 445–450.

Mei, N. and Nourigat, B. (1967) Etude electrophysiologique des neurons sensitifs du nerf larynge superieur. C. R. Seance Acad. Sci. Paris, 162: 149–153.

Melville, G. N. and Morris, D. (1972) Cold I: effect on airway resistance in health and disease. Environ. Physiol. Biochem., 2: 107–116.

Meyrick, B. and Reid, L. (1971) Nerves in rat intra-acinar alveoli: an electron microscopic study. Respir. Physiol., 11: 367–377.

Miller, A. J. (1982) Deglutition. Physiol. Rev., 62: 129–184.

Mills, J. E., Sellick, H. and Widdicombe, J. G. (1969) Activity of lung irritant receptors in pulmonary microembolism, anaphylaxis and drug-induced bronchoconstriction. J. Physiol., 203: 337–357.

Mills, J. E., Sellick, H. and Widdicombe, J. G. (1970) Epithelial irritant receptors in the lungs. In R. Porter (Ed.), Breathing: Hering-Breuer Centenary Symposium, Churchill, London, pp. 77–92.

Morton, D. R., Klassen, K. P. and Curtis, G. M. (1951) The clinical physiology of the human bronchi. II. The effect of vagus section upon pain of tracheobronchial origin. Surgery, 30: 800–809.

Mygind, N., Secher, C. and Kirkegaard, J. (1983) Role of histamine and antihistamine in the nose. Eur. J. Respir. Dis. Suppl., 128: 16–20.

Nadel, J. A. (1980) Autonomic relgulation of airway smooth muscle. In J. A. Nadel (Ed.), Physiology and Pharmacology of the Airways, Marcel Dekker, New York, pp. 217–257.

Nail, B. S., Sterling, G. M. and Widdicombe, J. G. (1969) Epipharyngeal receptors responding to mechanical stimulation. J. Physiol., 204: 91–98.

Newsom Davis, J. (1967) Contribution of somatic receptors in the chest wall to detection of added inspiratory airway resistance. Clin. Sci., 33: 249–260.

Noble, M. I. M., Eisele, J. H., Trenchard, D. and Guz, A. (1970) Effect of selective peripheral nerve blocks on respiratory sensations. In R. Porter (Ed.), Breathing: Hering-Breuer Centenary Symposium, Churchill, London, pp. 233–246.

Noble, M. I. M., Frankel, H. L., Else, W. and Guz, A. (1972) The sensation produced by threshold resistive loads to breathing. Eur. J. Clin. Invest., 2: 72–77.

Nolte, D. and Berger, D. (1983) On vagal bronchoconstriction in asthmatic patients induced by nasal irritation. Eur. J. Respir. Dis. Suppl., 128: 110–114.

Pack, R. J. and Widdicombe, J. G. (1984) Amine-containing cells of the lung. Eur. J. Respir. Dis., 65: 559–578.

Pack, R. J., Al-Ugaily, L. H. and Widdicombe, J. G. (1984) The innervation of the trachea and extrapulmonary bronchi of the mouse. Cell Tissue Res., 238: 61–68.

Paintal, A. S. (1955) Impulses in vagal afferent fibres from specific pulmonary deflation receptors. The response of these receptors to phenyl diguanide, potato starch, 5-hydroxytryptamine and nicotine, and their role in respiratory and cardiovascular reflexes. Q. J. Exp. Physiol., 40: 89–111.

Paintal, A. S. (1969) Mechanism of stimulation of type J pulmonary receptors. J. Physiol., 203: 511–532.

Paintal, A. S. (1973) Vagal sensory receptors and their reflex effects. Physiol. Rev., 53: 159–227.

Parker, G. H. (1922) Smell, Taste and Allied Senses in the Vertebrates. J. P. Lippincott, Philadelphia, PA.

Phillipson, E. A. and Bowes, G. (1986) Control of breathing during sleep. In N. S. Cherniack and J. G. Widdicombe (Eds.), Handbook of Physiology, The Respiratory System, II, American Physiological Society, Washington, DC, pp. 649–690.

Phipps, R. F. (1981) The airway mucociliary system. In J. G. Widdicombe (Ed.), Respiratory Physiology, III, University Park Press, Baltimore, pp. 213–260.

Roberts, J. L., Reed, W. R. and Thach, B. T. (1984) Pharyngeal airway stabilizing function of sternohyoid and sternothyroid muscles in the rabbit. J. Appl. Physiol., 57: 1790–1795.

Sampson, S. R. and Vidruk, E. H. (1978) Chemical stimulation of rapidly adapting receptors in the airways. Adv. Exp. Med. Biol., 99: 281–290.

Sant'Ambrogio, G. (1982) Information arising from the tracheobronchial tree of mammals. Physiol. Rev., 62: 531–569.

Sant'Ambrogio, G., Remmers, J. E., De Groot, W. J., Callas, G. and Mortola, J. P. (1978) Localization of rapidly adapting receptors in the trachea and main stem bronchus of the dog. Respir. Physiol., 33: 359–366.

Sant'Ambrogio, G., Mathew, O. P., Fisher, J. T. and Sant'Ambrogio, F. B. (1983) Laryngeal receptors responding to transmural pressure, airflow and local muscle activity. Respir. Physiol., 54: 317–333.

Sant'Ambrogio, G., Mathew, O. P., Sant'Ambrogio, F. B. and Fisher, J. T. (1985) Laryngeal cold receptors. Respir. Physiol., 59: 35–46.

Sellick, H. and Widdicombe, J. G. (1969) The activity of lung irritant receptors during pneumothorax, hyperpnoea and pulmonary vascular congestion. J. Physiol., 203: 359–381.

Sellick, H. and Widdicombe, J. G. (1970) Vagal deflation and inflation reflexes mediated by lung irritant receptors. Q. J. Exp. Physiol., 55: 153–163.

Sellick, H. and Widdicombe, J. G. (1971) Stimulation of lung irritant receptors by cigarette smoke, carbon dust, and histamine aerosol. J. Appl. Physiol., 31: 15–19.

Sheldon, R. E. (1909) The reactions of the dogfish to chemical stimuli. J. Comp. Neurol., 19: 273–311.

Szereda-Przestaszewska, M. and Widdicombe, J. G. (1973) Reflex effects of chemical irritation of the upper airways on the laryngeal lumen in cats. Respir. Physiol., 18: 107–115.

Tomori, Z. and Widdicombe, J. G. (1969) Muscular, bronchomotor and cardiovascular reflexes elicited by mechanical stimulation of the respiratory tract. J. Physiol., 200: 25–50.

Uddman, R. L., Malm, L. and Sundler, F. (1983) Substance P-containing nerve fibers in the nasal mucosa. Arch. Otorhinolaryngol., 238: 9–16.

Van Lunteren, E., Van de Graaff, W. B., Parker, D. M., Mitra, J., Haxhiu, M. A., Strohl, K. P. and Cherniack, N. S. (1984) Nasal and laryngeal reflex responses to negative upper airway pressure. J. Appl. Physiol., 56: 746–752.

Wells, R. E., Walker, J. E. C. and Hickler, R. B. (1960) Effects of cold air on respiratory airflow resistance in patients with respiratory tract disease. N. Engl. J. Med., 11: 268–273.

Widdicombe, J. G. (1954) Receptors in the trachea and bronchi of the cat. J. Physiol., 123: 71–104.

Widdicombe, J. G. (1981) Nervous receptors in the respiratory tract and lungs. In T. F. Hornbein (Ed.), Regulation of Breathing, Part II, Marcel Dekker, New York, pp. 429–472.

Widdicombe, J. G. (1986) Reflexes from the upper respiratory tract. In N. S. Cherniack and J. G. Widdicombe (Eds.), Handbook of Physiology, The Respiratory System, II, American Physiological Society, Washington, DC, pp. 363–394.

Winning, A. J., Hamilton, R. D., Shea, S. A., Kox, W. and Guz, A. (1985) The effects of stimulating lung afferents in man with intravenous capsaicin. Clin. Sci., 69, Suppl. 12: 34–35.

Wyke, B. D. and Kirchner, J. A. (1979) Neurology of the larynx. In R. Hinchcliffe and D. Harrison (Eds.), Scientific Foundations of Otolaryngology, Heinemann, London, pp. 546–574.

Yan, K. and Salome, C. (1983) The response of the airways to nasal stimulation in asthmatics with rhinitis, Eur. J. Resp. Dis. Suppl., 128: 105–108.

Zechman, F. W. Jr. and Wiley, R. L. (1986) Afferent inputs to breathing: respiratory sensation. In N. S. Cherniack and J. G. Widdicombe (Eds.), Handbook of Physiology, The Respiratory System, II, American Physiological Society, Washington, DC, pp. 449–474.

F. Cervero and J. F.B. Morrison
Progress in Brain Research, Vol. 67

CHAPTER 6

Vagal afferent innervation of the gastrointestinal tract

P. L. R. Andrews

Department of Physiology, St. George's Hospital Medical School, Cranmer Terrace, Tooting, London SW17 0RE, U.K.

Introduction

Systematic research on the vagus nerve probably started with Galen (129–199), whose dissections of pigs, Barbary apes and Roman gladiators revealed that it distributed to the viscera. More extensive studies by Vesalius (1543) and Willis (1664, quoted in Pick, 1970) demonstrated branches to a number of abdominal organs and an interchange of fibres between the dorsal and ventral vagi.

Although it was known at the turn of the century that the vagus nerve contained afferent fibres, their study was somewhat overshadowed by the more extensive investigations on the efferent functions of the vagus and splanchnic nerves by Langley (1903) and Gaskell (1916). Interest in vagal afferents was renewed when Adrian (1933) used the single-fibre dissection technique to record from vagal cardiac and respiratory afferents, and histological studies by Du Bois and Foley (1936) demonstrated that the vagus was predominantly an afferent nerve. In the 1950s these techniques were used by Paintal (1954), Iggo (1955), Evans and Murray (1954) and Agostoni et al. (1957) to investigate the properties and numbers of vagal afferents supplying the abdominal viscera. These and many other studies over the past quarter century have revealed that the abdominal vagus is composed of 80–90% afferent fibres (in non-ruminants) and that virtually all parts of the gastrointestinal tract are supplied by the vagus.

Vagal gastrointestinal afferents have been reviewed by Iggo (1966), Paintal (1973), Leek (1972a,b, 1977) and recently by Mei (1983). Whilst some degree of repetition is unavoidable, the aim of this review is to concentrate on a number of areas not dealt with previously and to examine whether activation of the abdominal afferents can evoke conscious sensations.

The abdominal vagus: distribution, fibre composition and routes to the CNS

Distribution

Descriptions of the thoracic and abdominal distribution of the vagi are available for a number of species (man, monkey, cat, dog, amphibia, fish, birds and reptiles, Pick, 1970; man and ferret, MacKay and Andrews, 1983; rat, Powley et al., 1983).

Several points arise from observations of the gross anatomy of the vagus. First, apart from the stomach and liver, the remaining abdominal viscera (e.g., pancreas) do not receive macroscopically identifiable discrete branches. This means that their afferent innervation can only be studied by either using tracer techniques or recording afferent activity at a distant site where the vagus is "contaminated" by afferents from other organs. Even in areas of the gut (e.g., small intestine) where discrete nerve bundles can be identified and activity recorded relatively easily the question of whether they are vagal remains, as the vagal and splanchnic nerves often share the same terminal course. Second, because it is so difficult to identify the peripheral course of the afferents, for example, supplying the duodenum, extreme care must be taken in the preparation of the animal to avoid accidental denervation of the relevant structure.

Third, the peripheral distribution of the vagus should be borne in mind when deciding which cervical trunk to record from. For example, in the rat the liver is innervated predominantly from the ventral vagus which in turn arises mainly from the left vagus; therefore, studies of hepatic afferents will be more fruitful if the left cervical vagus is used (Adachi, 1981). It remains to be investigated whether other visceral organs have a preferential projection.

Fibre composition

The afferent:efferent ratio for individual vagal branches is not known, but data are available for the dorsal and ventral trunks in several species and these are shown in Table I. In summary, about 80–90% of the fibres in the abdominal vagi are afferent and unmyelinated in non-ruminant animals and this has in general been confirmed by electrophysiological studies. Conduction velocity data from a number of gut regions and species are summarised in Table II. It is interesting that there is little relationship between the mass of abdominal visceral tissue innervated and the number of afferent (and also efferent) fibres. This may mean that the afferent fibres branch more profusely in the larger animals to give receptive fields of adequate size to cover the whole organ. Fibre counts are not yet available for the human abdominal vagus, but preliminary electromicroscopic and electrophysiological studies on isolated segments have shown that it is composed of predominantly unmyelinated fibres, with a few small-diameter myelinated fibres (Andrews and Taylor, 1982; MacKay and Andrews, 1983).

Myelinated fibres have been known to be present in the abdominal vagus from the earliest histological studies (Edgeworth, 1892) and, althought some contribution from sympathetic nerves cannot be excluded (see Lundberg et al., 1976; Liedberg et al., 1973), the majority are vagal. These small-diameter myelinated fibres are present in all species so far studied, and when supranodose vagotomy has been performed (cat, ferret) they appear to be almost all afferent (Table III). Whilst these fibres may represent axons which eventually lose their myelin as they approach their target (Iggo, 1958), they may form a specific sub-population of vagal fibres supplying a particular organ or subserving a specific afferent function. It is certainly of interest why these

TABLE I

Fibre number and composition of the abdominal vagi (dorsal and ventral combined) in a number of animals

Animal	Technique[a]	Fibre number (approx.)	% Afferent	Predominant type[b]	References
Cat	L.M.	31,000	90	UM	Agostoni et al. (1957)
	E.M.	40,000	90	UM	Mei et al. (1980)
Dog	L.M.	26,000	88	UM	Kemp (1973)
Ferret	E.M.	27,100	94	UM	Asala (1984)
Rabbit	L.M.	26,000	>90	UM	Evans and Murray (1954)
	E.M.	45,000	86	UM	Somerville and Bradley (1977)
Rat	L.M./E.M.	18,400	75–80	UM	Gabella and Pease (1973) Powley et al. (1983)
Sheep	L.M.	40,000	35	M	Dussardier (1960)

See references for details of fibre counting methods.
[a] L.M. = light microscopy; E.M. = electron microscopy.
[b] UM = unmyelinated; M = myelinated.

TABLE II

The conduction velocities of vagal afferents from receptors in a number of regions of the digestive tract

Organ	Receptor type	Conduction velocity (m/second)	Animal	References
Oesophagus	Muscle mechano-R	>C[a]	Rat	Clarke and Davison (1975)
		7.5–15	Ferret	Andrews and Lang (1982)
		9.3–27.7	Dog	Satchell (1984)
		2.7–12.8	Sheep	Falempin et al. (1978)
		5–18	Cat	Harding and Titchen (1975)
		1–14	Cat	Mei (1970)
		7.5	Cat	Iggo (1957a,b)
	Mucosal mechano/chemo-R	8–16	Cat	Harding and Titchen (1975)
	Thermo-R	0.7–1.5	Cat	El Ouazzani and Mei (1982)
LOS	Muscle mechano-R	0.8–1.2	Cat	Clerc and Mei (1983)
		1.0–1.3	Sheep	Falempin et al. (1978)
		2–12	Goat	Iggo (1955)
Stomach	Muscle mechano-R	1.0–1.7	Sheep	Falempin et al. (1978)
		5–23	Sheep	Leek (1969)
		<1	Rat	Clarke and Davison (1975)
		4.7	Cat	Mei (1970)
		~9	Cat	Paintal (1954)
		<1.3	Cat	Iggo (1957a,b)
		0.5–1.5	Ferret	Andrews et al. (1980c)
	Mucosal mechano/	0.9–6.0	Sheep	Harding and Leek (1972a,b)
	chemo/thermo-R	0.5–3.0	Rat	Clarke and Davison (1978)
		0.8–1.2	Cat	El Ouazzani and Mei (1981)
		1.0–5.0	Cat	Iggo (1957a,b)
		0.5–4.5	Cat	Davison (1972)
		0.7–1.5	Cat	El Ouazzani and Mei (1982)
Intestine	Muscle mechano-R	0.7 ± 0.26 (S.D.)	Sheep	Cottrell and Iggo (1984a)
		7.6 ± 1.6 (S.D.)		
		0.8–1	Cat	Mei (1970)
		<1.3	Cat	Iggo (1957a,b)
	Mucosal mechano/	0.73 ± 0.24 (S.D.)	Sheep	Cottrell and Iggo (1984c)
	chemo/thermo-R	3.3 ± 0.85 (S.D.)		
		0.5–3	Rat	Clarke and Davison (1978)
		>C	Cat	Paintal (1957)
		0.7–1.1	Cat	Garnier and Mei (1982)
		0.8–1.4	Cat	Jeanningros (1982)
		0.8–1.4	Cat	Mei (1978)
		0.5–4.5	Cat	Davison (1972)
		0.8–1.2	Cat	El Ouazzani and Mei (1981)
		0.8–1.4	Cat	El Ouazzani and Mei (1979)
	Serosal stretch	1.8 ± 0.5 (S.D.)	Sheep	Cottrell and Iggo (1984a)

[a] C = >2.5 m/second.

TABLE III

Myelinated fibres in the abdominal vagi from a number of animals

Animal	Myelinated fibres present	Diameter range (μm)	Number	References
Cat	√	2–6	200–400[a]	Agostoni et al. (1957)
Dog	√	<5	~ 200	Kemp (1973)
Ferret	√	1–6	160[b]	Asala (1984)
Guinea-pig	√	2–6	–	Diani et al. (1984)
Hedgehog	√	–	–	Toyota (1955)
Man	√	2–6	> 200	Andrews (unpublished data)
Rabbit	√	–	1000	Somerville and Bradley (1977)
Rat	√	1–14	150	Gabella and Pease (1973)

[a] Nearly all afferent.
[b] 95% afferent.

few fibres should retain their myelin at this level and also why they are rarely encountered in electrophysiological studies.

Pathways to the CNS

It is generally accepted that vagal afferents from the abdomen travel to the medulla via the thoracic and cervical vagi and have their cell bodies in the nodose ganglion. Whilst this is undoubtedly the major, if not the only pathway, I should like to draw the reader's attention to a paper published in 1935 which has largely been forgotten. In the early 1930s the distribution of vagal afferent fibres was mapped by studying the pupillary responses of the chloralose-anaesthetised cat to electrical stimulation of the central end of various branches of the abdominal vagus. Using this technique combined with selective nerve section, Harper et al. (1935) demonstrated that in addition to the "classical" pathway a second route was available for vagal afferents from the abdomen to the CNS. They suggested that the afferents left the thoracic vagal trunks and travelled with the intercostal nerves to enter the thoracic spinal cord via dorsal roots T2–T8. Their experiments did not allow them to determine whether the afferent synapsed in the spinal cord or projected centrally without synapsing. This pathway does not appear to have been investigated recently and is rarely considered in studies on the effects of vagotomy. Using modern electrophysiological and neuroanatomical tracing techniques the existence of this pathway could easily be studied. If the pathway does exist then it could have a number of implications for our understanding of visceral sensation, particularly in view of the degree of somato-visceral convergence which occurs in the thoracic spinal cord (see, e.g., Cervero, 1982a).

It can be seen that there are several basic neuroanatomical questions to be answered which have a direct bearing on the physiology of vagal afferent systems. The discussion below deals with the physiological characteristics of the vagal afferents found in each region of the gastrointestinal tract.

Properties of digestive tract vagal afferents

Any review of the properties of gastrointestinal afferents must take into account the differences in the gross anatomy of the alimentary tract between animals (e.g., see Oesophagus section) and regions of the tract and the wide variety of types of food and feeding habits employed, because the nature of the receptors may be influenced by such differences. The afferents from each organ will be described separately.

Oesophagus

In all animals the upper (cervical) portion of the oesophagus is composed of striated muscle. In its thoracic course it may be composed of predominantly either smooth or striated muscle, but the intra-abdominal portion is always smooth muscle (Christensen and De Carle, 1974). The cervical oesophagus is supplied by myelinated fibres in the superior laryngeal nerve whereas the thoracic and abdominal regions have a vagal innervation. See Christensen (1984) for review.

Muscle receptors

Recordings have been made from vagal afferents in animals with striated thoracic oesophagi (rat, Andrew, 1957; Clarke and Davison, 1975; ferret, Andrews and Lang, 1982; rabbit, Falempin and Rousseau, 1983; dog, Satchell, 1984; sheep, Falempin et al., 1978) and from the cat, which has a predominantly smooth muscle thoracic oesophagus (Mei, 1970; Harding and Titchen, 1975).

In the majority of studies the afferent fibres have a low level of spontaneous activity (e.g., 0.2–12 Hz in the dog, Satchell, 1984), usually modulated by respiration, and an increased discharge to moderate distension or muscle contractions evoked by vagal stimulation and distension. In response to a sustained inflation the discharge may reach a peak of 100 Hz and adapt slowly over the first 30 seconds, and more slowly thereafter. If the oesophagus is rapidly deflated units are often silent for several seconds before spontaneous activity returns. The muscle mechanoreceptors appear to be concentrated at the gastric and oral extremities of the thoracic oesophagus. Whilst the majority of afferent fibres supplying the abdominal viscera are unmyelinated, the thoracic oesophageal muscle appears to be supplied mainly by small-diameter myelinated fibres with conduction velocities up to 27 m/second (see Table II).

A quantitative study of oesophageal vagal afferents was undertaken by Satchell (1984) in the dog. The adapted discharge (23–44 Hz) of the afferents was linearly related to distension pressure over a relatively narrow range (up to 8 mmHg), above which it did not increase further. Using different rates of inflation Satchell (1984) obtained some evidence for a subdivision of the afferents. In response to sharp ramp inflations some units showed a pronounced burst of activity, and these fibres had a slightly faster conduction velocity than fibres having a more uniform response to inflation.

From the above studies it appears that oesophageal afferents with receptors in the muscle layers can signal the passage of a bolus by the distension it might produce or by the sequential contractions of the oesophagus which are used to propel it towards the stomach. However, care must be taken in interpreting the role of these afferents in view of observations by Falempin and Rousseau (1984) in the conscious sheep. Their studies showed that the afferents only discharged in response to a distension if the level of distension was sufficient to evoke a local contraction of the muscle and that it is the *response* to the bolus that is being monitored rather than the *presence* of the bolus. One of the problems with the latter study was that it was not possible to localise the receptors to the muscle layer, and Marie et al. (1984) have suggested that the receptors might be in the mucosal layer and during swallowing could respond to the movement of the bolus evoked by the contraction of the muscle.

It is possible that one role of the distension-sensitive afferents is to detect food which accumulates in the oesophagus if it is not completely cleared by the primary peristaltic wave. In animals with a smooth muscle oesophagus this distension should evoke a peristaltic wave to propel the bolus into the stomach. If the bolus cannot be moved, then the sustained distension and contractions evoked by its presence may give rise to pain (Payne and Poulton, 1927a,b).

Mucosal receptors

In response to balloon distension of the oesophagus rapidly-adapting receptors with high frequency (50–100 Hz) "on-off" discharges are observed (Mei, 1970; Harding and Titchen, 1975). The receptors are assumed to be in the mucosa and some units responded to HCl (50–100 mM), NaOH (50 mM), and hypertonic NaCl. The conduction velocity of these afferents was in the range for small-diameter myelinated fibres (Table II). These receptors would be ideally suited for detecting the presence of boli which produce very low levels of distension insufficient to activate the muscle receptors (e.g., saliva). Their mechanical and chemical sensitivity could allow the detection of refluxed gastric contents and reflexly exoke peristalsis to return them (Titchen and Wheeler, 1971). In addition to mucosal mechanoreceptors, recent studies in the cat by El Ouazzani and Mei (1982) have identified three types of slowly-adapting receptors responding to the temperature of the saline bathing the mucosa: (1) warm receptors discharged between 39 and 50°C, (2) cold receptors between 10 and 35°C, (3) mixed receptors responded to both temperature ranges. The response latency was 1–20 seconds. In the normal body temperature range the receptors were silent and they did not respond to stroking the musosa or superfusion with HCl or glucose. The discharge frequency (1–20 Hz) was in general related to the stimulus temperature; however, some units reached a maximum discharge before the extreme ends of the response range were reached.

Stomach

When considering gastric afferent activity we should bear in mind that whilst the stomach functions overall as one organ there is some separation of function: the gastric body serves as a reservoir in which the food is acted upon by acid and pepsin, whilst the antrum, which has little exocrine secretory capacity, does have powerful contractions which degrade large particles of food and propel the chyme into the duodenum. As in many other regions of the gut, there are receptors which monitor the luminal environment and activity of the muscle layers.

Mucosal stimulation

Three groups of stimuli have been used to investigate the properties of afferents in the gastric mucosa: mechanical, chemical and thermal.

Specific chemoreceptors

There appear to be only two examples of these, both described by El Ouazzani and Mei (1981) in the cat. One group responded to hydrochloric acid and the other to carbohydrates, particularly glucose. Some of the HCl-sensitive units also responded to acetic acid (cf. Cottrell and Iggo, 1984c). The response latencies were short (1–20 seconds) and comparable with latencies in other studies (e.g., Leek, 1977; Mei, 1978). The frequency of the discharge evoked by acid (2–14 Hz) was in general lower than that in the afferents which responded to glucose (2–30 Hz), but for both receptor types the discharge was very slowly adapting and usually outlasted application of the stimulus. Neither group was spontaneously active.

Specific thermoreceptors

Receptors sensitive only to the temperature of the fluid bathing the mucosa were reported by El Ouazzani and Mei (1979) in the cat. These receptors have characteristics identical to those found in the oesophageal mucosa (El Ouazzani and Mei, 1982) and duodenal mucosa (El Ouazzani and Mei, 1979). In a similar study Gupta et al. (1979) were unable to demonstrate "cold"-sensitive (12°C) vagal afferents in the stomach and duodenum, although they were present in the greater splanchnic nerves.

"Polymodal" receptors

In the sheep (Leek, 1972a; Harding and Leek, 1972a,b), rat (Clarke and Davison, 1978), and cat (Iggo, 1957b; Davison, 1972) rapidly adapting receptors responding to stroking of the gastric mucosa or epithelium were observed. Although there are a few reports of such fibres being insensitive to chemicals, the vast majority have a degree of chemosensitivity. At present, it is only possible to generalise about the properties of the receptors as in most studies only a few substances have been applied to *all* units at a range of concentrations and to the functionally different regions of the stomach. In non-ruminant animals the gastric antrum has been most studied whilst in the sheep all areas have been studied (Harding and Leek, 1972a,b).

Studies in the rat and sheep show a degree of agreement in that afferents responding to both acids (organic and inorganic) and alkalis (NaOH), hypertonic sodium chloride and water have been reported. In each case the response was relatively slowly adapting. Both studies concluded that the response to acids was not related to their pH value per se but rather their titratable acidity (cf. titratable alkalinity for the duodenal receptors, Cottrell and Iggo, 1984c) and molecular weight. In contrast, the receptors in the cat were sensitive to gentle stroking of the mucosa and either acid (HCl) or alkali (NaOH) but not hypertonic NaCl or water. They therefore appear to be very different from those in the sheep and rat across the spectrum of their properties. Clearly, more studies are required, particularly in carnviores, to elucidate whether these are species differences, presumably reflecting the differences in food composition, or whether they represent a technical artifact, as suggested by Leek (1977). In the ferret (carnivore) hypertonic sodium chloride applied to the gastric mucosa can evoke reflex changes in gastric motility and vomiting via vagal pathways (Andrews and Wood, 1984; P. L. R. Andrews and C. J. Davis, unpublished observations). The ferret therefore appears to have vagal afferents responding to hypertonic solutions, although confirmation awaits electrophysiological studies.

There are several problems which make the characteristation of mucosal afferent receptors particularly difficult: first, the mucosa must be maintained in a physiological condition after the stomach has been opened to permit topical application of chemicals. Second, a protective role has been ascribed to mucus covering the mucosa. The extent to which this acts as a mechanical and/or chemical barrier between the mucosa and the gastric contents is still a matter of controversy, and until this is resolved it is impossible to determine the natural environment of the receptors. Third, measurements are required to characterise the gastric environment so that the receptors can be studied using stimuli in the physiological range. This type of study would be particularly useful in determining whether the gastric environment ever becomes sufficiently alkaline to activate the alkali-sensitive receptors.

All the studies report that the mucosal receptors are not spontanously active even when gastric motility is present and that they only discharge when exogenous chemicals are applied. If there really are receptors sensitive to 50–100 mM HCl they should discharge when the stomach is stimulated to secrete as the acid is present under the mucus layer and hence closer to the receptors, and presumably in a higher concentration than when exogenously applied. The results from such a study might allow more justifiable conclusions to be drawn about the role of these receptors in the regulation of acid secretion. Other experiments that might help to elucidate their role are to examine the reflex effects caused by the application of chemicals known to activate thse afferents, and such studies have provided preliminary evidence for a role of the mucosal receptors in the regulation of gastric motility (Andrews and Wood, 1984).

Muscle stimulation

In response to distension and contraction of the stomach vagal afferents with receptors in the gastric muscle increase their discharge, and the response is usually very slowly adapting. It is now generally assumed that the receptors described above behave as if they are "in series" with the smooth muscle fibres, but this awaits histological confirmation. Many of the discrepancies between reports in the earlier literature appear to have resulted from the lack of spontaneous gastric activity and failure to evoke contractions in the cat stomach (Iggo, 1957a; Paintal, 1954). Whilst some of the discrepancies have been resolved, one interesting difference remains regarding conduction velocities. In Iggo's (1957a) experiments and those of subsequent workers using non-ruminants the muscle afferents have all had conduction velocities in the C-fibre range, but Paintal's (1954) "stretch afferents" have an estimated conduction velocity of 9 m/second, which would indicate small-diameter myelinated fibres such as are known to be present in the abdominal vagus. Therefore, it is still possible that Paintal's "stretch afferents" are a separate sub-group of muscle afferents.

In contrast to the study of gastrointestinal mucosal receptors, it has been rather easier to design physiological stimuli to study the muscle receptors. One way is to measure the volume of fluid ingested by an animal/unit time and mimic this rate and volume whilst recording afferent activity. This approach has revealed that whilst the receptors in the muscle are "in series" tension receptors, their discharge characteristics reflect the properties of the muscle in the different regions of the stomach and their response to gastric inflation. The stomach is able to accommodate relatively large volumes of fluid with only a small change in mean pressure (Andrews et al., 1980c). Approximately 80% of fluid resides in the fundus and corpus regions, provided the volume is within the physiological range. There are two main reasons for this. Firstly, the gastric body is more distensible than the antrum (Andrews et al., 1980b) and, secondly, as the stomach fills, the vagal non-adrenergic non-cholinergic inhibitory fibres supplying the gastric corpus are activated to cause relaxation (Andrews and Lawes, 1982, 1984, 1985). In contrast to the low level of rhythmic contractile activity in the gastric body, the antrum usually has a relatively high degree of spontaneous activity, which is enhanced by activation of a corpo-antral, vago-vagal reflex during gastric filling (Andrews et al., 1980a).

These differences in the behaviour of the two gastric regions to distension are reflected in the afferent discharges from receptors located in each area of the ferret stomach (Andrew et al., 1980b). Both groups of receptor are classified as "in series" tension receptors as they respond to gastric distension and spontaneous and evoked gastric contractions even in the empty stomach. However, when their response to physiological rates and volumes of distension is examined, they appear to signal two different types of information to the CNS. The receptors located in the gastric corpus have an irregular but continuous discharge (0.37–7.7 Hz) which presumably reflects the high degree of tension in the wall of the empty stomach. On inflation with saline the majority of units had a discharge (11–23 Hz) related to the gastric volume (50 ml) and intragastric pressure (6.0 cm H_2O). Once the inflation stopped the units showed a continuous very slowly adapting discharge that was only slightly modulated by gastric contractions. In contrast, units located in the antrum spontaneously discharged when contractions were present, and as the stomach was inflated the contractions were enhanced and the afferent units had a markedly enhanced discharge (up to 30 Hz) in phase with the antral contractions. Thus, whilst the receptors in both locations have the same general properties, their location determines their precise behaviour: afferents with receptors located in the antrum primarily signal the occurrence and magnitude of rhythmic contractions whilst those in the corpus and fundus indicate the overall level of distention of the stomach and could be involved in signalling pre-absorptive satiety. Whilst the afferents in the antrum can respond to distension of the antrum, this area is not usually subjected to gross sustained distension under physiological conditions.

In attempting to elucidate the properties of the gastric tension receptors, not only is the distension volume important but also the rate. Clearly, distensions of 150 ml in less than a second are unphysiological for a cat (Paintal, 1954), and whilst such stimuli are effective in activating the muscle afferents they are not very useful for understanding the afferent response to a meal. However, they may be useful for indicating which receptors *can* be activated by unphysiological stimuli, e.g., the mucosal and serosal mechanoreceptors. In the ferret the pressure at the peak of a "step" inflation is twice that for a physiological "ramp" inflation of the same volume (Andrews et al., 1980c), but after 2 minutes the plateau pressures are the same. Thus, after a "step" inflation intragastric pressure decreases rapidly to plateau whereas after a "ramp" inflation there is only a small decline in pressure. These changes (probably indicating decreases in wall tension) are reflected in the behaviour of the gastric tension receptors (Andrews et al., 1980b; see also Iggo, 1957a), particularly those in the antrum, where a physiologically evoked phasic discharge is replaced by an unphysiological continuous unmodulated discharge. Not only are step inflations unphysiological but their repeated use in one animal may lead to confusion over adaptation rates, as Andrews and Lawes (1982) have demonstrated that the $1/e$ decay time for peak to plateau pressures in the ferret stomach after a step inflation depended upon the number of inflations, the first inflation in a series having a longer adaptation time than the second; therefore, afferent activity may appear to adapt slowly or more rapidly depending upon the number of previous inflations.

Serosal stimulation

Iggo (1957a) describes a single receptor located in either the serosa or omentum in the region of the greater curve in the cat stomach. This receptor was activated by gastric distension, stretch and digital compression but not by gastric contractions. Further studies are required to determine whether this represents an as yet rarely identified group of afferents.

Intestine

Vagal afferents supply all parts of the small intestine and the proximal two-thirds of the colon (in the cat, Mei, 1970), paralleling the extent of the vagal efferent innervation. The most extentively studied parts of the intestine are the duodenum and jejunum.

Mucosal stimulation

Four types of receptor activity have been identified in the upper small intestine. The results are from a variety of species (rat, cat, sheep) and this must be borne in mind when interpreting the differences.

Specific mechanoreceptors

Receptors which respond only to stroking of the intestinal mucosa appear to be relatively rare (cf. stomach). In their recent extensive study in the sheep duodenum, Cottrell and Iggo (1984c) only found 20% of 61 units which did not respond to some chemical stimulus in addition to mechanical probing. This study provided some evidence for two populations of mucosal mechanoreceptors: "low threshold" requiring 132 mg weight for activation and receptive field area 1–5 mm^2 and spontaneously silent, "high threshold" activated by 750 mg, receptive field area 1 mm^2 and spontaneously active. The response of both types of unit was "slowly adapting", but the latter group had a characteristic sustained after discharge, suggesting that stroking initiated some local contraction of the muscularis mucosa or adjoining tissue which further activated the receptors (cf. rat, Clarke and Davison, 1978; cat, Paintal, 1957).

Paintal (1957) described vagal afferents which appear to act as mechanoreceptors, but instead of detecting material brushing against the mucosa they monitor contractions of the muscularis mucosa reflexly evoked by the presence of stimuli in the lumen. These receptors have a weak response to mucosal stroking and distension but are activated by strong compression and 30% NaCl in the lumen but not by other chemicals (e.g., sucrose, $MgSO_4$). The spontaneous and evoked activity of these afferents was rhythmical.

Specific chemoreceptors

These are mucosal receptors which respond to only one group of substances (carbohydrates or amino acids) and not to mechanical, osmotic or thermal stimuli. The two best characterised types are (i) Glucoreceptors: in the cat Mei (1978) described a group of vagal afferents which responded in a frequency-related manner to the luminal glucose concentration. Whilst the receptors have been called glucoreceptors, some respond to carbohydrates other than glucose (e.g., D-levulose, D-galatose, lactose, maltose), but glucose was the most potent. The discharge was prolonged and very slowly adapting and the latency of the response was 0.2–15 seconds. The receptors appeared to be more concentrated in the duodenum and proximal jejunum than more distal regions in the gut. (ii) Amino acid receptors: receptors responding only to amino acids in the lumen of the small intestine have been reported by Jeanningros (1982) in the cat. These afferents were not spontaneously active but responded either to a single amino acid or, more usually, to several amino acids (e.g., Arg, Leu). The latency of the response was 9 ± 0.7 seconds and the discharge prolonged and slowly adapting (cf. glucoreceptors). A single unit could respond to amino acids from each of the three groups (neutral, acidic, basic) of amino acids. Five of 36 amino acid units also responded to glucose, but none responded to osmotic or mechanical stimulation.

For both the amino acid and glucoreceptor afferents it is assumed that the substances must be transported by the enterocyte before they are detected (see Mei, 1978); however, direct proof is lacking. It would be interesting to know whether the response to glucose is abolished by pre-treatment with phlorizin or if the response is stereospecific, as are the transport mechanisms.

Specific thermoreceptors

In the cat duodenum El Ouazzani and Mei (1979) have identified vagal afferent which were silent until tonically activated by lumimal perfusion with warm (38–51°C) or cold (36–10°C) solutions. The receptors were insensitive to mechanical or chemical stimuli.

"Polymodal" receptors

These respond to mechanical stimulation of the mucosa and to one or more chemical stimuli. From the data available this type of receptor appears to be the most common, but it is difficult to classify these receptors because the same ranges of stimuli have not been used. For convenience discussion will be divided based on the animals used.

Cat and rat. Duodenal units have a rapidly-adapting response to mucosal stroking and slowly adapting response to acid (Davison, 1972; Clarke and Davison, 1978). Units in the rat also responded to water, and in the cat those not responding to acid, responded to alkalis (not tested in the rat). Garnier and Mei (1982) described vagal units in the cat small intestine which responded to mucosal stroking, strong distension, perfusion with HCl (pH 2), warm saline (48°C), hyper- and hypotonic solutions (NaCl, glucose, mannitol). These are considered to be polymodal receptors. It is of interest that they exhibit features of a number of the more "specific" receptors described by other workers, and one wonders whether some of the "specific" receptors might have been revealed as polymodal if a wider range of substances had been studied.

Sheep. 80% of the units which responded to mechanical stimulation of the duodenal mucosa also responded to a variety of chemicals, including sodium hydroxide (Cottrell and Iggo, 1984c). It was suggested that the receptors were responding to the titratable alkalinity rather than to the pH. Units were classified as sensitive to either potassium chloride or fatty acids (response related to titratable acidity). Other substances effective in activating some of these afferents were hydrochloric acid, sodium bicarbonate and papaverine, but none of the units exhibited specific thermo-, gluco- or osmosensitivity. The responses were considered to be slowly adapting. The authors discussed the possibility that some of these responses were secondary to contractions of the muscularis interna or externa, and this should always be borne in mind when interpreting the responses to mucosal applications of chemicals.

Muscle stimulation

Whilst there are discrepancies over exactly what the

mucosal receptors respond to (possibly because of the different species used and the different lengths to which various authors have gone to show that their particular receptors are specific), there is general agreement (so far) over the characteristics of the receptors in the muscle.

The vagal afferents have a relatively slowly adapting discharge which is evoked by distension of the intestine within the physiological range or by contraction of the muscle occurring spontaneously or evoked by electrical stimulation and drugs (Iggo, 1955, 1957b; Mei, 1970; Cottrell and Iggo, 1984a,b), and they also respond to compression of the muscle. The receptors therefore fulfil the criteria of being "in series" with the muscular elements, and in the sheep they appear to be located in the longitudinal muscle layer of the duodenum (Cottrell and Iggo, 1984a). In this study it was also demonstrated that chemicals applied to the mucosa (e.g., HCl, KCl, acetic acid, NaOH) evoked activity in the muscle tension receptors after a latency of 5–20 seconds and lasting up to 10 minutes. This was interpreted as a local reflex activation of the muscle by mucosal chemoreceptors. It was also demonstrated that tension receptor discharge could be reduced by simultaneous stroking of the mucosa, presumably via a local inhibitory reflex.

In addition to these receptors in the muscle, two other types of receptor were identified: one group located in the serosa responded to serosal probing, or stretching and distension of the duodenum with a balloon. Activity was only weakly stimulated by evoked duodenal contractions; the second group was located in the lesser omentum. These two groups of receptors have similar characteristics to splanchnic receptors described by Floyd and Morrison (1974) and Morrison (1977).

Whilst recording from a site close to the organ of interest, as in Cottrell and Iggo's studies, increases the chances of recording activity originating there, it does have the disadvantage that in the abdomen vagal and splanchnic nerves may travel together in their terminal portions, and therefore some care must be taken when considering the functional implications.

Colon

Although part of the colon is supplied by the vagus nerve there appears to be only one report of colonic vagal afferent activity. Mei (1970) described afferents responding to both distension and contraction of the colon in the cat. It is not known whether the colon has vagal mucosal mechano/chemoreceptors, although it would seem likely.

Pancreas

A vagal afferent supply to the pancreas has long been suspected, but its presence has only recently been confirmed. Sharkey and Williams (1983) using True Blue injections in the rat pancreas demonstrated the presence of labelled cells in the nodose ganglia. Interestingly, the left nodose ganglion preferentially supplies the duodenal lobe and the right the splenic lobe. The intra-pancreatic sites of termination of these vagal fibres are unknown. However, a preliminary electrophysiological study by Niijima (1981) showed that pancreatic vagal afferents responded to glucose, 2-deoxglucose, insulin, cholecystokinin and 5-hydroxytryptamine. These observations suggest that such afferents may be involved in vagal reflexes regulating the endocrine portion of the pancreas. It would be interesting to know whether there are any nerve endings in the ducts which could monitor the composition of the pancreatic juice, and hence be involved in reflexes regulating exocrine secretion.

Liver and biliary tree

The receptors described in the previous sections have all to some extent been involved in monitoring the state of digestion of the food in the gut lumen. Nutrients absorbed from the intestine are transported via the hepatic portal vein to the liver, and receptors located here would be in an ideal position to monitor the absorbed nutrient load and evoke appropriate reflexes (e.g., the hepato-pancreatic reflex, Sakaguchi and Yamaguchi, 1979). Electrophysiological studies in the guinea pig and rat have demonstrated three main types of vagal hepatic afferent. Their properties are described below, but some care must be taken in interpreting the results as the majority of recordings are from multi-fibre preparations.

Glucose-sensitive afferents

In the guinea-pig these afferents are spontaneously active at portal glucose levels of 120 mg/100 ml, and as the glucose level increased the afferent discharge decreased (Niijima, 1969b, 1980, 1982, 1983). The afferents are specific for D-glucose and do not respond to other hexoses (e.g., L-glucose, D-mannose), in contrast to the hepatic osmoreceptors. The fibres appear to have a relatively sustained discharge as long as the glucose level is constant. The decrease in discharge in response to glucose distinguishes these receptors from the "glucoreceptors" in the intestine (see above). In the rabbit Andrews and Orbach (1974, 1975) reported hepatic afferents (of unspecified orgin) that were spontaneously active but failed to respond to glucose in the range 0.2–5% but increased their discharge with 20% glucose. These results are very different from those of Niijima (1982) and indicate the need for further studies under similar experimental conditions in the guinea-pig and rabbit.

Whilst the above studies indicate that glucose is the major metabolite monitored, the work of Orbach and Andrews (1973) demonstrated afferents responding to the sodium salts of long-chain fatty acids, and this raises the possibility that a range of metabolites may be monitored at this site.

Osmoreceptors

For an afferent to be considered a true osmoreceptor it should have a discharge rate proportional to the osmolarity of the stimulus, irrespective of its nature (Mei, 1983). This criterion has been fulfilled for receptors described by Adachi et al. (1976) and Niijima (1969a), who demonstrated an increase in discharge rate in response to increasing osmotic loads of sodium chloride, glucose, and sucrose. In addition, Adachi (1984) reports that some afferents decreased their discharge as the osmotic pressure of a sodium chloride solution was increased from 220 to 340 mOsm/l, a response reminiscent of the glucose-sensitive afferents described above. In contrast to the above study, Andrews and Orbach (1974) concluded from their work in the rabbit that the hepatic afferents (of unknown origin) only responded to [Na^+], and therefore were not true osmoreceptors and should be considered to be sodium sensors. Whether this represents a species or technical difference awaits further studies.

Thermoreceptors

Adachi and Niijima (1982) demonstrated vagal afferents which increased their discharge in response to an increased temperature (35–39°C) of the Ringer's solution perfusing an isolated guinea-pig liver. These afferents have a low level of spontaneous activity at body temperature, and on warming the liver Q_{10} values between 4 and 16 were measured. The fibres did not respond to mechanical or osmotic stimuli. It is suggested that these thermoreceptors may be involved in the regulation of food intake by monitoring diet-induced thermogenesis (Adachi, 1984).

Although electrophysiological studies of hepatic vagal afferents are still at a relatively early stage, there is sufficient evidence that the liver is capable of monitoring a number of dietary components in the blood reaching it from the intestine. It is worth remembering that the existence and some properties of the hepatic afferents were predicted from behavioural studies of animals with denervated livers (see Sawchenko and Friedman, 1979). In studying visceral afferents the identification of behavioural deficits can provide a useful tool in establishing the physiological role of electrophysiologically identified afferents.

Biliary system

Vagal afferents responding to both contraction and

distension of the gall bladder have been reported (Crousillat and Ranieri, 1980), but such recordings are rare. More systematic studies of these afferents are required to investigate whether they can be divided into "high" and "low" threshold groups, like the biliary splanchnic afferents (Cervero, 1982b). Such a study might shed some light on whether vagal afferents could be involved in visceral nociception, a role suggested for the "high-threshold" splanchnic afferents.

Sphincters

Sphincters are located at several sites along the gastrointestinal tract and serve to regulate the flow of digesta from one gut region to another. Until relatively recently there had been few recordings from sphincter afferents, which is in some ways surprising as these might be expected to be key sites at which the progress of digestion could be monitored by signalling the progress of the food/chyme/faeces along the gut. Only two of the gut sphincters, the lower oesophageal and pyloric sphincters, have been studied and in general they have similar characteristics, but until recordings are made from afferents supplying the sphincter of Oddi, the ileocaecal and ileo-colic sphincters, it is not possible to state whether all sphincters have receptors with similar characteristics. The lower oesophageal sphincter has been most extensively studied and a discussion of its properties will serve as a guide to the expected characteristics of sphincter afferents.

Lower oesophageal sphincter (LOS)

Under resting conditions the LOS is held in a tonically constricted (but not completely closed) state and relaxes to allow the passage of a food bolus. Three types of receptor have been identified in the region of the LOS and the descriptions below are from the work of Clerc and Mei (1983) in the cat, Falempin et al. (1978) in the sheep and El Ouazzani and Mei (1982) in the cat.

Muscle mechanoreceptors

The majority of these receptors have a relatively high level of spontaneous discharge (40 Hz, sheep; 1–25 Hz, cat) which increased during distension (20–80 Hz, sheep). These receptors were also stimulated by contraction of the sphincter evoked by vagal stimulation. Discharges of 80–100 Hz were observed in the sheep, and in the cat they increased from 2.6 ± 1.1 to 10.1 ± 2.9 Hz ($n = 12$). In the cat, Clerc and Mei (1983) report that some of the afferents with high resting discharges decreased their discharge in response to LOS distension. All the receptors had discharges which were slowly adapting. When reflex relaxation of the sphincter was evoked by distension of more rostral regions of the oesophagus the resting discharge decreased.

Mucosal mechanoreceptors

These receptors rarely had a spontaneous discharge and did not directly respond to moderate distension or contraction of the sphincter. They were activated by "strong and rapid" balloon distension, "strong digital compression", stroking the mucosa, or "strong and rapid" saline injections. The discharge was usually a rapidly adapting burst of activity of less than 20 Hz. One of four receptors tested was sensitive to HCl (pH 2), but none to glucose (100 g/l). Units with similar responses to stroking the LOS mucosa were also reported by Davison (1972) in the cat.

Serosal mechanoreceptors

These appear to be the least frequently encountered type of receptor; of 62 mechanoreceptors only two were in the serosal layer. They were silent unless activated by stretching or stroking the serous membrane and were insensitive to contraction of the LOS or superfusion of the mucosa. Their discharge was rapidly adapting.

From their extensive study Clerc and Mei (1983) suggest the following functions for these receptors. The muscular mechanoreceptors serve to monitor the level of tone in the LOS, and hence play a role in its reflex control. The mucosal receptors may also be involved in this, but in addition they can monitor the consistency of food passing through the sphincter. All three types of mechanoreceptors are likely to be transiently stimulated by gastric contents entering the oesophagus during vomiting, and hence may play a role in its coordination.

Central projections of abdominal vagal afferents

For afferent impulses from the viscera to produce a sensation they must project to areas of the CNS involved in processing sensory information, and while the pathways for somatic afferents are relatively well known (e.g., Angel, 1977) those for visceral afferents, particularly abdominal vagal afferents, are not. The discussion below describes the results from some of the few studies which have examined abdominal vagal afferent influences on the CNS. For reviews of cervical vagal projections the reader is referred to Sawchenko (1983), Leslie et al. (1982) and Odekunle and Bower (1984).

Hindbrain

Vagal afferents from the gastrointestinal tract terminate in the nucleus tractus solitarus (NTS), including the area subpostrema (Leslie et al., 1982; Gwyn and Leslie, 1979). Interestingly, whilst Kalia and Mesulam (1980) demonstrated an abdominal vagal projection to the area postrema (AP) in the cat, no such projection was found in the rat (Leslie et al., 1982), and the lack of this pathway may contribute to the absence of the emetic reflex in the rat. These studies should be complemented by neurophysiological studies to determine whether there are viscerotopic projections from the gut into specific regions of NTS or whether functionally different afferents (e.g., mucosal and muscle) have discrete projections. Afferent activity has been recorded from the region of the NTS in the sheep (Harding and Leek, 1973) and rat (Barber and Burks, 1983) in response to gastric distension and hepatic afferent stimulation (Adachi, 1981).

Anatomical and neurophysiological evidence for an abdominal vagal input to the reticular formation is lacking; however, such information must reach parts of the reticular formation (probably the parvicellular region) as this area has been implicated in coordinating the act of vomiting evoked by activation of the AP and abdominal vagal afferents (see Brizzee and Mehler, 1986, for review).

Cerebellum

An input to the cerebellum from abdominal vagal afferents has not been directly tested, but Hennemann and Rubia (1978) have shown that vagal fibres in the cervical region with conduction velocities in the range 4–20 m/second project to a bilateral sagittal strip of lobe V and VI in the cat cerebellum. Some of these fibres may have originated from the gastrointestinal tract.

Midbrain

The NTS sends a large projection to the parabrachial nucleus, which itself gives rise to widespread projections, including the ventrobasal complex of the thalamus (Sawchenko, 1983). Although an abdominal vagal influence on cells in the parabachial nucleus has not been reported, such an input would be expected in the light of the large abdominal vagal input to NTS.

Forebrain

Of the forebrain regions the hypothalamus has been most studied, probably because of the evidence that it acts as a coordinating area for the autonomic nervous system. One of the earliest reports was by Anand and Pillai (1967), who demonstrated that gastric distension increased the discharge of neurones in the ventromedial nucleus (VMH, "satiety centre") and inhibited those in the lateral area (LHA, "feeding centre"). Whilst the change in firing was related to the degree of distension, only two levels were employed (15 and 30 mmHg). Electrical stimulation of gastric afferents had similar effects on hypothalamic activity. No attempt was made to determine the threshold level of distension required to activate these areas or whether other gut regions could influence their discharge.

Extensive studies in the rat by Barone et al. (1979) showed that units in the lateral preoptic, lateral hypothalamic-median forebrain bundle neuropil were markedly influenced by gastric inflation at a physiological rate and volume. In food-deprived animals neurones in this area were less sensitive to gastric distension than were animals fed ad libitum. Similar studies by Maddison and Horrell (rat, 1979) and Jeanningros (rat, cat, 1984) examined the influences of gastric and intestinal inflation and perfusion with nutrients on LHA cells. Gastric inflation increased or decreased the discharge in LHA cells (cf. Anand and Pillai, 1967) and similar responses were reported to duodenal inflation by Jeanningros (1984), but Maddison and Horrell (1979) found that this stimulus always decreased LHA discharge and increased that in the VMH. The studies also differ in the LHA responses to nutrient loads in the duodenum: Maddison and Horrell (1979) found no evidence for a visceral chemosensitive input to the LHA whereas Jeanningros (1984) found a high percentage (37%) of LHA units responded specifically to intestinal perfusion with an amino acid mixture (5% casein hydrolysate). Units in the LHA are also inhibited by the hepatic glucoreceptive afferents (see p. 76) (see Oomura and Yoshimatsu, 1984, for summary).

There seems little doubt that areas of the hypothalamus do receive information from the gut via vagal afferents, concerning the chemical nature of its contents, the degree of distension and absorbed glucose levels. This information presumably is used for such functions as the regulation of food intake and the control of autonomic outflow to the gut. It is not known whether some of this information projects to "higher centres", but vagal influences on other forebrain structures are discussed below.

Other forebrain regions

Whilst the pathways by which gastrointestinal afferent information may reach thalamic and cortical areas of the nervous system are relatively well described (see Sawchenko, 1983), direct neurophysiological evidence of such projections is lacking. Several workers have stimulated the cervical vagus and demonstrated evoked activity in the medial dorsal nucleus of the thalamus (e.g., Dell and Olsen, 1951; Hallowitz and MacLean, 1977), the orbital gyrus (Dell and Olsen, 1951) and cingulate cortex (Bachman et al., 1977). However, very few studies have attempted to study abdominal vagal inputs to these and other areas either to electrical or physiological stimuli. A study of the marsupial phalanger (Dunlop, 1958) showed that electrical or chemical stimulation of the gastric mucosa evoked slow wave activity in the hippocampus but not in the amygdala. It was assumed that the pathway was via vagal afferents. A projection of unmyelinated abdominal vagal afferents to the somatosensory cortex in the cat was demonstrated by Mei and Aubert (1972), but the type of information signalled was not determined.

From the above discussion it is clear that there is some evidence that vagal afferent information can access areas of the CNS which are involved either directly or indirectly in the conscious perception of sensory information. However, considerably more work is required before abdominal vagal afferent projections can be charted with the same degree of certainty as somatic afferents.

Abdominal vagal afferents and sensation

The extensive vagal afferent innervation of the gastrointestinal tract which monitors the nature and state of digestion of the luminal contents and activity of the muscle has been discussed in this chapter. Some evidence suggests that this information (or a subset) reaches CNS structures implicated in sensory processing. Whilst animal studies can demonstrate central projections it is only by well-controlled studies in conscious man that we can investigate whether vagal afferent activation evokes any sensations. Sensations associated with the gut are usually ill defined and poorly localised, and hence difficult to characterize and quantify. Furthermore, considerable variation in the degree of perception of visceral events exists between individuals. Thus, whilst retrospective studies of sensory deficits in patients with truncal vagotomies are of some use, patients should really be tested pre- and post-operatively with well-defined stimuli. Truncal vagotomy is an increasingly rare operation and, as it is usually combined with other procedures such as pyloroplasty, which modifies gut function, observations are difficult to interpret. In fact, vagotomy often leads to the development of a characteristic group of symptoms, including abdominal pain, nausea and bloating, which arise as a result of impaired gastric function and are presumably signalled via splanchnic afferents. Whilst such observations indicate that activation of splanchnic afferents in the disordered tract produces sensations, they do not preclude a role for vagal afferents in the genesis of sensations in the healthy gut. In contrast to vagotomy, spinal cord transection impairs gut function only slightly (Mathias and Frankel, 1983). Examination of patients with this lesion may show that abdominal vagal afferent stimulation can evoke sensations. Unfortunately, such studies have not been reported, and in their absence comments on the role of the abdominal vagus in visceral sensation are somewhat speculative. However, we can examine whether the afferents described above have properties which coincide with some of the characteristics of visceral sensation.

Gastrointestinal tract sensations

Lack of space does not permit a discussion of all the sensations associated with the gut, and therefore only some of the upper tract sensations will be described. The reader is referred to Beaumont (1833), Hertz (1911), Cannon and Washburn (1912), Payne and Poulton (1927a,b), Jones (1938), Lewis (1942) and Wolf (1965) for details of experiments on visceral sensation in man on which the discussion below is based.

Temperature

In his subject "Tom", Wolf (1965) reported that the gastric mucosa was temperature sensitive, and stimuli >40°C and <18°C were appreciated as hot or cold, respectively. The detection threshold was a change of 3°C and the latency 3–7 seconds. Several other studies have shown that the lower oesophagus is much more temperature sensitive than the stomach. The similarities between these subjective responses and the characteristics of the gut thermoreceptors described by El Ouazzani and Mei (1982) are striking and such afferents would be strong contenders for producing the above thermal sensations. Activation of the thermoreceptors can modify oesophageal and gastric motility (ibid), and hence there may be a contribution to the sensation from secondary activation of mechanoreceptors.

Touch and pressure

Light touch sensation is absent from the oesophageal and gastric mucosa, indicating that a stimulus which activates many of the mucosal receptors does not give rise to a sensation. Firm probing or squeezing of the mucosa produced a sensation of pressure comparable to that of skin stimulation. Such stimuli could evoke activity in mechanosensitive vagal afferents in all three gut layers, but Wolf (1965) demonstrated that these sensations could arise from a collar of mucosa devoid of muscle and peritoneal layers, and therefore receptors in the mucosa appear to be implicated. Mucosal mechanoreceptors with splanchnic afferents have not so far been reported from these regions, and if this is the case then sensations arising from mucosal stimulation alone should by default be ascribed to vagal afferent activation. Although the mucosal afferents appear to have a major role, some involvement of receptors in other layers cannot be excluded, as gentle stroking of the gastric mucosa modifies gastric motility (Andrews and Wood, 1984).

Emptiness and fullness

Of all the sensations associated with gut these

have probably received the most attention from a variety of fields and they are also probably the ones most often experienced. Rather than regarding them as two completely separate sensations they can be considered as part of a spectrum of information which an animal uses to regulate its feeding behaviour. Both sensations appear to derive from information from two sources: a peripheral input which indicates whether the upper gastrointestinal tract (particularly the stomach) contains food (but see below), and a central component which monitors the circulating level of absorbed nutrients, particularly glucose and amino acids. Only the peripheral inputs are relevant to this review and some of the possible mechanisms are described below.

The sensation of gastric emptiness arises some time after the stomach is empty and is an intermittent dull ache, gnawing sensation or tight feeling in the lower mid-chest or epigastrum. It is associated with gastric activity and is alleviated by food and non-food items in the stomach, e.g., in times of food shortage Indians on the banks of the Orinoco are reported to eat a pound of earth/day to stave off hunger (Cannon and Washburn, 1912). Non-food items, whilst they decrease the feeling of emptiness, obviously have little effect in the long term, as the blood glucose level does not change. This is analogous to thirst whereby wetting the buccal mucosa temporarily alleviates the sensation, but it only passes permanently when the body fluid composition is restored (Rolls and Rolls, 1982). To summarise, the empty stomach has a high level of muscle tone, particularly in the corpus region, and also if the animal is hypoglycaemic this is detected by hypothalamic glucoreceptors (Bulato and Carlson, 1924) which activate vagal efferents to enhance gastric motility markedly (the "hunger" contractions of Cannon and Washburn, 1912). This high level of motility can be detected by the "in series" tension receptors, particularly in the antrum. Andrews et al. (1980b) noted that the vagal tension receptors in the corpus region of the stomach in a starved animal had a relatively high level of tonic discharge, and this could contribute to the sensation of emptiness. Mucosal receptors may also play a role, as in the empty stomach the mocosal folds can rub against each other during contractions and activate the mucosal mechanoreceptors. It has often been reported that emptiness may be transiently alleviated by swallowing only a few mouthfuls of water insufficient to produce a significant distension. The most likely explanation is that swallowing evokes a vago-vagal reflex relaxation of the stomach via the vagal inhibitory fibres (Andrews and Lawes, 1985). This relaxation, which lasts several minutes, reduces the tension in the gastric wall (particularly the corpus), and hence decreases the drive to the "in series" tension receptors. The mucosal receptors may also contribute as stimulation of the mucosa can also produce relaxation of the underlying muscle (e.g., Cottrell and Iggo, 1984c).

Clinical studies on vagotomised humans have shown that the sensation of hunger is reduced but not abolished by this procedure. One interesting effect of abdominal vagotomy is that it modifies the perception of sweet and bitter solution (Kral, 1983).

The changes in gastric afferent discharge on inflating an empty stomach have been described (see p. 71) and the different patterns of firing presumably contribute to the sensation of fullness, and hence satiety. Because gastric distension by non-food items (e.g., a balloon) can produce a sensation of fullness, attention has focused on the gastric tension receptors and, although these certainly have a major role, a contribution from mucosal receptors in the stomach and duodenum (e.g., glucoreceptors) identifying the luminal contents as food cannot be excluded. Also, tension receptors in the duodenal wall may be involved.

Although the hypothalamus plays a significant role in monitoring the circulating level of nutrients, the liver is also capable of monitoring the level in the portal vein. The glucose-sensitive afferents have a tonic discharge when glucose levels are low and such information may contribute to the "hunger" signal. The reader is referred to Deutsch (1978) for a review of the role of the stomach in satiety and appetite.

Pain

Numerous clinical studies have shown that painful sensations from the gut are eliminated by section of the splanchnic nerves, and this has fostered the idea that vagal afferents play no part in nociception (Lewis, 1942). However, it would be unwise to dismiss the vagal afferents entirely, until more thorough electrophysiological experiments have been undertaken to determine, for example, if there are high-threshold mechanoreceptors, as have been found in the splanchnic afferents supplying the gallbladder, and which have been implicated in nociception (Cervero, 1982a,b). In many of the papers on gastric mechanoreceptors there are examples of afferents which are only activated by high levels of inflation, but as yet no study has systematically attempted to classify them based on their thresholds.

One of the major problems with studying gut pain is that the healthy gut responds quite differently from the diseased one. Wolf (1965) showed that vigorous gastric contractions and rapid overdistension of the stomach produced pain, but if it was inflamed or the prevailing tone was high then the threshold for pain was reduced. This was more marked for pain produced by irritation of the mucosa as he found that the healthy mucosa was insensitive to noxious stimuli, but if it became oedematous and hyperaemic the same stimuli now evoked pain. The implication from these experiments is that to study nociceptive afferents from the gut you must first modify the gut to mimic the diseased state, as this may fundamentally affect the characteristics of the receptor, and hence the nature of the afferent discharge.

Conclusions

It will be apparent from this review that there are many gaps in our knowledge of the abdominal vagal afferent system and some of them are highlighted here: (a) The mechanoreceptors in the wall of the gut are described as being "in series" with the muscle and signalling the tension, but the precise relationship between tension and discharge has not been quantified. Without these data it is difficult to decide whether there are sub-populations of tension receptors with different thresholds. (b) It is clear that the mucosa in most regions of the gut possesses mechano/chemo/thermoreceptors but our knowledge of their functional role is poor, particularly for the chemoreceptors. These need to be investigated more thoroughly under conditions which maintain the mucosa in a physiological state and attempt to relate the stimuli used to the normal contents of the lumen at different times after a meal. (c) Studies in anaesthetised animals have indicated the variety of receptors in the gut and the nature of the information reaching the CNS, but we can only speculate about the afferent discharge patterns during the course of digestion. The technique of Falempin and Rousseau (1983) permits recording of vagal afferent activity in conscious animals and offers the possibility of studying gastrointestinal afferents under more natural conditions. (d) Very little is known about the central projections of the abdominal vagus, particularly the pathways taken by the different types of afferents. These could be studied by using the 2-deoxyglucose autoradiography technique of Sokoloff et al. (1977), combined with physiological stimulation of the gut. This would also identify areas of interest for future neurophysiological studies. (e) There is reasonable circumstantial evidence that the vagal afferents are involved in visceral sensations such as gastric emptiness, but definitive studies are lacking. One of the few ways in which this problem could be tackled is by making carefully controlled studies of patients with high spinal cord lesions and comparing them with patients with truncal vagotomy. Such studies would also reveal whether the vagal afferents have any role in nociception.

Acknowledgements

I would like to thank Adele De Souza and Mike Lacey for typing the numerous versions of this manuscript and Louise Wood for her critical comments. Some of the work described in this review was supported by grants from the Wellcome Trust.

References

Adachi, A. (1981) Electrophysiological study of hepatic vagal projection to the medulla. Neurosci Lett., 24: 19–23.

Adachi, A. (1984) Thermosensitive and osmoreceptive afferent fibres in the hepatic branch of the vagus nerve. J. Auton. Nerv. System., 10: 269–273.

Adachi, A. and Niijima, A. (1982) Thermosensitive afferent fibres in the hepatic branch of the vagus nerve in the guinea pig. J. Auton. Nerv. System., 5: 101–109.

Adachi, A., Niijima, A. and Jacobs, H. L. (1976) An hepatic osmoreceptor mechanism in the rat: Electrophysiological and behavoural studies. Am. J. Physiol., 231: 1043–1049.

Adrian, E. D. (1933) Afferent impulses in the vagus and their effects on respiration. J. Physiol., 79: 332–358.

Agostoni, E., Chinnock, J. E., Daly, M. De B. and Murray, J. G. (1957) Functional and histological studies of the vagus nerve and its branches to the heart, lungs and abdominal viscera in the cat. J. Physiol., 135: 182–205.

Anand, B. K. and Pillai, R. V. (1967) Activity of single neurones in the hypothalamic feeding centres: Effects of gastric distension. J. Physiol., 192: 63–77.

Andrew, B. L. (1957) Activity in afferent nerve fibres from the cervical oesophagus. J. Physiol., 135: 54–55.

Andrews, P. L. R. and Lang, K. M. (1982) Vagal afferent discharge from mechanoreceptors in the lower oesophagus of the ferret. J. Physiol., 332: 29P.

Andrews, P. L. R. and Lawes, I. N. C. (1982) The role of vagal and intramural inhibitory reflexes in the regulation of intragastric pressure in the ferret. J. Physiol., 326: 435–451.

Andrews, P. L. R. and Lawes, I. N. C. (1984) Interactions between splanchnic and vagues nerves in the control of mean intragastric pressure in the ferret, J. Physiol., 473–490.

Andrews, P. L. R. and Lawes, I. N. C. (1985) Characteristics of the vagally driven non-adrenergic non-cholinergic inhibitory innervation of ferret corpus. J. Physiol., 363: 1–20.

Andrews, P. L. R. and Taylor, T. V. (1982) An electrophysiological study of the posterior abdominal vagus nerve in man. Clin. Sci., 63: 169–173.

Andrews, P. L. R. and Wood, K. L. (1984) The effects of chemical and mechanical stimuli applied to the gastric antral mucosa on corpus motility in the anaesthetised ferret. J. Physiol., 348: 63P.

Andrews, P. L. R., Grundy, D. and Scratcherd, T. (1980a) The reflex activation of antral motility by gastric distension in the ferret. J. Physiol., 298: 79–84.

Andrews, P. L. R., Grundy, D. and Scratcherd, T. (1980b) Vagal afferent discharge from mechanoreceptors in different regions of the ferret stomach. J. Physiol., 298: 513–524.

Andrews, P. L. R., Grundy, D. and Lawes, I. N. C. (1980c) The role of the vagus and splanchinic nerves in the regulation of intra-gastric pressure in the ferret. J. Physiol., 307: 401–411.

Andrews, W. H. and Orbach, J. (1974) Sodium receptors activating some nerves of perfused rabbit livers. Am. J. Physiol., 227: 1273–1275.

Andrews, W. H. and Orbach, J. (1975) Effects of osmotic pressure on spontaneous afferent discharges in the nerves of the perfused rabbit liver. Pflugers Arch., 361: 89–94.

Angel, A. (1977) Processing of sensory information. Prog. Neurobiol., 9: 1–122.

Asala, S. A. (1984) A multidisciplinary study into changes in the vagus nerve following partial chronic vagotomy. Ph.D. Thesis, University of Sheffield.

Bachman, D. S., Hallowitz, R. A. and MacLean, P. D. (1977) Effects of vagal volleys and serotonin on units of cingulate cortex in monkeys. Brain Res., 130: 253–269.

Barber, W. D. and Burks, T. F. (1983) Brain stem response to phasic gastric distension. Am. J. Physiol., 245: G242–G248.

Barone, F. C., Wayner, M. J., Weiss, C. S. and Almli, C. R. (1979) Effects of intragastric water infusion and gastric distension on hypothalamic neuronal activity. Brain Res. Bull., 4: 267–282.

Beaumont, E. (1833) Experiments and Observations on the Gastric Juice and the Physiology of Digestion, F. P. Allen, Plattsburg, pp. 178.

Brizzee, K. R. and Mehler, W. R. (1986) The central nervous connections involved in the vomiting reflex. In C. J. Davis, G. D. Lake-Bakaar and D. G. Grahaeme-Smith (Eds.), Nausea and Vomiting: Mechanisms and Treatment, ch. 4. Advances in Neurological Sciences, Vol. 3, Springer Verlag, Heidelberg, pp. 210.

Bulato, E. and Carlson, A. J. (1924) Contributions to the physiology of the stomach. Influence of experimental changes in blood sugar level on gastric hunger contractions. Am. J. Physiol., 69, 107–115.

Cannon, W. B. and Washburn, A. L. (1912) An explanation of hunger. Am. J. Physiol., 24: 441–454.

Cervero, F. (1982a) Noxious intensities of visceral stimulation are required to activate viscero-somatic multireceptive neurons in the thoracic spinal cord of the cat. Brain Res., 240: 350–352.

Cervero, F. (1982b) Afferent activity evoked by natural stimulation of the biliary system in the ferret. Pain, 13: 137–151.

Christensen, J. (1984) Origin of sensation in the oesophagus. Am. J. Physiol., 246: G221–G225.

Christensen, J. and De Carle, D. J. (1974) Comparative anatomy of the oesophagus. Gastroenterology, 67: 407–408.

Clarke, G. D. and Davison, J. S. (1975) Tension receptors in the oesophagus and the stomach of the rat. J. Physiol., 244: 41P–42P.

Clarke, G. D. and Davison, J. S. (1978) Mucosal receptors in the gastric antrum and small intestine of the rat with afferent fibres in the cervical vagus. J. Physiol., 284: 55–67.

Clerc, N. and Mei, N. (1983) Vagal mechanoreceptors in the lower oesophageal sphincter of the cat. J. Physiol., 336: 487–498.

Cottrell, D. F. and Iggo, A. (1984a) Tension receptors with vagal afferent fibres in the proximal duodenum and pyloric sphincter of sheep. J. Physiol., 354: 457–475.

Cottrell, D. F. and Iggo, A. (1984b) The response of duodenal tension receptors in sheep to pentagastrin, cholecystokinin and some other drugs. J. Physiol., 354: 477–495.

Cottrell, D. F. and Iggo, A. (1984c) Mucosal enteroreceptors with vagal afferent fibres in the proximal duodenum of sheep. J. Physiol., 354: 497–522.

Crousillat, J. and Ranieri, F. (1980) Mechanoreceptors splanchniques de la voie biliare et de son peritoni. Exp. Brain Res., 40: 146–153.

Davison, J. S. (1972) Responses of single vagal afferent fibres to mechanical and chemical stimulation of gastric and duodenal mucosa in cats. Q. J. Exp. Physiol., 57: 405–416.

Dell, P. and Olsen, R. (1951) Projections thalamique, corticales, et cerebelleuses des afferences viscerals vagales. C. R. Soc. Biol., 145: 1084–1088.

Deutsch, J. A. (1978) The stomach in food satiation and the regulation of appetite. Prog. Neurobiol., 10: 133–153.

Diani, A., West, C., Vidmar, T., Peterson, T. and Gerritsen, G. (1984) Morphometric analysis of the vagus nerve in the non-diabetic and ketonuric diabetic chinese hamster. J. Comp. Pathol., 94: 495–503.

Du Bois, F. S. and Foley, J. O. (1936) Experimental studies on the vagus and spinal accessory nerves in the cat. Anat. Rec., 64: 285–307.

Dunlop, C. W. (1958) Viscero-sensory and somato-sensory representation in the rhinencephalon. Electroenceph. Clin. Neurophysiol., 10: 297–304.

Dussardier, M. (1960) Recherches sur le controle bulbaire de la motricite gastrique chez les ruminants. Therses Docteur es. Sciences Naturelles, Université de Paris.

Edgeworth, F. H. (1892) On a large fibered sensory supply of the thoracic and abdominal viscera. J. Physiol., 13: 260–271.

El Ouazzani, T. and Mei, N. (1979) Mise en evidence electrophysiologique des thermorecepteurs vagaux dans la region gastrointestinale. Leur role dans la regulation de la moticite digestive. Exp. Brain Res., 39: 419–434.

El Ouazzani, T. and Mei, N. (1981) Acido- et glucoreceptors vagaux de la region gastroduodenale. Exp. Brain Res., 42: 442–452.

El Ouazzani, T. and Mei, N. (1982) Electrophysiologic properties and role of the vagal thermoreceptors of lower esophagus and stomach of cat. Gastroenterology, 83: 995–1001.

Evans, D. H. L. and Murray, J. G. (1954) Histological and functional studies on the fibre composition of the vagus nerve of the rabbit. J. Anat., 88: 320–337.

Falempin, M. and Rousseau, S. P. (1983) Reinnervation of skeletal muscles by vagal sensory fibres in the sheep, cat, and rabbit, J. Physiol., 335: 367–479.

Falempin, M. and Rousseau, J. P. (1984) Activity of lingual, laryngeal oesophageal receptors in conscious sheep. J. Physiol., 347: 47–58.

Falempin, M., Mei, N. and Rousseau, J. P. (1978) Vagal mechanoreceptors of the inferior thoracic oesophagus, the lower oesophageal sphincter and the stomach in the sheep. Pflugers Arch., 373: 25–30.

Floyd, K. and Morrison, J. F. B. (1974) Splanchinic mechanoreceptors in the dog. Q. J. Exp. Physiol., 59: 359–364.

Gabella, G. and Pease, H. L. (1973) Number of axons in the abdominal vagus of the rat. Brain Res., 58: 465–469.

Galen, C. (129–199) De usu partium corporis humani: Liber IX, Lugduni, Nicolao Regio Calabre (1550).

Garnier, L. and Mei, N. (1982) Do true osmoreceptors exist at intestinal level? J. Physiol., 327: 97–98.

Gaskell, W. H. (1916) The Involuntary Nervous System, Longmans, Green and Co., London, pp. 178.

Gupta, B. N., Nier, K. and Hensel, H. (1979) Cold-sensitive afferents from the abdomen. Pflugers Arch., 380: 203–204.

Gwyn, D. G. and Leslie, R. A. (1979) A projection of the vagus nerve to the area subpostrema in the cat. Brain Res., 161: 335–341.

Hallowitz, R. A. and MacLean, P. D. (1977) Effects of vagal volleys on units of intralaminar and juxtalaminar thalamic nuclei in monkeys. Brain Res., 130: 271–286.

Harding, R. and Leek, B. F. (1972a) Gastro-duodenal receptor responses to chemical and mechanical stimuli, investigated by a single fibre technique. J. Physiol., 222: 139P–140P.

Harding, R. and Leek, B. F. (1972b) Rapidly adapting mechanoreceptors in the reticulorumen which respond to chemicals. J. Physiol., 223: 32P–33P.

Harding, R. and Leek, B. F. (1973) Central projections of gastric vagal inputs. J. Physiol., 228: 73–90.

Harding, R. and Titchen, D. A. (1975) Chemosensitive vagal endings in the oesophagus of the cat. J. Physiol., 247: 52P–53P.

Harper, A. A., McSwiney, B. A. and Suffolk, S. F. (1935) Afferent fibres from the abdominal in the vagus nerve. J. Physiol., 85: 267–276.

Hennemann, H. E. and Rubia, J. (1978) Vagal representation in the cerebellum of the cat. Pflugers Arch., 375: 119–123.

Hertz, A. F. (1911) The Sensibility of the Alimentary Canal, Hodder and Stroughton, London, pp. 83.

Iggo, A. (1955) Gastrointestinal tension receptors in the stomach and the urinary bladder. J. Physiol., 128: 593–607.

Iggo, A. (1957a) Gastrointestinal tension receptors with unmyelinated afferent fibres in the vagus of the cat. Q. J. Exp. Physiol., 42: 130–143.

Iggo, A. (1957b) Gastric mucosal chemoreceptors with vagal afferent fibres in the cat. Q. J. Exp. Physiol., 42: 389–409.

Iggo, A. (1958) The electrophysiological identification of single nerve fibres, with particular reference to the slowest-conducting vagal afferent fibres in the cat. J. Physiol., 142: 110–126.

Iggo, A. (1966) Physiology of visceral afferent systems. Acta Neuroveg., 28: 121–134.

Jeanningros, R. (1982) Vagal unitary responses to intestinal amino-acid infusions in the anaesthetised cat: a putative signal for protein induced satiety. Physiol. Behav., 28: 9–21.

Jeanningros, R. (1984) Lateral hypothalamic responses to preabsorptive and post-absorptive signals related to amino acid ingestion. J. Auton. Nerv. System, 10: 261–268.

Jones, C. M. (1938) Digestive Tract Pain, The MacMillan Company, New York.

Kalia, M. and Mesulam, M. M. (1980) Brain stem projections of sensory and motor components of the vagus complex in the cat. II. Laryngeal, tracheobronchial, pulmonary, cardiac and gastrointestinal branches. J. Comp. Neurol., 193: 467–508.

Kemp, D. R. (1973) A histological and functional study of the gastric mucosal innervation of the dog. The quantification of the fibre content of the normal subdiaphragmatic vagal trunks and their abdominal branches. Aust. N.Z. J. Surg. 43: 289–294.

Kral, J. G. (1983) Behavioural effects of vagotomy in humans. In J. G. Kral, T. L. Powley and C. McC. Brooks (Eds.), Vagal Nerve Function: Behavioural and Methodological Considerations, Elsevier Science Publishers B.V., Amsterdam, pp. 273–282.

Langley, J. N. (1903) The autonomic nervous system. Brain, 26: 1–26.

Leek, B. F. (1969) Reticiulo-ruminal mechanoreceptors in the sheep. J. Physiol., 202: 585–609.

Leek, B. F. (1972a) The innervation of sheep forestomach papillae from which combined chemoreceptors and rapidly adapting mechanoreceptor responses are obtainable. J. Physiol., 227: 22P–23P.

Leek, B. F. (1972b) Abdominal visceral receptors. In E. Neil (Ed.), Enteroreceptors, Handbook of Sensory Physiology, Vol III, Springer, Berlin, pp. 113–160.

Leek, B. F. (1977) Abdominal and pelvic visceral receptors. Br. Med. Bull., 33: 163–168.

Leslie, R. A., Gwyn, D. G. and Hopkins, D. A. (1982) The central distribution of the cervical vagus nerve and gastric afferent and efferent projections in the rat. Brain Res. Bull., 8: 37–48.

Lewis, T. (1942) Pain, Macmillan, New York, pp. 192.

Liedberg, G., Nielsen, K. C., Owman, C. H. and Sjoberg, N. O. (1973) Adrenergic contribution to the abdominal vagus nerve in the cat. Scand. J. Gastroenterol., 8: 177–180.

Lundberg, J., Ahlman, H., Dahlstrom, A. and Kewewter, J. (1976) Catecholamine-containing nerve fibres in the human abdominal vagus. Scand. J. Gastroenterol., 70: 472–475.

MacKay, T. W. and Andrews, P. L. R. (1983) A comparative study of the vagal innervation of the stomach in man and the ferret. J. Anat., 136: 449–481.

Maddison, S. and Horrell, R. I. (1979) Hypothalamic unit responses to alimentary perfusions in the anaesthetised rat. Brain Res. Bull., 4: 259–260.

Marie, A., Falempin, M. and Rousseau, J. P. (1984) Activity of esophageal and gastric receptors in conscious sheep. Can. J. Anim. Sci., 64 (Suppl.): 1–2.

Mathias, C. J. and Frankel, H. L. (1983) Clinical manifestations of malfunctioning sympathetic mechanisms in tetraplegia. J. Auton. Nerv. System, 7: 303–312.

Mei, N. (1970) Mechanorecepteurs vagaux digestifs chez le chat. Exp. Brain Res., 11: 502–514.

Mei, N. (1978) Vagal glucoreceptors in the small intestine of the cat. J. Physiol., 282: 485–506.

Mei, N. (1983) Sensory structures in the viscera. In D. Ottoson (Ed.), Progress in Sensory Physiology, Vol. 4, Springer Verlag, New York, Heidelberg, Berlin, pp. 1–42.

Mei, N. and Aubert, M. (1972) Modifications de l'activite unitaire du cortex somatosensoriel provoques chez le chat par le excitation des fibres vagales anyeliniques. J. Physiol., 65: 147A.

Mei, N., Condamin, M. and Boyer, A. (1980) The composition of the vagus nerve of the cat. Cell Tissue Res., 209: 423–431.

Morrison, J. F. B. (1977) The afferent innervation of the gastrointestinal tract. In F. P. Brooks and P. W. Evers (Eds.), Nerves and the Gut, Charles B. Slack, Inc, NJ, pp. 297–326.

Niijima, A. (1969a) Afferent discharges from osmoreceptors in the liver of the guinea pig. Science, 166: 1519–1520.

Niijima, A. (1969b) Afferent impulse discharges from glucoreceptors in the liver of the guinea pig. Ann. N.Y. Acad. Sci., 157: 690–700.

Niijima, A. (1980) Glucose sensitive afferent fibres in the liver and regulation of blood glucose. Brain Res. Bull., 5, Suppl. 4: 175–179.

Niijima, A. (1981) Visceral afferents and metabolic function. Diabetologia, 20: 325–330.

Niijima, A. (1982) Glucose-sensitive afferent nerve fibres in the hepatic branch of the vagus nerve in guinea pig. J. Physiol., 332: 315–323.

Niijima, A. (1983) Glucose sensitive afferent nerve fibres in the liver and their role in food intake and blood glucose regulation. In J. G. Kral, T. L. Powley and C. McC. Brooks (Eds.), Vagal Nerve Function: Behavioural and Methodological Considerations, Elsevier Science Publishers B.V., Amsterdam, pp. 207–220.

Odekunle, A. and Bower, A. (1985) Brainstem connections of vagal afferent nerves in the ferret: an autoradiographic study. J. Anat., 140: 461–469.

Oomura, Y. and Yoshimatsu, H. (1984) Neural network of glucose monitoring system. J. Auton. Nerv. System, 10: 359–372.

Orbach, J. and Andrews, W. H. H. (1973) Stimulation of afferent nerve terminals in the perfused rabbit liver by sodium salts of some long-chain fatty acids. Q. J. Exp. Physiol., 58: 267–274.

Paintal, A. S. (1954) A study of gastric stretch receptors. Their role in the peripheral mechanism of satiation of hunger and thirst. J. Physiol., 126: 255–270.

Paintal, A. S. (1957) Responses from mucosal mechanoreceptors in the small intestine of the cat. J. Physiol., 139, 353–368.

Paintal, A. S. (1973) Vagal sensory receptors and their reflex effects. Physiol. Rev., 53: 159–227.

Payne, W. W. and Poulton, E. P. (1927a) Experiments on visceral sensation. Part I. The relation of pain to activity in the human oesophagus. J. Physiol., 63: 217–241.

Payne, W. W. and Poulton, E. P. (1927b) Experiments on visceral sensation. Part II. The sensation of "nausea" and "sinking"; oesophageal reflexes and counter-irritation. J. Physiol., 65: 157–172.

Pick, J. (1970) The Autonomic Nervous System, Morphological Comparative and Surgical Aspects, J. B. Lippincott, Philadelphia.

Powley, T. L., Prechtl, J. C., Fox, E. A. and Berthoud, H. R. (1983) Anatomical considerations for surgery of the rat abdominal vagus: distribution, paraganglia and regeneration. In J. G. Kral, T. L. Powley and C. McC. Brooks (Eds.), Vagal Nerve Function: Behavioural and Methodological Considerations, Elsevier Science Publishers B.V., Amsterdam, pp. 79–98.

Rolls, B. J. and Rolls, E. T. (1982) Thirst, Cambridge University Press, pp. 194.

Sakaguchi, T. and Yamaguchi, K. (1979) Effects of electrical stimulation of the hepatic vagus nerve on the plasma insulin concentration in the rat. Brain Res., 164: 314–316.

Satchell, P. M. (1984) Canine oesophageal mechanoreceptors. J. Physiol., 346: 587–300.

Sawchenko, P. E. (1983) Central connections of the sensory and motor nuclei of the vagus nerve. In J. G. Kral, T. L. Powley and C. McC. Brooks (Eds.), Vagal Nerve Function: Behavioural and Methodological Considerations, Elsevier Science Publishers B.V., Amsterdam, pp. 13–26.

Sawchenko, P. E. and Friedman, M. J. (1979) Sensory functions of the liver — a review. Am. J. Physiol., 236: R5–R20.

Sharkey, K. A. and Williams, R. G. (1983) Extrinsic innervation of the rat pancreas: Demonstration of vagal sensory neurones in the rat by retrograde tracing. Neurosci. Lett., 42: 131–135.

Sokoloff, L., Reivich, M., Kennedy, C., Rosiers, D., Patlak, C. S., Pettigrew, K. D., Sakurada, O. and Shinohara, M. (1977) The [^{14}C]deoxyglucose method for the measurement of local cerebral glucose utilization: Theory, procedures and normal values in conscious and anaesthetised albino rat. J. Neurochem., 28: 897–916.

Somerville, M. and Bradley, W. G. (1977) Axoplasmic flow in myelinated and unmyelinated nerves. Brain Res., 124: 393–402.

Titchen, D. A. and Wheeler, J. S. (1971) Contractions of the caudal region of the oesophagus of the cat. J. Physiol., 215: 119–137.

Toyota, T. (1955) On innervation of stomach of hedgehog. Archiv. Hist. Jpn., 7: 573–584.

Vesalius, A. (1543) De Humani Corporis, Fabricia, Basel.

Wolf, S. (1965) The Stomach, Oxford University Press, New York, pp. 321.

F. Cervero and J. F.B. Morrison
Progress in Brain Research, Vol. 67
© 1986 Elsevier Science Publishers B.V. (Biomedical Division)

CHAPTER 7

Functional properties of spinal visceral afferents supplying abdominal and pelvic organs, with special emphasis on visceral nociception

W. Jänig[1] and J. F. B. Morrison[2]

[1] *Physiologisches Institut, Christian-Albrechts Universität, Olshausenstrasse 40, D-2300 Kiel, F.R.G.* and [2] *Department of Physiology, University of Leeds Medical School, Leeds LS2 9TJ, U.K.*

Introduction

Organs in the abdominal and pelvic cavities have a dual extrinsic afferent innervation which travels to the central nervous system in the autonomic nerve trunks; the cell bodies of afferents that run with the parasympathetic fibres are concentrated in the vagal nodose ganglia and in the sacral dorsal root ganglia, whereas those of afferents in the main sympathetic nerve trunks have a thoraco-lumbar distribution. Both sets of visceral afferents participate in a number of reflexes and in visceral sensations. Noxious sensations from viscera probably depend mainly on spinal visceral afferents that enter thoraco-lumbar and sacral segments of the cord. The stimuli that elicit these sensations include excessive distension and contraction of hollow viscera, traction on mesenteries, and inflammation or chemical stimuli within the peritoneal cavity.

Many vagal afferent neurones from the gastrointestinal tract react quite selectively to mechanical stimuli to the mucosa or muscle, and to chemicals within the lumen, and can be divided into separate populations with different functional properties (Leek, 1977; Mei, 1983, 1985).

This may apply also to some spinal visceral afferent neurones (Mei, 1983). However, for the majority of spinal visceral afferents, it is not at all clear whether they can be excited specifically by a particular physical or chemical stimulus, and whether the excitation of these afferents is linked more or less selectively to one visceral sensation or reflex. Certain sacral visceral afferents may be involved in maintaining continence and/or in emptying of the urinary bladder or the colon; whether these afferents are also specifically linked to the corresponding sensations during micturition or defaecation, and to other sensations, such as pain, is unknown. For example, it is known that slow passive distension of the urinary bladder can elicit a variety of vague sensations in humans that span from feelings of slight pressure "deep in the mid-perineum or faint pressure from within" to fullness and then to pain (Denny-Brown and Robertson, 1933). These and other sensations from the urinary bladder can probably be elicited from the sacral afferents as well as hypogastric afferents (Riddoch, 1921; Denny-Brown and Robertson, 1933; White and Sweet, 1969).

Are the different qualities of sensation that originate from one viscus elicited by the excitation of different types of afferents, or are they all subserved by a single category of afferents? This important question leads to one of the main problems we will deal with in this review: to what extent can spinal visceral afferents from abdominal and pelvic organs be excited specifically by one or a few of the types of mechanical or chemical stimuli that can occur in the visceral domain?

Theoretically, there are several ways in which

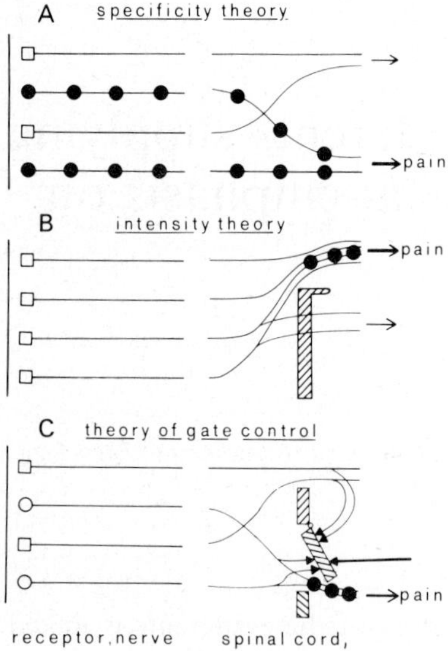

Fig. 1. Schematic representation of theories of neuronal encoding of peripheral events which lead to pain. A. The "specificity theory" postulates specific nociceptive primary afferent neurones which synapse specifically with second-order neurones, etc., thus establishing nociceptive pathways from the periphery to the cortex. B. The intensity theory is based on the assumption that nocuous and non-nocuous peripheral events are encoded in the intensity of the discharge of the same population of primary afferent neurones. Pain appears when the intensity of the discharge reaches a certain height; this theory postulates a central "pain threshold". C. "Theories of gate control" have their origin in the "pattern theory", which assumed that nocuous and non-nocuous events are encoded by different patterns of discharge in the same population of primary afferent neurones. The gate control in its modern form postulates that the event "pain" is the result of the balance of the activity in large- and small-diameter afferent fibres and of central impulses which operate at a neuronal gate in the spinal cord or in supraspinal brain structures. The gate control is principally compatible with the stimulus specificity of the primary afferent neurones. Modified from Handwerker (1984). For details, see text.

different peripheral stimuli in the visceral domain could be encoded by primary afferent and central neurones so as to elicit different sensations: (1) Primary afferents from an organ react specifically to certain stimuli and not to others. These afferents are more or less specifically linked synaptically to neurones in the spinal cord and lead, when excited, to characteristic sensations and reflexes (Fig. 1A). This is the simplest theory and can be traced back to Johannes Müller and Max von Frey (see Sinclair, 1981). The specificity theory is compatible with the idea of an "adequate stimulus", i.e., "that the sensorial end-organ is an apparatus by which an afferent nerve fibre is rendered distinctly amenable to some particular physical agent, and at the same time rendered less amenable to other excitants ..." (Sherrington, 1900, 1906). It is generally — though not universally — believed that this theory applies to the cutaneous sensations (Burgess and Perl, 1973; Lynn, 1984; Perl, 1984). (2) Primary afferents from an organ encode the peripheral stimuli that can elicit various sensations and reflexes in the intensity of their discharge. In this case, one must assume that the major decoding process leading to different sensations, including visceral pain, occurs centrally, e.g., by way of a central threshold. This theory is called the "intensity theory" or "summation hypothesis" (see Fig. 1B) and was particularly propagated by the German clinician Goldscheider (1920), the great opponent of von Frey, and some physiologists believe it to apply to visceral sensations (Morrison, 1977, 1981; Malliani and Lombardi, 1982). (3) The third theory, which was created in the first half of this century and particularly favoured by psychologists, is the "pattern theory" (Nafe, 1929; see Kenshalo, 1984). In its original, extreme form this theory postulated that sensations result from different spatio-temporally dispersed patterns of afferent discharges, and that there is no stimulus specificity of these afferents at all. This theory did not survive since ample evidence had accumulated proving the existence of many afferents which were stimulus-specific, particularly in skin. Whether or not it is also valid for the spinal afferent innervation of viscera and deep somatic tissues (Mense, 1985) is a matter of debate. In a modern form, the "pattern theory" reappeared in the "gate control theory" of pain by Melzack and Wall (1965). This theory states that the discharges in small myelinated and unmyelinated fibres converge on second-order neurones in the dorsal horn of the spinal cord, and that pain results, depending on the balance of excitation in small- and large-diameter fibres, keeping a hypothetical neuronal gate in the spinal cord open by activity in small-diameter fibres (allowing pain to appear) and closed by activity in large-diameter fibres or by central impulses. This theory is also compatible with the stimulus-specificity theory of primary afferents (Fig. 1C); however, scientifically it can barely be proved or disproved. In this sense, its value is more heuristical, as it initiated a large body of experimental work (for discussion see Nathan, 1976; Wall, 1978; Sinclair, 1981).

This review focusses on the functional properties of spinal afferent neurones supplying abdominal and pelvic viscera and, in particular, on the problem of how physical and chemical stimuli that lead to visceral pain in humans and equivalent reactions in animals are encoded. Data obtained on spinal visceral afferents from various organs in animals, using neurophysiological and morphological techniques, will be discussed and compared with information obtained from the literature concerning the conditions which evoke visceral sensations and reflexes in humans. Finally, the whole complex will be discussed in the framework of the theories outlined above, in order to get some idea of the possible ways in which the peripheral events in the visceral organs are encoded in the discharge of visceral afferents.

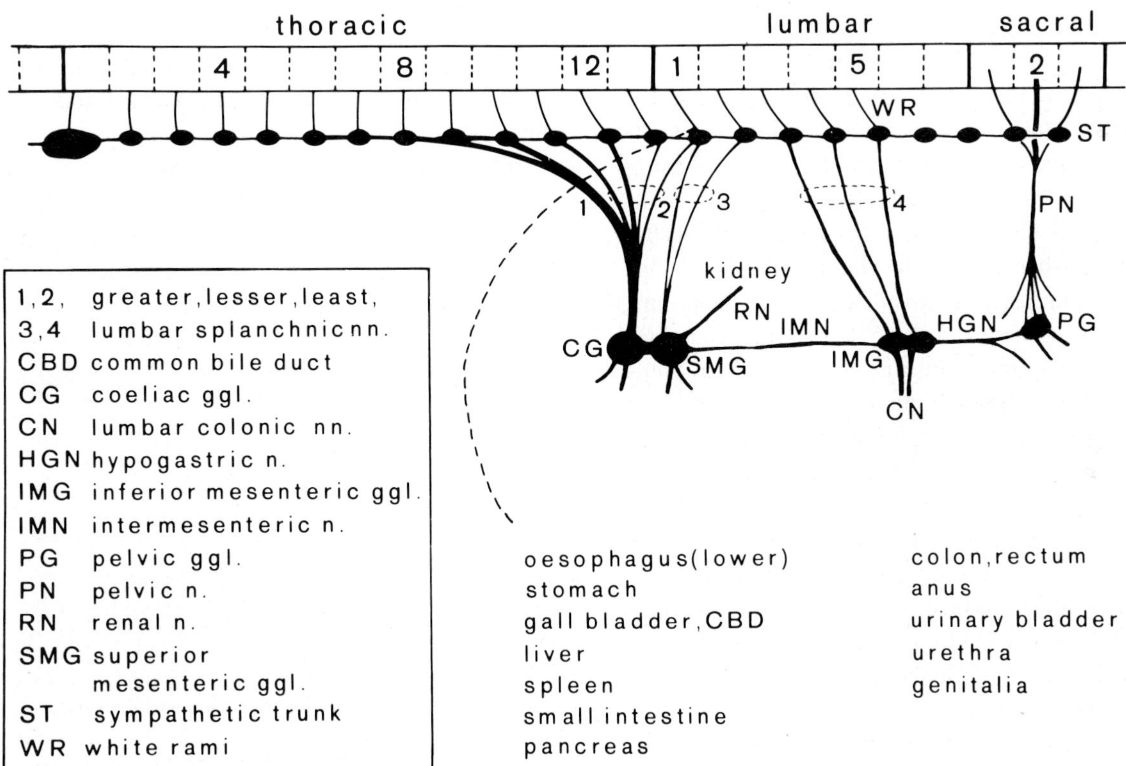

Fig. 2. Schematic arrangement of visceral nerves in the cat which contain spinal afferent fibres from abdominal and pelvic organs. Sympathetic trunk (ST) and white rami (WR) are indicated. There are only a very few pelvic afferent fibres which travel through the sympathetic trunks and have their cell bodies in the dorsal root ganglia rostral to L7. Most electrophysiological and morphological studies reported in this review were conducted on afferents running in these nerves. The diaphragm is indicated by the interrupted line. The nomenclature greater, lesser, least and lumbar splanchnic nerves (1, 2, 3, 4) is equivalent to the officially accepted anatomical nomenclature N. splanchnicus major, N. splanchnicus minor, N. splanchnicus imus and Nn. splanchnici lumbales. The pelvic nerve is officially named Nn. splanchnici pelvini (Williams and Warwick, 1980).

The methods employed in the morphological and neurophysiological studies on animals and the sensory studies in humans have been described extensively in the literature referred to in this review. Details of procedures will be described if necessary, as results are presented.

Numerical and spatial aspects of the spinal innervation of viscera

Numbers of spinal visceral afferents

The last decade has seen a considerable improvement in the quality and quantity of information available concerning the numbers of afferents that innervate the abdominal and pelvic viscera of the cat (see Fig. 3). Quantitative studies on neuronal somata identified by retrograde tracing methods, particularly the horseradish peroxidase (HRP) technique, and on axons in peripheral nerves using the electron microscope have been largely responsible for this change. The advantage of the HRP technique, when applied to visceral nerves, is that one can obtain with relative ease, in the *same* animal, quantitative estimates of numbers, segmental distributions, dimensions and locations of afferent and pre- and postganglionic neurones projecting in the labelled nerve (e.g., Baron et al., 1985a–d). Electron microscopy is not so easy, but it does allow precise numbers and sizes of axons in peripheral nerves to be obtained. Recent studies on the greater splanchnic nerve, for instance (Kuo et al., 1982), have used more appropriate nerve sections than previously (Foley, 1948; Ranieri et al., 1975) to establish the numbers of afferent preganglionic and postganglionic fibres in this nerve. They estimated a total of 6000–7000 fibres (bilaterally), which included about 600–700 myelinated axons, the largest of which are connected to mesenteric Pacinian corpuscles. Kuo and De Groat (1985), using HRP, found an even lower number of afferent neurons (about 2400, unilaterally) projecting in the left greater splanchnic nerve. This estimate may be too low since it is based on the average of four animals and not on the best preparations; furthermore, the authors may have overcorrected their numbers using Abercrombie's correction (Abercrombie, 1946; cf. McLachlan and Jänig, 1983).

The lesser (or minor) splanchnic nerve is estimated to be approximately half the size of the major splanchnic nerve (Kuntz et al., 1957). No estimate can be made of the number of afferent fibres in the least splanchnic nerves, which originate from the first and second lumbar sympathetic ganglia in the cat. These nerves are about the same size as the lumbar splanchnic nerves (Baron et al., 1985a). Thus, it would not be surprising if they contained another 1000–2000 afferent axons, the majority probably supplying the kidney (Kuo et al., 1983).

The afferent fibre numbers of the hypogastric, lumbar splanchnic, lumbar colonic and pelvic nerves (see Fig. 2) have now been studied adequately, and the lumbar innervation uses about 4600 afferents (Baron et al., 1985b–d) and the sacral innervation about 7350 afferents (Morgan et al., 1981). In total, about 22,000–25,000 primary afferent neurones appear to be responsible for signalling afferent information from the abdominal and pelvic

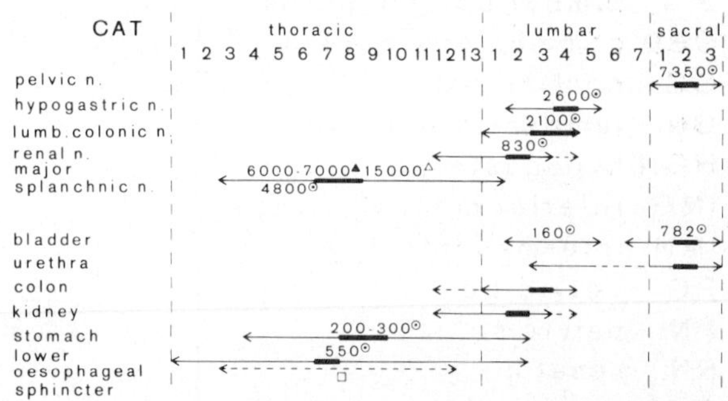

Fig. 3. Segmental distributions and numbers (both sides) of visceral afferent neurones projecting in different visceral nerves and to abdominal and pelvic organs of the çat. For techniques used see inset in Fig. 4. Data from: pelvic n., Morgan et al. (1981); hypogastric n. and lumbar colonic n., Baron et al. (1985b,d); renal n., Kuo et al. (1983); major splanchnic n., Foley (1948), Ranieri et al. (1973, 1975), Kuo et al. (1982), Kuo and De Groat (1985); urinary bladder, Applebaum et al. (1980); urethra, Downie et al. (1984); colon, Hazarika et al. (1964), Baron et al. (1985d); kidney, Kuo et al. (1983); stomach, El-Quazzani (1981, quoted by Cervero et al., 1984); lower oesophageal sphincter, Clerc (1983).

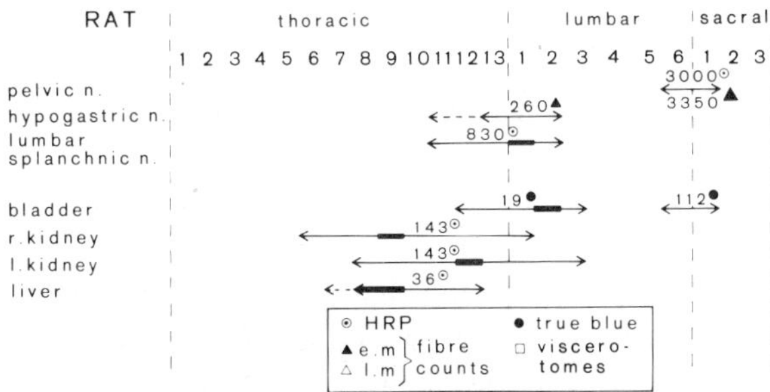

Fig. 4. Segmental distributions and numbers of visceral afferent neurones projecting in different visceral nerves and to abdominal and pelvic organs of the rat. Data from: pelvic n., Hulsebosch and Coggeshall (1982), Nadelhaft and Booth (1984); hypogastric n., Hulsebosch and Coggeshall (1982); lumbar splanchnic n., Neuhuber (1982); urinary bladder, Applebaum et al. (1980), Sharkey et al. (1983); right (r.) kidney, left (l.) kidney, Ciriello and Calaresu (1983); liver, Magni and Carobi (1983).

viscera of the cat. To this number, another 1000 afferents from T1–T7, that innervate the heart, thoracic large vessels and lungs (Oldfield and McLachlan, 1978; Rühle et al., 1985), may be added. In the cat, the estimated total number of spinal visceral afferents is about 1.5–2.5% of the total number of spinal afferent neurones supplying the periphery, which may amount to about 1–1.5 million (Holmes and Davenport, 1940). This low percentage is slightly less than that for individual dorsal root ganglia T8 and T9 (Cervero et al., 1984). The numbers of fibres in the pelvic, lumbar splanchnic and renal nerves of the rat appear to be about 40, 20 and 33%, respectively, of those in the cat (see Fig. 4).

Segmental distribution of spinal visceral afferents

Afferents from different intra-abdominal nerve trunks enter different segments of the cord: there is a degree of overlap between these groups of afferents in the dorsal roots, but each nerve shows a peak of afferent innervation in one or two adjacent segments. For example, Baron et al. (1985b–d) and Kuo et al. (1983) have demonstrated peak innervations from the hypogastric, lumbar colonic and renal nerves in the fourth, third and second lumbar dorsal root ganglia, respectively, while the majority of afferents in the pelvic nerve have cell bodies in the second sacral segment in the cat (Morgan et al., 1981). The segmental innervation of different viscera also shows considerable overlap, as would have been predicted by physiological studies of viscerotomes (Hazarika et al., 1964). However, observations on the numbers of filled cells in dorsal root ganglia following injection of HRP or True Blue into a viscus shows that the innervation of each organ is most dense in only one or two segments; thus, Applebaum et al. (1980) have shown that the bladder afferents enter the cord in greatest numbers through the third lumbar and second sacral dorsal roots in the cat, and the second and sixth lumbar segments in the rat. Sharkey et al. (1983) found peaks at L1 and L6 in the rat using True Blue as a marker. Bladder innervation is thus at a higher segmental level in the rat than in the cat, and, in particular, the majority of pelvic nerve afferents enter the lumbar rather than the sacral cord. In this species the density of the afferent input from the left and right kidneys and the liver/biliary tract is maximal at T12, T9, and T8/T9, respectively, with the liver being represented predominantly on the right side, and the kidneys being innervated unilaterally (Applebaum et al., 1980; Magni and Carobi, 1983; Ciriello and Calaresu, 1983). The liver and biliary tract also have a significant vagal innervation.

Thus, the relationship between a viscus and the spinal cord can be described in terms of the spinal segments that receive the majority of the afferent fibres and the degree of lateralisation of this afferent pathway. True visceral sensation (arising from a viscus without any involvement of the parietal peritoneum) is felt in the midline of the abdomen if the viscus receives a bilateral afferent input of roughly equal size; or to one side of the midline if the viscus is innervated either predominantly or completely from one side of the neuraxis (see Bentley and Smithwick, 1940). Thus, the kidney, gallbladder and ovary are the main abdominal viscera giving true visceral sensations that are lateralised. True visceral sensations from the gut tube and bladder are normally felt in the midline, but there are reports of localized stimulation within the bladder being lateralised by subjects (Langworthy et al., 1940, p. 129). Applebaum et al. (1980) calculated that less than 10% of afferent fibres from one side of the bladder cross over to the opposite side of the cord, and Baron et al. (1985b) found that approximately 20% of hypogastric nerve afferents do.

Ventral root afferents

There are some reports that unmyelinated afferent fibres exist in the lumbo-sacral ventral roots of cats and that many of these have receptive fields in the viscera (Coggeshall et al., 1974; Applebaum et al., 1976; Clifton et al., 1976; Coggeshall and Ito, 1977). It now appears that few of these enter the spinal cord through the ventral roots; most appear to loop back into the dorsal roots or innervate the pia mater (Risling et al., 1984a), but some have been traced to the dorsal horn (Light and Metz, 1978). There are few reports of functional studies on reflexes induced by "ventral root" afferents. Longhurst et al. (1980) concluded that they have a minor role to play in the hindlimb pressor reflex in cats.

Spinal afferent neurones branching to visceral and somatic tissues

Recently, it has been proposed that some afferent neurones send axon collaterals into two different somatic nerves or into a somatic and a visceral nerve. This idea is supported by some neurophysiological and histological experiments (Bahr et al., 1981; Pierau et al., 1982; Taylor and Pierau, 1982), but the evidence of these groups deals with different neuronal populations. Bahr et al. (1981) studied unmyelinated axons in the lumbar splanchnic nerves of the cat that followed stimuli to the white ramus and to somatic nerves at 50 Hz, and could have been afferent. Antidromic stimulation from the dorsal root was not performed and receptive fields were not located because both visceral and somatic nerves were cut. All of these fibres were unmyelinated, had no ongoing discharge and could not be activated reflexly via spinal or supraspinal pathways. Evidence of branching was present in 18% of 84 unmyelinated afferents studied in the lumbar splanchnic nerves.

In contrast, Pierau et al. (1982) studied intracellular recordings from cells in the L6 dorsal root ganglion of the rat that had evidence of axon collaterals in the sciatic and pudendal nerves. All of these axons were myelinated and the majority conducted at 30–60 m/second. 44% of cells were found to respond to stimulation of both nerves, but high-stimulus voltages were used and it is possible that some stimulus spread may have occurred. A later study by Taylor and Pierau (1982) demonstrated double fluorescence in L6 dorsal root ganglion cells following the application of bisbenzimide or Nuclear Yellow to the pudendal nerve and of propidium iodide or Fast Blue to the sciatic nerve.

Branching of sensory axons distal to sacral dorsal root ganglia in the rat appears to be a relatively common occurrence (Langford and Coggeshall, 1979, 1981). These authors compared the number of dorsal root ganglion cells with the number of fibres in the nerve 0.2 mm distal to the end of the dorsal root ganglion; they found about 2.3 times more axons than dorsal root ganglion cells and concluded that individual sacral primary afferent neurones may send several axons to the periphery. As interesting as these results and the interpretation may appear, it must be kept in mind that the counts were made 5–7 days after cutting the sciatic nerve and the ventral roots and after sympathectomy. These surgical procedures might well have induced regenerative changes (sprouting!) of the primary afferent neurones (Risling et al., 1983, 1984b). Unfortunately, no control data (obtained on rats without surgery) have been reported by Langford and Coggeshall (1981). Furthermore, it must be kept in mind that looping of primary afferent fibres into the ventral roots may occur (Coggeshall, 1980), resulting theoretically in the possibility that the same axon is counted three times. Finally, it would seem that the percentage of neurones that have axon collaterals in two somatic nerves is very low, judging by the electrophysiological studies of Devor et al.

(1984), who found only 14 of such neurones in 6400 neurones studied, including over 2700 neurones with unmyelinated axons. Similar negative electrophysiological results were obtained on neurones with unmyelinated fibres in rat hindlimb nerves by W. Jänig (unpublished observations), who recorded from axon bundles that had been sectioned distally: of 300–400 neurones, which projected in the sural or superficial peroneal or tibial nerve, no neurone could be activated by electrical stimulation of the other two nerves. In the trigeminal system, Borges and Moskowitz (1983) found only two doubly labelled cells out of 852 studied following application of different retrograde tracers to the intracranial and extracranial branches of the trigeminal nerve.

A major weakness of all the experimental evidence is that two functional receptive fields have never been found in neurones that show branching, and suggestions that they participate in referred pain must be tentative until functional information of this sort is available.

Properties of visceral afferents

Methods

The main body of experimental evidence on which the arguments in this review are based has been obtained in neurophysiological experiments on visceral spinal afferent neurones in cats; some experiments were also conducted on dogs, sheep and ferrets. In these experiments animals were anaesthetised, usually with alpha-chloralose or sodium pentobarbitone, and were often artificially ventilated and immobilised; various monitors of physiological conditions were used, so as to maintain the physiological state of the animal.

Afferent activity was recorded from single units dissected from visceral nerves, white rami, or sacral dorsal roots in a pool of paraffin oil, using standard techniques.

Mechanical and chemical stimuli were used to characterise the receptors: (1) Glass or nylon rods with fine tips, or cat's whiskers were used to determine the location and extent of the mechanosensitive receptive fields. (2) Passive distension of hollow organs with fluid (or air) at constant pressure, or by repeated injection of small volumes. (3) Isovolumetric or isotonic contraction of muscular viscera, either occurring naturally after filling, or elicited by nerve stimulation. (4) Tension applied to vessels and mesenteries, either manually or by means of a pulley system. (5) Vascular changes induced by injection of drugs, occlusion of the common carotid arteries, by occlusion of intra-abdominal arteries or veins, or by infusions into intra-abdominal veins. (6) Chemical stimuli applied intra-arterially, or by superfusion over the receptive fields of receptors; the chemicals included bradykinin, KCl, HCl and hypertonic saline. (7) Temperature changes could be applied by a thermode or superfusion of saline at different temperatures.

Receptive fields

The majority of mechanoreceptors in the spinal afferent pathway from viscera have receptive fields in a mesentery or peritoneal ligament and/or the adjacent viscus, and consist of between one and nine mechanosensitive spots distributed along the course of the nerves (periarterial nerves) innervating the viscera. Probing these endings, using forces often less than 10 mN, gives rise to a slowly adapting discharge. In compliant tissues with large surface area the receptive fields are sometimes larger than those described by Bessou and Perl (1966) and Morrison (1973). In the mesentery, the receptive endings occur particularly at sites where vessels divide, and are also common in the serosa, at the point where a vessel enters the wall of the viscus. Occasionally, mechanosensitive endings may be present within a solid viscus such as the liver, but they are usually confined to the mesenteric or peritoneal attachments. The endings can occur around veins, when these are not accompanied by arteries, such as along the portal vein as it passes through the pancreas.

Receptors with these properties have been found

throughout the abdomen, along vessels supplying all parts of the gastrointestinal and urogenital tracts, the lymph nodes, spleen, peritoneum and large vessels in cats, dogs and sheep (Bessou and Perl, 1966; Ranieri et al., 1973; Morrison, 1973, 1977, 1980; Floyd and Morrison, 1974; Cervero, 1982; Blumberg et al., 1983; Bahns et al., 1985a,b). About 120–350 Pacinian corpuscles are present in the mesenteries and pancreas of the cat; these sense organs have large myelinated fibres, and are extremely sensitive to vibrations transmitted from outside the animal.

Thermoreceptors and chemoreceptors have also been described in the spinal afferent pathway from viscera (Riedel, 1976; Hardcastle et al., 1978; Recordati et al., 1978, 1980, 1981; Perrin et al., 1981). Little is known of their receptive fields; their properties will be discussed later.

Adaptation

Bessou and Perl (1966) reported that most units adapted rapidly, but Ranieri et al. (1973), Morrison (1973, 1977), Floyd et al. (1976a), Blumberg et al. (1983) and Bahns et al. (1986a,b) found that local pressure usually produced slowly adapting responses. The probing of mechanosensitive sites with forces of 0.1 N or less produces responses which adapt with half-times of 2–8, 20–30 and 200–250 seconds (Morrison, 1977). During distension of viscera, the response of the units depends on the position of the ending with respect to the visceral movement, and adaptation can be rapid, lasting 2–3 seconds (Bessou and Perl, 1966), or slow (Morrison, 1973; Floyd et al., 1976a,b). Blumberg et al. (1983) found that 48% of colonic units adapted to a steady-state discharge, while most of the remainder adapted to the pre-existing resting discharge within 10–30 seconds; only 2% of the units responded by a very rapid, short-lasting burst of activity.

Conduction velocities

Apart from the mesenteric Pacinian corpuscles which have large-diameter axons, the remainder of the mechanoreceptors have fibres with Aδ- and C-fibre conduction velocities. Both groups of fibres are present in the thoraco-lumbar supply to all abdominal viscera (Ranieri et al., 1973; Morrison 1973, 1977; Floyd et al., 1976a; Blumberg et al., 1983; Bahns et al., 1986a,b). Nothing appears to be known about the properties of Aβ-fibres in renal nerves reported by Calaresu et al. (1978), but it seems likely that they originate from Pacinian or Paciniform corpuscles.

The conduction velocities of most sacral visceral afferent fibres which pass through the pelvic nerves and enter the spinal cord through the dorsal roots are also in the Aδ- and C-fibre range. The fastest conducting axons come from the urethra (range, 10–45 m/second; mean $\pm$ S.D., 25.2 $\pm$ 11.2 m/second, n = 12). Sacral afferents from the urinary bladder conduct at 12.7 $\pm$ 9.7 m/second (n = 31). No unmyelinated pelvic fibres responding to distension and contraction of the urinary bladder have been found. Afferents from the anal canal conduct at 9.8 $\pm$ 5 m/second (n = 35) and sacral afferents from the colon are the slowest conducting, some of them being unmyelinated (4.8 $\pm$ 5 m/second, n = 12) (Bahns et al., 1985a).

Most sacral ventral root afferents supplying pelvic organs are unmyelinated (Applebaum et al., 1976; Clifton et al., 1976; Coggeshall and Ito, 1977). Whether or not these fibres are collaterals of visceral neurones which also have a branch in the dorsal roots, is unclear (for further discussion, see p. 92).

Ongoing activity

Thoraco-lumbar visceral afferents

Many papers report that mesenteric Pacinian corpuscles in the cat commonly show cardiovascular rhythms, as might be expected of receptors that are specialised to pick up low-amplitude, high-frequency vibrations (Talaat, 1937; Gernandt and Zotterman, 1946; Winter, 1971; Ranieri et al., 1973). The Aδ- and C-fibre mechanoreceptors in the thoraco-lumbar afferent pathway from the bladder, colon, small intestine, kidney, renal pelvis, liver, billiary tract, the thermoreceptors in the dorsal abdominal wall, and one group of renal chemoreceptors also show ongoing activity. In some units the discharges are not related to any obvious mechanical event of the viscera, while others are modulated by arterial, respiratory or gastrointestinal movements (Talaat, 1937; Bessou and Perl, 1966; Andrews and Palmer, 1967; Beacham and Kunze, 1969; Winter, 1971; Ranieri et al., 1973; Riedel, 1976; Recordati et al., 1980; Cervero, 1982; Blumberg et al., 1983; Bahns et al., 1986a,b). The rhythms probably indicate that sensitive receptors are located near arteries, veins or visceral muscle. In some instances it is possible to modify the rhythm by moving the tissue in which the sensory endings are present. Other rhythms are probably not explained by local movements, e.g., the activity in pre-renal and retroperitoneal receptors (Ranieri et al., 1973; Bahns et al., 1986b).

The rates of ongoing activity vary from 1 spike every 2–10 seconds (Coggeshall and Ito, 1977; Blumberg et al., 1983; Bahns et al., 1986a,b) to 10–25 impulses per second (Ranieri et al., 1973). More than 50% of units exhibit ongoing activity (Bessou and Perl, 1966; Ranieri et al., 1973; Blumberg et al., 1983; Bahns et al., 1986a,b).

It may be argued that the ongoing activity in thoraco-lumbar visceral afferents does not normally occur in physiological (non-painful) conditions, and that it is due to the experimental, surgical and stimulation procedures used. Though the latter cannot be denied completely, there is, at least from some studies, ample evidence showing that the ongoing activity — in its rhythm as well as in its spike rate — also occurs with the visceral organs being in situ in their natural environment, with the peritoneum intact (Floyd et al., 1976b; Morrison, 1977; Blumberg et al., 1983; Bahns et al., 1986a,b).

Sacral visceral afferents

In contrast, there are few reports of ongoing activity in the pelvic nerve afferents. Talaat (1937), Iggo (1955) and Floyd and Lawrenson (1979) did not report any activity. Bahns et al. (1985a,b) did not find any afferent units with ongoing activity from the urinary bladder and urethra, but occasionally observed some from the anus.

Responses to distension and contraction

Mechanical considerations

The response of afferent neurones to distension of viscera has to be considered in relation to the normal capacity and function of the organs. The pressure-volume curves of most viscera show that they are compliant within the physiological range, but that small increases in volume within the supraphysiological range cause pressure to rise sharply. To some extent the gradient of this part of the curve and the volume at which the gradient increases are dependent on the tone of smooth muscle and the actions of its motor nerve supply (Gjone, 1966; Edvardsen, 1968). In addition, the rate of inflation can influence the gradient of the filling phase of the pressure-volume curve, and in normal situations the bladder accomodates to increased volume with little change in intravesical pressure (Klevmark, 1974, 1977). In man, the speed of fast cystometry prevents accomodation from occurring and there is a significant rise in pressure at physiological levels of distension, and the maximum volume subjects can tolerate in these conditions is less than the volume they would normally void (Abrams and Torrens, 1979). Finally, low levels of distension can induce changes in motility in most viscera; sensation is commonly associated with these reflex contractions (Schuster, 1968; Turner-Warwick, 1979), and the size of the contractions and intensity of the sensation increase if the movement of the visceral contents is resisted by some obstruction. Thus, the change from isotonic to isovolumetric recording conditions abolishes flow and increases the pressure developed in the closed system (Mellanby and Pratt, 1940) and the responses of visceral afferents that respond to contractions (Iggo, 1955, 1966). In some viscera the occurrence of contractions can be irregular in time and force, and may be localised, propagated, or involve the whole organ. In isovolumetric conditions, contractions are inevitably accompanied by stretch of in series elastic elements in the viscus, such as elastic tissue or inactive smooth muscle. Thus, during isovolumetric conditions, bladder contractions cause distension of the proximal urethra, and endings opposed to this part of the viscus can be excited by displacement of fluid from the bladder. This local change may be minimal in isotonic conditions, in which there are large changes in the volume of the bladder itself (see Lapides, 1958). Distension of the proximal urethra may be associated with a sensation that micturition is imminent, which is sometimes referred to as urgency.

Urinary bladder and urethra

Distension of the bladder can excite receptors in the pelvic (PN) and hypogastric (HGN) nerves. The urethra is innervated in addition by the pudendal nerve (Todd, 1964; Downie et al., 1984) and the main electrophysiological studies on urethral afferents are by Bahns et al. (1985a,b, 1986a) and Todd (1964).

Pelvic nerve

Fig. 6 shows that several workers have found the range of pressure thresholds in afferents from the bladder to be within the physiological range; attempts to find units with high thresholds have been unsuccessful (Floyd and Lawrenson, 1979, and unpublished data; Bahns et al., 1985a). G. Lawrenson (unpublished data) found that the pressure thresholds all fell on the flat compliant part of the pressure-volume curve, at about 25–75% of the pressure at which the curve became steep. These thresholds are quite consistent with the conditions under which humans report the first sensation of filling during cystometry (Torrens and Abrams, 1979). The stimulus-response relationships during distensions have been examined in conditions which abolish reflex bladder contractions, either by adding 5–20 ml of saline to the viscus every 3–5 minutes (Floyd and Lawrenson, 1979) or by increasing the head of pressure applied to the organ from zero to a constant level for 90 seconds (Bahns et al., 1985a; see also Bahns et al., 1986a). In the former conditions, the relationship between discharge rate and intravesical pressure becomes less steep or plateaus at pressures that correspond to the steep part of the pressure-volume curve. In the latter experiments, spike rate increased almost linearly with rise in pressure. The difference can probably be attributed to adaptation in Floyd and Lawrenson's experiments, as it could take 20 or more minutes to reach high intravesical pressures using that protocol. Slow filling is more physiological than rapid distension (Klevmark, 1974, 1977). Winter (1971) attempted to record from bladder afferents during slow filling. His recordings were from a mixed population of PN and HGN units and were dominated by excitation due to reflex contractions, which occur at low volumes in anaesthetised, but not in awake cats (Klevmark, 1980).

PN afferents can also register the size and timing of bladder contractions (Evans, 1936; Talaat, 1937; Iggo, 1955, 1966; Arlhac, 1971; Winter, 1971; Floyd and Lawrenson, 1979; Bahns et al., 1985b). Iggo (1966) reported that the responses during contractions could be variable, due to the relative positions of receptive endings and contracting muscle, and that the responses were larger in isovolumetric than in isotonic conditions. By changing from isotonic to isovolumetric recording conditions during a contraction, Mellanby and Pratt (1940) observed a marked increase in intravesical pressure, which was accompanied, in Iggo's experiments (1955, 1966), by a marked increase in the rate of discharge of PN afferents. In humans, these conditions are simulated during rapid voluntary interruption of micturition; Turner-Warwick (1979) reports that under these conditions a sensation of desire to void occurs as soon as urine flow stops and lasts until the smooth muscle of the bladder relaxes.

The thresholds of PN afferents during bladder contractions have been studied by Bahns et al. (1985b), using irregular contractions that occurred either spontaneously or were evoked. The thresholds were within the range 5–15 mmHg (see Fig. 6). These thresholds are within the physiological range for contractions: during micturition in normal humans the bladder pressure reaches 30–40 mmHg. Morrison (1981) reported that sympathetic stimulation could reduce the responses of PN afferents and of spontaneous bladder contractions in the cat. It is clear that PN afferents provide the cord with accurate information concerning the size and timing of bladder contractions.

All of the PN recordings mentioned above were from myelinated fibres, and the only reports of unmyelinated bladder afferents that enter the sacral cord were from Applebaum et al. (1976) and Coggeshall and Ito (1977) in sacral ventral roots. However, it must be kept in mind that they determined the conduction velocities between two pairs of recording electrodes which were positioned about 4–8 mm apart at the ventral root filaments. Thus, it might well be that some of their unmyelinated units were branches of myelinated fibres. The majority of their units responded to distensions, but not to contractions; however, a few responded to both. The receptive fields of these units were not investigated and may have been extravesical; also, no information on stimulus-response relations is available for these units.

Hypogastric nerve

Recent work on HGN afferents from the bladder suggests that they behave similarly to those in the PN (Floyd et al., 1976a; Morrison, 1981; Bahns et al., 1986). In these studies, 50% of afferent units had thresholds of 8–15 mmHg (see Fig. 6). Earlier studies by Talaat (1937) suggested the presence of high-threshold afferents, but these recordings were complicated by previous denervation of the PN supply to the bladder, and by the lack of unitary recordings: Talaat's conclusions about HGN afferents were based on studies of "slow waves" that he observed at high volumes. The stimulus-response relationship during contractions is linear (Floyd et al., 1976a; Bahns et al., 1986a); contractions have been studied either by stimulating the sacral cord after a transection at L6, so as to obtain an adapted discharge rate at a constant intravesical pressure, or by observing responses to irregular contractions, produced during recovery from spinal anaesthesia. No functional differences were observed between the Aδ- and C-fibre populations in the HGN, except that the spike rates in the latter group were lower.

Colon and anus

Pelvic nerve

Little information is available about the sacral afferent pathway from the colon, and most of that derives from studies of ventral root afferents. Threshold pressures of 11 mmHg upwards have been reported, and some units were insensitive to distension (Clifton et al., 1976; Coggeshall and Ito, 1977; Floyd et al., 1976c; Morrison and McMahon, 1982). U. Halsband and W. Jänig (unpublished data) have recently found that colonic afferents in S1 and S2 dorsal roots usually have thresholds of 20–40 mmHg.

The mucosal skin of the anus is supplied by sacral afferent fibres that pass through the pelvic nerves and dorsal roots. These afferents have unique functional properties, probably indicating their special role in eliciting reflexes and sensations. They respond vigorously to mechanical shearing stimuli of the mucosal skin and less vigorously or not at all to distension and noxious stimuli (Bahns et al., 1985a). This class of spinal visceral afferents appears to be quite distinct from most other types of spinal visceral afferents; exciting them by shearing stimuli elicits most powerful spinal reflexes in lumbar preganglionic "motility-regulating" neurones (Bahr et al., 1986; Bartel et al., 1986).

Hypogastric and lumbar splanchnic nerves

Blumberg et al. (1983) have reported that lumbar splanchnic afferents from the colon usually have thresholds of around 25 mmHg, and the histogram of thresholds tailed off at high pressures, where a few units responded to 50–75 mmHg. Most units showed ongoing activity, and excitation during distension. The units that did not respond probably were postganglionic efferents (they could not be activated by any mechnical or chemical stimulus

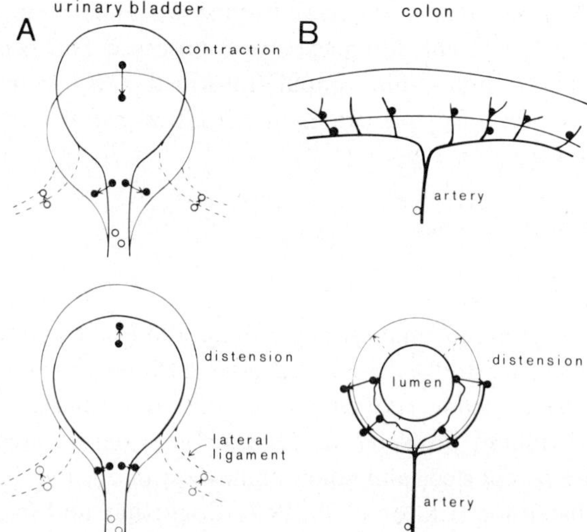

Fig. 5. Change of position of visceral receptors during contraction and distension of visceral organs. Positions of receptors which are excited by these procedures are indicated by dots. Positions of receptors which are not excited or only weakly excited with a few spikes at the beginning of a distension or a contraction are indicated by circles.

(Blumberg et al., 1983; Haupt et al., 1983)) or did not respond because of the position of their receptive field in relation to the distended portion of colon. Many of these units were in the mesentery rather than on the colonic wall. For less than half of the units only, which responded to distension, the receptive fields were localized because of the inaccessibility of one side of the colon. These positional factors may be responsible for the variation between units in their rates of adaptation: four classes were identified according to their behaviour during distensions lasting 60 seconds. Positional factors may also be responsible for the low slope of some of the stimulus-response curves from this organ shown in Fig. 6. Fig. 5B indicates some of the mechanical changes that occur during distension of the colon that affect the transmission of forces to receptive endings.

The studies of Floyd et al. (1976a), Morrison (1977, 1982) and Blumberg et al. (1983) suggest that the thresholds of these units during contractions are low, and that the units respond to spontaneous peristaltic contractions; no stimulus-response curves are available however.

Biliary tract

Reports on the effects of distension of the biliary tract on spinal afferents have been made by Morrison (1981) in the cat and Cervero (1982, 1983) in

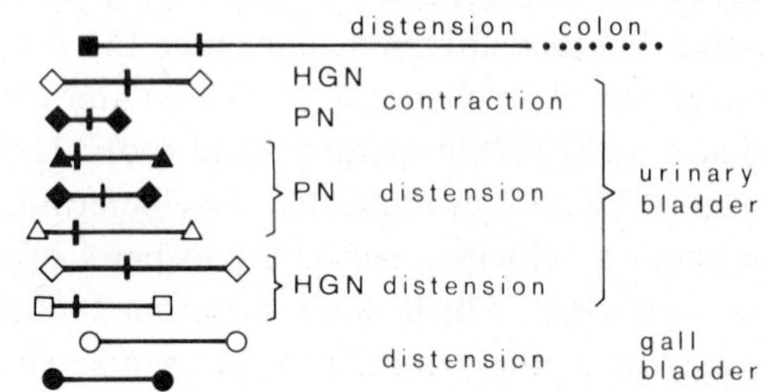

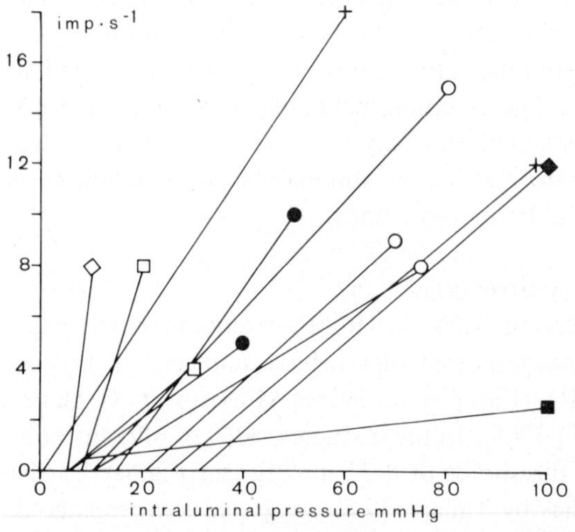

Fig. 6. Thresholds and stimulus-response relations of thoracolumbar and pelvic visceral afferents to contraction and distension of colon, urinary bladder and gallbladder. Upper part: range of thresholds of primary afferents to distension and contraction. The medians are indicated by the vertical bars. HGN, hypogastric nerve; PN, pelvic nerve. Data from: colon (■), Blumberg et al. (1983); HGN (□), Floyd et al. (1976a), (◇), Bahns et al. (1986a); PN (◆), Bahns et al. (1985b), (▲), Talaat (1937), (△), Morrison (1981); gallbladder (○), Cervero (1983), (●), Morrison (1980). Lower part: representative simplified stimulus-response relations of visceral afferent units from urinary bladder, colon and gallbladder to distension. +, pelvic nerve units to colon distension (Morrison, 1982), otherwise symbols as above.

the ferret. The published data indicated thresholds in the range 5–20 mmHg and stimulus-response curves that were not dissimilar to those from other viscera (see Fig. 6). Units along the portal vein and bile duct did not always respond to a rise in biliary pressure, probably because of their position. Cervero divided his units into low- and high-threshold groups depending on the relationship of the activity of his units to opening of the sphincter of Oddi or to a rise in arterial pressure. Little information was provided about the absolute pressures necessary for activation, and the data used in Fig. 6 are taken from one of Cervero's figures. We can see no clear reason for attempting to divide these units into separate groups as they represent, in our view, different parts of the spectrum of properties shown by afferents from most viscera. These variable properties can be attributed to differences in compliance of the tissues, and to differences in the position of receptive endings. In Morrison's (1981) report, some endings that responded to an increase in venous pressure also gave meagre responses at high biliary tract pressures, and this is again probably due to the position of the endings rather than to basic differences in transducer function.

Stomach and small intestine

It is clear that some afferent units in these viscera have thresholds as low as 5–8 mmHg, although many small intestinal units need at least 25 mmHg, to be excited; they have not been studied as systematically as those innervating the bladder and colon. Ranieri et al. (1973) found that afferents from the stomach discharge during the rising phase of, or throughout, gastric contractions. Units in the lesser omentum and diaphragmatic surface can also be activated by gastric movements, either because of spread of forces into local structures or because of friction between peritoneal surfaces. In the small intestine, peristaltic movements also excite spinal afferents (Gernandt and Zotterman, 1946; Bessou and Perl, 1966; Ranieri et al., 1973).

Ureter and renal pelvis

At the upper end of the ureter and at the renal hilum there is a dense plexus of nerves (Gosling, 1969, 1970; Dixon and Gosling, 1971). Beacham and Kunze (1969) found sensitive mechanoreceptors that responded to increased venous pressure or ureteric pressure at this site. The thresholds for venous pressure could be as low as a few mmHg, but were usually greater than 15 mmHg for ureteric pressure. At the lower end of the ureter sensitive mechanoreceptors can respond phasically to increases in bladder pressure (Floyd et al., 1976a) and sometimes to the passage of a peristaltic wave along the ureter (E. Bahns and W. Jänig, unpublished observations).

Tension on mesenteries; vascular factors

Most workers agree that the application of forces that distort the mesentery and its perivascular endings causes a discharge whose intensity is related to the force applied (Bessou and Perl, 1966; Ranieri et al., 1973; Morrison, 1973, 1977; Blumberg et al., 1983; Bahns et al., 1986a). Forces of a few tens of mN are necessary to activate the endings, and the stimulus-response curves are approximately linear; Floyd and Lawrenson (1979) reported thresholds of 0.007–0.4 N/mm in the bladder and colon. It is not surprising that sensitive receptors within a compliant structure, such as the mesentery, respond to local forces produced by biological events, such as repiratory movement (Andrews and Palmer, 1967; Morrison, 1973; Ranieri et al., 1973; Cervero, 1982), arterial pulsation (Bessou and Perl, 1966; Morrison, 1973, 1977; Ranieri et al., 1973; Bahns et al., 1986b), venous distension (Andrews and Palmer, 1967; Beacham and Kunze, 1969; Morrison, 1973, 1980) or gastrointestinal movement (Bessou and Perl, 1966; Morrison, 1973; Ranieri et al., 1973; Blumberg et al., 1983), depending on the position of the ending. They often show ongoing activity that is modulated by these events (see above). Some also respond to sliding of one peritoneal surface over another.

Sensitivity to chemicals

Injection of bradykinin (BK), one of the most potent algogenic substances known to man, into the peritoneal cavity or the splenic artery produces pseudoaffective reflexes and antinociceptive actions in animals (Lim, 1960, 1970; Lim et al., 1962, 1964, 1967; Le Bars et al., 1979). The peptide is known to excite fine myelinated or unmyelinated afferents that may be involved in nociceptive functions from skin, muscle and viscera (Beck and Handwerker, 1974; Uchida and Murao, 1974; Franz and Mense, 1975; Handwerker, 1976; Floyd et al., 1977; Kumazawa and Mizumura, 1977, 1980; Mense, 1977, 1985; Nishi et al., 1977; Baker et al., 1980; Lombardi et al., 1981; Haupt et al., 1983; Bahns et al., 1986b) and also afferent fibres that are probably not involved in nociception (Fjällbrandt and Iggo, 1961; Beck and Handwerker, 1974).

Floyd et al. (1977), Haupt et al. (1983) and Bahns et al. (1986b) found that mechanoreceptive afferent units from the bladder, colon, uterus, pancreas, spleen, small intestinal mesentery and peritoneal lining of the posterior abdominal wall were usually excited by BK, administered intra-arterially or by superfusion of the receptor site. No Aδ- or C-fibre afferents were found that showed chemosensitivity without mechanosensitivity, but this view is not held by Longhurst et al. (1984), who maintain that visceral afferent C-fibres in the thoracic white rami that responds to BK are not mechanosensitive. Their A-fibre population must have included Pacinian corpuscles as the range of conduction velocities was up to 84 m/second.

It seems likely that BK can have some direct action on at least some visceral nerve endings, because superfusion of mesenteric receptors with the drug causes excitation. However, muscular contraction probably plays a part in most situations, and in some viscera, such as the bladder, the responses to BK are reduced or abolished if contractions are prevented from occurring (Floyd et al., 1977). Paralysis of the colon, however, does not abolish the response to BK (Haupt et al., 1983).

Other intraperitoneal chemical stimuli, such as KCl, HCl, acetic acid and hypertonic saline, elicit pupillary dilatation in chloralosed cats and writhing in rats (Downman et al., 1948; Giesler and Liebeskind, 1976; Le Bars et al., 1979). Haupt et al. (1983) found that lumbar colonic afferents responded to intra-arterial KCl by producing short-lasting, high-frequency bursts, particularly if the units exhibited ongoing activity in the absence of external stimuli, whereas hypertonic saline (injected intra-arterially) had little effect. The effects on the units were highly correlated with their responses to colonic distension and BK. Schmitt (1973) reported that the portal injection of hypertonic solutions modulated the discharge of hypothalamic neurones in rats, and depended on a splanchnic afferent pathway. More than 90% of lumbar afferent units from vessels, nerves, lymph nodes, fat and parietal peritoneum responded to local application of hypertonic NaCl solution (4.5 or 9%) and about 75% responded to local KCl (60 and 155 mmol/l) (Bahns et al., 1985b).

Beacham and Kunze (1969) recorded from renal nerve afferents in the cat and found that they responded to small elevations of renal venous pressure (1–2 mmHg) and to increasing ureteral pressure by more than 15 mmHg. These units, like the renal "baroreceptors" described by Niijima (1971, 1972, 1975), also responded to probing the renal hilum, and appeared to be mechanoreceptors: the relationship between these units and the renal chemoreceptors in the rat is unclear (Recordati et al., 1978, 1980, 1981). One group of renal chemoreceptors (Recordati et al., 1980) are excited by backflow of non-diuretic urine into the renal pelvis, apparently because of a change in the chemical composition of the renal interstitium produced by ions crossing the papillary epithelium, leakage from ischaemic cells, or alterations in renal blood flow or excretion of fluid and electrolytes. These units show ongoing activity in the non-diuretic state and respond to elevation of ureteral pressure, apparently by modifying the chemical environment around the nerve endings. However, Recordati et al. (1980) appear not to have tested directly for mechanosensitivity, and it is unclear whether they accept the existence of a separate population of renal mechanoreceptors or whether they believe that all units that respond to raised ureteric pressure are specific chemoreceptors.

Temperature and ischaemia

Heating the wall of the small intestine to over 46°C dilates the pupil of the chloralosed cat and elicits an intestino-intestinal inhibitory reflex (Chang and Hsu, 1942; Downman et al., 1948). The sensitivity of spinal visceral afferents to thermal stimuli has not been studied in detail, but mechanosensitive units in the retroperitoneal space which respond to local application of BK, KCl and hypertonic saline may also respond to heat stimuli of more than 42–44°C (Bahns et al., 1986b). Thus, responses to intra-abdominal heating need not depend on a specific group of afferent units excited by heat.

Intra-abdominal heating to 42–44°C using a thermode causes thermoregulatory changes in sheep, and these can be abolished by splanchnic nerve section (Rawson and Quick, 1970, 1972). The role of these receptors in sensation is unknown, but observations in rabbits have suggested the existence of specific thermoreceptors with unmyelinated fibres in the dorsal abdominal wall. These units were unaffected by mechanical stimuli, and two populations, with static and dynamic maxima at 40 and 46°C, respectively, were identified (Riedel, 1976).

The effects of ischaemia on spinal afferents have been studied in the colon and in the kidney. Haupt et al. (1983) found that colonic units that responded to distension and to BK were also excited by ischaemia; a bursting pattern of discharge was induced, and potentiation of the reponse to colonic distension was observed, along with an increase in cardiovascular reflex effects of distension and BK. Recordati et al. (1980) found renal receptors that were insensitive to changes in arterial, venous or ureteral pressure, but were excited by renal ischaemia. These endings produced bursts of impulses during occlusion of the renal artery, severe hypotension or prolonged renal venous stasis.

Sensations and visceral afferent activity

Types of pain and other sensations elicited from viscera

Some perceived visceral sensations provide relatively precise information upon which the brain can act and initiate an appropriate behaviour. The information relayed by a relatively small number of afferents from the lower urogenital and gastrointestinal tracts confers the ability to distinguish not only between fullness of different viscera, e.g., the bladder or rectum, or between the presence of flatus or faeces in the latter, or between different stages of sexual activity, but also to assess to some extent the degree of filling of one of the reservoir organs. The site, intensity, timing and nature of these normal visceral stimuli can be perceived. Certain stimuli, such as heat, do not elicit sensation, when applied to the bladder (Nathan, 1952b). In contrast, during overdistension, discomfort or overt pain occur, and differ in that they are vague and diffusely localized (usually), and the source of the pain commonly has to be deduced from observations of how the pain changes with different motor acts, such as defaecation or micturition. On the first occurrence of a visceral pain, the patient has no framework of reference to decide on its origin: the site of the pain often bears no relation to the site of the organ from which it originates. The pain is described as abdominal rather than visceral, and the patient has usually to rely on a trained observer to discern the source of the pain; that diagnosis depends, at least partly, on an understanding of the peripheral organisation of spinal visceral afferent pathways. Therefore, visceral pain is a diagnosis rather than a symptom.

The relationship between the location of true visceral sensation and segmental innervation

Figs. 3 and 4 summarise the available information on the size and segmental distribution of the afferent innervation of different viscera in the cat and rat. The density of the spinal innervation of each viscus is maximal in one or two adjacent segments, and there are a few segments of the lower lumbar cord that do not participate in visceral innervation; the somatic structures innervated by these segments, i.e., structures below the knee, are usually not involved in referred pain. In the cat, the peak density of neurones innervating the kidney, colon and bladder occurs in the second, third and fourth lumbar segments, respectively; the colon and bladder are also innervated by sacral afferent neurones that are most numerous in the second sacral segment. In man, the sacral innervation is more caudal, whereas in the rat it is more rostral and extends into the lumbar cord. The afferent innervation of viscera may be entirely unilateral, as in the kidney, predominantly unilateral, as in the liver, or bilateral, as in the colon.

The site of true visceral pain (see Lewis, 1942) appears to be determined by the segmental origin of the afferent innervation of the viscus and its degree of lateralisation; the higher the segmental origin of the afferent fibres, the more rostral the abdominal pain. The importance of these factors was emphasised by White (1943) and White and Sweet (1969). These neurosurgeons transected white rami at different segmental levels to treat pain of visceral origin, and were able to map the distribution of "pain pathways" from the viscera. Fig. 7 summarises the denervations that were necessary to relieve pain originating from different viscera. The major afferent pathways that subserve pain from a viscus enter the cord in a relatively small group of segments, the distribution of which is remarkably similar to those that are principally concerned with the afferent innervation of the viscus in the cat or rat (Figs. 3 and 4), given minor rostro-caudal adjustments in the different species. In the case of the colon, the lumbar denervations were insufficient to relieve pain, probably due to the integrity of the sacral innervation of this viscus. Ruch (1979) describes a "pelvic pain line" which delineates viscera, in which pain sensation depends on a sacral afferent pathway. This concept, based largely on the work of White (1943), is quite consistent with modern neurosurgical experience; Torrens and Hald (1979) report that a selective neurectomy in the third sacral segment in man abolished painful frequency and urgency in patients whose lower urinary tract physiology had been well investigated. Pain arising from viscera that receive an afferent supply from lumbar and sacral segments may be located both suprapubically (upper lumbar innervation) and in the perineum (sacral innervation). Distension of balloons in the upper, middle and lower thirds of the gastrointestinal tract gives rise to pain above, around or below the umbilicus (Lipkin and Sleisenger, 1958). These pains are usually felt in the midline, either in the front or, less commonly, in the back of the abdomen. However, if the innervation of the viscus is entirely from one side of the cord, the sensation is ipsilateral; viscera that are innervated mainly from one side tend also to give rise to pain on the side of the body that has the greatest innervation. Evidence that the degree of lateralisation of the innervation determines the side of the abdomen in which pain is perceived comes from experiments on humans who have the afferent pathway from the viscera sectioned surgically on one

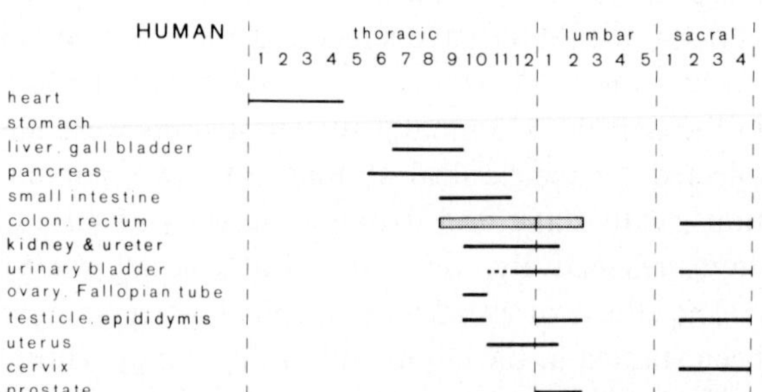

Fig. 7. Relief of visceral pain by transection of white rami and sacral dorsal roots. Section of the number of white rami and sacral dorsal roots indicated by the length of the black horizontal lines. The stippled area indicates the lesions which did not relieve colonic pain, presumably due to the integrity of the sacral innervation. From White (1943) and White and Sweet (1969).

side of the body: in these patients, distension of the jejunum gives rise to pain, not in the midline as would occur in normal individuals, but on the side of the body that still receives afferent information from the viscus (Bentley and Smithwick, 1940). In normal individuals some viscera are innervated mainly from one side of the spinal cord, and the distribution of visceral pain is lateralised. Thus, kidney pain is invariably lateralised to the loin or flank, and biliary tract pain is commonly lateralised to the right upper quadrant (Gaensler, 1951; Risholm, 1954). (Two-thirds of the spinal innervation of the liver and biliary tract in the rat is from the right side of the cord.) Pain referred from the biliary tract to the right shoulder tip can also be explained by the innervation of the biliary tract from the right phrenic nerve (Hazarika et al., 1964). Thus, the site of abdominal pain that arises from a viscus depends partly on the level of the spinal segments that innervate the viscus, and the degree of lateralisation of that nerve supply.

The involvement of sacral as well as thoracolumbar spinal segments in visceral pain mechanisms can also be deduced from studies of the distribution of cutaneous hyperalgesia, deep tenderness and referred pain in visceral disease (see McKenzie, 1909; Lewis, 1942). Fig. 8 shows the distribution of cutaneous hyperalgesia (Head, 1893), deep tenderness (Hansen, 1963) and the distribution of referred pain

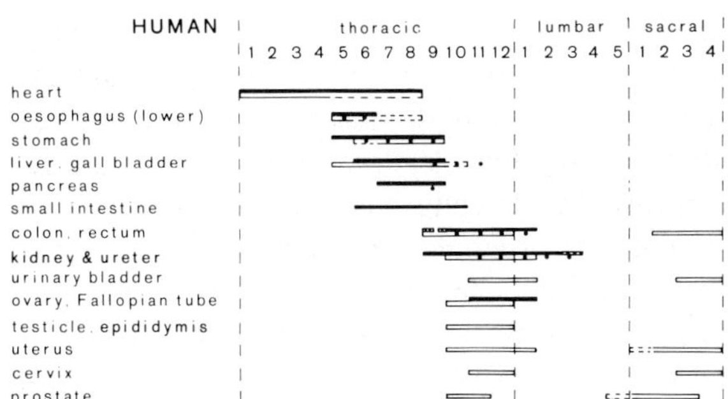

Fig. 8. Segmental distribution of cutaneous and subcutaneous hyperalgesia occurring spontaneously or elicited by pressure, and of tenderness during affection of visceral organs. Solid bars, Hansen (1963); open bars, Head (1893); dots, relief of referred pain by paravertebral blocks (from Flowers and Kappis, in Hansen, 1963; Läwen, 1922, 1923).

that could be abolished by cutting different spinal roots (see Flowers and Kappis, in Hansen, 1963). The similarity of these distributions with those known to mediate true visceral pain (Fig. 7) is remarkable.

The relation between sensation, reflexes and afferent activity: adequate stimuli

Fig. 9 summarises the available information on the levels of distending pressures that evoke innocuous and noxious sensations in man, and reflex activity in spinal afferent neurones in animals, principally cats. There can be considerable variation in different reports, which seems to depend on the methodology employed; e.g., the thresholds depend on the time for which distension is applied (Lipkin and Sleisenger, 1958), the length of the distended segment (of bowel) (Peterson and Youmans, 1945) and the occurrence of reflex contractions (Payne and Poulton, 1923; Denny-Brown and Robertson, 1933: Schuster, 1968). This figure demonstrates the differences in regional sensitivity to visceral distension that were demonstrated by Irving et al. (1937) in the chloralosed cat, and by other workers who studied sensory thresholds in man. Sensitivity to distension decreases in the following order: pylorus, biliary tract, upper ureter, oesophagus, colon, small intestine and terminal ileum. The extent to which these regional differences in sensitivity depend upon the density of innervation of the organs is unknown. The terminal ileum and middle ureter are apparently insensitive to pressures of 100–200 mmHg (Irving et al., 1937; Risholm, 1954). The position of the urethra in this sequence is unclear: the urethral sphincter normally exerts a pressure of 80–100 cm H_2O, and distension of the proximal urethra with 100 cm H_2O in Denny-Brown and Robertson's (1933) experiments did not elicit sensation. As a general rule, the reflex thresholds are less than the noxious sensory thresholds, and can be as low as the innocuous sensory threshold in viscera such as the bladder and colon. The latter is not surprising since numerous investigators have noted

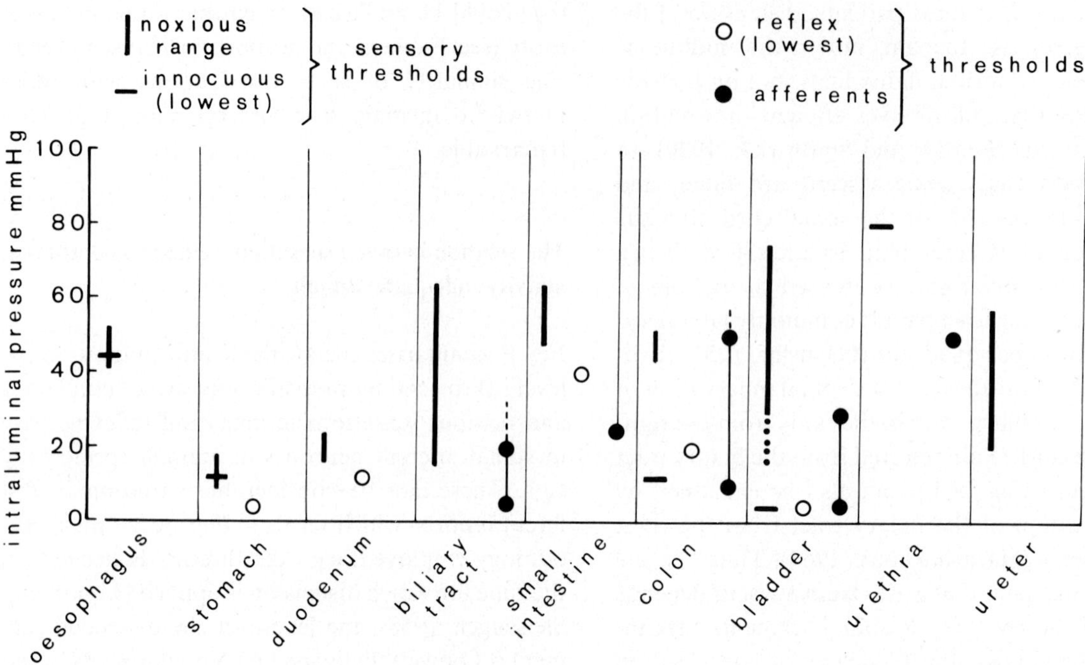

Fig. 9. Summary of data on intraluminal pressures that elicit innocuous and noxious sensations in humans, pupillary and visceral reflexes, and excitation of spinal afferents from viscera. Data on innocuous and noxious sensations in humans from: Payne and Poulton (1923), Denny-Brown and Robertson (1933, 1935), Gaensler (1951), Nathan (1952a, 1956), Risholm (1954), Lipkin and Sleisenger (1958), Murphy and Schoenberg (1960), Scott et al. (1964), Code and Carlson (1968), Cohen and Wolff (1968), Hightower (1968), Schuster (1968). Data on pupillary and visceral reflexes from: Irving et al. (1937), Ravdin et al. (1942), Youmans (1944), Peterson and Youmans (1945), Abrahamsson (1973), Floyd et al. (1982), McMahon and Morrison (1982), McMahon et al. (1982). Data on excitation of spinal afferents from viscera from: Floyd et al. (1976), Morrison (1980, 1981, 1982), Cervero (1982, 1983), Blumberg et al. (1983), Bahns et al. (1986a), Bahns, unpublished observation.

the occurrence of sensation in association with contractions (see later). The thresholds of the afferent units in cats, and the "specific nociceptors" from the biliary tract in ferrets (Cervero, 1982) were usually below the range of noxious thresholds reported in man. These interpretations depend on the assumption that no species differences occur between cats and humans with respect to these thresholds: the parallel nature of the regional variations in cats and humans suggests that they may be similar. In the absence of good behavioural data on animals, the choice is between this correlation: observations on cardiovascular reflexes in animals (see Cervero, 1982) or measurements of the visceral pressure that is necessary to induce DNIC-like (diffuse noxious inhibitory control) activity (see Lumb, this volume).

Most visceral receptors are directly or indirectly associated with smooth muscles of the gastrointestinal and urogenital tracts and vascular system: contraction of smooth muscle can modulate the excitability or may lead to excitation of visceral receptors, by changing visceral compliance or by altering the spatial arrangement of receptive structures and smooth muscles (see Fig. 3). These muscles are controlled by extrinsic sympathetic and/or parasympathetic nerves, and — as far as the gastrointestinal tract is concerned — by the activity of neurones in the enteric nervous system. Thus, the excitability of many visceral receptors not only depends on the adequate stimuli acting in the periphery and on the "tone" and activity of smooth muscle, but also on extrinsic and intrinsic neuronal ac-

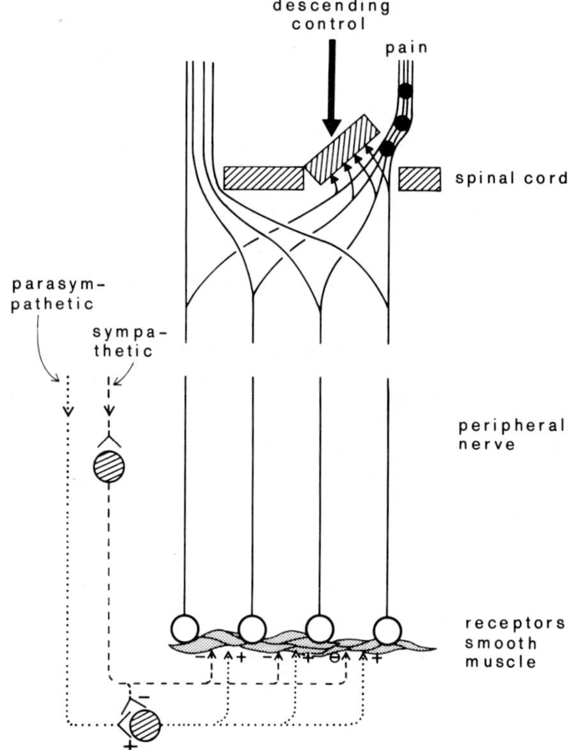

Fig. 10. Functional scheme on the interposition of most spinal visceral afferent neurones between peripheral visceral tissues and the second-order neurones in the spinal cord. At the level of the receptors, the excitation of the afferent neurones depends not only on the adequate physical and chemical stimuli but also indirectly on the activity of the extrinsic and intrinsic autonomic nervous systems and on the state of the smooth muscles (viscero-elastic properties, myogenic activity). The central decoding process of spinal visceral afferent information, for inducing sensations and reflexes, is indicated by a hypothetical gating mechanism. This mechanism must not be restricted to the spinal cord and may consist of multiple gates. For details see text.

tivity (see Fig. 10) (Iggo, 1955, 1966; Morrison, 1977, 1981; Blumberg et al., 1983; Bahns et al., 1986b). The role of the inhibitory efferent supply to the viscera in suppressing sensations of desire to void (McDowall, 1960), for example, is not known, but it cannot be assumed that the sites of interactions which exert some control over visceral sensation occur only within the central nervous system. Furthermore, since activities such as micturition and defaecation are separated by hours or days, it would need receptors that show extremely slow adaptation to monitor the fullness of viscera on a continuous basis; it is possible that voluntary or involuntary contractions play a part in bringing receptors into action in such a way as to allow the degree of distension to be sensed, possibly by comparing afferent activity with the efferent command signal, in a manner similar to that proposed for proprioception (McCloskey, 1981). Thus, contractions need not be regarded simply as reflex events, and could play a part in eliciting visceral sensation.

The top of the range of pressures exerted during spontaneous contractions of viscera may exceed the bottom of the range of noxious sensory thresholds, e.g., in the colon. These contractions are of short duration, and the thresholds given are the minimum pressures that can elicit pain after a period in excess of 20 seconds (Lipkin and Sleisenger, 1958). Contractions accompanied by movement of visceral contents or voiding may not sustain an adequate level of receptor excitation for a long enough period to elicit sensation, but there is little doubt that contractions of viscera themselves evoke sensations that may be uncomfortable, e.g., colic (Payne and Poulton, 1923; Connel et al., 1965; Schuster, 1968). During normal micturition, the isotonic contraction causes intravesical pressure to rise to around 30 mmHg (Murphy and Schoenberg, 1960; Shah, 1984). Voluntary interruption of voiding when the bladder is half full gives rise to a sensation of desire to void until sufficient time has passed for the detrusor to relax (Turner-Warwick, 1979). Isovolumetric contractions, however, give rise to severe pain if the bladder is overdistended (Denny-Brown and Robertson, 1933). In contrast, high pressures can occur in the bladder during micturition, say as a consequence of outlet obstruction, but these pressures do not elicit pain; in these circumstances intravesical pressure may rise to over 90 cm H_2O during voiding, the bladder muscle is often hypertrophied, and the lack of sensation may be due to a change in the compliance of the viscus (see Shah, 1984).

One of the commonest sensory disturbances involving the lower urinary tract is the urge syndrome, characterised by either a constant desire to void, or a desire to void at low bladder volumes, and occurring particularly in women. In some of these patients the sensation is associated with involuntary detrusor contractions, whereas in others the sensations are not accompanied by any abnormality that can be demonstrated by bacteriological, radiological, urodynamic or endoscopic investigation (Mundy and Stephenson, 1984). Pain is uncommon in this condition, and the patho-physiological basis of the sensation of urgency is uncertain. In some patients the sensation of urgency occurs when the urethra relaxes and becomes distended, sometimes at low pressure (McGuire, 1984). This aetiology could be associated with the activation of endings outside the urethra itself during the distension that accompanied muscular relaxation. Therefore, the possibility exists that some of the sensations that can be elicited from the lower urinary tract may be due to excitation of localized groups of receptors.

Encoding of events in the visceral domain by spinal visceral afferents

Spinal visceral afferents supplying abdominal and pelvic organs are involved in a variety of functions: neural regulation of continence or evacuation of the bladder or colon, reflexes (viscero-visceral, viscero-somatic) and sensations (painful and non-painful). The messages which trigger these diverse activities must be derived entirely from the information passed to the central nervous system by visceral afferent pathways, and we have to address the problem of how central neurones decode these messages in order to elicit appropriate reflexes, sensations and behaviours. Does any part of the decoding process depend on differentation of visceral afferent neurones with respect to different (adequate) stimuli? Can we, as quasi-objective observers, classify the spinal visceral afferent neurones according to their discharge characteristics and assign them hypothetically to different functions? If not, how are different visceral events encoded by afferents? These questions will now be discussed, and particular attention will be paid to events which are potentially painful.

The spinal cord extracts information about events in viscera by way of (1) the segmental organisation of the afferent inflows from various target organs (see Figs. 3, 4 and 7), (2) the discharge patterns in the visceral afferents initiated by naturally occurring stimuli, and (3) there may be preprogrammed specific synaptic connections between visceral primary afferents and spinal second-order neurones; there may be special biochemical mechanisms (in which the neuropeptides may be involved) which regulate the establishment and maintenance of these functional synaptic connections. The first point is well established and does not require further discussion. The segmental width of the visceral afferent inflow from the organs finds its counterpart in the inaccuracy of the projected true visceral sensations. The third point, as interesting as it may be, is pure speculation and cannot be supported by experimental evidence.

The second point does deserve some special discussion: from the experimental studies which have been reviewed in this paper, it appears likely that the spinal afferent supply to the pelvic and abdominal viscera is, cum grano salis, functionally homogeneous. This may also apply to the spinal visceral afferent innervation of thoracic organs (Malliani, 1982, this volume; see Bahns et al., 1985b). Possibly not included are the afferent fibres of mesenteric Pacinian corpuscles (Gammon and Bronk, 1935), pelvic nerve afferents from the anal canal (Bahns et al., 1985a), lumbar and pelvic afferents from the urethra (Bahns et al., 1985b, 1986a) and thoracic afferents from the oesophagus. These afferent neurones probably serve very special sensory and other functions, and therefore exhibit distinct discharge characteristics to applied stimuli. The function of mesenterial Pacinian corpuscles is presumably concerned with sensing transmitted vibration.

Functional homogeneity means that no subdivision of the visceral afferents into functionally homogeneous types can be made on the basis of their discharge patterns or other properties, such as the stimulus-response relations to natural stimuli (distension and contraction, see Fig. 6), the distributions of the thresholds to natural stimuli, the ongoing activity, responses to chemical stimuli and the distribution of the conduction velocity of the axons. The studies which have tried to establish a subclassification of spinal visceral afferents into those with nociceptive function and those with other functions (gallbladder: Cervero, 1982; heart: Baker et al., 1980) are probably open to alternative interpretations. Afferents from the gallbladder that respond to high distending pressures may either be the extreme cases of a continuous spectrum of afferent thresholds or their mechanosensitive sites might not have been situated in the wall of the viscus, but close by (see Morrison, 1980; Blumberg et al., 1983; Bahns et al., 1986a,b). The same arguments may apply to the small percentage of spinal visceral afferents from the heart and large thoracic vessels which Baker et al. (1980) claimed to have primarily nociceptive function: these afferents had irregular ongoing activity, high thresholds to mechanical probing and responded vigorously to local application of bradykinin. Though the point of Baker et al. (1980) cannot be refuted, it appears to us that this small fraction of afferents designated as "nociceptive" merely exhibits some minor quantitative differences, in their reactions to the stimuli used, from the so-called "cardiovascular" spinal visceral afferents.

If no functional subclassification of spinal visceral afferents can be made, it must be concluded that the reflexes, regulations and sensations associated with a viscus are produced by the excitation of the same population of visceral afferents, and that no specialised function can be assigned to subpopulations of visceral spinal afferents. This means that these afferents cannot be labelled functionally as "nociceptive" (Baker et al., 1980; Cervero, 1982), "micturition" or "defaecation", etc., but only according to the viscus that is innervated.

A subclassification of visceral receptors based partly on gross anatomy and partly on function has arisen by default, as a result of the historical development of information about visceral afferents; many investigators studied the innervation of individual viscera rather than visceral afferents as a group, and many of the descriptions refer to nerves that sense changes in the state of one viscus. Thus, the movement receptors of the small intestine (Bessou and Perl, 1966), the "in series" tension receptors in the bladder (Iggo, 1955), the specific nociceptors in the biliary tract (Cervero, 1982), the cardiovascular receptors (Malliani, 1982), the renal baroreceptors (Niijima, 1971, 1972, 1975), the adrenal baroreceptors (Niijima and Winter, 1968), the portal venous receptors (Andrews and Palmer, 1967), the renal venous receptors (Beacham and Kunze, 1969), the gastric and mesenteric receptors (Ranieri et al., 1973), and the colonic and retroperitoneal receptors (Blumberg et al., 1983; Bahns et al., 1986a) have been regarded as quite separate functional groups. Indeed, they are separate groups in that they innervate structures with different functions. The differences between receptors that exist in these structures can probably be explained by regional variations in the structures themselves, e.g., in compliance, the amount of smooth muscle present, and the position of receptive endings relative to the viscus will also modify the responses of units. Nevertheless, the results shown in Fig. 6 show a remarkable similarity between the ranges of pressure thresholds of afferents from different abdominal viscera. The unimodal nature of the distribution of thresholds and the fact that the majority of units have stimulus-response functions that cover the normal and supra-normal ranges of visceral pressures point to the existence of a fairly uniform population of receptors in the viscera. No systematic differences appear to exist between Aδ- and C-fibre afferents. Furthermore, the conclusion that there is no substantial evidence for a functional subdivision of spinal visceral afferents means that the specificity theory in its classical sense (see Fig. 1) does not hold for spinal visceral afferents. Therefore, the spinal cord must extract its important information from the intensity of discharge in the visceral primary afferent population. Therefore, we conclude that the "intensity theory" or "summation hypothesis" (Goldscheider, 1920; see Fig. 1) must be applied to spinal visceral afferents.

Fig. 9 summarises the data on sensory and reflex thresholds to visceral distension in man and the cat, and of afferent thresholds in the cat and ferret. The afferent thresholds are lower than the noxious sensory thresholds, and often less than the reflex thresholds. There is some disagreement in the literature regarding the innocuous and noxious sensory thresholds in the oesophagus and stomach, which are probably due to methodological considerations. However, our overall conclusion from Fig. 9 is that noxious sensations are not due to activation of a specific group of visceral receptors, but to a more intense activation of a population of low-threshold receptors, consistent with the electrophysiological evidence presented earlier.

We do not know the actual neuronal mechanisms of central decoding of visceral afferent activity which leads to different sensations, reflexes and regulations (see Nathan, 1952a; Floyd et al., 1982; McMahon and Morrison, 1982; McMahon et al., 1982; McMahon, this volume; Willis, this volume), but it most probably involves neuronal gating processes (see Morrison, 1982). These gates could be influenced by the intensity of discharge in visceral afferent neurones and by various central influences, such as activity in systems which descend from the brainstem, hypothalamus and telencephalon (Fig. 10) and activity in afferents arising from other structures (see Lumb, this volume). The gating mechanism can hardly be explained in the way that Melzack and Wall (1965) and Wall (1978) explained the generation of cutaneous pain in their "gate control theory". The latter theory presupposes the differentiation of the primary afferent inflow into large and small fibres. This differentiation is missing in the visceral domain. However, the gating mechanisms for visceral functions (sensations, reflexes, etc.) may be influenced by afferent inflows from the skin and deep somatic domain (see Cervero and Tattersall, this volume; Lumb, this volume).

Summary

Functional and morphological properties of spinal visceral afferent neurones supplying abdominal and pelvic organs have been reviewed. These neurones are involved in the regulation of visceral functions, in sensations and in various spinal and supraspinal reflexes. Special emphasis has been placed on visceral nociception and pain. (1) Visceral organs in the thoracic abdominal and pelvic cavities of the cat are supplied by about 22,000–25,000 spinal afferent neurones which amounts to about 1.5–2.5% of the total spinal afferent input. Thus, the density of innervation of the viscera by spinal afferents is small when compared to the density of afferent innervation in the skin and probably in many deep somatic tissues. (2) The spatial resolution of the sensations which can be elicited from the viscera is relatively vague and can be fully explained by the segmental width of the afferent inflow from each viscus. (3) Most spinal visceral afferent units have various common functional properties: they are silent or display a low rate of ongoing activity; their axons are unmyelinated or thinly myelinated (conduction velocity below 2 m/second and mostly below 20 m/second, respectively); their receptive fields consist of from one to nine mechanosensitive sites located in the mesenteries, on the serosal surface or in the walls of the organs; local pressure in their receptive fields elicits slowly adapting responses; they respond to distensions and contractions of the viscera and to stretching of their mechanosensitive endings; they respond to various chemical stimuli applied in their receptive fields. (4) Graded distension and contraction of hollow organs (colon, urinary bladder, gallbladder) lead to graded responses of the visceral afferent neurones. The stimulus-response relationships and distributions of intraluminal threshold pressures for the afferent units show that the thoraco-lumbar and sacral visceral afferents from the hollow organs are largely homogeneous. No distinct population of high-threshold afferents which would qualify as "visceral nociceptive" could be separated from the whole population of spinal visceral afferents. (5) Afferents from mesenteric Pacinian corpuscles have been excluded from this consideration of visceral afferents. Their function in the viscera is not very well understood, and there is considerable variation in their numbers in different species. Furthermore, spinal afferent neurones that supply the distal parts of the urinary and gastrointestinal tract (urethra and anus), and the oesophagus may show some functional specialisation. (6) The functional homogeneity of the spinal visceral afferent neurones suggests that the same population of afferents encodes various events that give rise to non-nocuous and noxious sensations, a number of reflexes, and to the regulation of viscera. No convincing experimental data exist which justify a subclassification into visceral "nociceptive" and other functional subgroups. It is hypothesised that noxious and innocuous events in the visceral domain are encoded in the intensity of the discharge of the same population of visceral afferent neurones.

Acknowledgements

This work was supported by the Deutsche Forschungsgemeinschaft (F.R.G.) and by the Medical Research Council (U.K.)

References

Abercrombie, M. (1945) Estimation of nuclear population from microtome sections. Anat. Rec., 94: 239–247.

Abrahamsson, H. (1973) Studies on the inhibitory nervous control of gastric motility. Acta Physiol. Scand. Suppl., 390: 5–38.

Abrams, P. and Torrens, M. (1979) Cystometry. In R. Turner-Warwick and C. G. Whiteside (Eds.), Clinical Urodynamics, The Urological Clinics of North America, Vol. 6, W. B. Saunders, Philadelphia, pp. 79–84.

Andrews, W. H. H. and Palmer, J. F. (1967) Afferent nervous discharge from the canine liver. Q. J. Exp. Physiol., 52: 269–276.

Applebaum, M. L., Clifton, G. L., Coggeshall, R. E., Coulter, J. D., Vance, W. H. and Willis, W. D. (1976) Unmyelinated fibres in the sacral 3 and caudal 1 ventral roots of the cat. J. Physiol., 256: 557–572.

Applebaum, A. E., Vance, W. H. and Coggeshall, R. E. (1980) Segmental localization of sensory cells that innervate the bladder. J. Comp. Neurol., 192: 203–209.

Arlhac, A. (1971) Données nouvelles sur la décharge des mécanorécepteurs vésicaux. Pflügers Arch., 333: 258–270.

Bahns, E., Halsband, U. and Jänig, W. (1985a) Functional characteristics of sacral afferent fibres from the urinary bladder, colon and the anus. Pflügers Arch., 405, Suppl. 2: R51.

Bahns, E., Halsband, U. and Jänig, W. (1985b) Reaction of visceral afferents in the pelvic nerve to distension and contraction of the urinary bladder in the cat. Neurosci. Lett., Suppl. 22: S86.

Bahns, E., Ernsberger, U., Jänig, W. and Nelke, A. (1986a) Functional characteristics of lumbar visceral afferent fibres from the urinary bladder and the urethra in the cat. Plügers Arch., in press.

Bahns, E., Ernsberger, U., Jänig, W. and Nelke, A. (1986b) Discharge properties of mechanosensitive afferents supplying the retroperitoneal space. Pflügers Arch., in press.

Bahr, R., Blumberg, H. and Jänig, W. (1981) Do dichotomising afferent fibres exist which supply visceral organs as well as somatic structures? A contribution to the problem of referred pain. Neurosci. Lett., 24: 25–28.

Bahr, R., Bartel, B., Blumberg, H. and Jänig, W. (1986) Functional characterization of preganglionic neurons projecting in the lumbar splanchnic nerves: neurons regulating motility. J. Auton. Nerv. System, 15: 109–130.

Baker, D. G., Coleridge, H. M., Coleridge, J. C. G. and Nerdrum, T. (1980) Search for a cardiac nociceptor: stimulation by bradykinin of sympathetic afferent nerve endings in the heart of the cat. J. Physiol., 306: 519–536.

Baron, R., Jänig, W. and McLachlan, E. M. (1985a) On the anatomical organization of the lumbosacral sympathetic chain and the lumbar splanchnic nerves of the cat — Langley revisited. J. Auton. Nerv. System, 12: 289–300.

Baron, R., Jänig, W. and McLachlan, E. M. (1985b) The afferent and sympathetic components of the lumbar spinal outflow to the colon and pelvic organs in the cat: I. The hypogastric nerve. J. Comp. Neurol., 238: 135–146.

Baron, R., Jänig, W. and McLachlan, E. M. (1985c) The afferent and sympathetic components of the lumbar spinal outflow to the colon and pelvic organs in the cat: II. The lumbar splanchnic nerves. J. Comp. Neurol., 238: 147–157.

Baron, R., Jänig, W. and McLachlan, E. M. (1985d) The afferent and sympathetic components of the lumbar spinal outflow to the colon and pelvic organs in the cat: III. The colonic nerves, incorporating an analysis of all components of the lumbar prevertebral outflow. J. Comp. Neurol., 238: 158–168.

Bartel, B., Blumberg, H. and Jänig, W. (1986) Discharge patterns of motility-regulating neurons projecting in the lumbar splanchnic nerves to visceral stimuli in spinal cats. J. Auton. Nerv. System, 15: 153–163.

Beacham, W. S. and Kunze, D. L. (1969) Renal receptors evoking a spinal vasomotor reflex. J. Physiol., 201: 73–85.

Beck, P. W. and Handwerker, H. O. (1974) Bradykinin and serotonin effects on various types of cutaneous nerve fibres. Pflügers Arch., 347: 209–222.

Bentley, F. H. and Smithwick, R. H. (1940) Visceral pain produced by balloon distension of the jejunum. Lancet, 2: 389–391.

Bessou, P. and Perl, E. R. (1966) A movement receptor of the small intestine. J. Physiol., 182: 404–426.

Blumberg, H., Haupt, P., Jänig, W. and Kohler, W. (1983) Encoding of visceral noxious stimuli in the discharge patterns of visceral afferent fibres from the colon. Pflügers Arch., 398: 33–40.

Borges, L. F. and Moskowitz, M. A. (1983) Do intracranial and extracranial trigemincal afferents represent divergent axon collaterals? Neurosci. Lett., 35: 265–270.

Burgess, P. R. and Perl, E. R. (1973) Cutaneous mechanoreceptors and nociceptors. In A. Iggo (Ed.), Handbook of Sensory Physiology, Vol. II, Somatosensory System, Springer-Verlag, Berlin, pp. 29–78.

Calaresu, F. R., Kim, P., Nakamura, H. and Sato, A. (1978) Electrophysiological characteristics of renorenal reflexes in the cat. J. Physiol., 283: 141–154.

Cervero, F. (1982) Afferent activity evoked by natural stimulation of the biliary system in the ferret. Pain, 13: 137–151.

Cervero, F. (1983) Mechanisms of visceral pain. In S. Lipton and J. Miles (Eds.), Persistent Pain, Vol. 4. Academic Press, London, pp. 1–19.

Cervero, F., Connell, L. A. and Lawson, S. N. (1984) Somatic and visceral primary afferents in the lower thoracic dorsal root ganglia of the cat. J. Comp. Neurol., 228: 422–431.

Chang, P. Y. and Hsu, F. Y. (1942) The localization of the intestinal inhibitory reflex arc. Q. J. Exp. Physiol., 31: 311–318.

Ciriello, J. and Calaresu, F. R. (1983) Central projections of afferent renal fibers in the rat: an anterograde transport study of horseradish peroxidase. J. Auton. Nerv. System, 8: 273–286.

Clerc, N. (1983) Afferent innervation of the lower oesophageal sphincter of the cat. An HRP study. J. Auton. Nerv. System, 9: 623–636.

Clifton, G. L., Coggeshall, R. E., Vance, W. H. and Willis, W. D. (1976) Receptive fields of unmyelinated ventral root afferent fibres in the cat. J. Physiol., 256: 573–600.

Code, C. F. and Carlson, H. C. (1968) Motor activity of the stomach. In Handbook of Physiology, Alimentary Canal, Vol. IV, Motility, American Physiological Society, Washington, DC, pp. 1903–1916.

Coggeshall, R. E. (1980) Law of separation of function of the spinal roots. Physiol. Rev., 60: 716–755.

Coggeshall, R. E. and Ito, H. (1977) Sensory fibres in ventral roots L7 and S1 in the cat. J. Physiol., 267: 215–235.

Coggeshall, R. E., Coulter, J. D. and Willis, W. D. (1974) Unmyelinated axons in the ventral roots of the cat lumbosacral enlargement. J. Comp. Neurol., 153: 39–58.

Cohen, B. R. and Wolff, B. S. (1968) Cineradiographie and intraluminal pressure correlations in the pharynx and oesophagus. In Handbook of Physiology, Alimentary Canal, Vol. IV, Motility, American Physiological Society, Washington, DC, pp. 1841–1860.

Connell, A. M., Avery-Jones, F. and Rowlands, E. N. (1965) The motility of the pelvic colon. IV. Abdominal pain associated with colonic hypermotility after meals. Gut, 6: 105–112.

Denny-Brown, D. and Robertson, E. G. (1933) On the physiology of micturition. Brain, 56: 149–190.

Denny-Brown, D. and Robertson, E. G. (1935) An investigation of the nervous control of defaecation. Brain, 58: 256–310.

Devor, M., Wall, P. D. and McMahon, S. B. (1984) Dichotomizing somatic nerve fibers exist in rats but they are rare. Neurosci. Lett., 49: 187–192.

DeWolf, W. C. and Fraley, E. E. (1975) Renal pain. J. Urol., 6: 403–408.

Dixon, J. S. and Gosling, J. A. (1971) Histochemical and electron-microscopic observations on the innervation of the upper segment of the mammalian ureter. J. Anat., 110: 57–66.

Downie, J. W., Champion, J. A. and Nance, D. M. (1984) A quantitative analysis of the afferent and extrinsic efferent innervation of specific regions of the bladder and urethra in the cat. Brain Res. Bull., 12: 735–740.

Downman, C. B. B., McSwiney, B. A. and Vass, C. C. N. (1948) Sensitivity of the small intestine. J. Physiol., 107: 97–106.

Edvardsen, P. (1968) Nervous control of the urinary bladder in cats. I. The collecting phase. Acta Physiol. Scand., 72: 157–171.

El-Quazzani, T. (1981) Contribution à l'étude de la sensibilité digestive. Approche histologique histochimique et électrophysiologique chez le chat. Thèse Doctorat d'Etat ès — Sciences Naturelles. Marseilles, France: Aix-Marseille Université III, p. 269.

Evans, J. P. (1936) Observations on the nerves of supply to the bladder and urethra of the cat, with a study of their action potentials. J. Physiol., 86: 396–414.

Fjällbrant, N. and Iggo, A. (1961) The effect of histamine, 5-hydroxytryptamine and acetylcholine on cutaneous afferent fibres. J. Physiol., 156: 578–590.

Floyd, K. and Lawrenson, G. (1979) Mechanosensitive afferents in the cat pelvic nerve. J. Physiol., 290: 51–52P.

Floyd, K. and Morrison, J. F. B. (1974) Splanchnic mechanoreceptors in the dog. Q. J. Exp. Physiol., 59: 359–364.

Floyd, K., Hick, V. E. and Morrison, J. F. B. (1976a) Mechanosensitive afferent units in the hypogastric nerve of the cat. J. Physiol., 259: 457–471.

Floyd, K., Hick, V. E. and Morrison, J. F. B. (1976b) The discharge of splanchnic nerve afferents in dogs with intact abdomen. J. Physiol., 263: 221–222P.

Floyd, K., Koley, J. and Morrison, J. F. B. (1976c) Afferent discharges in the sacral ventral roots of cats. J. Physiol., 259: 37–38P.

Floyd, K., Hick, V. E., Koley, J. and Morrison, J. F. B. (1977) The effects of bradykinin on afferent units in intra-abdominal sympathetic nerve trunks. Q. J. Exp. Physiol., 62: 19–25.

Floyd, K., Hick, V. E. and Morrison, J. F. B. (1982) The influence of visceral mechanoreceptors on sympathetic efferent discharge in the cat. J. Physiol., 323: 65–76.

Foley, J. O. (1948) The functional types of nerve fibres. Anat. Rec., 100: D34, P166.

Franz, M. and Mense, S. (1975) Muscle receptors with group IV afferent fibres responding to application of bradykinin. Brain Res., 92: 369–383.

Gaensler, E. A. (1951) Quantitative determination of the visceral pain threshold in man. J. Clin. Invest., 30: 406–420.

Gammon, G. D. and Bronk, D. W. (1935) The discharges of impulses from Pacinian corpuscles in the mesentery and its relation to vascular changes. Am. J. Physiol., 114: 77–84.

Gernandt, B. and Zotterman, Y. (1946) Intestinal pain: an electrophysiological investigation on mesenteric nerves. Acta Physiol. Scand., 12: 56–72.

Giesler, G. J. and Liebeskind, J. C. (1976) Inhibition of visceral pain by electrical stimulation of the periaqueductal gray matter. Pain, 2: 43–48.

Gjone, R. (1966) Peripheral autonomic influence on the motility of the urinary bladder in the cat. II. Tone. Acta Physiol. Scand., 66: 72–80.

Goldscheider, A. (1920) Das Schmerzproblem, Springer-Verlag, Berlin, pp. 77–91.

Gosling, J. A. (1969) Observations on the distribution of intrarenal nervous tissues. Anat. Rec., 163: 81–88.

Gosling, J. A. (1970) The innervation of the upper urinary tract. J. Anat., 106: 51–61.

Handwerker, H. O. (1976) Influences of algogenic substances and prostaglandins on the discharges of unmyelinated cutaneous nerve fibers identified as nociceptors. In J. J. Bonica and D. G. Albe-Fessard (Eds.), Advances in Pain Research and Therapy, Vol. 1, Raven Press, New York, pp. 41–51.

Handwerker, H. O. (1984) Experimentelle Schmerzanalyse beim Menschen. In M. Zimmermann and H. O. Handwerker (Eds.), Schmerz, Springer-Verlag, Berlin, pp. 87–123.

Hansen, K. (1963) Visceraler Schmerz (segmentale Projektionen). In M. Monier (Ed.), Physiologie und Pathophysiologie des Vegetativen Nervensystems, Band II: Pathophysiologie, Hippokrates-Verlag, Stuttgart, pp. 760–770.

Hardcastle, J., Hardcastle, P. T. and Sandford, P. A. (1978) Effect of actively transported hexoses on afferent nerve discharge from rat small intestine. J. Physiol., 285: 71–84.

Haupt, P., Jänig, W. and Kohler, W. (1983) Response pattern of visceral afferent fibres, supplying the colon, upon chemical and mechanical stimuli. Pflügers Arch., 398: 41–47.

Hazarika, N. H., Coote, J. and Downman, C. B. B. (1964) Gastrointestinal dorsal root viscerotomes in the cat. J. Neurophysiol., 27: 107–116.

Head, H. (1893) On disturbances of sensation, with special reference to the pain of visceral diseases. Brain, 16: 1–133.

Hightower, N. C. (1968) Motor action of the small bowel. In Handbook of Physiology, Alimentary Canal, Vol. IV, Motility, American Physiological Society, Washington, DC, pp. 2001–2024.

Holmes, F. W. and Davenport, H. A. (1940) Cells and fibres in spinal nerves. J. Comp. Neurol., 73: 1–5.

Hulsebosch, C. E. and Coggeshall, R. E. (1982) An analysis of the axon populations in the nerves to the pelvic viscera in the rat. J. Comp. Neurol., 211: 1–10.

Iggo, A. (1955) Tension receptors in the stomach and the urinary bladder. J. Physiol., 128: 593–607.

Iggo, A. (1966) Physiology of visceral afferent systems. Acta Neuroveg., 28: 121–134.

Irving, J. T., McSwiney, B. A. and Suffolk, S. F. (1937) Afferent fibres from the stomach and small intestine. J. Physiol., 89: 407–420.

Kenshalo, D. R. (1984) Cutaneous temperature sensitivity. In W. W. Dawson and J. M. Enoch (Eds.), Foundations of Sensory Science, Springer-Verlag, Berlin, pp. 419–464.

Klevmark, B. (1974) Motility of the urinary bladder in cats during filling at physiological rates. I. Intravesical pressure patterns studied by a new method of cystometry. Acta Physiol. Scand., 90: 565–577.

Klevmark, B. (1977) Motility of the urinary bladder in cats during filling at physiological rates. II. Effects of extrinsic bladder denervation on intraluminal tension and intravesical pressure patterns. Acta Physiol. Scand., 101: 176–184.

Klevmark, B. (1980) Motility of the urinary bladder in cats during filling at physiological rates. III. Spontaneous rhythmic bladder contractions in the conscious and anaesthetised animal. Influence of distension and innervation. Scand. J. Urol. Nephrol., 14: 219–224.

Kumazawa, T. and Mizumura, K. (1977) Thin-fibre receptors responding to mechanical, chemical, and thermal stimulation in the skeletal muscle of the dog. J. Physiol., 273: 179–194.

Kumazawa, T. and Mizumura, K. (1980) Chemical responses of polymodal receptors of the scrotal contents in dogs. J. Physiol., 299: 219–231.

Kuntz, A., Hoffman, H. H. and Schaefer, E. M. (1957) Fibre components of the splanchnic nerves. Anat. Rec., 128: 139–146.

Kuo, D. C. and De Groat, W. C. (1985) Primary afferent projections of the major splanchnic nerve to the spinal cord and gracile nucleus of the cat. J. Comp. Neurol., 231: 421–434.

Kuo, D. C., Yang, G. C. H., Yamasaki, D. S. and Krauthamer, G. M. (1982) A wide field electron microscopic analysis of the fiber constituents of the major splanchnic nerve in the cat. J. Comp. Neurol., 210: 49–58.

Kuo, D. C., Nadelhaft, I., Hisamitsu, T. and De Groat, W. C.

(1983) Segmental distribution and central projections of renal afferent fibers in the cat studied by transganglionic transport of horseradish peroxidase. J. Comp. Neurol., 216: 162–174.

Langford, L. A. and Coggeshall, R. E. (1979) Branching of sensory axons in the dorsal root and evidence for the absence of dorsal root efferent fibers. J. Comp. Neurol., 184: 193–204.

Langford, L. A. and Coggeshall, R. E. (1981) Branching of sensory axons in the peripheral nerve of the rat. J. Comp. Neurol., 203: 745–750.

Langworthy, O. R., Kolb, L. C. and Lewis, L. G. (1940) Physiology of Micturition, The Williams and Wilkins Company, Baltimore, p. 129.

Lapides, J. (1958) Structure and function of the internal vesical sphincter. J. Urol., 80: 341–353.

Läwen, A. (1922) Ueber segmentäre Schmerzaufhebung durch paravertebrale Novocaininjektionen zur Differentialdiagnose intraabdominaler Erkrankungen. Münchener Med. Wochenschr., 40: 1423–1426.

Läwen, A. (1923) Weitere Erfahrungen über paravertebrale Schmerzaufhebung zur Differentialdiagnose von Erkrankungen der Gallenblase, des Magens, der Niere und des Wurmfortsatzes sowie zur Behandlung postoperativer Lungenkomplikationen. Zentralblatt f. Chir., 12: 461–465.

Le Bars, D., Dickenson, A. H. and Besson, J.-M. (1979) Diffuse noxious inhibitory controls (DNIC). I. Effects on dorsal horn convergent neurones in the rat. Pain, 6: 283–304.

Leek, B. F. (1977) Abdominal and pelvic visceral receptors. Br. Med. Bull., 33: 163–168.

Lewis, T. (1942) Pain, The Macmillan Company, New York, pp. 128–172.

Light, A. R. and Metz, C. B. (1978) The morphology of the spinal cord efferent and afferent neurons contributing to the ventral roots of the cat. J. Comp. Neurol., 179: 501–516.

Lim, R. K. S. (1960) Visceral receptors and visceral pain. Am. N.Y. Acad. Sci., 86: 73–89.

Lim, R. K. S. (1970) Pain. Annu. Rev. Physiol., 32: 269–288.

Lim, R. K. S., Liu, C. N., Guzman, F. and Braun, C. (1962) Visceral receptors concerned in visceral pain and the pseudoaffective response to intra-arterial injection of bradykinin and other algesic agents. J. Comp. Neurol., 118: 269–277.

Lim, R. K. S., Rodgers, D. W., Goto, K., Braun, C., Dickerson, C. D. and Engle, R. J. (1964) Site of action of narcotic and non-narcotic analgesics determined by blocking bradykinin-evoked visceral pain. Arch. Int. Pharmacodyn., 152: 25–58.

Lim, R. K. S., Miller, D. G., Guzman, F., Rodgers, D. W., Rodgers, R. W., Wang, S. K., Chao, P. Y. and Shih, T. Y. (1967) Pain and analgesia evaluated by the intraperitoneal bradykinin-evoked pain method in man. Clin. Pharmacol. Ther., 8: 521–542.

Lipkin, M. and Sleisenger, M. H. (1958) Studies of visceral pain: Measurements of stimulus intensity and duration associated with the onset of pain in esophagus, ileum and colon. J. Clin. Invest., 37: 28–34.

Lombardi, F., Della Bella, P., Casati, R. and Malliani, A. (1981) Effects of intracoronary administration of bradykinin on the impulse activity of afferent sympathetic unmyelinated fibers with left ventricular endings in the cat. Circ. Res., 48: 69–75.

Longhurst, J. C., Mitchell, J. H. and Moore, M. B. (1980) The spinal cord ventral root: an afferent pathway of the hindlimb pressor reflex in cats. J. Physiol., 301: 467–476.

Longhurst, J. C., Kaufman, M. P., Ordway, G. A. and Musch, T. I. (1984) Effects of bradykinin and capsaicin on endings of afferent fibers from abdominal visceral organs. Am. J. Physiol., 247: R552–R559.

Lynn, B. (1984) The detection of injury and tissue damage. In P. D. Wall and R. Melzack (Eds.), Textbook of Pain, Churchill Livingstone, Edinburgh, pp. 19–33.

Magni, F. and Carobi, C. (1983) The afferent and preganglionic parasympathetic innervation of the rat liver demonstrated by the retrograde transport of horseradish peroxidase. J. Auton. Nerv. System, 8: 231–260.

Malliani, A (1982) Cardiovascular sympathetic afferent fibers. Rev. Physiol. Biochem. Pharmacol., 94: 11–74.

Malliani, A. and Lombardi, F. (1982) Consideration of the fundamental mechanisms eliciting cardiac pain. Am. Heart J., 103: 575–578.

McCloskey, D. I. (1981) Corollary discharges: motor commands and perception. In J. M. Brookhart and V. B. Mountcastle (Eds.), Handbook of Physiology, Section 1, The Nervous System, Vol. II, Motor Control, Part I, American Physiological Society, Bethesda, pp. 1415–1448.

McDowall, R. J. S. (1960) Handbook of Physiology, Micturition, 43rd Edn., John Murray, London, pp. 415–418.

McGuire, E. J. (1984) The neuropathic urethra. In A. R. Mundy, T. P. Stephenson and A. J. Wein (Eds.), Urodynamics, Churchill Livingstone, Edinburgh, pp. 288–296.

McKenzie, J. (1909) Symptoms and their Interpretation, Shaw and Sons, London, pp. 1–206.

McLachlan, E. M. and Jänig, W. (1983) The cell bodies of origin of sympathetic and sensory axons in some skin and muscle nerves of the cat hindlimb. J. Comp. Neurol., 214: 115–130.

McMahon, S. B. and Morrison, J. F. B. (1982) Factors that determine the excitability of parasympathetic reflexes to the cat bladder. J. Physiol., 322: 35–43.

McMahon, S. B., Morrison, J. F. B. and Spillane, K. (1982) An electrophysiological study of somatic and visceral convergence in the reflex control of the external sphincter. J. Physiol., 328: 379–388.

Mei, N. (1983) Sensory structures in the viscera. In A. Aütrüm, D. Ottoson, E. R. Perl, R. F. Schmidt, H. Shimazu and W. D. Willis (Eds.), Progress in Sensory Physiology, Vol. 4, Springer-Verlag, Berlin, pp. 1–42.

Mei, N. (1985) Intestinal chemosensitivity. Physiol. Rev., 65: 211–237.

Mellanby, J. and Pratt, C. L. (1940) The reaction of the urinary bladder under conditions of constant volume. Proc. Roy. Soc.

London B., 128: 186–201.

Melzack, R. and Wall, P. D. (1965) Pain mechanisms: a new theory. Science, 150: 971–979.

Mense, S. (1977) Nervous outflow from skeletal muscle following chemical noxious stimulation. J. Physiol., 267: 75–88.

Mense, S. (1985) Slowly conducting afferent fibers from deep tissues: neurobiological properties and central nervous actions. In H. Aütrüm, D. Ottoson, E. R. Perl, R. F. Schmidt, H. Shimazu and W. D. Willis (Eds.), Progress in Sensory Physiology, Vol. 6, Springer-Verlag, Berlin, pp. 139–219.

Morgan, C., Nadelhaft, I. and De Groat, W. C. (1981) The distribution of visceral primary afferents from the pelvic nerve to Lissauer's tract and the spinal gray matter and its relationship to the sacral parasympathetic nucleus. J. Comp. Neurol., 201: 415–440.

Morrison, J. F. B. (1973) Splanchnic slowly adapting mechanoreceptors with punctate receptive fields in the mesentery and gastrointestinal tract of the cat. J. Physiol., 233: 349–362.

Morrison, J. F. B. (1977) The sensory innervation of the gastro-intestinal tract. In F. P. Brooks and P. Evers (Eds.), Nerves and the Gut, Charles Slack, Thorofare, NJ, pp. 297–326.

Morrison, J. F. B. (1980) The spinal afferent innervation of liver, biliary tract and portal vein. In H. Popper, L. Bianchi, F. Gudat and W. Reutter (Eds.), Communications of Liver Cells, MTP Press, Lancaster, pp. 139–149.

Morrison, J. F. B. (1981) Sensory processing in spinal afferent pathways from the bladder. In E. Grastyán and P. Molnár (Eds.), Advances in Physiological Science, Vol. 16, Sensory Functions, Akadémiai Kiadó, Budapest; Pergamon Press, Oxford, pp. 325–333.

Morrison, J. F. B. (1982) The neural control of the bladder. In S. R. Bloom, J. M. Polak and E. Lindenlaub (Eds.), Systemic Role of Regulatory Peptides, Symposia Medica Hoechst, Vol. 18, F. K. Schattauer Verlag, Stuttgart, pp. 381–396.

Morrison, J. F. B. and McMahon, E. B. (1982) Colonic afferents and their reflexes. In M. Wienbeck (Ed.), Motility of the Digestive Tract, Raven Press, New York, pp. 19–30.

Mundy, A. R. and Stephenson, T. P. (1984) The urge syndrome. In A. R. Mundy, T. P. Stephenson and A. J. Wein (Eds.), Urodynamics, Churchill Livingstone, Edinburgh, pp. 212–218.

Murphy, J. J. and Schoenberg, H. W. (1960) Observations on intravesical pressure changes during micturition. J. Urol., 84: 106–110.

Nadelhaft, I. and Booth, A. M. (1984) The location and morphology of preganglionic neurons and the distribution of visceral afferents from the rat pelvic nerve: a horseradish peroxidase study. J. Comp. Neurol., 226: 238–245.

Nafe, J. P. (1929) A quantitative theory of feeling. J. Gen. Psychol., 2: 199–211.

Nathan, P. W. (1952a) Micturition reflexes in man. J. Neurol. Neurosurg. Psychiat., 15: 148–149.

Nathan, P. W. (1952b) Thermal sensation in the bladder. J. Neurol. Neurosurg. Psychiat., 15: 150–151.

Nathan, P. W. (1956) Sensations associated with micturition. Br. J. Urol., 28: 126–131.

Nathan, P. W. (1976) The gate-control theory of pain. A critical review. Brain, 99: 123–158.

Neuhuber, W. (1982) The central projections of visceral primary afferent neurons of the inferior mesenteric plexus and hypogastric nerve and the location of the related sensory and preganglionic sympathetic cell bodies in the rat. Anat. Embryol., 164: 413–425.

Niijima, A. (1971) Afferent discharges from arterial mechanoreceptors in the kidney of the rabbit. J. Physiol., 219: 477–485.

Niijima, A. (1972) The effect of efferent discharges in renal nerves on the activity of arterial mechanoreceptors in the kidney of the rabbit. J. Physiol., 222: 335–343.

Niijima, A. (1975) Observation on the localization of mechanoreceptors in the kidney and afferent nerve fibres in the renal nerves in the rabbit. J. Physiol., 245: 81–90.

Niijima, A, and Winter, D. L. (1968) Baroreceptors in the adrenal gland. Science, 159: 434–435.

Nishi, K., Sakanashi, M. and Takenaka, F. (1977) Activation of afferent cardicac sympathetic nerve fibers of the cat by pain-producing substances and by noxious heat. Pflügers Arch., 372: 53–61.

Oldfield, B. J. and McLachlan, E. M. (1978) Localization of sensory neurons traversing the stellate ganglion of the cat. J. Comp. Neurol., 182: 915–922.

Payne, W. W. and Poulton, E. P. (1923) Experiments on visceral sensation: the relation of pain to activity in the human oesophagus. J. Physiol., 63: 217–241.

Perl, E. R. (1984) Characterization of nociceptors and their activation of neurons in the superficial dorsal horn: first steps for the sensation of pain. In: L. Kruger and J. C. Liebeskind (Eds.), Advances in Pain Research and Therapy, Vol. 6, Raven Press, New York, pp. 23–51.

Perrin, J., Crousillat, J. and Mei, N. (1981) Assessment of true splanchnic glucoreceptors in the jejuno-ileum of the cat. Brain Res. Bull., 7: 625–628.

Peterson, C. G. and Youmans, W. B. (1945) The intestino-intestinal inhibitory reflex: threshold variations, sensitization and summation. Am. J. Physiol., 143: 407–412.

Pierau, F. K., Taylor, D. C. M., Abel, W. and Friedrich, B. (1982) Dichotomizing peripheral fibres revealed by intracellular recording from rat sensory neurones. Neurosci. Lett., 31: 123–128.

Ranieri, F., Mei, N. and Crousillat, J. (1973) Les afférences splanchniques provenant des mécanorécepteurs gastrointestinaux et péritonéaux. Exp. Brain Res., 16: 276–290.

Ranieri, F., Crousillat, J. and Mei, N. (1975) Étude électrophysiologique et histologique des fibres afférentes splanchniques. Arch Ital. Biol., 113: 354–373.

Ravdin, I. S., Royster, H. P. and Sanders, G. B. (1942) Reflexes originating in the common bile duct give rise to pain simulating angina pectoris. Am. J. Surg., 115: 1055–1062.

Rawson, R. O. and Quick, K. P. (1970) Evidence of deep-body thermoreceptor response to intra-abdominal heating of the ewe. J. Appl. Physiol., 28: 813–820.

Rawson, R. O. and Quick, K. P. (1972) Localization of intraabdominal thermoreceptors in the ewe. J. Physiol., 222: 665–677.

Recordati, G. M., Moss, N. G. and Waselkov, L. (1978) Renal chemoreceptors in the rat. Circ. Res., 43: 534–543.

Recordati, G. M., Moss, N. G., Genovesi, S. and Rogenes, P. R. (1980) Renal receptor in the rat sensitive to chemical alterations of their environment. Circ. Res., 46: 395–405.

Recordati, G., Moss, N. G., Genovesi, S. and Rogenes, P. (1981) Renal chemoreceptors. J. Auton. Nerv. System, 3: 237–251.

Riddoch, G. (1921) Conduction of sensory impulses from the bladder by the inferior hypogastrics and the central afferent connection of these nerves. J. Physiol., 54: 134–135P.

Riedel, W. (1976) Warm receptors on the dorsal abdominal wall of the rabbit. Pflügers Arch., 361: 205–206.

Risholm, L. (1954) Studies on renal colic and its treatment by posterior splanchnic block. Acta Chir. Scand. Suppl., 184: 1–64.

Risling, M., Aldskogius, H., Hildebrand, C. and Remahl, S. (1983) Effects of sciatic nerve resection on L7 spinal roots and dorsal root ganglia in adult cats. Exp. Neurol., 82: 568–580.

Risling, M., Dalsgaard, C.-J., Cukierman, A. and Cuello, A. C. (1984a) Electronmicroscopic and immunohistochemical evidence that unmyelinated ventral root axons make U-turns or enter the spinal pia mater. J. Comp. Neurol., 225: 53–63.

Risling, M., Hildebrand, C. and Cullheim, S. (1984b) Invasion of the L7 ventral root amd spinal pia mater by new axons after sciatic nerve division in kittens. Exp. Neurol., 83: 84–97.

Ruch, T. C. (1979) Pathophysiology of pain. In T. Ruch and H. D. Patton (Eds.), Physiology and Biophysics, W. B. Saunders Company, Philadelphia, pp. 272–324.

Rühle, W., Dembowsky, K., Czachurski, J. and Seller, H. (1985) Segmental distribution of afferent fibres in the left inferior cardiac nerve of the cat studied by anterograde transport of horseradish peroxidase. Neurosci. Lett., 56: 353–358.

Schmitt, M. (1973) Influences of hepatic portal receptors on hypothalamic feeding and satiety centers. Am. J. Physiol., 225: 1089–1095.

Schuster, M. M. (1968) Motor action of rectum and anal sphincter in continence and defaecation. In Handbook of Physiology: Alimentary Canal, Vol. IV, Motility, American Physiological Society, Washington, DC, pp. 2121–2139.

Scott, F. B., Quesada, E. M. and Cardus, D. (1964) Studies on the dynamics of micturition: observations on healthy men. J. Urol., 92: 455–463.

Shah, P. J. R. (1984) The assessment of patients with a view to urodynamics. In A. R. Mundy, T. P. Stephenson and A. J. Wein (Eds.), Urodynamics, Churchill Livingstone, Edinburgh, pp. 53–61.

Sharkey, K. A., Williams, R. G., Schultzberg, M. and Dockray, G. J. (1983) Sensory substance P — innervation of the urinary bladder possible site of action of capsaicin in causing urine retention in rats. Neuroscience, 10: 861–868.

Sherrington, C. S. (1900) Cutaneous sensations. In E. A. Schäfer (Ed.), Textbook of Physiology, Vol. 2, Young J. Pentland, Edinburgh, pp. 920–1001.

Sherrington, C. S. (1906) The Integrative Action of the Nervous System, Yale University Press, New Haven, p. 413.

Sinclair, D. (1981) Mechanisms of Cutaneous Sensation. Oxford University Press, Oxford, New York, Toronto, p. 363.

Talaat, M. (1937) Afferent impulses in the nerves supplying the urinary bladder. J. Physiol., 89: 1–13.

Taylor, D. C. M. and Pierau, F. K. (1982) Double fluorescent labelling supports electrophysiological evidence for dichotomizing peripheral sensory nerve fibres in rats. Neurosci. Lett., 33: 1–6.

Todd, J. K. (1964) Afferent impulses in the pudendal nerves of the cat. Q. J. Exp. Physiol., 49: 258–267.

Torrens, M. and Abrams, P. (1979) Urine flow studies. In R. Turner-Warwick and C. G. Whiteside (Eds.), Clinical Urodynamics, The Urological Clinics of North America, Vol. 6, W. B. Saunders, Philadelphia, pp. 71–78.

Torrens, M. and Hald, T. (1979) Bladder denervation procedures. In R. Turner-Warwick and C. G. Whiteside (Eds.), Clinical Urodynamics, The Urological Clinics of North America, Vol. 6, W. B. Saunders, Philadelphia, pp. 283–294.

Turner-Warwick, R. (1979) Observations on the function and dysfunction of the sphincter and detrusor mechanisms. In R. Turner-Warwick and C. G. Whiteside (Eds.), Clinical Urodynamics, The Urological Clinics of North America, Vol. 6, W. B. Saunders, Philadelphia, pp. 13–30.

Uchida, Y. and Murao, S. (1974) Bradykinin-induced excitation of afferent cardiac sympathetic nerve fibers. Jpn. Heart J., 15: 84–91.

Wall, P. D. (1978) The gate control theory of pain mechanisms. A re-examination and re-statement. Brain, 101: 1–18.

White, J. C. (1943) Sensory innervation of the viscera. Studies on visceral afferent neurones in man based on neurosurgical procedures for the relief of intractable pain. Res. Publ. Ass. Nerv. Ment. Dis., 23: 373–390.

White, J. C. and Smithwick, R. H. (1948) The Autonomic Nervous System, 2nd edn., Macmillan, New York, pp. 131–147.

White, J. C. and Sweet, W. H. (1969) Pain and the Neurosurgeon; A. Forty-Year Experience, Charles C. Thomas, Springfield, IL, pp. 525–559, 560–585.

Williams, P. L. and Warwick, R. (Eds.) (1980) Gray's Anatomy, 36th Edn., Churchill Livingstone, Edinburgh, p. 1131.

Winter, D. L. (1971) Receptor characteristics and conduction velocities in bladder afferents. J. Psychiat. Res., 8: 225–235.

Wyatt, A. P. (1967) The relationship of the sphincter of Oddi to the stomach, duodenum and gall-bladder. J. Physiol., 193: 225–243.

Youmans, W. B. (1944) The intestino-intestinal inhibitory reflex. Gastroenterology, 3: 114–118.

F. Cervero and J. F.B. Morrison
Progress in Brain Research, Vol. 67

CHAPTER 8

Sensory innervation of reproductive organs

Takao Kumazawa

Department of Nervous and Sensory Functions, The Research Institute of Environmental Medicine, Nagoya University, Furo-cho, Chikusa-ku, Nagoya, 464, Japan

Visceral afferent innervation of reproductive organs

Development of reproductive organs is quite complicated, for they involve tissues originating from the cranial as well as the caudal region of the abdominal cavity, and, furthermore, the organs derived from the cranial segments migrate caudally in a complex manner. Reflecting the history of the development of the organs, the innervation is also complicated, because it is generally considered that nervous innervation begins in an early stage of development, a stage of somite differentiation.

The reproductive organs can be grossly divided into four parts on the basis of the developmental aspects: the urogenital ridge containing the gonads, the part derived from the duct system (Wolffian or Muellerian duct), the part derived from the urogenital sinus, and the external genitals. The innervation of the individual organ has a fairly clear relationship to the original location of its primordium.

Female reproductive organs

Respiratory and circulatory responses to stimulation of the ovarian plexus demonstrate that the afferent pathway from the ovary ascends along the ovarian artery and enters the main sympathetic chain at the 4th lumbar sympathetic ganglion, and ascends further rostral along with the main chain to reach the cord at the level of the 10th thoracic segment. Neither the superior hypogastric plexus, the inferior mesenteric ganglia nor the lower aortic plexus contains afferents from the ovary (Labate and Reynolds, 1937).

The afferent fibres supplying the uterine tube reach the spinal cord through the 11th and 12th thoracic and lumbar nerves via the hypogastric nerve (Kuntz, 1947).

Intensive studies on the management of labour pains have contributed much information on the afferent pathways from the female reproductive organs. A convergent line of data shows that most of the pain in the first stage of labour is due to dilatation and the consequent stretching or tearing of the cervix. Pathways for labour pains at this stage were at one time assumed to involve sensory nerves contained in the nervi erigentis, which pass through the spinal cord via the 2nd, 3rd and 4th sacral nerves. This notion was chiefly deduced from the findings of Head (1893) on the distribution of referred pain in this stage. However, the contribution of the nervi erigentis to the pain of this stage is strongly questioned by the results of nervous block to relieve the pain of this stage (Cleland, 1933; Routledge and Elliott, 1962; Bonica, 1975) and also by the results of the utero-somatic reflex induced by raising the intra-uterine pressure or by stimulation of the uterine nerve in dogs (Cleland, 1933). According to Bonica (1967), the pathway for the pain of this stage is as follows: the uterine plexus — the pelvic (inferior hypogastric) plexus — the middle hypogastric plexus or "nerve" — the superior hypogastric plexus — the lumbar and lower thoracic sympathetic chain — the white rami communicantes associated with the 11th and 12th nerve — the dorsal roots of these nerves. Although the pain is referred to the skin overlying the lower lumbar and upper and middle sacral area, this fact is explained by the migration of the cutaneous branches of the posterior division of the lower thoracic and the upper lumbar nerves to these areas (Bonica, 1975).

Towards the end of the second stage, when perineal distension causes stretching and possibly tearing of the surrounding tissues, blocking of the pudendal nerve, a somatic sacral nerve, virtually eliminates the pain (Bonica, 1975). Recordings from the pelvic nerve of cats show that this nerve rarely carries afferents from the vagina (Abrahams and Teare, 1969).

However, at least a part of the vagina is embryologically derived from the endoderm of the urogenital sinus. This portion is also the origin of the urinary bladder, which is known to be innervated also by sensory fibres of the pelvic nerve. The following findings suggest an implication of the visceral sacral afferents in the vagina. After bilateral pelvic nerve neurectomies in rats, all of the intravaginal mucosa become anaesthetic and analgesic, and pinching of the vaginal mucosa and other intense noxious stimuli fail to elicit a response of "pseudopregnancy" (Kollar, 1953). The vagina-gastrointestinal reflexes are completely abolished only when both of the hypogastric and pelvic nerves are bilaterally sectioned (Mori, 1967). The pelvic nerve is activated by stimulation of the vaginal wall, rectal wall, or cervix (Komisaruk et al., 1972). Thus, involvement of the sacral visceral afferents of the female reproductive organs in sensation is still an open question.

Male reproductive organs

The absence of any intact nerve fibres in the testis after degeneration of the superior spermatic nerve indicates that the afferent innervation of the testis is exclusively via this nerve (Kuntz and Morris, 1946). By means of nerve blockade, Woollard and Carmichael (1933) determined that the pathway of painful sensation from the testis accompanied the spermatic artery, entering the spinal cord at the 10th thoracic segment. This finding is confirmed by their observations on clinical cases with crush fractures of the spinal cord. The tunica albuginea and tunica vasculosa of the testis are abundantly innervated, and at least some of them are undoubtedly afferent. Direct innervation of the seminal epithelium and the interstitial secretory tissue of the testis is regarded as extremely doubtful (Yamashita, 1939; Kuntz, 1947).

Mitchell (1953) in man and Kuntz and Morris (1946) in cats and rats found no anatomical evidence that any fibres from the superior spermatic nerve supplied the epididymis. Electrophysiological investigation of the superior spermatic nerve in dogs reveals that a large number of sensory afferent units recorded from this nerve have their receptive fields at the epididymis or at both the testis and epididymis (Kumazawa and Mizumura, 1980a).

The nerve supply to the seminal vesicle and ductus deferens is derived from the hypogastric plexus. The subepithelial plexus in the lamina propria of the ductus deferens is made up of afferent nerve fibres derived via the inferior mesenteric plexus and afferent components of the pelvic nerve (Kuntz and Morris, 1946).

Histology of sensory endings in reproductive organs

According to Seto's review (1957) on the morphology of the sensory endings in the human reproductive organs, simple bifurcated or non-bifurcated free nerve endings of spine-like or node-like form are found in the connective tissue surrounding the rete testis and in the superficial layer of the tunica albuginea. In the ductus deferens, especially at the ampulla portion, glomerular endings which are similar to the genital corpuscles are also found besides bifurcated endings. Kreutz (1964) described encapsulated endings which resemble the genital corpuscles and Meissner's corpuscles in the tunica albuginea. A few simple bifurcated endings are found in the seminal vesicle and the ductus ejaculatorius. Complicated bifurcated endings derived from large nerve fibres are often found in the prostate (Seto, 1957).

In contrast to the testis, sensory endings are found also inside the ovary. They are complicated bifurcated spine-like or node-like endings. Simple bifurcated or non-bifurcated endings are found in the uterine tube and mesosalpinx and in the mucous membrane of the uterus. The endings are densest at the cervix, less so at the corpus and least at the fundus (Seto, 1957). According to Pallie et al. (1954), no specific sensory end-organs are found in the uterine horn of rabbits.

Peptidergic nerves in reproductive organs

In addition to well known cholinergic and adrenergic innervations, recent immunohistochemical studies have revealed the existence of various kinds of peptidergic nerves containing enkephalin, vasoactive intestinal polypeptide (VIP) and substance P in the reproductive organs (Larsson et al., 1977; Alm et al., 1978, 1981; Ottesen, 1981; Fahrenkrug and Ottesen, 1982; Traurig et al., 1984).

Localization of the enkephalin-immunoreactive nerve fibres among the cell bodies in the paraurethral and cervical ganglia as well as in the smooth muscle layer suggests that these nerves are not sensory types but play a neuromodulator role on the function of the organ (Alm et al., 1981). Some of sensory afferent nerves certainly contain VIP, because VIP immunoreactivity has been demonstrated in the central branches of primary sensory afferents at the dorsal horn or in the dorsal root ganglion cells, and it is markedly reduced by neonatal capsaicin treatment (Lundberg et al., 1978; Jancsó et al., 1981). VIP-containing nerve fibres were found in the smooth muscle wall and in the endometrium of the genito-urinary organs (Larsson et al., 1977; Ottesen, 1981). However, the origin of the uterine VIPergic nerves seems to be cell bodies located in ganglia of the paracervical tissue at the uterovaginal junction (Alm et al., 1977), and the release of VIP induced by stimulation of the hypogastric or the pelvic nerve is blocked by hexamethonium (Fahrenkrug and Ottesen, 1982). These results suggest that the VIP neurons observed in these organs are not sensory but intrinsic.

Convergent lines of experimental results reveal that small-fibre primary sensory afferents contain substance P (SP) at both central and peripheral branches: SP immunoreactivity is confined to small cells of the dorsal root ganglia and at the dorsal part of the dorsal horn (Hökfelt et al., 1975); strong stimulation of the peripheral nerve causes the release of SP in the spinal cord (Otsuka and Konishi, 1976; Yaksh et al., 1980); nociceptive reflexes in the isolated spinal cord-tail preparation are reduced by the application of an SP-antagonist (Yanagisawa and Otsuka, 1984); and capsaicin, which causes depletion of SP, selectively degenerates primary small fibres (Jancsó et al., 1980).

SP-nerves are found also in the reproductive organs (Alm et al., 1978; Hökfelt et al., 1978; Brodin and Nilsson, 1981). The density of SP-nerve innervation varies much depending on the species, but the distribution of this type of nerve is definitely different from that of adrenergic, cholinergic and VIPergic nerves (Alm et al., 1978). In the female reproductive organs the vagina receives the richest supply of SP-containing nerve fibres: single nerve terminals are found beneath the surface epithelium of the vagina. Fewer fibres are found in the cervix uterine horn, uterine tube and ovary. In contrast to the case of cholinergic or adrenergic nerves (Adham and Schenk, 1969), the amount of SP immunoreactivity contained in the whole organ of the uterus, cervix, or vagina does not vary according to the oestrus cycle or the term of pregnancy and is markedly reduced by capsaicin treatment, suggesting their presence in primary afferent fibres (Traurig et al., 1984). In the male, SP-nerves are scarcer than in the female. In the testis, epididymis and seminal vesicle they are found in the organ capsule and in the interstitial connective tissue; in the ductus deferens single fibres occur beneath the epithelium as well as in the smooth muscle layer and in the adventitial connective tissue (Alm et al., 1978).

Roles of afferents from reproductive organs

In general, visceral afferents may have a role in transmitting information to build up sensation and/or to induce reflexive modulations on the functions of their innervating and the other organs. Sensations other than "discomfort" or "pain" might be evoked by activation of sensory afferents of the reproductive organs, for example, sexual orgasm, but the mechanism for this is not clear yet. Also, only little is known as to whether these afferents play important roles in regulating the functions of reproductive organs, probably because powerful hormonal influences on these organs mask the role of the nervous system. Ever since the work of Goltz and Freusberg in 1874, it has been known that well-organized activities such as pregnancy and parturition can progress without the central nervous system. Clinically, parturition is normally processed under blocking of the nerves to the reproductive organs.

Pain and discomfort

Pain of an indefinite nature, and usually poorly localized, may be produced by expanding growth of the ovary. Normal ovulation may at times causes some discomfort or pain. This "intermenstrual pain" occurs on one side of the body only in any cycle, although in other cycles it may occur on the opposite side. Cysts and tumours may also give rise to pain, but severe pain is not usual unless there are additional contributing factors, such as the twisted pedicle of a cyst or sudden distension by haemorrhage into a cyst.

Javert and Hardy (1950) attempted quantitative measurements of labour pain expressed in "dols", by comparing the pain with that measured at the skin with the Hardy-Wolff-Goodell dolorimeter at periods between uterine contractions. The intermittent Braxton Hicks contractions occurring at the end of pregnancy or uterine contractions produced by intravenous oxytocin are painless, unless the cervix is dilating. During the second stage of labour, the pain intensity has been measured at 10.5 dols; this is the "ceiling pain" which is evoked by heat producing a third-degree burn on the skin. Allowing for individual patient variation, the pain intensity in dols is approximately equal to the degree of dilatation of the cervix in centimetres.

The cervix is considered to be more or less insensitive, and may be grasped with a forceps with sharp hooks and cauterized without any anaesthetic. Application of a stick of silver nitrate causes pain in patients who suffer from dysmenorrhoea, but not in normal postnatal clinic patients (Theobald, 1936). These observations suggest that mechanical and chemical stimulation of the sensory receptors in the cervix may cause pain only when they are stimulated summatively, either temporally and/or spatially, for example, by the distension of the whole cervical canal simultaneously, or by pre-existing irritation of the neighbouring organs.

The valuable observations by Woollard and Carmichael (1933) mentioned above reveal that the weight applied to the scrotum causes no sensation, uncomfortable feeling, discomfort of various degree, and definite pain, in that order, when increasing the weight, and that the pain threshold is raised by blocking the nerves one after another.

Clinically, pains from the scrotal contents are often caused by torsion of the testis or of testicular appendages: the appendix testis — a remnant of the Muellerian duct — and the appendix epididymis — a vestige of the most cranial Wolffian duct (Barker and Raper, 1964; Skoglund et al., 1970).

Reflex activities induced by afferents of reproductive organs

Afferent inputs from the reproductive organs cause various viscero-visceral and -somatic reflexes. In some mammalian species, ovulation occurs after the stimulus of coitus. Mechanical or electrical stimulation of the cervix during oestrus in rats causes prolongation of the life of the corpus luteum, "pseudopregnancy" (Shelesnyak, 1931; Haterius, 1937; Greep and Hisaw, 1938). Distension of the cervix and vagina elicits a secretion of posterior pituitary hormone (Ferguson, 1941; Roberts and

Share, 1968), and responses of paraventricular and supraoptic neurons by vaginal distension have been reported (Negoro et al., 1973; Dreifuss et al., 1976; Myers and Jennings, 1985). During oestrus, when a periodic increase of spontaneous activity of the uterus is greatest, the latency of the Achilles tendon reflex becomes longer; this effect is abolished after abdominal sympathectomy (Herren and Haterius, 1931, 1932). Cervical stimulation of female rats prolongs lordosis after intromission and immobilizes them longer compared with rats whose pelvic nerves are bilaterally sectioned (Diakow, 1970). Mechanical stimulation of the vaginal cervix in rats suppresses vocalization responses to noxious tail shock in parallel to the increase in the intensity of genital stimulation (Crowley et al., 1976). The analgesic effect of this stimulation is confirmed by a marked suppression of the nociceptive responses of the neurons in the ventrobasal complex of the thalamus (Komisaruk and Wallman, 1977).

Electrophysiological studies on the primary afferent fibres of reproductive organs

Female reproductive organs

Unit-responses to genital stimuli have been reported in extensive brain areas, the hypothalamus, limbic system, thalamus, midbrain, pons and medulla (Barraclough and Cross, 1963; Kawakami and Saito, 1967; Chhina and Anand, 1969; Kawakami and Kubo, 1971; Rose and Sutin, 1971; Rose, 1975). However, limited information is available on the characteristics of the peripheral sensory afferents. Responses to digital pressure and traction of the uterus, uterine tube and broad ligament or distension of the uterus with a balloon have been recorded from the uterine nerve of the rabbit (Bower, 1959, 1966). Mainly based on the size of the action potential, Bower classified these afferents into two groups: one with larger spikes from the broad ligament and another with smaller spikes from the uterus. In general, it is quite difficult and risky to use the size of action potential as a basis for classification. Floyd et al. (1976, 1977) have also described the characteristics of receptors associated with the uterus and broad ligament recorded from the hypogastric nerve of the cat. These sensory units have several punctate receptive sites, mechanical stimulation of which causes tonic discharges. Distension of an intrauterine balloon elicits both tonic and phasic responses. There is no clear separation between receptors of the uterus and those of the broad ligament, and some units have mechanosensitive sites associated with both tissues (Floyd et al., 1976). Although the features of mechanical responses and receptive fields of these sensory receptors reported by Floyd et al. are quite similar to those of the testicular afferents described in the next section, bradykinin, one of the most consistent chemical stimulants for the testicular polymodal receptors, does not give consistent responses for the uterus units (Floyd et al., 1977).

Male reproductive organs

More than 95% of the fibres of the superior spermatic nerve have been found to be nonmyelinated. Studies of electrically evoked compound action potentials after degeneration of afferent fibres by dorsal rhizotomy have shown that almost all myelinated fibres involved in this nerve are afferent, while some portion of the unmyelinated fibres are also afferent (Peterson and Brown, 1973).

Our studies on several hundred single units recorded from canine superior spermatic nerve have revealed that the great majority of these units are of the polymodal receptor, although a few (about 3%), rapidly adapting mechanoreceptors are also found. The latter are characterized as follows: A weak mechanical stimulus moving across the receptive field is the most effective stimulation. Therefore, it is difficult to define the size of the receptive field, but several sensitive areas of a few mm in diameter are found at the testis and/or epididymis. These receptors rarely respond to chemical and heat stimulation. Conduction velocities range between 17.5 and 50.1 m/second, and the mean is 31.9 ± 4.4 m/second, which is faster than those of the poly-

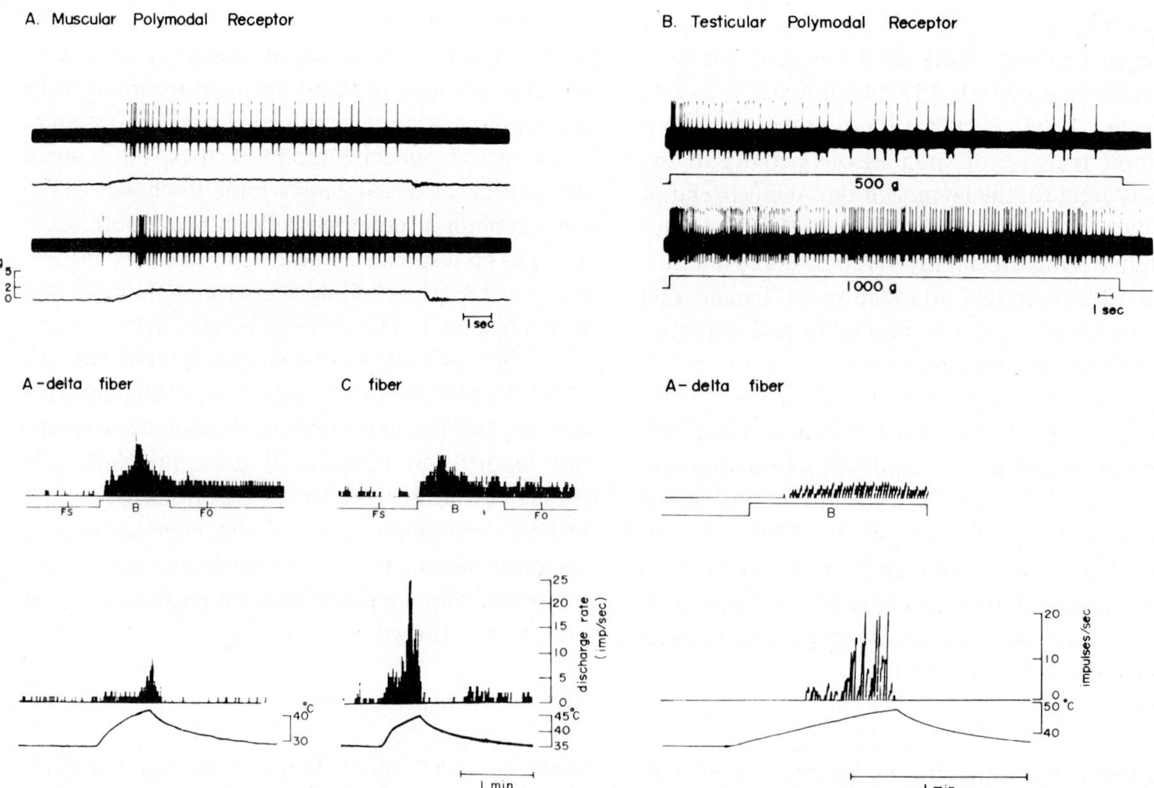

Fig. 1. Mechanical, chemical, and heat responses of the muscular and testicular polymodal receptor. A, responses of an Aδ- and a C-fibre muscular unit; for C-fibre only chemical and heat responses are shown. B, responses of an Aδ-fibre testicular unit. Top traces, responses to mechanical stimulation of two intensities; middle traces, peristimulus histograms of discharge responses to application of bradykinin, indicated by B at the lower bar deflexion; bottom traces, responses to heat.

modal receptors (Kumazawa, Mizumura and Sato, unpublished data).

Polymodal receptors

The testicular polymodal receptors respond to all of the mechanical, chemical and heat stimuli in a similar manner as found in the muscular thin fibre afferents shown in Fig. 1 (Kumazawa and Mizumura, 1977a, 1980a,b). A slowly adapting response is evoked by mechanical stimulation on the sensitive points less than 1 mm in diameter. When the stimulus is applied but not exactly to the sensitive point, it does not evoke a slowly-adapting response but often causes an apparently rapidly-adapting response. This might explain the comparatively great population of the rapidly adapting mechanoreceptors in the testicular afferents reported by Peterson and Brown (1973). As shown in Fig. 2, the collision test reveals that one unit has multiple sensitive points separated clearly from each other at the testis and epididymis or both. Conduction velocities measured from the spermatic cord range between 0.1 and 39.4 m/second, and the mean is 10.2 ± 0.3 m/second (n = 466). About 90% of the recorded units are of conduction velocity above 2.5 m/second. The latencies measured from the receptive site are much longer than those measured from the spermatic cord, as shown in Fig. 2. Although the actual course of the nerves innervating these receptive sites is not known and the real conduction velocities at the receptive region could not be de-

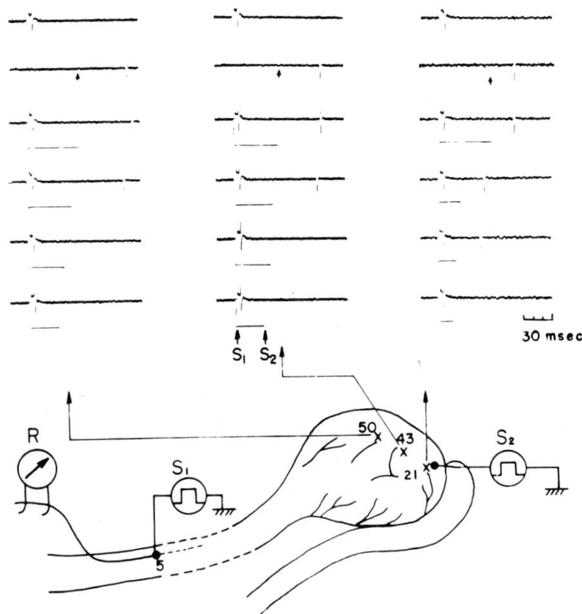

Fig. 2. Several receptive sites of a single testicular polymodal receptor unit, identified by the collision test. × and numbers on the drawing at the bottom show the location of receptive sites and latencies of the response evoked by electrical stimulation at each site, respectively. In each of three panels, the first trace, the response to stimulation at the nerve trunk (S1); the second trace, that at the receptive site (S2); the third to sixth traces, S2 was stimulated after S1 with an interval shown by a bar under each trace. From Kumazawa and Mizumura (1980a).

termined, this remarkable elongation of latency at the receptive region suggests that a myelinated fibre at the spermatic cord sends out unmyelinated branches in the receptive site.

The mechanical threshold measured by Von Frey type, calibrated nylon hair shows a tendency for the stimulator with the larger tip diameter to give lower thresholds (Kumazawa and Mizumura, 1980a). Those measured by the tip diameter of 0.4 mm^2 range between 0.9 and 270 g/mm^2 and about 80% of the total 475 units have thresholds less than 17 g/mm^2, which is quite innocuous when applied to the human skin. This wide range of the mechanical thresholds might be attributed to the depth of the real receptive site from the surface or to a difference of the physical nature of the surface over the receptive site. For example, the mean of the mechanical threshold at the testis (21 g/mm^2) is significantly higher than that at the epididymis (11 g/mm^2), which is covered by a thinner surface membrane. The mean mechanical threshold of A-fibre units is significantly lower than that of C-fibre units, and there is a rough tendency for the faster fibres to have a lower mechanical threshold.

Fig. 3 shows the response to various weights applied on the testicular surface through a round disk of 10 mm in diameter. Most of the units respond to 50 g (as low as 0.4 g/mm^2) and increase their discharges monotonously to an enormously high intensity as 2 kg weight. Discharges after the cessation of high-intensity stimulation are very often observed, as shown in Fig. 3. As described above, Woollard and Carmichael (1933) reported that an overt pain sensation is evoked with several hundred grams on the scrotum applied in a similar way as used in our experiment. Thus, the polymodal receptors respond to mechanical stimuli of well below the intensity required to cause human pain, in addition to signaling information of definitely noxious range. This wide dynamic range property is one of the conspicuous characteristics of the polymodal receptor.

Participation of the polymodal receptors in nociceptive functions is also suggested from their responses to chemical stimuli. Algesic substances such as bradykinin, hypertonic saline and potassium ions consistently evoke discharges of the receptor; sensitizing substances such as prostaglandins or serotonin augment responses of the receptor; peripherally-acting analgesics such as aspirin suppress the response to a certain kind of chemical stimulus (Kumazawa and Mizumura, 1984a,b).

Fig. 4 shows the responses to three algesic substances described above. Although these substances consistently evoke dose-dependent responses of the polymodal receptors, the discharge pattern to each substance is quite different, suggesting the involvement of different exciting mechanisms. There is no significant difference in the responses to chemical stimulations between A-fibre units and C-fibre units. Repetition of bradykinin application with an

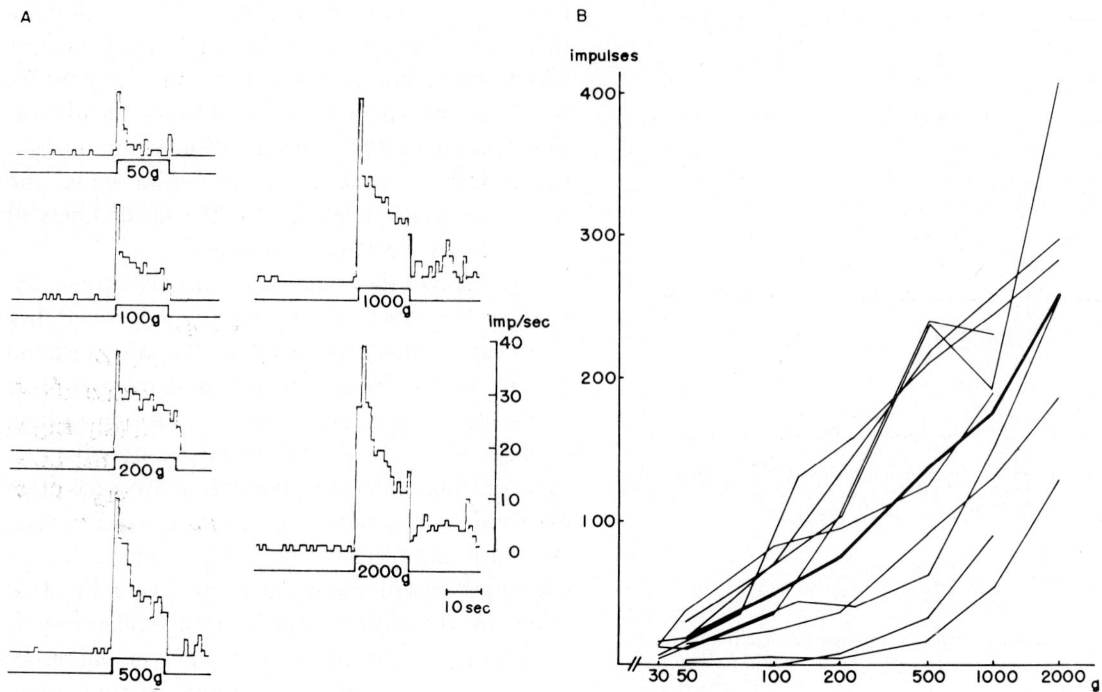

Fig. 3. Mechanical responses of the testicular polymodal receptor. A, response patterns of a single unit to application of various weights (shown by the numbers at the lower bar deflexion) on the testis. B, total numbers of impulses evoked during 15-second periods of stimulations with various intensities. The thick line represents a mean value obtained from these nine units. From Kumazawa and Mizumura (1980a).

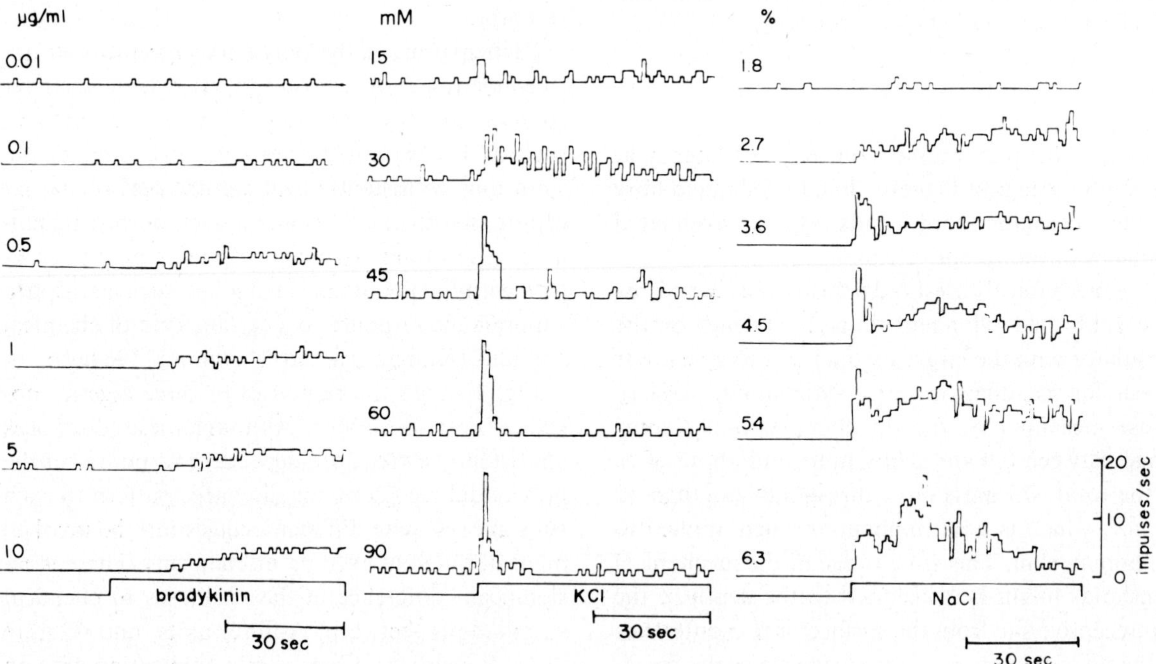

Fig. 4. Response patterns of the testicular polymodal receptor to bradykinin, KCl and NaCl solutions of various concentrations. Concentrations used are shown at the left of each panel.

interval less than 15 minutes causes a marked reduction of the response in the subsequent trials, "tachyphylaxis"; conversely, if the repetition interval is long (more than 30 minutes), an augmented response is observed. The mechanisms causing "tachyphylaxis" with a short repetition interval or "sensitization" with a long interval are not known. An occurrence of and recovery from a hypothesized internalization of drug-receptors or different time courses of depletion and synthesis-acceleration of sensitizing substances, and other mechanisms might explain these phenomena. The response to hypertonic saline also indicates tachyphylactic behaviour but of only slight degree. Acetylcholine, histamine, and synthetic substance P have an inconsistent and much weaker stimulating effect, if any, for the polymodal receptors (Kumazawa and Mizumura, 1979). Prostaglandins E_2 and I_2, and serotonin are also inconsistent stimulants. However, these substances potentiate the responses of the polymodal receptors to algesic substances without having any apparent direct stimulating effects on these receptors.

The action of an aspirin-like drug such as indomethacin or acetylsalicylic acid is due to inhibition of prostaglandin synthesis (Vane, 1971). Indomethacin suppresses or abolishes the response to bradykinin without significant influence on the response to KCl at the same receptive site of the polymodal receptor, as shown in Fig. 5 (Kumazawa and Mi-

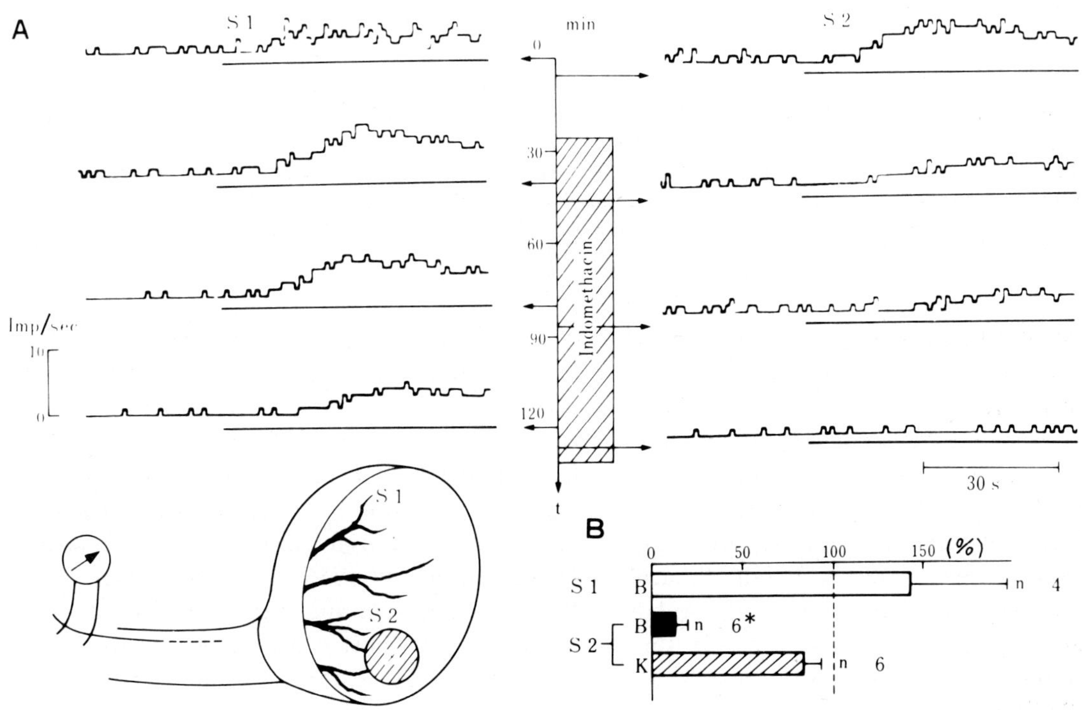

Fig. 5. Suppression of bradykinin response by indomethacin. A. Two receptive sites of a testicular polymodal receptor unit (depicted in the schematic drawing at the bottom left) were used, the one for control response shown on the left half (S1), the other for testing indomethacin effect on bradykinin responses shown on the right half (S2). The vertical bar in the centre is a time axis, and the period of indomethacin (10 μg/ml) application is shown as an obliquely hatched column. B. The mean changes in discharge rates after indomethacin are shown as the percentage to the first response. White column, bradykinin response at the control site; black column, bradykinin response at the indomethacin site; hatched column, KCl response tested at the indomethacin site. Modified from Kumazawa and Mizumura (1980b).

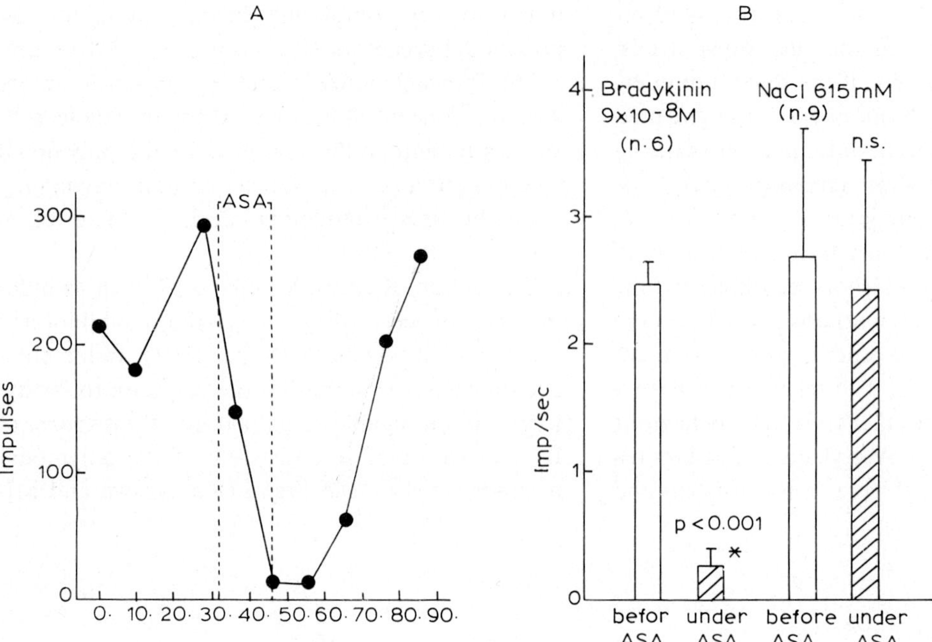

Fig. 6. Effects of acetylsalicylic acid (ASA) on the response of the polymodal receptor to bradykinin and hypertonic saline. A, time course of suppressive effect of acetylsalicylic acid on bradykinin responses of a polymodal receptor. Ordinate, total impulse number evoked by a 1-minute application of bradykinin (9×10^{-8} M); abscissa, time after the beginning of the first bradykinin application, in minutes. The period of acetylsalicylic acid application (5.5×10^{-4} M) is marked by broken lines. B, responses to bradykinin (left two columns) and to hypertonic saline (right two columns) before and under administration of acetylsalicylic acid. Ordinate, net mean discharge rate during 60 (bradykinin) and 30 (hypertonic saline) seconds of stimulation. From Mizumura et al. (1984).

zumura, 1980b). Thus, it is suggested that afferent discharges of polymodal receptors evoked by bradykinin partly involve activation of bradykinin-induced release of prostaglandins reported in various tissues (McGiff et al., 1972; Ferreira et al., 1973; Moncada et al., 1975; Lembeck et al., 1976). In another series of experiment using in vitro preparation, it was confirmed that acetylsalicylic acid suppresses the response to bradykinin but not that to hypertonic saline (Fig. 6), and that the suppressed bradykinin responses were reversed by exogenous application of prostaglandin E_2 (Mizumura and Kumazawa, 1984). These results provide clear electrophysiological evidence at the sensory receptor level that explains why aspirin is effective for inflammatory pains but not for experimentally induced mechanical or heat pains (Beecher, 1957; Lim et al., 1964).

Activity of this receptor is enhanced in a pathological condition such as inflammation. Our study using an in vitro preparation (Kumazawa and Mizumura, 1984b) has revealed that abnormal burst-like activities of the polymodal receptors are elicited by application of clioquinol, which has been known as the causal agent of subacute myelo-optico-neuropathy (SMON) (Shigematsu, 1975). Peculiar unpleasant and very often painful dysesthesiae are the most conspicuous sensory disturbances of this disease (Sobue, 1979). Irregular burst activities shown in Fig. 7A are elicited a few to 30 minutes after application of clioquinol (1–100 μM), and they last long after removal of the drug with interposed silent periods. At higher concentrations, clioquinol tended to excite the receptor activity consistently with a shorter latency and to evoke discharges of a higher rate. It is also noteworthy that

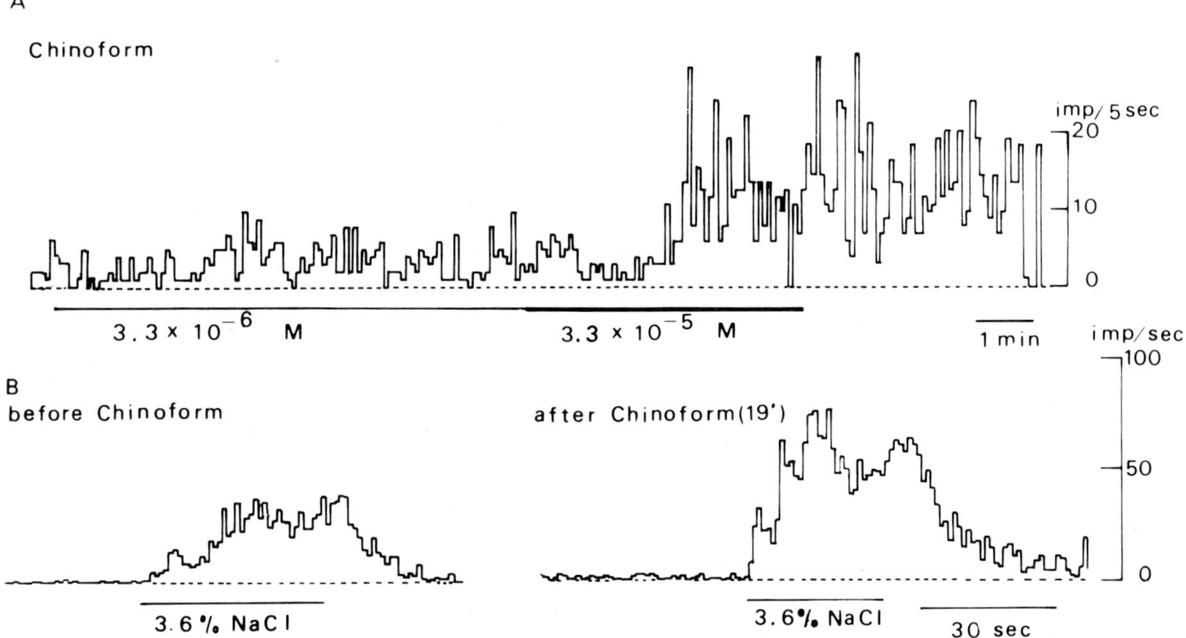

Fig. 7. Effects of clioquinol on a testicular polymodal unit activity. A, abnormal bursting activity induced by clioquinol (chinoform). B, response to hypertonic saline before and after application of clioquinol.

this drug treatment causes changes in receptor characteristics of the polymodal receptors. After activation by clioquinol, the polymodal receptors become sensitive to cold and the response to hypertonic saline becomes much larger than before (Fig. 7B).

The importance of Ca^{2+} in transduction mechanisms in some sensory receptors is well known. When the receptive region of the polymodal receptors is exposed to Ca^{2+}-depleted (+1 mM EGTA) Krebs solution, responses to hypertonic saline and high potassium-ion solution are augmented to 2–3 times the level before Ca^{2+}-depletion. Burst-like activities after application of clioquinol are suppressed by increasing the Ca^{2+} concentration and enhanced by its depletion. Since these enhancing effects of Ca^{2+}-depletion on the activity of the polymodal receptors are reversed by addition of Mg^{2+}, these phenomena presumably depend on depolarization of the receptor membrane by Ca^{2+}-depletion. On the contrary, Ca^{2+}-depletion suppresses responses to bradykinin and also the sensitizing effects of prostaglandin E_2. In this case, Mg^{2+} is not effective as a substitute for Ca^{2+}. A specific role of Ca^{2+} might be implicated in the intermediary steps in the action of bradykinin: for example, Ca^{2+} is needed for activation of phospholipase A_2, an enzyme for the synthesis of prostaglandins (T. Kumazawa, M. Mizumura and J. Sato, unpublished results).

Another characteristic of the polymodal receptor is its response to heat stimulation, as has been reported in the skin (Iggo, 1959; Bessou and Perl, 1969; Beck et al., 1974; Beitel and Dubner, 1976; Croze et al., 1976; Kumazawa and Perl, 1977), muscle (Kumazawa and Mizumura, 1976, 1977a), and visceral organs (Nishi et al., 1977; Kumazawa and Mizumura, 1977b, 1980a). In response to heating above around 45°C, the testicular polymodal receptors give irregular discharges that increase roughly in parallel to temperature rise. Repetition of heating lowers the threshold temperature and increases

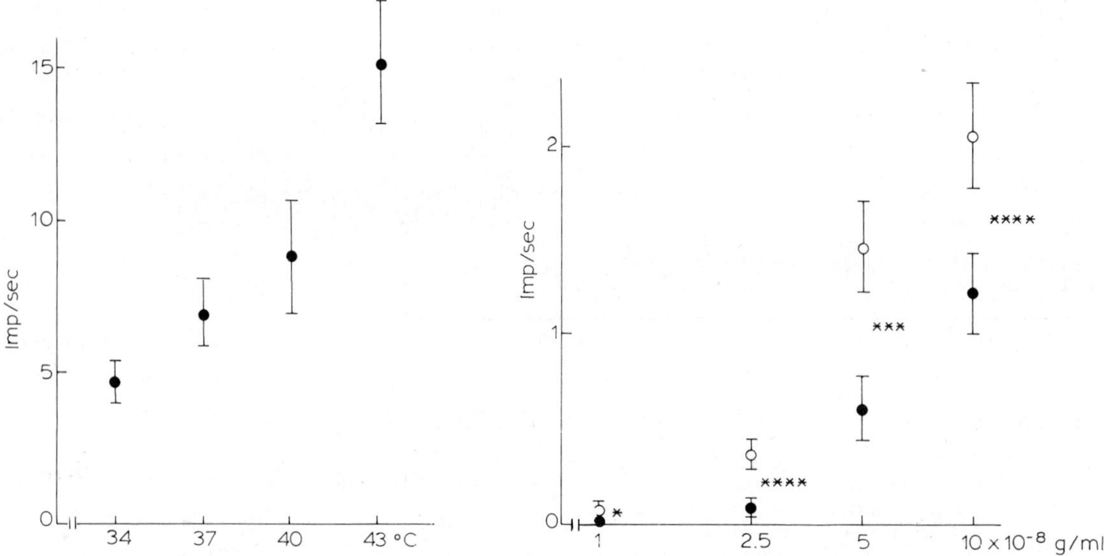

Fig. 8. Effects of temperature rise subthreshold to the polymodal receptors on responses to hypertonic saline and bradykinin. Left, ordinate gives mean discharge rate during a 1-minute application of a 4.5% NaCl solution; abscissa, temperature of the test solution. Right, concentration-response relation of bradykinin at 30 and 36°C. Ordinate, mean discharge rate during a 1-minute application of bradykinin; abscissa, concentration of bradykinin. Black circles, response at 30°C; white circles, response at 36°C. Modified from Kumazawa and Mizumura (1983).

discharges in the subsequent heating in some units (sensitization), but reverse effects are also observed in another units (desensitization). Desensitization tends to be more frequently induced in units which have relatively lower heat thresholds and thus are heated to a temperature far beyond the threshold, as has been reported in the cutaneous polymodal receptors (Bessou and Perl, 1969; Beitel and Dubner, 1976; Kumazawa and Perl, 1977). In the sensitized units, responses to hypertonic saline are also augmented after heating (Mizumura and Kumazawa, 1983).

Although the polymodal receptors are excited by heating above a noxious range, whether the temperature rise subthreshold to the receptors has any effect on the activity of the receptor might be an interesting question, since our ordinary experiences show that cooling an inflamed region alleviates spontaneous pain while warming strengthens it. As shown in Fig. 8, responses to the same concentration of hypertonic saline are increased in parallel with the rise of temperature by 3°C in a range between 34°C (ordinary temperature of testis surface) and 43°C (just subthreshold to most of the units). Responses to different concentrations of bradykinin tested at 36°C are significantly larger and have a lower threshold than those tested at 30°C (Fig. 8) (Kumazawa and Mizumura, 1983).

General considerations

Visceral afferents of the reproductive organs might be characterized by their complex innervation reflecting the developmental process of these organs and by the fact that sensory receptors reported in these organs so far, show much less variety than those found in the skin. It might be teleologically reasonable that there are only a few kinds of sensory afferents in the organs which are located deep within the body and are normally exposed to fewer and less varied stimuli compared with those on the body surface.

The studies by the present authors on the sensory

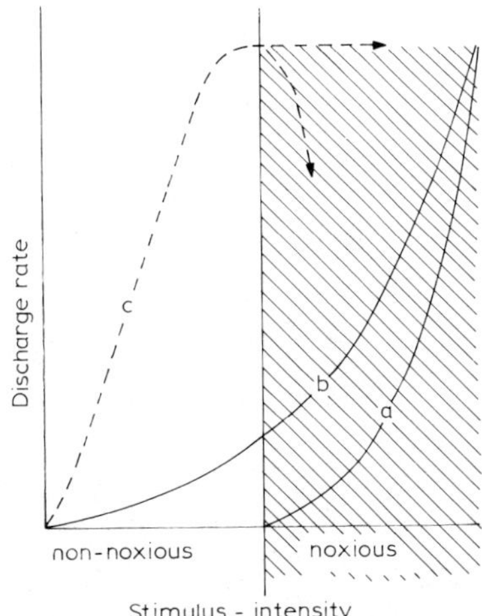

Fig. 9. Schematic representation of nociceptors and non-nociceptors.

afferents in visceral and somatic deep tissues reveal that the great majority of sensory afferents in the superior spermatic nerve as well as in the gastrocnemius muscle nerve are of the polymodal receptor type (Kumazawa and Mizumura, 1976, 1977a,b, 1980a). A wide distribution of this type of receptor in the body may be suggested from the data described in other chapters of this book. The name "polymodal" is derived from the fact that this receptor can respond to various (poly) modes of stimuli: mechanical, chemical and thermal stimuli, showing the not well differentiated or primitive nature of the receptor. Presumably, these polymodal receptors play important roles in nociceptive functions and also autonomic nervous regulation, both of which are considered to be developed at quite an earlier stage of nervous system evolution (Kumazawa, 1981). Activation of the muscular polymodal receptors causes circulatory responses and respiratory responses of dose-dependent facilitation and inhibition via the endogenous opiate system (Mizumura and Kumazawa, 1976; Kumazawa et al., 1980, 1981; Kumazawa and Tadaki, 1983).

Although the classification of nociceptors has not been completed, a tentative one is shown schematically in Fig. 9. Nociceptors are defined by the ability to send information on the intensity of the stimulus in the noxious range. They are divided into two groups: one responds exclusively to noxious stimuli (Fig. 9a), such as the high-threshold mechanoreceptor, and the other responds intensity-dependently to noxious stimuli but also responds to stimuli of the non-noxious level (Fig. 9b), such as the polymodal receptor. As far as the testicular afferents are concerned, the high-threshold mechanoreceptors have not been found. Thus, the nociceptor in this organ, and probably in the other visceral organs, may be the polymodal receptor.

Nociceptive information is transmitted by special sets of sensory receptors and central pathways to build up pain sensation. In this sense the "specificity theory" of pain seems to be quite valid. However, temporally and spatially summated excitation of the polymodal receptors induced by stimulation of a high intensity may be needed to evoke visceral pain sensations. The "intensity theory" may be valid in this sense but not in the sense that pain sensations can be evoked by every kind of sensory receptors when they are stimulated excessively. The notion that summated inputs are needed for evoking visceral pain from the reproductive organs is supported from observations mentioned previously: the weight on the scrotum necessary to evoke testicular pain increases to about 800 g after blocking the posterior scrotal nerve, ileo-inguinal nerve, and genito-femoral nerve, compared to 200–300 g with the nerves intact (Woollard and Carmichael, 1933); application of silver nitrate to the cervix causes pain only in patients suffering from dysmenorrhoea (Theobald, 1936).

As mentioned previously, vaginal stimulation modulates various neuroendocrine functions. Convergence of the inputs of vaginal distension and of noxious stimulation of the foot is found in the paraventricular nucleus neurons (Negoro et al., 1973). Khayutin et al. (1976) differentiated two components in the responses of blood pressure induced by intra-arterial injection of bradykinin to the visceral area: a non-nociceptive and a nociceptive response (Fig. 10A, B). Fig. 10C shows the dose-response relationship of the testicular polymodal receptors to bradykinin (Kumazawa and Mizumura 1980b),

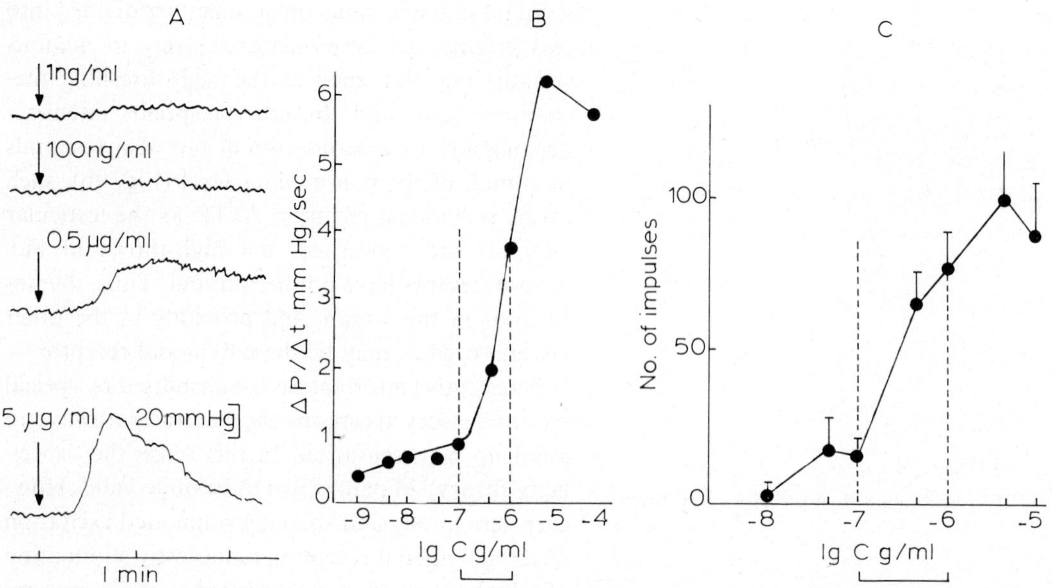

Fig. 10. Dose relationship of the pressor response to bradykinin applied to the small intestine of the cat, compared with that of the testicular polymodal receptor unit activity. A, responses on the arterial blood pressure to bradykinin injected intra-arterially to the small intestine of the cat. B, relationship between the rate of arterial pressure rise and the concentration of bradykinin injected. Modified from Khayutin et al. (1976). C, the mean of discharges of testicular polymodal receptor units evoked by various concentrations of bradykinin. Modified from Kumazawa and Mizumura (1980b).

indicating a similar dose relationship to the reflex response shown in Fig. 10B. The above-mentioned results might suggest that the sensory receptor which plays a role in nociceptive functions could also play an important role in reflex responses, including non-nociceptive ones. Therefore, the term "polymodal receptor" is employed instead of the polymodal nociceptor which had originally been designated (Bessou and Perl, 1969).

References

Abrahams, V. C. and Teare, J. I. (1969) Peripheral pathways and properties of uterine afferents in the cat. Can. J. Physiol. Pharmacol., 47: 576–577.

Adham, N. and Schenk, E. A. (1969) Autonomic innervation of the rat vagina, cervix, and uterus and its cyclic variation. Am. J. Obst. Gynecol., 104: 508–516.

Alm, P., Alumets, J., Håkanson, R. and Sundler, F. (1977) Peptidergic (vasoactive intestinal peptide) nerves in the genito-urinary tract. Neuroscience, 2: 751–754.

Alm, P., Alumets, J., Brodin, E., Håkanson, R., Nilsson, G., Sjöberg, N.-O. and Sundler, F. (1978) Peptidergic (substance P) nerves in the genito-urinary tract. Neuroscience, 3: 419–425.

Alm, P., Alumets, J., Håkanson, R., Owman, Ch., Sjöberg, N.-O., Stjernqvist, M. and Sundler, F. (1981) Enkephalin-immunoreactive nerve fibers in the feline genito-urinary tract. Histochemistry, 72: 351–355.

Barker, K. and Raper, F. P. (1964) Torsion of the testis. Br. J. Urol., 36: 35–41.

Barraclough, C. A. and Cross, B. A. (1963) Unit activity in the hypothalamus of the cyclic female rat: effect of genital stimuli and progesterone. J. Endocrinol., 26: 339–359.

Beck, P. W., Handwerker, H. O. and Zimmermann, M. (1974) Nervous outflow from the cat's foot during noxious radiant heat stimulation. Brain Res., 67: 373–386.

Beecher, H. K. (1957) The measurement of pain. Prototype for quantitative study of subjective response. Pharmacol. Rev., 9: 59–209.

Beitel, R. F. and Dubner, R. (1976) Response of unmyelinated (C) polymodal nociceptors to thermal stimuli applied to monkey's face. J. Neurophysiol., 39: 1160–1175.

Bessou, P. and Perl, E. R. (1969) Response of cutaneous sensory units with unmyelinated fibers to noxious stimuli. J. Neurophysiol., 32: 1025–1043.

Bonica, J. J. (1967) Principles and Practice of Obstetric Analgesia and Anesthesia, F. A. Davis, Philadelphia, p. 107.

Bonica, J. J. (1975) Clinics in Obstetrics and Gynaecology, W. B. Saunders Co. Ltd., London, pp. 499–516.

Bower, E. A. (1959) Action potentials from uterine sensory nerves. J. Physiol. (Lond.), 148: 2P–3P.

Bower, E. A. (1966) The characteristics of spontaneous and evoked action potentials recorded from the rabbit's uterine nerves. J. Physiol. (Lond.), 183: 730–747.

Brodin, E. and Nilsson, G. (1981) Concentration of substance P-like immunoreactivity (SPLI) in tissues of dog, rat and mouse. Acta Physiol. Scand., 112: 305–312.

Chhina, G. S. and Anand, B. K. (1969) Responses of neurones in the hypothalamus and limbic system to genital stimulation in adult and immature monkeys. Brain Res., 13: 511–521.

Cleland, J. G. P. (1933) Paravertebral anesthesia in obstetrics. Surg. Gynecol. Obstet., 57: 51–62.

Crowley, W. R., Jacobs, R., Volpe, J., Rodriguez-Sierra, J. F. and Komisaruk, B. R. (1976) Analgesic effect of vaginal stimulation in rats; modulation by graded stimulus intensity and hormones. Physiol. Behav., 16: 483–488.

Croze, S., Duclaux, R. and Kenshalo, D. R. (1976) The thermal sensitivity of the polymodal nociceptors in the monkey. J. Physiol. (Lond.), 263: 539–562.

Diakow, C. (1970) Effects of genital desensitization on the mating pattern of female rats as determined by motion picture analysis. Am. Zool., 10: 486.

Dreifuss, J. J., Tribollet, E. and Baertschi, A. J. (1976) Excitation of supraoptic neurones by vaginal distension in lactating rats; correlation with neurohypophysial hormone release. Brain Res., 113: 600–605.

Fahrenkrug, J. and Ottesen, B. (1982) Nervous release of vasoactive intestinal polypeptide from the feline uterus: pharmacological characteristics. J. Physiol. (Lond.), 331: 451–460.

Ferguson, J. K. (1941) Study of motility of the intact uterus at term. Surg. Gynecol. Obst., 73: 359–366.

Ferreira, S. H., Moncada, S. and Vane, J. R. (1973) Prostaglandins and the mechanism of analgesia produced by aspirin-like drugs. Br. J. Pharmacol., 49: 86–97.

Floyd, K., Hick, V. E. and Morrison, J. F. B. (1976) Mechanosensitive afferent units in the hypogastric nerve of the cat. J. Physiol. (Lond.), 259: 457–471.

Floyd, K., Hick, V. E., Koley, J. and Morrison, J. F. B. (1977) The effects of bradykinin on afferent units in intra-abdominal sympathetic nerve trunks. Q. J. Exp. Physiol., 62: 19–25.

Goltz, F. and Freusberg, A. (1874) Ueber den Einfluss des Nervensystems auf die Vorgänge während der Schwangerschaft und des Gebörakh. Pflügers Arch., 9: 552–565.

Greep, R. O. and Hisaw, F. L. (1938) Pseudopregnancies from electrical stimulation of the cervix in the diestrum. Proc. Soc. Exp. Biol. Med., 39: 359–360.

Haterius, H. O. (1937) Studies on a neuro-hypophyseal mechanism influencing gonadotrophic activity. Q. Biol., 5: 280–288.

Head, H. (1893) On disturbances of sensation with special reference to the pain of visceral disease. Brain, 16: 1–132.

Herren, R. Y. and Haterius, H. O. (1931) The relation of ovarian hormones to electromyographically determined Achilles reflex time. Am. J. Physiol., 96: 214–220.

Herren, R. Y. and Haterius, H. O. (1932) On the mechanism of certain ovarian hormonal influences on the central nervous system. Am. J. Physiol., 100: 533–536.

Hoekfelt, T., Kellerth, J.-O., Nilsson, G. and Pernow, B. (1975) Experimental immunohistochemical studies on the localization and distribution of substance P in cat primary sensory neurons. Brain Res., 100: 235–252.

Hoekfelt T., Schulzberg, M., Elde, R., Nilsson, G., Terenius, L., Said, S. and Goldstein, M. (1978) Peptidergic neurones in peripheral tissues including the urinary tract: immunohistochemical studies. Acta Pharmacol. Toxicol., 43: 79–89.

Iggo, A. (1959) Cutaneous heat and cold receptors with slowly conducting C afferent fibres. Q. J. Exp. Physiol., 44: 362–370.

Jancsó, G., Király, E. and Jancsó-Gábor, A. (1980) Chemosensitive pain fibres and inflammation. Int. J. Tissue Reac., 2: 57–66.

Jancsó, G., Hoekfelt, T., Lundberg, J. M., Király, E., Halász, N., Nilsson, G., Terenius, L., Rehfeld, J., Steinbusch, H., Verhobstad, A., Elde, R., Said, S. and Brown, M. (1981) Immunohistochemical studies on the effect of capsaicin on spinal and medullary peptide and monoamine neurons using antisera to substance P, gastrin/CCK, somatostatin, VIP, enkephalin, neurotensin and 5-hydroxytryptamine. J. Neurocytol., 10: 963–980.

Javert, C. T. and Hardy, J. D. (1950) Measurement of pain intensity in labor and its physiologic, neurologic and pharmacologic implications. Am. J. Obst. Gynecol., 60: 552–563.

Kawakami, M. and Kubo, K. (1971) Neuro-correlate of limbic-hypothalamo-pituitary-gonadal axis in the rat: change in limbic-hypothalamic unit activity induced by vaginal and electrical stimulation. Neuroendocrinology, 7: 65–89.

Kawakami, M. and Saito, H. (1967) Unit activity in the hypothalamus of the cat: effect of genital stimuli, luteinizing hormone and oxytocin. Jpn. J. Physiol., 17: 466–486.

Khayutin, V. M., Baraz, L. A., Lukoshkova, E. V., Sonia, R. S. and Chernilovskaya, P. F. (1976) Chemosensitive spinal afferents: thresholds of specific and nociceptive reflexes as compared with thresholds of excitation for receptors and axons. In A. Iggo and O. B. Ilyinsky (Eds.), Progress in Brain Research, Vol. 43, Elsevier, Amsterdam, pp. 293–306.

Kollar, E. J. (1953) Reproduction in the female rat after pelvic nerve neurectomy. Anat. Rec., 115: 641–658.

Komisaruk, B. R. and Wallman, J. (1977) Antinociceptive effects of vaginal stimulation in rats: neurophysiological and behavioral studies. Brain Res., 137: 85–107.

Komisaruk, B. R., Adler, N. T. and Hutchison, J. (1972) Genital sensory field: enlargement by estrogen treatment in female rats. Science, 178: 1295–1298.

Kreutz, W. (1964) Ueber das Vorkommen korpuskulaerer Nervenendigungen in der Tunica albuginea Testis des Menschen. Anat. Anz., 115: 27–34.

Kumazawa, T. (1981) Nociceptors and autonomic nervous control. Asian Med. J., 24: 632–656.

Kumazawa, T. and Mizumura, K. (1976) The polymodal C-fiber receptor in the muscle of the dog. Brain Res., 101: 589–593.

Kumazawa, T. and Mizumura, K. (1977a) Thin-fibre receptors responding to mechanical, chemical and thermal stimulation in the skeletal muscle of the dog. J. Physiol. (Lond.), 273: 179–194.

Kumazawa, T. and Mizumura, K. (1977b) The polymodal receptors in the testis of dogs. Brain Res., 136: 553–558.

Kumazawa, T. and Mizumura, K. (1979) Effects of synthetic substance P on unit-discharges of testicular nociceptors of dogs. Brain Res., 170: 553–557.

Kumazawa, T. and Mizumura, K. (1980a) Mechanical and thermal responses of polymodal receptors recorded from the superior spermatic nerve of dogs. J. Physiol. (Lond.), 299: 233–245.

Kumazawa, T. and Mizumura, K. (1980b) Chemical responses of polymodal receptors of the scrotal contents in dogs. J. Physiol. (Lond.), 299: 219–231.

Kumazawa, T. and Mizumura, K. (1983) Temperature dependency of the chemical responses of the polymodal receptor units in vitro. Brain Res., 278: 305–307.

Kumazawa, T. and Mizumura, K. (1984a) Functional properties of the polymodal receptors in the deep tissues. In W. Hamann and A. Iggo (Eds.), Sensory Receptor Mechanisms, World Scientific Publ. Co., Singapore, pp. 193–202.

Kumazawa, T. and Mizumura, K. (1984b) Abnormal activity of polymodal receptors induced by clioquinol (5-chloro-7-iodo-8-hydroxyquinoline). Brain Res., 310: 185–188.

Kumazawa, T. and Perl, E. R. (1977) Primate cutaneous sensory units with unmyelinated (C) afferent fibers. J. Neurophysiol., 40: 1325–1338.

Kumazawa, T. and Tadaki, E. (1983) Two different inhibitory effects on respiration by thin-fiber muscular afferents in cats. Brain Res., 272: 364–367.

Kumazawa, T., Tadaki, E. and Kim, K. (1980) A possible participation of endogenous opiates in respiratory reflexes induced by thin-fiber muscular afferents. Brain Res., 199: 244–248.

Kumazawa, T., Tadaki, E. and Kim, K. (1981) Naloxone effects on the blood pressure responses induced by thin-fiber muscular afferents. Brain Res., 205: 452–456.

Kuntz, A. (1947) The Autonomic Nervous System, Lea and Febiger, Philadelphia, pp. 304–323.

Kuntz, A. and Morris, R. E., Jr. (1946) Components and distribution of the spermatic nerves and the nerves of the vas deferens. J. Comp. Neurol., 85: 33–44.

Labate, J. S. and Reynolds, S. R. M. (1937) Sensory pathways of the ovarian plexus. Am. J. Obst. Gynecol., 34: 1–11.

Larsson, L.-I., Fahrenkrug, J. and De Muckadell, O. B. S. (1977) Vasoactive intestinal polypeptide occurs in nerves of the female genitourinary tract. Science, 197: 1374–1375.

Lembeck, F., Popper, H. and Juan, H. (1976) Release of prostaglandins by bradykinin as an intrinsic mechanism of its algesic effect. Naunyn-Schmiedeberg's Arch. Pharmacol., 294: 69–73.

Lim, R. K. S., Gutzman, F., Rodgers, D. W., Goto, K. and Braun, C. (1964) Site of action of narcotic and non-narcotic analgesics determined by blocking bradykinin evoked visceral pain. Arch. Int. Pharmacodyn., 152: 25–58.

Lundberg, J. M., Hökfelt, T., Nilsson, G., Terenius, L., Rehfeld, D., Elde, R. and Said, S. (1978) Peptide neurons in the vagus-splanchnic and sciatic nerves. Acta Physiol. Scand., 104: 499–501.

McGiff, J. C., Terragno, N. A., Malik, K. U. and Lonigro, A. J. (1972) Release of a prostaglandin E-like substance from canine kidney by bradykinin. Circ. Res., 31: 36–43.

Mitchell, G. A. G. (1953) Anatomy of the Autonomic Nervous System, Livingston, Edinburgh.

Mizumura, K. and Kumazawa, T. (1976) Reflex respiratory response induced by chemical stimulation of muscle afferents. Brain Res., 109: 402–406.

Mizumura, K. and Kumazawa, T. (1983) Sensitization effect of heat stimulation on heat response and on response to hypertonic saline of testicular polymodal receptors in vitro. Environ. Med., 27: 75–78.

Mizumura, K., Sato, J. and Kumazawa, T. (1984) Acetylsalicylic acid suppresses the response to bradykinin but not to hypertonic saline of testicular polymodal receptors in vitro. Environ. Med., 28: 37–40.

Moncada, S., Ferreira, S. H. and Vane, J. R. (1975) Inhibition of prostaglandin biosynthesis as the mechanism of aspirin-like drugs in the dog knee joint. Eur. J. Pharmacol., 31: 250–260.

Mori, T. (1967) The vagina-gastrointestinal reflex. J. Physiol. Soc. Jpn., 29: 315–319 (in Japanese).

Myers, L. J. and Jennings, D. P. (1985) Effects of intrajugular hypertonic saline, vaginal distension and vulvar massage on activity of supraoptic neuroendocrine cells. Brain Res., 326: 366–369.

Negoro, H., Visessuwan, S. and Holland, R. C. (1973) Reflex activation of paraventricular nucleus units during the reproductive cycle and in ovariectomized rats treated with oestrogen or progesterone. J. Endocrinol., 59: 559–567.

Nishi, K., Sakanashi, M. and Takenaka, F. (1977) Activation of afferent cardiac sympathetic nerve fibers of cats by pain producing substances and by noxious heat. Pflügers Arch., 372: 53–61.

Otsuka, M. and Konishi, S. (1976) Release of substance P-like immunoreactivity from isolated spinal cord of newborn rat. Nature, 264: 83–84.

Ottesen, B. (1981) Vasoactive intestinal polypeptide (VIP): effect on rabbit uterine smooth muscle in vivo and in vitro. Acta Physiol. Scand., 113: 193–199.

Pallie, W., Corner, G. W. and Weddell, G. (1954) Nerve terminations in the myometrium of the rabbit. Anat. Rec., 118: 789–812.

Peterson, D. F. and Brown, A. M. (1973) Functional afferent innervation of testis. J. Neurophysiol., 36: 425–433.

Roberts, J. S. and Share, L. (1968) Oxytocin in plasma of pregnant, lactating and cycling ewes during vaginal stimulation. Endocrinology, 83: 272–278.

Rose, J. D. (1975) Response properties and anatomical organization of pontine and medullary units responsive to vaginal stimulation in the cat. Brain Res., 97: 79–93.

Rose, J. D. and Sutin, J. (1971) Responses of single thalamic neurons to genital stimulation in female cats. Brain Res., 33: 533–539.

Routledge, J. H. and Elliott, H. (1962) Pain studies in pelvic viscera. Am. J. Obst. Gynecol., 83: 701–709.

Seto, H. (1957) Studies of the Sensory Innervation, Igaku Shoin Ltd., Tokyo (in Japanese), pp. 196–220.

Shelesnyak, M. C. (1931) The induction of pseudopregnancy in the rat by means of electrical stimulation. Anat. Rec., 49: 179–183.

Shigematsu, I. (1975) Subacute myelo-optico-neuropathy (SMON) and clioquinol. A response to doubts about clioquinol causation theory. Jpn. J. Med. Sci. Biol. Suppl., 28: 35–55.

Skoglund, R. W., McRoberts, J. W. and Ragde, H. (1970) Torsion of testicular appendages: presentation of 43 new cases and a collective review. J. Urol., 104: 598–600.

Sobue, I. (1979) Clinical aspects of subacute myelo-optico-neuropathy (SMON). In P. J. Vinken and G. W. Bruyn (Eds.), Handbook of Clinical Neurology, Vol. 37, North-Holland Publishing Company, Amsterdam, pp. 115–139.

Theobald, G. W. (1936) Referred pain and in particular that associated with dysmenorrhoea and labour. A preliminary report. Br. Med. J., 2: 1307–1308.

Traurig, H., Saria, A. and Lembeck, F. (1984) Substance P in primary afferent neurons of the female rat reproductive system. Naunyn-Schmiedeberg's Arch. Pharmacol., 326: 343–346.

Vane, J. R. (1971) Inhibition of prostaglandin synthesis as a mechanism of action for aspirin-like drugs. Nature New Biol., 231: 232–235.

Woollard, H. H. and Carmichael, E. A. (1933) The testis and referred pain. Brain, 56: 293–303.

Yaksh, T. L., Jessell, T. M., Gamse, R., Mudge, A. W. and Leeman, S. E. (1980) Intrathecal morphine inhibits substance P release from mammalian spinal cord in vivo. Nature, 286: 155–157.

Yamashita, K. (1939) Histological studies on the innervation of human testis and epididymis. J. Oriental Med., 30: 367–394 (in Japanese).

Yanagisawa, M. and Otsuka, M. (1984) The effect of a substance P antagonist on chemically induced nociceptive reflex in the isolated spinal cord-tail preparation of the newborn rat. Proc. Jpn. Acad., 60, Ser. B: 427–430.

F. Cervero and J. F.B. Morrison
Progress in Brain Research, Vol. 67

CHAPTER 9

Neurochemistry of visceral afferent neurones

G. J. Dockray and K. A. Sharkey

MRC Secretory Control Research Group, Physiological Laboratory, University of Liverpool, Brownlow Hill, P.O. Box 147, Liverpool L69 3BX, U.K.

Introduction

Until quite recently, almost nothing was known of the transmitters that might be used by visceral afferent neurones. This has now changed, with the identification by radioimmunoassay and immunohistochemistry of a number of biologically active peptides in primary sensory neurones, including visceral afferents. The evidence indicates that these peptides are synthesized within small-diameter afferents, transported to both their central and peripheral terminations, and can be released at these sites. The neurotoxin capsaicin has proved a valuable tool for analysing the organisation and functions of sensory peptide-containing neurones. When given to neonatal rats it produces permanent loss of small-diameter unmyelinated primary afferent fibres (Jancso et al., 1977) and, in high doses, some thin myelinated fibres (Lawson and Nickels, 1980; Nagy et al., 1983). Local application of capsaicin to sensory nerves in adult animals blocks axonal transport of neuropeptides, stimulates the release of neuropeptides from nerve endings, and then produces a long-lasting insensitivity to further stimulation (see Nagy, 1982; Fitzgerald, 1983).

It is proposed to review here present knowledge of the organization and chemistry of peptidergic visceral afferents with particular reference to the innervation of the gastrointestinal tract and to the distribution of peripheral terminals. Although it may be possible to identify afferents on the basis of other neurochemical properties, e.g., fluoride-resistant acid phosphatase histochemistry (Nagy and Hunt, 1982; Dalsgaard et al., 1984), serotonin uptake (Gaudin-Chazal et al., 1981), tyrosine hydroxylase activity (Price and Mudge, 1983; Katz et al., 1983) and adenosine deaminase (Nagy et al., 1984), the physiology of these sub-types of afferent neurones is less clear than that of the peptidergic afferents.

Identification of neuropeptides in visceral afferents

General aspects

The idea that biologically active peptides might be localized in afferent fibres can be traced to the identification by bioassay of substance P in dorsal root (Lembeck, 1953) and vagal nerve extracts (Pernow, 1953). Much of the recent progress has depended on the use of radioimmunoassay and immunohistochemistry. However, these experimental approaches are not sufficient for the unequivocal identification of a particular peptide. In radioimmunoassay, it is necessary to establish the chromatographic properties of the material being assayed and where possible to use a variety of antibodies that react with different regions of the peptide. Similarly, the importance of absorption controls in immunohistochemistry needs no emphasis, but even allowing for the rigorous application of controls it is seldom, if ever, possible to make a definitive identification by immunohistochemistry alone. Within the last 2 years the elucidation of gene sequence for several peptides found in primary afferent neurones, notably the preprotachykinins and calcitonin gene-related peptide (CGRP) (Nawa et al., 1983, 1984; Amara et al., 1982; Rosenfeld et al., 1983), has greatly extended our perception of the chemistry and localization of these substances. The importance of applying these methods to other peptides is obvious.

All the peptides so far localized to primary afferents are also known to occur in nerves or endocrine cells elsewhere in the body. All of them also belong to families of related peptides that are united by shared evolutionary or biosynthetic origins (Dockray, 1979, 1985). It is not surprising then, to find that a particular peptide has a wide spectrum of biological actions, neither is it surprising to find similar patterns of biological activities amongst members of the same structural family. Therefore, appropriate caution must be applied in interpreting the physiological significance of studies on the biological effects of different peptides.

Vagal afferents

Nerve cell bodies of the nodose ganglia have been stained in immunohistochemical studies using antibodies to substance P, cholecystokinin (CCK)/gastrin, somatostatin, and vasoactive intestinal polypeptide (VIP) (Lundberg et al., 1978; Helke et al., 1980a,b; Katz and Karten, 1980; Mantyh and Hunt, 1984). It is also possible that calcitonin gene-related peptide (CGRP) is produced in vagal afferents (Rosenfeld et al., 1983). There is immunohistochemical evidence for the transport of these peptides in afferent fibres since an accumulation of immunoreactive material occurs central to ligatures of the nerve trunk (Lundberg et al., 1978; Gamse et al., 1979; Brimijoin et al., 1980). Chemical evidence, in the form of radioimmunoassay and column chromatography, also provides direct support for the identification of substance P, somatostatin 14, and CCK-8 in extracts of vagal nerve (Gamse et al., 1979; Dockray et al., 1981; MacLean and Lewis, 1984a). The distinction between CCK-8 and gastrin in the vagus has, in the past, posed problems. These peptides share a common C-terminal pentapeptide, and C-terminal specific antibodies react with both peptides. The presence of heptadecapeptide gastrin (G17) in cat vagus was first suggested by Uvnas-Wallensten et al. (1977). Initial attempts by ourselves to confirm this in dog were unsuccessful. Instead, material with the immunochemical and chromatographic properties of CCK-8 was found in all samples. Later, it became clear that vagal nerve extracts of about 20–30% of the animals (dog and cat) examined possessed low concentrations of gastrin (Dockray et al., 1981). This has since been confirmed (Rehfeld and Lundberg, 1983). It seems that in the earlier study (Uvnas-Wallensten et al., 1977), samples had been subject to initial screening and only those containing gastrin were selected for the further studies that were subsequently reported.

Spinal afferents

Hökfelt et al. (1975, 1976) were the first to report that antibodies to substance P revealed 10–20% of dorsal root ganglia neurones in the rat, and that somatostatin antibodies revealed a separate population of about 10% of total neurones; it is now thought that these proportions may vary at different segmental levels (Tuchscherer and Seybold, 1985). Subsequently, CCK-, VIP-, bombesin/gastrin-releasing peptide (GRP)- and CGRP-like immunoreactivities have also been localized by immunohistochemistry to dorsal root ganglia cell bodies (Dalsgaard et al., 1982b; Panula et al., 1983; Kawatani et al., 1983; Gibson et al., 1984; Tuchscherer and Seybold, 1985). It is not yet clear if all these peptides occur in visceral afferents. Experiments involving ligation of the guinea pig lumbar splanchnic nerve indicate the transport of substantial quantities of substance P-like immunoreactivity toward the viscera in afferent fibres; by comparison, there appeared to be little or no CCK-, somatostatin- or VIP-like immunoreactivity transported towards the periphery (Dalsgaard et al., 1983). However, VIP may occur in a proportion of pelvic nerve afferents (Kawatani et al., 1983). The case for substance P, bombesin/GRP and CGRP in dorsal root ganglia is supported by radioimmunoassay and chromatographic evidence (Panula et al., 1983; Gibson et al., 1984). However, there are problems with the identification of CCK-like material. In capsaicin-treated rats there is depletion of CCK-immunoreactive material visualized by immunohistochemistry in dorsal root ganglia and dorsal horn (Jancso et al., 1981; Priestley et al., 1982), but no change in concentrations of the peptide (mainly CCK-8) measured by radioimmunoassay of extracts of dorsal spinal cord (Schultzberg et al., 1982; Marley et al., 1982). The results indicate that the material in rat dorsal root ganglia visualized by immunohistochemistry is unlikely to be authentic CCK-8, but is probably a substance with relatively low affinity for CCK antibodies (Schultzberg et al., 1982).

There is now immunohistochemical evidence that in many parts of the nervous system two or more peptides or classical transmitters occur in the same neurone. In the case of the substance P neurones of the dorsal root ganglia, it seems that in addition to substance P and substance K (see below) these also contain a CCK-like peptide (Dalsgaard et al., 1982b) and CGRP-like immunoreactivity (Gibson et al., 1984).

Quantitative aspects

Substance P is the most abundant of the vagal peptides, it occurs in concentrations (50–250 pmol g^{-1}) roughly ten times higher than those of CCK-8, somatostatin and VIP (each 1–10 pmol · g^{-1}) in the cervical vagus of several mammals (Fig. 1). The differences in concentration are not simply a reflection of different rates of axonal transport, because transport velocities are similar for the different peptides (see below).

Retrograde tracing using fluorescent dyes has been used, together with immunohistochemistry, to determine quantitatively the proportion of substance P-containing neurones in the afferent innervation of a variety of structures (Fig. 2, Table I).

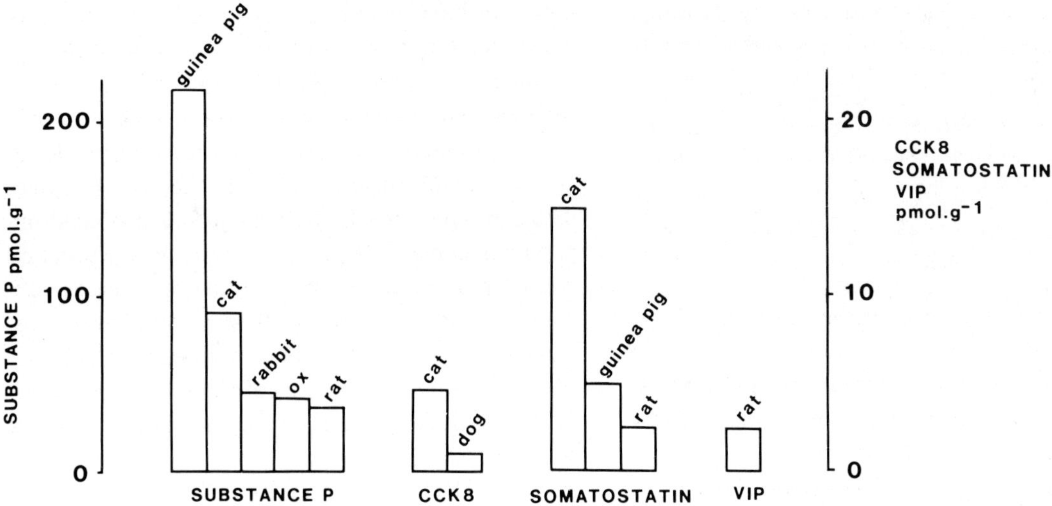

Fig. 1. Concentrations of four peptides in the cervical vagus nerve trunk of several species. Note that the concentrations of substance P are 10–20 times higher than those of CCK-8, somatostatin and VIP-like immunoreactivity. Compiled from the data of Gamse et al. (1979), Gilbert et al. (1980), Dockray et al. (1981), MacLean and Lewis (1984a) and Rehfeld and Lundberg (1983).

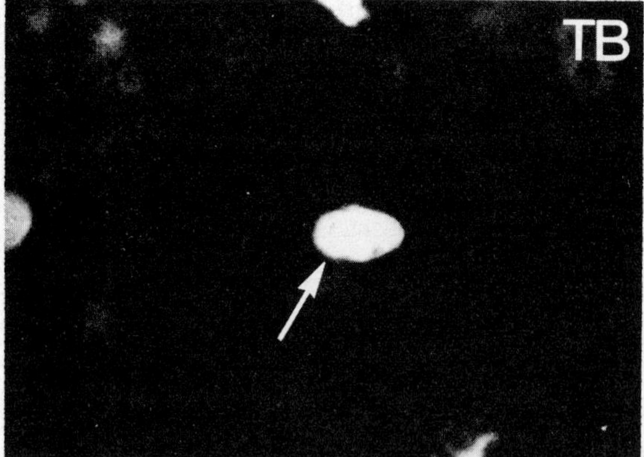

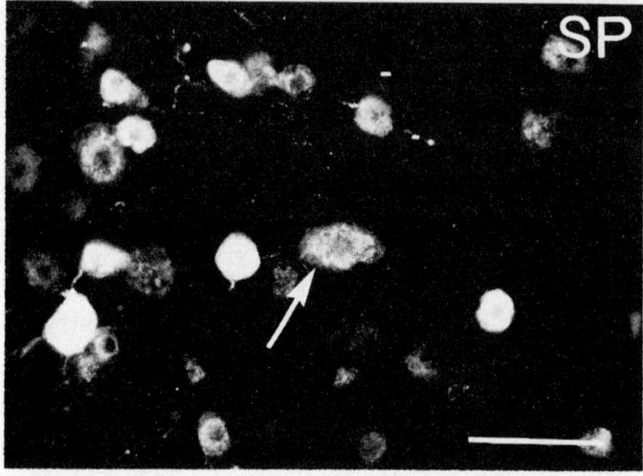

Fig. 2. Localization of the fluorescent dye True Blue in T10 dorsal root ganglion neurones following injection into the splenic lobe of the pancreas. Anaesthetized rats received True Blue (4 μl aqueous suspension) and after 5 days, to allow uptake and retrograde transport to ganglion cells, the animals were re-anaesthetized and perfused-fixed with paraformaldehyde. Upper panel shows True Blue, the lower one substance P localized by immunohistochemistry. Note the cell containing both True Blue and substance P (arrowed), while others contain substance P alone. Scale bar, 50 μm.

The experimental approach depends on the uptake of a fluorescent tracer, for example, True Blue, by nerve terminals and its subsequent transport to nerve cell bodies where it can be visualized. Simultaneous processing of the tissue for the localization of peptides by immunohistochemistry allows the identification and quantification of neurochemically defined neurones projecting to a particular tissue (Skirboll et al., 1984). It is essential to minimize leakage of the fluorescent dye from the site of injection to adjacent tissues. This can be achieved by using fine needles, low injection volumes (less than 5 μl of 5% suspension) and thorough swabbing of the area with saline after injection. In some cases it may be advantageous to use a physical barrier to prevent diffusion of the tracer (see, for example, Karim et al., 1984). When injected into the ventral face of the rat stomach, True Blue is taken up by nerve terminals and retrogradely transported to neurones in the dorsal root ganglia (T6–L1), nodose ganglia, dorsal motor nuclei of the vagus, and coeliac ganglion (Sharkey et al., 1984). Labelled cells are found predominantly in the left nodose ganglion and left side of the vagal nucleus. Similarly, injection into the splenic lobe of the pancreas labels nodose ganglion cells (predominantly on the right), as well as spinal, sympathetic and parasympathetic neurones. Substance P immunoreactivity is found in some of the True Blue-labelled spinal afferents (Fig. 2).

In rat and guinea pig, 40–60% of the spinal afferent neurones to the stomach, and portal vein/hepatic artery contain immunoreactive substance P (Lindh et al., 1983; Barja and Mathison, 1984; Sharkey et al., 1984). In contrast, a lower proportion (10–24%) of the spinal afferents to the pancreas, urinary bladder, skin or kidney react with substance P antibodies (Table I). Although there is abundant substance P in the vagus nerve, there is little evidence to indicate a vagal substance P supply to the stomach, pancreas, or portal vein in the rat (Barja and Mathison, 1984; Sharkey et al., 1984). Thus, in our hands True Blue injected into rat stomach or pancreas labelled cells in the mid region and caudal pole of the nodose ganglion, whereas substance P-containing neurones were found at the rostral end of the ganglion, and there was scarcely any overlap in the distribution of the two populations of cells. Similar studies in the guinea pig revealed only occasional nodose ganglion cells containing substance P (Lindh et al., 1983). Therefore, it seems that the upper gastrointestinal tract is an unlikely destination for vagal substance P fibres. There is, however, evidence to suggest a vagal substance P

TABLE I

The percentage contribution of substance P-containing neurones to the afferent innervation of visceral and other structures

Tissue	Species	Ganglion	Percentage substance P-containing afferents	References
Pylorus	Guinea pig	T7–T9	60	Lindh et al. (1983)
Stomach	Rat	T10	41.4 ± 4.7	Sharkey et al. (1984)
Hepatic artery/portal vein	Rat	T7–13	40	Barja and Mathison (1984)
Kidney	Rat	L1–L3	24	Kuo et al. (1984)
Middle cerebral artery	Cat	Trigeminal	20 ± 6	Liu-Chen et al. (1984)
Urinary bladder	Rat	L6	16.2 ± 4.2	Sharkey et al. (1983)
Skin				
Hind paw	Rat	L5	15.6 ± 0.4	Unpublished observations
Neck	Rat	C2	8.4	Neuhuber et al. (1981)
Pancreas	Rat	T11	11.3 ± 0.9	Sharkey et al. (1984)
Parotid	Rat	Trigeminal	6.5 ± 1.0	Sharkey and Templeton (1984)
Stomach	Rat	Nodose	<2	Sharkey et al. (1984)

innervation of various thoracic structures, including the bronchi, trachea and baro- and chemoreceptors (Helke et al., 1980a,b; Lundberg et al., 1984b).

Precise data for the other peptides are still needed, but using combined retrograde tracing and immunohistochemistry we found little evidence that somatostatin-containing spinal afferents contribute to the sensory innervation of the bladder (Sharkey et al., 1983). Taking the available data as a whole, it is clear that there are marked differences between tissues in the relative proportions of substance P-containing afferents, and probably other peptides too.

Biosynthesis

It is well established that biologically active peptides are produced as large precursors that are then cleaved to give smaller active products (Docherty and Steiner, 1982). They are also subject to other post-translational modifications, e.g., sulphation of tyrosine residues (as in CCK-8), C-terminal amidation, glycosylation. Cleavage sites are frequently at pairs of basic residues, but this is not a rule, and, for example, in CCK-8 only a single basic residue occurs at the main cleavage points. Direct studies of biosynthesis of substance P have been made in rat dorsal root ganglia, and guinea pig nodose ganglion, by following incorporation of [^{35}S]methionine or [^{3}H]proline (Harmar et al., 1981; MacLean and Lewis, 1984b). Radioactively labelled peptide can be detected 2–4 hours after exposure to the labelled amino acid, indicating the time taken for incorporation and processing.

The pathways of biosynthesis are not invariant. There are two important ways in which different cell types expressing the same gene may subsequently produce different peptides. First, at the transcriptional level there may be alternative splicing pathways that yield different mRNA species. Second, at the level of post-translational processing, different patterns of cleavage or other modification can yield peptides varying in chain length. The former is well illustrated by CGRP, which is produced by alternative splicing of the calcitonin gene (Amara et al., 1982; Rosenfeld et al., 1983), and by the substance P gene (preprotachykinin gene) (Nawa et al., 1983,

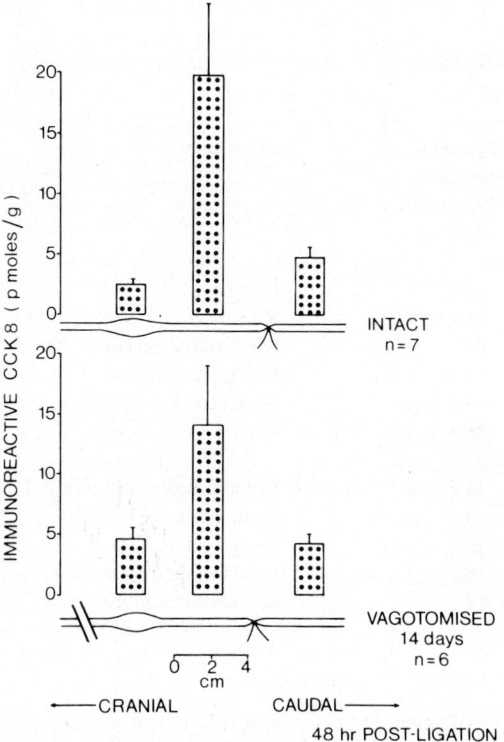

Fig. 3. Accumulation of CCK-8-like immunoreactivity in the cat vagus following ligation below the nodose ganglion (upper panel). The accumulation was still seen in animals in which the nerve had been transected above the nodose ganglion 14 days before ligation (lower panel). Below the ligature, there is only a modest depletion (<30%) of immunoreactivity compared with control sections of nerve, indicating that most of the activity behaves as if it is stationary. From Dockray et al. (1981).

1984). The latter gives rise to two mRNA species, one encodes substance P and a second tachykinin, substance K, whereas the other lacks the segment corresponding to substance K. Therefore, cells expressing this gene may give rise to two sorts of polypeptide precursor: both contain the substance P sequence, but only one also contains substance K. Several lines of evidence indicate that primary afferent neurones contain both substance K as well as substance P. (1) Substance K (also known as neuromedin L and neurokinin α) has been isolated from spinal cord and chemically characterized (Kimura et al., 1983; Minamino et al., 1984). (2) Radioimmunoassays for the amphibian skin peptide kassinin, which react with substance K, reveal material in extracts of dorsal root ganglia and spinal cord, and show decreases in concentration of this material in rats treated neonatally with capsaicin (Maggio and Hunter, 1984). (3) Biosynthesis of substance K has been demonstrated directly in dorsal root ganglia by incorporation of ^{3}H-labelled Val, Ser, Phe and His (Harmar and Keen, 1984). It is not yet clear if both mRNA species are produced in the same primary sensory neurone and, if so, whether their proportions vary in different subpopulations of afferents. Neither is it clear if a third member of the tachykinin family isolated from spinal cord (neuromedin K, or neurokinin β) also occurs in dorsal root ganglia (Kimura et al., 1983; Kangawa et al., 1983).

Cell-specific patterns of post-translational processing are illustrated by CCK. In the cat and dog vagus, as in other central and peripheral neurones, the octapeptide, CCK-8, is the predominant form (Dockray et al., 1981). However, in gut endocrine cells there are also relatively high concentrations of the larger forms, consisting of N-terminal extension to CCK-8, i.e., CCK-33, -39, -58 (Dockray, 1982). In neurones there is evidently more complete cleavage than in endocrine cells. In the case of CCK, all the main products are biologically active. But in other cases it is possible that different patterns of post-translational processing may fail to liberate all the peptides with potential bioactivity. This applies, at least in principle, to the substance P/substance K precursor, and also to the VIP precursor. Studies of the cDNA sequence (Itoh et al., 1983) encoding VIP in human neuroblastoma cells reveal, in addition to VIP, the sequence of a related peptide corresponding to the peptide PHI (peptide histidine isoleucine amide) first isolated from pig intestine by Tatemoto and Mutt (1981). Providing the appropriate processing steps are completed, the VIP-containing afferents ought therefore to contain PHI as well; however, it is not known if post-translational processing always proceeds in this way.

One approach to the study of post-translational

TABLE II

Rates of axonal transport of neuropeptides in the vagus nerve

Peptide	Species	Rate of transport ($mm \cdot hour^{-1}$)	References
Substance P	Cat	2.5	Gamse et al. (1979)
	Cat	0.6 ± 0.1	MacLean and Lewis (1984a)
	Rat	1.9 ± 0.2	MacLean and Lewis (1984a)
	Rat	1.3 ± 0.2	Gilbert et al. (1980)
	Guinea pig	1.6 ± 0.2	MacLean and Lewis (1984a)
	Guinea pig	1.25	Brimijoin et al. (1980)
	Rabbit	4.0 ± 0.8	Gilbert et al. (1980)
CCK	Cat	2.0	Dockray et al. (1981)
	Cat	2.0	Rehfeld and Lundberg (1983)
	Dog	2.2	Dockray et al. (1981)
Somatostatin	Rat	2.7 ± 0.7	Gilbert et al. (1980)
	Rat	1.7 ± 0.3	MacLean and Lewis (1984a)
	Guinea pig	1.3 ± 0.2	MacLean and Lewis (1984a)
	Cat	1.9 ± 0.2	MacLean and Lewis (1984a)
VIP	Rat	0.8	Gilbert et al. (1980)

processing mechanisms is to systematically seek all the main peptides predicted to exist from the gene sequence. For example, we have developed antibodies to the four main peptides that are produced from progastrin by cleavage at pairs of basic residues (Dockray, 1984). These antibodies have been used to re-examine the vagal origins of the gastrins. On the cranial side of ligatures of the cervical vagus in the ferret, C-terminal-specific G17 antibodies consistently showed a large accumulation of immunoreactive material that could be either gastrin or CCK. In about 40% of all ferrets we were able to find an accumulation of immunoreactive material with antibodies to the other progastrin-derived peptides. The fibres were scattered and plainly less numerous than those revealed by C-terminal G17 antibodies (Dockray et al., 1985), suggesting that CCK-8 occurs in a higher proportion of vagal afferents than does gastrin. The combined presence of immunoreactive material corresponding to all four of the major peptides predicted to arise from progastrin is strong evidence for the biosynthesis of gastrin in a population of vagal afferents.

Axonal transport

Direction

The peptides synthesized in the cell bodies of afferent neurones are transported to both central terminals, e.g., in dorsal horn or nucleus of the solitary tract, and towards the periphery. Attempts have been made to estimate quantitatively the relative proportions of substance P transported centrally and peripherally in guinea pig vagal afferents and in rat dorsal root ganglion neurones. The estimates vary from "about 35%" to 6–8% going centrally (Brimijoin et al., 1980; Harmar and Keen, 1982; MacLean and Lewis, 1984a); in both vagal and

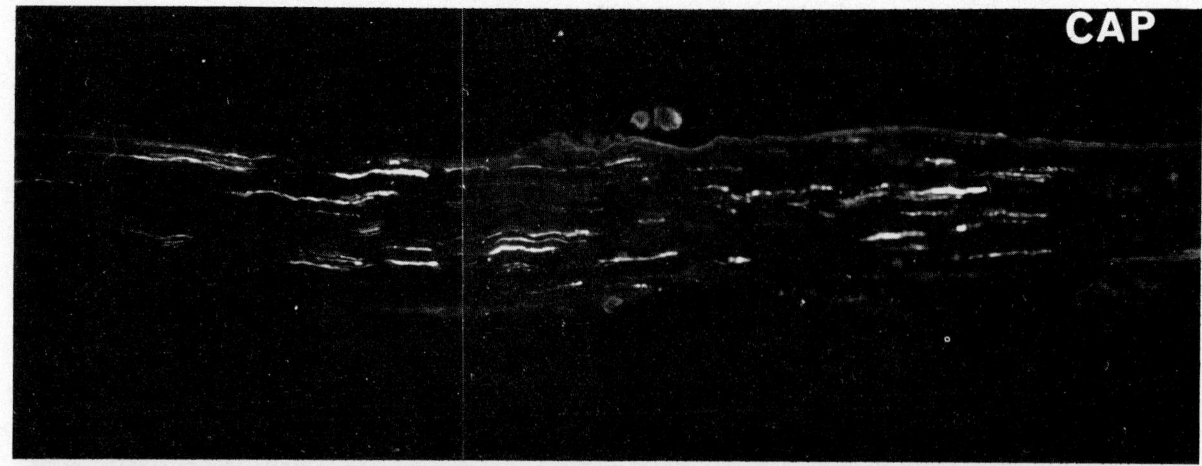

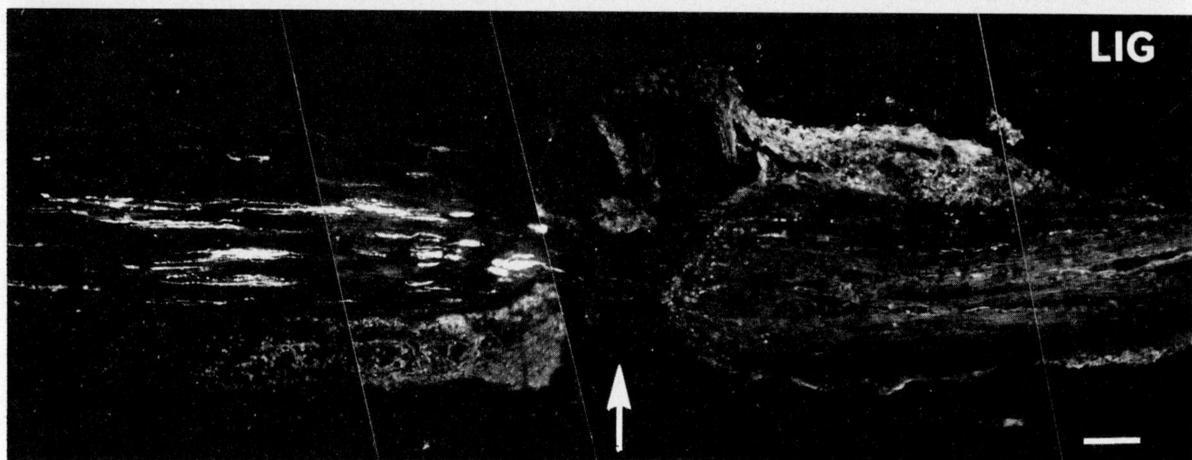

Fig. 4. Inhibition of axonal transport of substance P immunoreactivity in the rat cervical vagus. In the lower panel, the nerve was ligated (arrow) for 24 hours. In the upper panel, capsaicin had been applied locally to the nerve (1% solution in olive oil) 24 hours previously; application of olive oil alone had no effect. In both cases, substance P fibres are visible, while in control sections of nerve they were not. Scale bar, 100 μm.

spinal afferents, therefore, it is clear that the greater part of the material is transported towards the periphery. It seems reasonable to suppose that similar proportions of the other peptides are transported centrally.

Rates

The axonal transport velocities of substance P, CCK-8, somatostatin and VIP have been determined in the vagus nerve in various species. The experimental approach usually employed involves ligation or crushing the nerve, followed after 6–48 hours by estimating the accumulation of immunoreactivity in extracts on the proximal side, and depletion on the distal side (Fig. 3). There is general agreement that only a proportion of the peptide behaves as if it were moving. Thus, in experiments in which two ligatures are placed on the same nerve, there may be a depletion of only 30%, or less, on the peripheral side of the first ligature, suggesting that about 70% of total activity acts as if it were

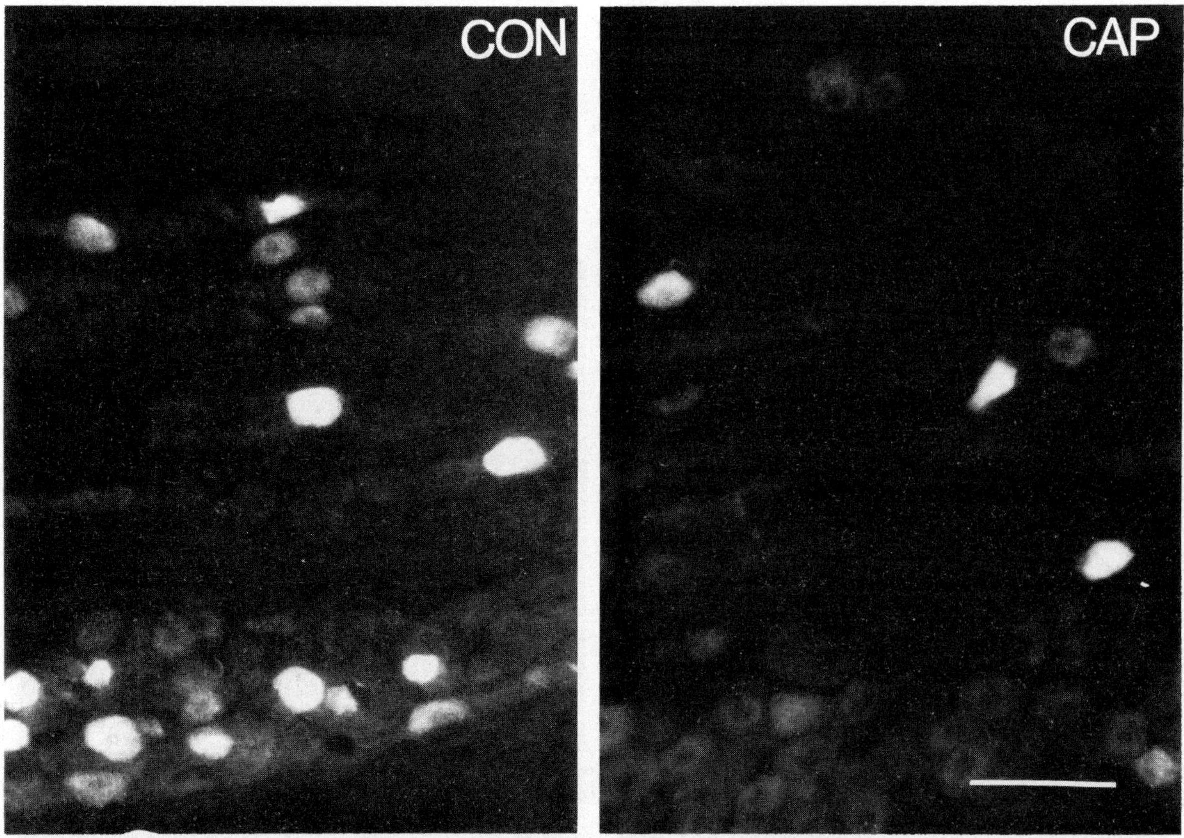

Fig. 5. Localization of True Blue in nodose ganglia of rats following injection into the stomach. On the left is shown a ganglion from a control rat, and on the right from a rat treated with capsaicin applied locally to the cervical vagus. Note the decrease in True Blue-labelled cells after capsaicin. Scale bar, 50 μm.

stationary. The mean rate of transport for CCK-8, substance P, VIP and somatostatin is closely similar for different species and varies from 0.8 to 4.0 mm $\cdot$ hour^{-1} (Table II). Allowing for the fact that only about 30% is moving, the true rate is probably closer to 10 mm $\cdot$ hour^{-1}, which is within the range for fast axonal transport. The mitotic inhibitor, colchicine, has been shown to block axonal transport (Gamse et al., 1979). Capsaicin applied locally to the cervical vagus also inhibits the transport of substance P and produces an accumulation resembling that caused by ligation (Fig. 4). Local application of capsaicin to the cervical vagus nerve also inhibits the retrograde transport of True Blue to the nodose ganglion following administration of dye into the stomach (Fig. 5). Thus, 7 days after capsaicin there was a reduction of 70% in the numbers of True Blue-labelled cells on the treated side compared with the control side (unpublished observations).

Peripheral terminations

Distribution

A variety of different approaches has been used to identify the peripheral terminals of visceral afferents. These include studies of the effects on peripheral peptide systems of lesion or ligation of the splanchnic and vagal nerves, extirpation of the sensory ganglia, and the administration of capsaicin. The results reveal the distribution of peripheral terminals of afferent fibres, and also the presence of collaterals from spinal afferents on nerve cell bodies in the prevertebral ganglia, through which visceral afferents pass (Gamse et al., 1981; Dalsgaard et al., 1982a; Matthews and Cuello, 1984).

In the gastrointestinal tract there are particular problems with the identification of peptide-containing afferent terminals because the same pep-

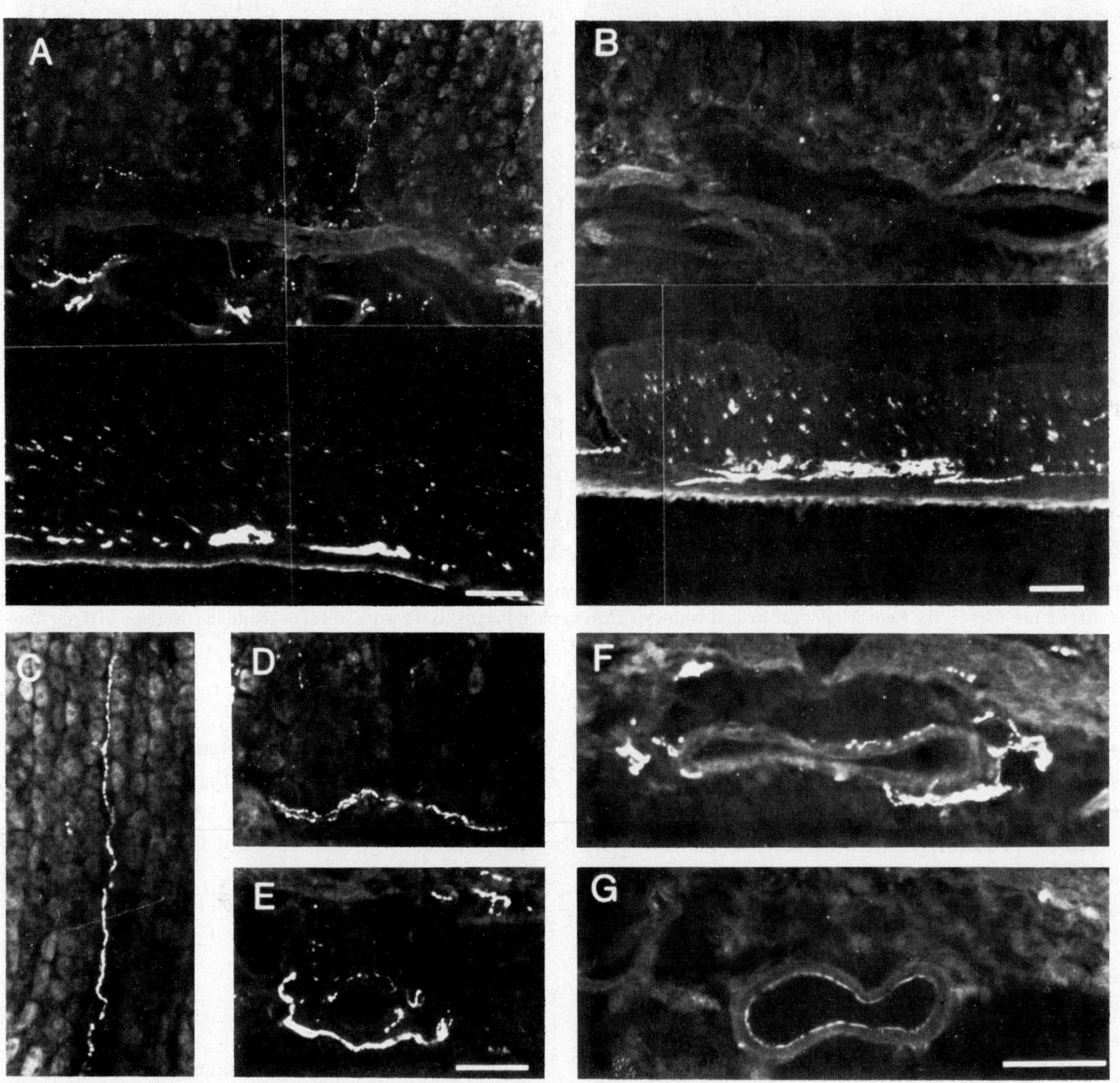

Fig. 6. Substance P localized by immunohistochemistry to nerve fibres in submucosa and mucosa of the stomach in capsaicin-treated rats (panels B and G), and control rats (panels A, C, D, E and F). Whole stomach is shown in A and B, mucosa in C–E and submucosal blood vessels in F and G. Note the loss of peptide around blood vessels of capsaicin-treated rats. Scale bar, 50 μm. Taken from Sharkey et al. (1984).

tides also occur in intrinsic neurones. However, in cat, Hayashi et al. (1982) reported that spinal ganglionectomy (T5–L2 bilateral) greatly reduced substance P-immunoreactive fibres in the myenteric plexus. Similarly, in rat, splanchnic (although not vagal) lesions reduced a population of substance P-immunoreactive fibres in the myenteric plexus (Minagawa et al., 1984). Lesioning the extrinsic innervation of the guinea pig ileum also reduced a population of substance P fibres projecting to the sub-mucosa and to blood vessels (Costa et al., 1981). It appears, however, that intrinsic substance P neurones account for the bulk of the peptide found in extracts of the gut. For example, in rats treated neonatally with capsaicin, both spinal and vagal substance P is depleted, but there is little or no difference in concentrations of substance P in stomach extracts (Holzer et al., 1980). In other visceral structures, however, there is no difficulty in identifying a decrease in substance P concentrations in capsaicin-treated rats, e.g., in skin, urinary bladder, lungs, trachea (Holzer et al., 1982). In the stomach of capsaicin-treated rats, we were able to show a loss of substance P-immunoreactive fibres around blood vessels in the sub-mucosa and in the mucosa (Fig. 6). There was also a marked loss of immunoreactive fibres in the pancreas, bladder and parotid, although the situation in the latter is complicated by the presence of substance P in parasympathetic efferents (Sharkey et al., 1983, 1984; Sharkey and Templeton, 1984). In these and other visceral structures, the afferent substance P fibres are frequently associated with blood vessels (Furness et al., 1982).

Peripheral actions

It is well established that substance P causes vasodilatation. It is of interest that other peptides in afferents, e.g., VIP and CGRP, also exert powerful vasodilator actions (Brain et al., 1985). In skin and probably other tissues, substance P is released by capsaicin or antidromic nerve stimulation and in turn stimulates histamine secretion, and evokes an increase in capillary permeability and plasma extravasation (Lembeck and Gamse, 1982). These effects are consistent with the idea that substance P plays a part in local defense mechanisms following tissue injury. The upper gastrointestinal tract appears to differ from many other tissues in that capsaicin, or antidromic afferent stimulation, does not induce plasma extravasation (Saria et al., 1983; Lundberg et al., 1984a). However, several types of gastrointestinal response are attributable to substance P release from afferent nerve endings. Effects on gut motility and blood flow have been relatively well studied, but there may also be effects on secretion, e.g., gastric mucosal bicarbonate secretion (Fandriks and Delbro, 1983).

In both guinea pig small intestine in vitro, and cat stomach in vivo, electrical stimulation of the splanchnic innervation produces a contractile response (Szolcsanyi and Bartho, 1978; Delbro and Lisander, 1980). The effect is seen most clearly after blockade of adrenergic sympathetic fibres, for example, with guanethidine. Hexamethionum does not inhibit the response so that cholinergic-nicotinic transmission is not involved. Atropine blocks the response in the cat stomach and reduces it in the guinea pig ileum, indicating the involvement of a cholinergic-muscarinic synapse. Desensitization to substance P, and substance P antagonists, block the effect in both cat stomach in vivo and guinea pig ileum in vitro, which is consistent with the idea that this peptide is released by antidromic stimulation of primary afferents (Bartho et al., 1982; Delbro et al., 1983). In the guinea pig ileum, capsaicin exerts similar effects to antidromic nerve stimulation; at a dose of 10^{-6} M it also produces desensitization to antidromic stimulation, although the responses to exogenous acetylcholine or substance P are not affected (Szolcsanyi and Bartho, 1978; Bartho and Szolcsanyi, 1978; Bartho et al., 1982). Totgether, these results strongly suggest that substance P from the collaterals of spinal afferents may, in different regions of the gut, act either on cholinergic nerve cell bodies, or directly on smooth muscle. Nociceptive stimulation of the mucosa, e.g., warming to 45–52°C, may normally activate these axon reflexes (Delbro et al., 1984).

Injection of small doses of capsaicin into the superior mesenteric artery of the anaesthetized dog produces a transient increase in blood flow (Rozsa et al., 1984). Providing low doses are used, the effect is reproducible. Hexamethonium or adrenergic antagonists had no effect on this response, but atropine partly diminished it. Rozsa et al. (1985) have shown that passive immunization by close arterial injection of antibodies to substance P, VIP or CCK-8 each reduces the increase in blood flow caused by subsequent administration of these peptides alone, or by subsequent administration of capsaicin. In contrast, somatostatin antibodies enhance the vasodilator response to capsaicin. Simultaneous administration of atropine and antibodies to CCK-8, VIP and substance P almost completely abolished the response to capsaicin. Therefore, each of these peptides may play a part in mediating the vasodilator actions of capsaicin in the splanchnic bed. Because they have all been localized to afferent fibres it is reasonable to suggest that they are involved at an early stage in mediating the response to capsaicin. However, it remains possible that capsaicin acts on afferents that in turn stimulate intrinsic neurones of the gut, or even gut endocrine cells, to release some or all these peptides (Fig. 7).

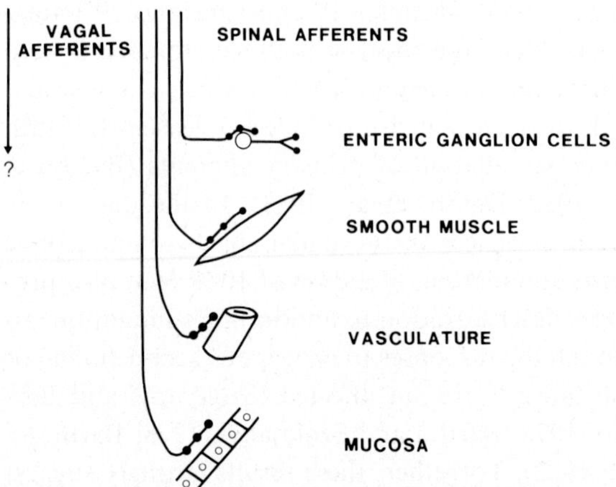

Fig. 7. Schematic representation of the sites of termination of afferent substance P-containing fibres in the stomach and intestine, based on evidence derived from immunohistochemical and pharmacological studies, nerve lesions, electrical stimulation, and capsaicin (see text for details).

In addition to peripheral actions attributable to substance P released at terminals of visceral afferents in the gut, there is also electrophysiological evidence to indicate substance P produces the noncholinergic slow excitatory postsynaptic potential (EPSP) seen in prevertebral ganglion cells following pre- or post-ganglionic nerve stimulation. In particular, substance P antagonists have been shown to block the long, slow EPSP in guinea pig inferior mesenteric ganglion cells, but hexamethonium had no effect; moreover, capsaicin treatment mimicked and then blocked the effects of pre- and postganglionic stimulation (Tsunoo et al., 1982; Jiang et al., 1982; Konishi et al., 1983).

Perspectives

It is now clear that several biologically active peptides, of which substance P is best studied, occur in visceral afferents. The patterns of their biosynthesis are complex and at the transcriptional and posttranslational level there may be differences between cells expressing the same gene. In any case, it is certain that simple generalizations, such as one peptide-one neurone, cannot be justified. Different populations of peptidergic afferents vary in their contribution to the innervation of different organs. Although the flow of information in afferent neurones is towards the CNS, the bulk of the peptides in these cells is transported to the periphery. This material is releasable, and may contribute to axonal reflexes. The responses of a variety of different cells and tissues can be attributed to peripheral release of peptides from visceral afferents, including the vasculature, cholinergic and adrenergic ganglion cells, smooth muscle and the gut mucosa. The elucidation of the physiological significance of these actions will depend on the ability to relate neurochemically identified afferents to electrophysiologically characterized cells.

References

Amara, S. G., Jonas, V., Rosenfeld, M. G., Ong, E. S. and Evans, R. M. (1982) Alternative RNA processing in calcitonin gene expression generates mRNA's encoding different polypeptide products. Nature, 298: 240–244.

Barja, F. and Mathison, R. (1984) Sensory innervation of the rat portal vein and the hepatic artery. J. Auton. Nerv. System, 10: 117–125.

Bartho, L. and Szolcsanyi, J. (1978) The site of action of capsaicin on the guinea pig isolated ileum. Naunyn-Schmeideberg's Arch. Pharmacol., 305: 75–81.

Bartho, L., Holzer, P., Lembeck, F. and Szolcsanyi, J. (1982) Evidence that the contractile response of the guinea pig ileum to capsaicin is due to release of substance P. J. Physiol., 332: 157–167.

Brain, S. D., Williams, T. J., Tippins, J. R., Morris, H. R. and MacIntyre, J. (1985) Calcitonin-gene related peptide is a potent vasodilator. Nature, 313: 54–56.

Brimijoin, S., Lundberg, J. M., Brodin, E., Hökfelt, T. and Nilsson, G. (1980) Axonal transport of substance P in the vagus and sciatic nerves of the guinea pig. Brain Res., 191: 443–447.

Costa, M., Furness, J. B., Llewellyn-Smith, I. J. and Cuello, A. C. (1981) Projections of substance P-containing neurons within the guinea pig small intestine. Neuroscience, 6: 411–424.

Dalsgaard, C.-J., Hökfelt, T., Elfvin, L.-G., Skirboll, L. and Emson, P. (1982a) Substance P-containing primary sensory neurones projecting to the inferior mesenteric ganglion: evidence from combined retrograde tracing and immunohistochemistry. Neuroscience, 7: 647–654.

Dalsgaard, C.-J., Vincent, S. R., Hökfelt, T., Lundberg, J. M., Dahlstrom, A., Schultzberg, M., Dockray, G. J. and Cuello, A. C. (1982b) Co-existence of cholecystokinin- and substance P-like peptides in neurons of the dorsal root ganglia of the rat. Neurosci. Lett., 33: 159–163.

Dalsgaard, C.-J., Hökfelt, T., Schultzberg, M., Lundberg, J. M., Terenius, L., Dockray, G. J. and Cuello, A. C. (1983) Origin of peptide-containing fibres in the inferior mesenteric ganglion of the guinea pig: immunohistochemical studies with antisera to substance P, enkephalin, vasoactive intestinal polypeptide, cholecystokinin and bombesin. Neuroscience, 9: 191–211.

Dalsgaard, C.-J., Ygge, J., Vincent, S. R., Ohrling, M., Dockray, G. J. and Elde, R. (1984) Peripheral projections and neuropeptide coexistence in a subpopulation of fluoride-resistant acid phosphatase reactive spinal primary sensory neurons. Neurosci. Lett., 51: 139–144.

Delbro, D. and Lisander, B. (1980) Non-ganglionic cholinergic excitatory pathways in the sympathetic supply to the feline stomach: an afferent system or afferents with excitatory axon collaterals? Acta Physiol. Scand., 110: 137–144.

Delbro, D., Fandriks, L., Rosell, S. and Folkers, K. (1983) Inhibition of antidromically induced stimulation of gastric motility by substance P receptor blockade. Acta Physiol. Scand., 118: 309–316.

Delbro, D., Lisander, B. and Andersson, S. A. (1984) Atropine-sensitive smooth muscle excitation by mucosal nociceptive stimulation — the involvement of an action reflex? Acta Physiol. Scand., 122: 621–627.

Docherty, K. and Steiner, D. F. (1982) Post-translational proteolysis in polypeptide hormone biosynthesis. Annu. Rev. Physiol., 44: 625–638.

Dockray, G. J. (1979) Comparative biochemistry and physiology of gut hormones. Annu. Rev. Physiol., 41: 83–95.

Dockray, G. J. (1982) The physiology of cholecystokinin in brain and gut. Br. Med. Bull., 38: 253–258.

Dockray, G. J. (1984) New perspectives in the identification, distribution and processing of peptide hormones and neurotransmitters: the gastrins. In W. Paton, J. Mitchell and P. Turner (Eds.), Proceedings of the IUPHAR 9th International Congress, Macmillan Press, London, pp. 163–168.

Dockray, G. J. (1985) Evolutionary aspects of gastrointestinal hormones. In V. Mutt (Ed.), Advances in Metabolic Disorders, Vol. II, Academic Press, New York, in press.

Dockray, G. J., Gregory, R. A., Tracy, H. J. and Zhu, W.-Y. (1981) Transport of cholecystokinin-octapeptide-like immunoreactivity towards the gut in afferent vagal fibres in cat and dog. J. Physiol., 314: 501–511.

Dockray, G. J., Desmond, H., Gayton, R. J., Jonsson, A.-C., Raybould, H., Sharkey, K. A., Varro, A. and Williams, R. G. (1985) Cholecystokinin and gastrin forms in the nervous system. Ann. New York Acad. Sci., 448: 32–43.

Fandriks, L. and Delbro, D. (1983) Neuronal stimulation of gastric bicarbonate secretion in the cat. An involvement of vagal axon-reflexes and substance P? Acta Physiol. Scand., 118: 301–304.

Fitzgerald, M. (1983) Capsaicin and sensory neurons — a review. Pain, 15: 109–130.

Furness, J. B., Papka, R. E., Della, N. G., Costa, M. and Eskay, R. L. (1982) Substance P-like immunoreactivity in nerves associated with the vascular system of guinea-pigs. Neuroscience, 7: 447–459.

Gamse, R., Lembeck, F. and Cuello, A. C. (1979) Substance P in the vagus nerve: Immunochemical and immunohistochemical evidence for axoplasmic transport. Naunyn-Schmiedeberg's Arch. Pharmacol., 306: 37–44.

Gamse, R., Wax, A., Zigmond, R. E. and Leeman, S. E. (1981) Immunoreactive substance P in sympathetic ganglia: distribution and sensitivity towards capsaicin. Neuroscience, 6: 437–441.

Gaudin-Chazal, G., Segu, L, Seyfritz, N. and Puizillout, J. J. (1981) Visualization of serotonin neurones in the nodose ganglia of the cat. An autoradiographic study. Neuroscience, 6: 1127–1137.

Gibson, S. J., Polak, J. M., Bloom, S. R., Sabate, I. M., Mulderry, P. M., Ghatei, M. A., McGregor, G. P., Morrison, J. F. B., Kelly, J. S., Evans, R. M. and Rosenfeld, M. G. (1984)

Calcitonin gene-related peptide immunoreactivity in the spinal cord of man and eight other species. J. Neurosci., 4: 3101–3111.

Gilbert, R. F. T., Emson, P. C., Fahrenkreg, J., Lee, C. M., Penman, E. and Wass, J. (1980) Axonal transport of neuropeptides in the cervical vagus nerve of the rat. J. Neurochem., 34: 108–113.

Harmar, A. and Keen, P. (1982) Synthesis and central and peripheral axonal transport of substance P in a dorsal root ganglion-nerve preparation in vitro. Brain Res., 231: 379–385.

Harmar, A. J. and Keen, P. (1984) Rat sensory ganglia incorporate radiolabelled aminoacids into substance K (neurokinin) in vitro. Neurosci. Lett., 51: 387–391.

Harmar, A., Schofield, J. G. and Keen, P. (1981) Substance P biosynthesis in dorsal root ganglia: an immunochemical study of [^{35}S]methionine- and [^{3}H]proline incorporation in vitro. Neuroscience, 6: 1917–1922.

Hayashi, H., Ohsumi, K., Ueda, M., Fujiwara, M. and Mizuno, M. (1982) Effect of spinal ganglionectomy on substance P-like immunoreactivity in the gastroduodenal tract of cats. Brain Res., 232: 227–230.

Helke, C. J., O'Donohue, T. L. and Jacobowitz, D. M. (1980a) Substance P as a baro- and chemoreceptor afferent neurotransmitter: immunocytochemical and neurochemical evidence in the rat. Peptides, 1: 1–9.

Helke, C. J., Goldman, W. and Jacobowitz, D. M. (1980b) Demonstration of substance P in aortic nerve afferent fibres by combined use of fluorescent retrograde neuronal labelling and immunocytochemistry. Peptides, 1: 359–364.

Hökfelt, T., Kellerth, J.-O., Nilsson, G. and Pernow, B. (1975) Substance P: localization in the central nervous system and in some primary sensory neurones. Science, 190: 889–890.

Hökfelt, T., Elde, R., Johansson, O., Luft, R., Nilsson, G. and Arimura, A. (1976) Immunohistochemical evidence for separate populations of somatostatin-containing and substance P-containing primary afferent neurons in the rat. Neuroscience, 1: 131–136.

Holzer, P., Gamse, R. and Lembeck, F. (1980) Distribution of substance P in the rat gastrointestinal tract — lack of effect of capsaicin pretreatment. Eur. J. Pharmacol., 61: 303–307.

Holzer, P., Bucsics, A. and Lembeck, F. (1982) Distribution of capsaicin-sensitive nerve fibres containing immunoreactive substance P in cutaneous and visceral tissues of the rat. Neurosci. Lett., 31: 253–257.

Itoh, N., Obata, K.-I., Yanaihara, N. and Okamoto, H. (1983) Human preprovasoactive intestinal polypeptide contains a novel PHI-27-like peptide, PHM-27. Nature, 304: 547–549.

Jancso, G., Kiraly, E. and Jancso-Gabor, A. (1977) Pharmacologically induced selective degeneration of chemosensitive primary sensory neurones. Nature, 270: 741–743.

Jancso, G., Hökfelt, T., Lundberg, J. M., Kiraly, E., Halasz, N., Nilsson, G., Terenius, Z., Rehfeld, J. M., Steinbusch, H., Verhofstad, A., Elde, R., Said, S. and Brown, M. (1981) Immunohistochemical studies on the effect of capsaicin on spinal and medullary peptide and monoamine neurons using antisera to substance P, gastrin/CCK, somatostatin, VIP, enkephalin, neurotensin, and 5-hydroxytryptamine. J. Neurocytol., 10: 963–980.

Jiang, Z.-G., Dun, N. J. and Karczmar, A. G. (1982) Substance P: A putative sensory transmitter in mammalian autonomic ganglia. Science, 217: 739–741.

Kangawa, K., Minamino, N., Fukuda, A. and Matsuo, H. (1983) Neuromedin K: A novel mammalian tachykinin identified in porcine spinal cord. Biochem. Biophys. Res. Commun., 114: 533–540.

Karim, M. A., Shaikh, E., Tan, J. and Ismail, Z. (1984) The organization of the gastric efferent projections of brainstem of monkey: an HRP study. Brain Res., 293: 231–240.

Katz, D. M. and Karten, H. J. (1980) Substance P in the vagal sensory ganglia: localization in cell bodies and percellular aborizations. J. Comp. Neurol., 193: 549–564.

Katz, D. M., Markey, K. A., Goldstein, M. and Black, I. B. (1983) Expression of catecholaminergic characteristics by primary sensory neurones in the normal adult rat in vivo. Proc. Natl. Acad. Sci. U.S.A., 80: 3526–3530.

Kawatani, M., Low, I. P., Nudelhaft, I., Morgan, C. and De Groat, W. C. (1983) Vasoactive intestinal polypeptide in visceral afferent pathways to the sacral spinal cord of the cat. Neurosci. Lett., 42: 311–316.

Kimura, S., Okada, M., Sugita, Y., Kanagawa, I. and Munekata, E. (1983) Novel neuropeptides, neurokinin alpha and beta, isolated from porcine spinal cord. Proc. Jpn. Acad., 59: 101–104.

Konishi, S., Otsuka, M., Folkers, K. and Rosell, S. (1983) A substance P antagonist blocks non-cholinergic slow excitatory postsynaptic potential in guinea pig sympathetic ganglia. Acta Physiol. Scand., 117: 157–160.

Kuo, D. C., Oravitz, J. J., Eskay, R. and De Groat, W. C. (1984) Substance P in renal afferent perikarya identified by retrograde transport of fluorescent dye. Brain Res., 323: 168–171.

Lawson, S. N. and Nickels, S. M. (1980) The use of morphometric techniques to analyse the effect of neonatal capsaicin treatment on dorsal root ganglia and dorsal roots. J. Physiol., 303: 12P.

Lembeck, F. (1953) Zur Frage der zentralen Ubertragung afferenter Impulse III Mitteilung. Dus Vorkommen und die Bedeutung der Substanz P in der dorsalen Wurzeln des Ruckenmarks. Naunyn-Schmiedelberg's Arch. Exp. Pathol. Pharmacol., 219: 197–213.

Lembeck, F. and Gamse, R. (1982) Substance P in peripheral sensory processes. Ciba Foundation Symp., 91: 35–54.

Lindh, B., Dalsgaard, C.-J., Elfvin, L.-G., Hökfelt, T. and Cuello, A. C. (1983) Evidence of substance P-immunoreactive neurones in dorsal root ganglion and vagal ganglia projecting to the guinea pig pylorus. Brain Res., 269: 365–369.

Liu-Chen, L.-Y., Gillespie, S. A., Norregaard, T. V. and Moskowitz, M. A. (1984) Co-localization of retrogradely transported wheat germ agglutinin and putative neurotransmitter substance P within trigeminal ganglion cells projecting to the cat middle cerebral artery. J. Comp. Neurol., 225: 187–192.

Lundberg, J. M., Hökfelt, T., Nilsson, G., Terenius, L., Rehfeld, J., Elde, R. and Said, S. (1978) Peptide neurones in the vagus, splanchnic and sciatic nerves. Acta Physiol. Scand., 104: 499–501.

Lundberg, J. M., Brodin, E., Hua, X. and Saria, A. (1984a) Vascular permeability changes and smooth muscle contraction in relation to capsaicin-sensitive substance P afferents in the guinea pig. Acta Physiol. Scand., 120: 217–227.

Lundberg, J. M., Hökfelt, T., Martling, C.-R., Saria, A. and Cuello, C. (1984b) Substance P immunoreactive sensory nerves in the lower respiratory tract of various mammals including man. Cell Tissue Res., 235: 251–261.

MacLean, D. B. and Lewis, S. F. (1984a) Axoplasmic transport of somatostatin, and substance P in the vagus nerve of the rat, guinea pig and cat. Brain Res., 307: 135–145.

MacLean, D. R. and Lewis, S. F. (1984b) De novo synthesis and axoplasmic transport of [^{35}S]methionine-substance P in explants of nodose ganglion/vagus nerve. Brain Res., 310: 325–335.

Maggio, J. E. and Hunter, J. C. (1984) Regional distribution of kassinin-like immunoreactivity in rat central and peripheral tissues and the effect of capsaicin. Brain Res., 307: 370–373.

Mantyh, P. W. and Hunt, S. P. (1984) Neuropeptides are present in projection neurones at all levels in visceral and taste pathways: from periphery to sensory cortex. Brain Res., 299: 297–311.

Marley, R. D., Nagy, J. I., Emson, P. C. and Rehfeld, J. F. (1982) Cholecystokinin in the rat spinal cord: distribution and lack of effect of neonatal capsaicin treatment and rhizotomy. Brain Res., 230: 494–498.

Matthews, M. R. and Cuello, A. C. (1984) The origin and possible significance of substance P immunoreactive networks in the prevertebral ganglia and related structures in the guinea pig. Phil. Trans. Roy. Soc. B, 306: 247–276.

Minagawa, H., Shiosaka, S., Inoue, H., Hayashi, N., Kasahara, A., Kamata, T., Tohyama, M. and Shiotani, Y. (1984) Origins and three-dimensional distribution of substance P-containing structures on the rat stomach using whole-mount tissue. Gastroenterology, 85: 51–59.

Minamino, N., Kangawa, K., Fukuda, A. and Matsuo, H. (1984) Neuromedin L: A novel mammalian tachykinin identified in porcine spinal cord. Neuropeptides, 4: 157–166.

Nagy, J. I. (1982) Capsaicin: a chemical probe for sensory neuron mechanisms. In L. L. Iversen, S. D. Iversen and S. H. Snyder (Eds.), Handbook of Psychopharmacology, Vol. 15, Plenum Press, New York, pp. 185–235.

Nagy, J. I. and Hunt, S. P. (1982) Fluoride-resistant acid phosphatase-containing neurones in dorsal root ganglia are separate from those containing substance P or somatostatin. Neuroscience, 7: 89–97.

Nagy, J. I., Iversen, L. L., Goedert, M., Chapman, D. and Hunt, S. P. (1983) Dose-dependent effects of capsaicin on primary sensory neurones in the neonatal rat. J. Neurosci., 3: 399–406.

Nagy, J. I., Buss, M., Labella, L. A. and Daddona, P. E. (1984) Immunohistochemical localization of adenosine deaminase in primary afferent neurons of the rat. Neurosci. Lett., 48: 133–138.

Nawa, H., Hirose, T., Takashima, H., Inayama, S. and Nakanishi, S. (1983) Nucleotide sequences of cloned cDNA's for two types of bovine brain substance P precursor. Nature, 306: 32–36.

Nawa, H., Kotani, H. and Nakanishi, S. (1984) Tissue-specific generation of two preprotachykinin mRNAs from one gene by alternative RNA splicing. Nature, 312: 729–734.

Neuhuber, W., Groh, V., Gottschall, J. E. and Celio, M. R. (1981) The cornea is not innervated by substance P-containing primary afferent neurones. Neurosci. Lett., 22: 5–9.

Panula, P., Hadjiconstantinou, M., Yang, H. Y. T. and Costa, E. (1983) Immunohistochemical localization of bombesin/gastrin-releasing peptide and substance P in primary sensory neurons. J. Neurosci., 3: 2021–2029.

Pernow, B. (1953) Studies on substance P purification, occurrence and biological actions. Acta Physiol. Scand., 29: Suppl. 105.

Price, J. and Mudge, A. W. (1983) A subpopulation of rat dorsal root ganglion neurones is catecholaminergic. Nature, 301: 241–243.

Priestley, J. V., Bramwell, S., Butcher, L. L. and Cuello, A. C. (1982) Effect of capsaicin on neuropeptides in areas of termination of primary sensory neurones. Neurochem. Int., 4: 57–65.

Rehfeld, J. F. and Lundberg, J. M. (1983) Cholecystokinin in feline vagal and sciatic nerves: concentration, molecular form and transport velocity. Brain Res., 275: 341–347.

Rosenfeld, M. G., Mermod, J.-J., Amara, S. G., Swanson, L. W., Sawchenko, P. E., Rivier, J., Vale, W. W. and Evans, R. M. (1983) Production of a novel neuropeptide encoded by the calcitonin gene via tissue specific RNA processing. Nature, 304: 129–135.

Rozsa, Z., Jancso, G. and Varro, V. (1984) Possible involvement of capsaicin-sensitive sensory nerves in the regulation of intestinal blood flow in the dog. Naunyn-Schmiedeberg's Arch. Pharmacol., 326: 352–356.

Rozsa, Z., Varro, A. and Jancso, G. (1985) Use of immunoblockade to study the involvement of peptidergic afferent nerves in the intestinal vasodilatory response to capsaicin in the dog. Eur. J. Pharmacol., 115: 59–64.

Saria, A., Lundberg, J. M., Skofitsch, G. and Lembeck, F. (1983) Vascular protein leakage in various tissues induced by substance P, capsaicin, bradykinin, serotonin, histamine and by antigen challenge. Naunyn-Schmiedeberg's Arch. Pharmacol., 324: 212–218.

Schultzberg, M., Dockray, G. J. and Williams, R. G. (1982) Capsaicin depletes CCK-like immunoreactivity detected by immunohistochemistry, but not that measured by radioimmunoassay in rat dorsal spinal cord. Brain Res.,235: 198–204.

Sharkey, K. A. and Templeton, D. (1984) Substance P in the rat parotid gland: evidence for a dual origin from the otic and trigeminal ganglia. Brain Res., 304: 392–396.

Sharkey, K. A., Williams, R. G., Schultzberg, M. and Dockray, G. J. (1983) Sensory substance P-innervation of the urinary bladder: possible site of action of capsaicin in causing urine retention in rats. Neuroscience, 10: 861–868.

Sharkey, K. A., Williams, R. G. and Dockray, G. J. (1984) Sensory substance P-innervation of the stomach and pancreas: demonstration of capsaicin-sensitive sensory neurons in the rat by combined immunohistochemistry and retrograde tracing. Gastroenterology, 87: 914–921.

Skirboll, L., Hökfelt, T., Norell, G., Phillipson, O., Kuypers, H. G. M., Bentivoglio, M., Catsman-Berrevoets, C. E., Visser, T. J., Steinbusch, H., Verhofstad, A., Cuello, A. C., Goldstein, M. and Brownstein, M. (1984) A method for specific transmitter identification of retrogradely labelled neurons: Immunofluorescence combined with fluorescence tracing. Brain Res. Rev., 8: 99–127.

Szolcsanyi, J. and Bartho, L. (1978) New type of nerve-mediated cholinergic contraction of the guinea pig ileum and its selective blockade by capsaicin. Naunyn-Schmiedeberg's Arch. Pharmacol., 305: 83–90.

Tatemoto, K. and Mutt, V. (1981) Isolation and characterization of the intestinal peptide porcine PHI (PHI-27), a new member of the glucagon-secreting family. Proc. Natl. Acad. Sci. U.S.A., 78: 6603–6607.

Tsunoo, A., Konishi, S. and Otsuka, M. (1982) Substance P as an excitatory transmitter of primary afferent neurones in guinea-pig sympathetic ganglia. Neuroscience, 7: 2025–2037.

Tuchscherer, M. M. and Seybold, V. S. (1985) Immunohistochemical studies of substance P, cholecystokinin-octapeptide and somatostatin in dorsal root ganglia of the rat. Neuroscience, 14: 593–606.

Uvnas-Wallensten, K., Rehfeld, J. F., Larsson, L. I. and Uvnas, B. (1977) Heptadecapeptide gastrin in the vagal nerve. Proc. Natl. Acad. Sci. U.S.A., 74: 5707–5710.

F. Cervero and J. F.B. Morrison
Progress in Brain Research, Vol. 67

CHAPTER 10

Pharmacological aspects of visceral sensory receptors

H. Higashi

Department of Physiology, Kurume University, School of Medicine, Kurume 830, Japan

Introduction

In the tissue, noxious stimuli produce and release algogenic substances, such as 5-hydroxytryptamine (5-HT), histamine (Hst), acetylcholine (ACh), bradykinin (BK), substance P (SP), prostaglandin (PG) and some others. It is well known that these substances excite the free endings of sensory nerve fibres, particularly Aδ- and C-fibers arising from the skin (Douglas and Ritchie, 1960; Fjällbrant and Iggo, 1961; Beck and Handwerker, 1974), muscles (Mense and Schmidt, 1974; Fock and Mense, 1976; Hiss and Mense, 1976; Kumazawa and Mizumura, 1977; Mense, 1977, 1982; Franz and Mense, 1978; Foreman et al., 1979) and viscera (Douglas and Ritchie, 1957; Armett and Richie, 1961; Kumazawa and Mizumura, 1980; Niijima, 1980; Delpierre et al., 1981). Cottrell and Iggo (1984a,b) have also reported that local intra-arterial bolus injections of the algogenics and some other autocoids (pentagastrin, cholecystokinin, etc.) arouse or enhance activity in the duodenal tension receptors with vagal afferent fibres of sheep. However, these results have not established whether the mechanism of receptor excitation by these substances involves direct or indirect mechanisms. Even if the substances directly alter the sensitivity of the nerve ending, it is not yet clearly known how the substances induce generator potentials that trigger afferent impulses in the sensory nerve terminals, owing to the difficulty in measuring the membrane potential changes in the terminals.

In 1974, Nishi et al. found that the cell bodies of somatic primary afferent nerves (dorsal root ganglion) are endowed with GABA receptors, similar to those on their central terminals (Fig. 1B). They showed that activation of the GABA receptors produces a depolarization that is associated with a selective increase in chloride permeability of the receptor membrane. They proposed that the same mechanism might underlie the GABA-mediated depolarization of primary afferent terminals. In support of this concept, the similarities in electrical and pharmacological characteristics of the GABA receptors at the somata and the central terminals of spinal primary afferent neurones have been confirmed experimentally (Levy, 1977; Gallagher et al., 1978; Higashi and Nishi, 1982b). Higashi (1977), using an intracellular record map, demonstrated that the visceral primary afferent somata (nodose ganglion cells) possess 5-HT receptors of an excitatory type, which might be similar to those of the nerve ending (Fig. 1A). A variety of excitatory receptors susceptible to BK, Hst or ACh and some inhibitory receptors sensitive to opiate substances have since been found in visceral primary afferent neurones (Higashi et al., 1982a,b). These findings have suggested the ideas that both the somata and the terminals of primary afferent neurones are equipped with similar, if not identical, receptors and that the properties of the terminal receptors that are inaccessible with the current techniques may be investigated indirectly by studying the somatic receptors using conventional microiontophoresis techniques.

This chapter deals with the chemosensitivities of

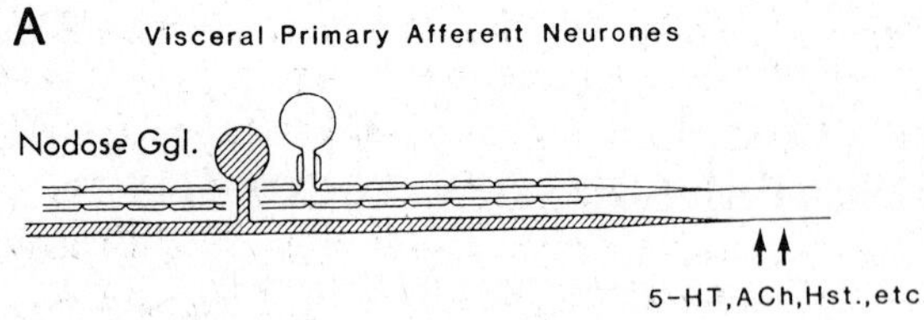

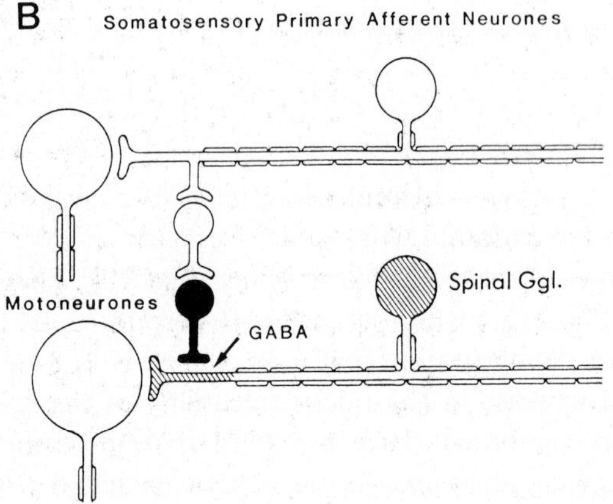

Fig. 1. The chemoreceptors located with primary afferent sensory neurones. Both the somata and terminals of visceral (A) and somatosensory (B) afferent neurones are endowed with similar, if not identical, chemoreceptors (see text). Ggl, ganglions.

visceral primary afferent neurones (nodose ganglion cells) to intrinsic algesic agents, and shows that no essential chemosensitive differences exist between the somatic and visceral primary afferent neurones. Also described are the specific firing patterns of sensory fibres to each algesic agent which can be related to the characteristics of the potential changes in the nodose ganglion cells to individual algogenics. The effects of analgesics on visceral primary afferent neurones are also included in this chapter.

Electrical properties of nodose ganglion cells

The nodose ganglion of the vagus nerve contains the cell bodies of afferent fibres innervating the respiratory, cardiovascular and gastrointestinal systems. Approximately 80% of the 30,000 fibres in the cervical vagus are sensory, and of these 70% are unmyelinated afferent fibres from abdominal viscera (Evans and Murray, 1954; Agostoni et al., 1957; see also Leek, 1972). The cell bodies in the nodose ganglion are devoid of synapses (Cajal, 1909).

In 1978, Gallego and Eyzaguirre measured the electrical properties of mammalian nodose ganglion cells identified as type A or type C by the conduction velocities and the threshold of their axons. The ratio of type A to type C neurones was in good agreement with the ratio of myelinated to nonmyelinated sensory fibres of the cervical vagus. This observation has been confirmed recently, as shown in Fig. 2 (Higashi and Nishi, 1982a). Thus, type A neurones have myelinated axons while the type C have non-myelinated axons.

Our results obtained in studies on the electrical properties of the rabbit nodose ganglion cells were generally in agreement with those of Gallego and Eyzaguirre (1978). Type A neurones had processes conducting at about 8 m/second (range, 6–12 m/second). The action potential evoked by direct depolarization of the soma membrane was abolished completely by tetrodotoxin (TTX, 0.1–0.3 μM). Type C neurones had action potentials with a shoulder on the falling phase. An action potential in the soma followed a stimulus to the vagus nerve

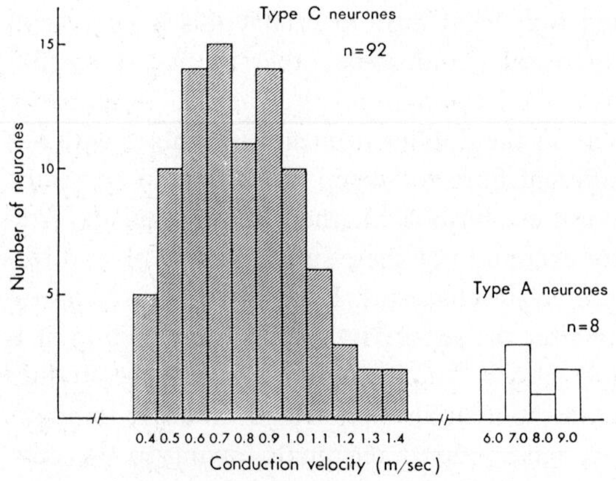

Fig. 2. Distribution of neuronal types within the rabbit nodose ganglion (Higashi and Nishi, 1982a). 100 neurones are characterized, according to their axonal conduction velocity.

with a latency appropriate to conduction at 0.4–1.4 m/second. The action potential evoked by direct depolarization of the soma membrane was much reduced in amplitude and rate of rise, but not abolished, by TTX. The residual action potential in the presence of TTX was abolished by removal of Ca^{2+}, or addition of cobalt to the extracellular solution (Higashi et al., 1982a, 1984; Ito, 1982). Thus, type C neurones exhibited a regenerative Ca^{2+} system in addition to the sodium spike-producing system while type A neurones lacked the former. Moreover, Stansfeld and Wallis (1983, 1984) have suggested that nodose type C neurones may possess TTX-insensitive Na^+ channels, besides regenerative Ca^{2+} and TTX-sensitive Na^+ channels.

In rabbit type C neurones the action potentials were followed by a fast (up to 50 mseconds) after-hyperpolarization and a subsequent long-lasting (90 mseconds–4 seconds) after-hyperpolarization (Higashi et al., 1982a). The slowly developing after-hyperpolarization was associated with an increase in the membrane conductance to K^+; it reversed polarity at about −90 mV and the reversal potential was dependent on extracellular K^+ concentration. The increase in K^+ conductance during the slow after-hyperpolarization was blocked in a Ca^{2+}-free or Co^{2+} (1–2 mM) -containing solution. Intracellular injection of EGTA abolished the after-hyperpolarization; intracellular injection of Ca^{2+} mimicked the after-hyperpolarization (Higashi et al., 1984). These results suggest that the Ca^{2+} entry during the action potential leads to a long-lasting increase in K^+ conductance in type C neurones. This observation may be compatible with the finding from in vivo or in vitro preparations of cat and rabbit nodose ganglia that repetitive action potentials cause a persistent hyperpolarization lasting up to several seconds (Jaffe and Sampson, 1976).

Harper and Lawson (1985a,b) have recently demonstrated the subdivisions and electrical properties of rat dorsal root ganglion cells. Neurones were divided into four groups, based on the conduction velocity of their peripheral axons (Aα, 30–50 m/second; Aβ, 14–30 m/second; Aδ, 2.2–8 m/second; C, 1.4 m/second). The fast-conducting (Aα) and slowly conducting (Aδ) myelinated fibres had short-duration somatic spikes within the ranges of 0.49–1.35 and 0.5–1.7 mseconds, respectively. The Aβ and C cells had longer action potential durations, in the range of 0.6–2.9 and 0.6–7.4 mseconds, respectively. The longer durations were related to the presence of an inflexion on the repolarizing phase seen in one-third of A neurones and all C neurones (Harper and Lawson, 1985b). An inward Ca^{2+} current has previously been proposed to underlie the presence of an inflexion in cultured dorsal root ganglion neurones of the chick (Dichter and Fischback, 1977) and mouse (Yoshida et al., 1978). Thus, the Aβ and C cells would have a Ca^{2+}-dependent regenerative spike with a Na^+ component. The action potential overshoot and the after-hyperpolarization were greater in C neurones than in A neurones. These characteristics of electrical properties in the dorsal root ganglion cells are consistent with those in the nodose ganglion cells.

Chemosensitivities of nodose ganglion cells

Visceral afferent A and C nerve terminals differ in their chemosensitivities to various endogenous algesics (see Paintal, 1963, 1964), i.e., both 5-HT and ACh cause firing of unmyelinated C-fibres, but only weakly excited myelinated A-fibres. Neto (1978) demonstrated that 5-HT depolarized non-myelinated C-fibres but not myelinated A-fibres of the rabbit cervical vagus and sciatic nerves. As shown in Table I, the somata of visceral afferent type C neurones are depolarized by algogenic substances (such as 5-HT, BK or Hst) while type A neurones are less sensitive to these algogenics (Higashi et al., 1982a). These results indicate that somata and axons of type C visceral afferent neurones are excited by algogenics, while type A neurones are less sensitive to algogenic substances.

On the other hand, Fjällbrant and Iggo (1961) and Beck and Handwerker (1974) demonstrated that 5-HT not only stimulated group IV (C) fibres but also excited slowly adapting, groups II to IV

TABLE I

Sensitivity of type A and C neurones in nodose ganglion to endogenous substances (10 μM)

Neurone type	5-HT-sensitive	BK-sensitive	ACh-sensitive	Hst-sensitive	GABA-sensitive	
A (14)	2 (14%)	0	1 (7%)	0	14 (100%)	
C (42)	39 (93%)[a]	15 (36%)	14 (33%)	10 (24%)	33 (79%)	
	5-HT depolarization (mV)	BK depolarization (mV)	ACh depolarization (mV)	Hst depolarization (mV)	GABA depolarization (mV)	Resting potential (mV)
A	4.5 ± 2.1	0	7.0	0	14.4 ± 8.7	−58.0 ± 5.5
C	23.8 ± 10.9	8.4 ± 5.7	12.5 ± 6.9	6.7 ± 7.0	6.6 ± 7.0	−57.7 ± 5.5

Each response is the mean ± S.D. in mV of the responses tabulated above. Data are from Higashi et al. (1982b).
[a] Of these 39 neurones, 34 were depolarized and five hyperpolarized.

inclusive, fibres. In this latter report (see Table 1 in Beck and Handwerker, 1974), 5-HT was found to be particularly active on group IV fibres which innervate cutaneous heat receptors. Morita et al. (1983a) suggested that the majority of type C and half of type A neurones of the bullfrog dorsal root ganglia were responsive to 5-HT or ACh. Altogether, these results may imply that the differences in the sensitivities of type A and type C sensory neurones to endogenous algesic substances are due to the relative differences in the densities of pertinent receptors rather than to the absolute existence or absence of certain receptors.

What follows is the description of the response of the somata of the visceral or somatic primary afferent neurones to several endogenous algesics.

5-Hydroxytryptamine (5-HT)

When blood platelets disintegrate, they release 5-HT and Hst. 5-HT (0.1 μM) applied to the nerve endings in an exposed blister base elicits a severe pain in man (see Keele et al., 1982).

The cell bodies of vagal primary afferents which are located in the nodose ganglion are excited and produce action potentials in response to application of 5-HT (Sampson and Jaffe, 1974; De Groat and Simonds, 1976). Thereafter, a direct depolarizing action of 5-HT on the neurones has been demonstrated (Higashi, 1977, 1980; Simonds and De Groat, 1980; Wallis et al., 1982). The majority of type C neurones, in response to 5-HT applied by superfusion (≥1 μM) or by ionophoresis (≥5 nA, 50 mseconds), showed a rapid depolarization of about 30 mV in amplitude which was followed by a hyperpolarization of 5–15 mV (Higashi and Nishi, 1982a). This after-hyperpolarization was occasionally followed by a long-lasting depolarization of a few mV. All three of these 5-HT-induced responses were associated with a reduction in membrane resistance (Fig. 3A). The initial depolarization induced by 5-HT was abolished by Na^+-free Krebs solution and was reduced by a few mV in K^+-free Krebs solution. The response in normal Krebs solution was reversed at a membrane potential level of +7.3 mV. The after-hyperpolarization disappeared in Na^+-free or Ca^{2+}-free Krebs solution while it was markedly enhanced in K^+-free Krebs solution. This after-hyperpolarization was reversed in normal Krebs solution at a membrane potential of −88.7 mV; it was abolished at membrane potentials more positive than −20 mV. The

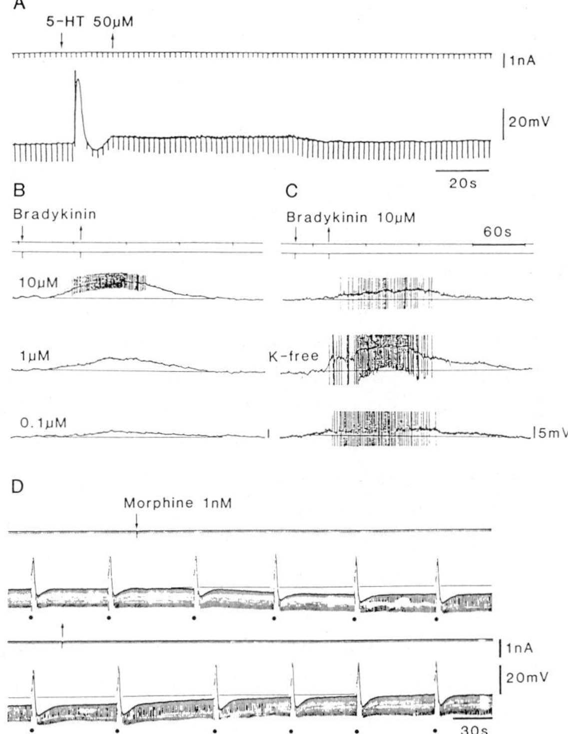

Fig. 3. The algogenic and analgesic induced responses in type C visceral afferent neurones. A, during superfusion with 5-HT (50 μM) a triphasic potential change is recorded. All the responses are accompanied by a decrease in input resistance. B, bradykinin (0.1–10 μM) produces dose-related depolarizations in normal Krebs solution. C, bradykinin (10 μM) depolarization induced in normal Krebs solution, K^+-free solution and normal Krebs solution, from top to bottom. D, morphine (1 nM) produces a hyperpolarization associated with a decrease in input resistance. In addition, the Ca^{2+}-dependent after-hyperpolarizations of 5-HT responses evoked by ionophoresis (filled circles) are markedly prolonged during superfusion with morphine.

second, slower-in-onset depolarization was abolished by removal of external Na^+ but was not altered by either K^+-free or low Cl^- media. These results suggest that the initial depolarization is due mainly to simultaneous increases in Na^+ and K^+ conductances that the after-hyperpolarization is brought about by an increase of K^+ conductance which is triggered by a voltage-dependent influx of Ca^{2+}, and that the long-lasting, slow-in-onset depolarization is associated with a small, but sustained increase in Na^+ conductance. In a small number of type C neurones, 5-HT applied by superfusion ($\leqslant 1$ μM) or by ionophoresis (0.5–20 nA, 50 mseconds), evoked a simple hyperpolarizing response of 3–8 mV without any associated pre- and post-depolarization (also see Higashi, 1977; Stansfeld and Wallis, 1984). Since removal of K^+ enhanced this hyperpolarization and since displacement of the membrane potential to a level more negative than -90 mV reversed its polarity, an increased K^+ conductance may constitute the ionic mechanism responsible for this hyperpolarization. When the same neurones were superfused with a higher concentration (10 μM) of 5-HT, applied iontophoretically with larger currents (50–100 nA, 50 mseconds), the hyperpolarizing response was preceded by a rapid depolarization of 5–15 mV; both the hyperpolarizing and depolarizing components were associated with a decrease in membrane resistance. A majority of type A neurones did not respond to 5-HT, whether applied by superfusion or by ionophoresis; the few type A neurones that did respond to 5-HT, showed a depolarization of only a few mV (Higashi et al., 1982a,b; Stansfeld and Wallis, 1984).

Wallis et al. (1982) investigated the depolarizing action of 5-HT analogues on the rabbit nodose ganglion and discovered that for activation of 5-HT receptors of nodose ganglion cells the ligand must possess a hydroxyl moiety at position 5 of the indole nucleus. Absence from the ligand of a hydroxyl group, as in tryptamine, or the presence of a bulky substituent group, as in 5-methoxytryptamine, leads to a marked reduction in activity. Amongst the compounds tested in which the side-chain was *N*-methylated, only bufotenine showed substantial depolarizing ability. Psilocin, which is *N*-methylated but exhibits the hydroxyl group in position 4 of the nucleus, was inactive. Methysergide and LSD-25, both recognized as specific 5-HT antagonists, did not produce any significant antagonism of 5-HT depolarization (Higashi et al., 1982a; Wallis et al., 1982). Neto (1978) reported also that methysergide does not affect 5-HT depolarization of rabbit cervical vagal fibres. Nishi

(1975) noted that LSD-25 or methysergide do not alter the excitatory effect of 5-HT on the cat carotid body, which causes firing recorded from the carotid nerve. On the other hand, quipazine, which is reputed to act centrally by mimicking the action of 5-HT, reduced 5-HT depolarization without exhibiting any agonist activity (Wallis et al., 1982).

Higashi et al. (1982a) demonstrated that *d*-tubocurarine (*d*TC, 0.2–5 μM) depressed 5-HT-induced inward currents of nodose ganglion neurones without altering their resting membrane properties, and caused a parallel shift to the right of the concentration response curves for 5-HT. At concentrations greater than 10 μM, *d*TC caused a non-parallel shift to the right and depression of the maximum peak response to 5-HT. In addition, the time course of the 5-HT currents at these higher concentrations was altered significantly, i.e., the falling phase was frequently shortened and became biphasic (Higashi et al., 1982a). Besides antagonizing the 5-HT effect on the nodose ganglion cells, *d*TC (0.2–5 μM) blocked both ACh- and GABA-induced depolarization. Picrotoxin (1–10 μM) also blocked 5-HT as well as GABA- and ACh-induced depolarizations (see below). However, picrotoxin was 6 to 10 times less potent than *d*TC in blocking ACh- and 5-HT-induced depolarizations (Higashi et al., 1982b). Also, picrotoxin blocked in vivo 5-HT as well as GABA depolarizations of cat nodose ganglion (De Groat and Simonds, 1976; Simonds and De Groat, 1980).

Morita and Katayama (1986) reported that the 5-HT receptors located on the somata of the bullfrog dorsal root ganglion cells might be similar to those located on the rabbit nodose ganglion cells. Thus, in response to 5-HT applied by superfusion (< 1 μM), approximately 80% of type C neurones showed a hyperpolarization ranging from 3–10 mV in amplitude. The 5-HT-induced hyperpolarization was often preceded by a rapid depolarization of a few mV, as previously seen in the rabbit nodose ganglion cells. The hyperpolarizing response reversed its polarity near the K^+ equilibrium potential, which was estimated from the reversal potential of the after-hyperpolarization of the soma spikes. This hyperpolarization was blocked by removal of Ca^{2+} or addition of Co^{2+} to the extracellular solution. These results suggest that Ca^{2+} influx during the activation of the 5-HT receptor may lead to a long-lasting increase in K^+ conductance. When 5-HT was applied by superfusion at high concentrations (≥ 6 μM), 55% of type C neurones showed a rapid depolarization, amounting to about 10 mV, which was accompanied by a decreased input resistance. The depolarization was followed by a hyperpolarization and/or a small depolarization. Since 5-HT depolarization disappeared in Na^+-free solution and reversed its polarity at -10 mV, this depolarization was probably due to an increase in membrane conductance to both Na^+ and K^+. In response to 5-HT applied by superfusion (10 nM–30 μM), the minority of type C neurones (10%) showed a slow-in-onset depolarization accompanied by an increase in input resistance. Since this response reversed its polarity at -90 mV, it is presumably due to K^+ inactivation. On the other hand, half of the type A neurones also responded to 5-HT with a slow depolarization which was associated with a decrease in input resistance. The slow depolarization reversed its polarity at about -65 mV. The reversal potential was dependent on the external K^+ concentration. The response, however, was reduced in its amplitude in Na^+-free solution and completely abolished by removal of external Ca^{2+}. These results suggest that the slow depolarizing response in type A neurones may be due to a simultaneous increase in Ca^{2+} and K^+ conductance which is possibly regulated by extracellular Na^+ (Morita and Katayama, 1986, also see Morita et al., 1983a). Both *d*TC (0.1–30 μM) and picrotoxin (≥ 1 μM) abolished three 5-HT responses, the rapid depolarizing and hyperpolarizing responses in type C neurones and the slow depolarization in type A neurones, all of which were associated with an increase in membrane conductance. Methysergide (0.1 μM) reversibly blocked the hyperpolarization in type C neurones and the slow depolarization in type A neurones, but had no significant effect on the rapid and the slow depolarization in type C neurones (Morita and Katayama, 1986).

Acetylcholine (ACh)

Of several endogenous algogenics (BK, SP, ACh, 5-HT, ATP and KCl) which stimulate paravascular nociceptors, BK, SP and ACh were found to be far more active than the other substances (Juan and Lembeck, 1974).

In response to ACh applied by superfusion ($\geqslant 10$ μM) or by iontophoresis ($\geqslant 5$ nA, 50 mseconds), approximately 30% of type C neurones in rabbit nodose ganglia show a rapid depolarization, amounting to about 10 mV, which is accompanied by decreased input resistance. ACh depolarization disappeared in low Na^+ (11.7 mM) Krebs solution and reversed its polarity at 0 mV (Higashi, 1980). These data indicate that the ACh-induced depolarization may be due to a simultaneous increase in Na^+ and K^+ conductance. ACh depolarization was blocked by *d*TC (10–50 μM), but unaffected by atropine (1 μM), suggesting that ACh depolarization was generated by nicotinic receptors (Higashi, 1980; Higashi et al., 1982b). In agreement with these findings, Wallis et al. (1982) reported that a nicotinic receptor ligand, 1,1-dimethyl-4-phenyl piperazinium iodide (DMPP), depolarizes nodose ganglion cells of the rabbit.

The effect of ACh on dorsal root ganglion cells seems to be compatible with those in the nodose ganglion cells. ACh (10 μM–1 mM) caused a fast depolarization associated with a decrease in input resistance in the bullfrog dorsal root ganglion cells (Morita and Katayama, 1984). The ACh depolarization reversed its polarity at the membrane potential of about -30 mV. The reversal potential was dependent on both Na^+ and K^+ concentrations in the superfusing solution. Nicotinic receptor antagonists (nicotine, *d*TC, hexamethonium) reversibly blocked the ACh response, suggesting that the fast depolarization was generated by the activation of nicotinic receptors. This response was observed in a particular group of cells (presumably type C neurones) which were characterized with relatively slow conduction velocity (0.3–1.0 m/second), long-lasting after-hyperpolarization and TTX-resistant action potential. On the other hand, ACh and muscarine caused a slowly developing depolarization in other groups of cells (presumably type A neurones) whose action potentials were sensitive to TTX. The slow depolarization was associated with an increase in membrane resistance (Morita and Katayama, 1984). These results suggest that bullfrog dorsal root ganglion cells are capable of producing nicotinic and muscarinic responses.

Histamine (Hst)

Most cells contain Hst, which in high concentrations (>100 μM) produces pain, but in low concentrations (1–100 μM) arouses itch (see Keele et al., 1982).

About 25% of type C neurones in rabbit nodose ganglia respond to the depolarizing action of Hst (10–100 μM). In a majority of the type C neurones which respond to Hst, the behaviour of Hst-induced slow depolarization at different levels of membrane potential and in a K^+-free medium is similar to that of BK-induced depolarization, suggesting that both share the same ionic mechanism, that is, both are due to reduction in K^+ conductance (Higashi et al., 1982b). In a small number of type C neurones, Hst caused a rapid depolarization which was accompanied by a decrease in input resistance. The response disappeared in low-Na^+ Krebs solution and reversed its polarity at -10 to 0 mV (Higashi, unpublished observation). It is still unknown whether Hst_1 or Hst_2 receptors are involved in these Hst-induced responses.

Morita et al. (1983a) reported that in bullfrog dorsal root ganglion cells Hst produced a slow depolarization associated with a decreased membrane conductance, probably to K^+.

Bradykinin (BK)

Plasma kinins are powerful algesic agents. The kinins, chief of which is BK ($\geqslant 0.1$ μM), cause an intense, burning pain when applied to the exposed base of a blister. When the kinins are injected into arteries supplying skin, muscle or various viscera, nociceptive responses or pain occurs in animals and in man (see Armstrong, 1970).

BK (0.1–10 μM) depolarized the membrane and increased the input resistance of about one-third of type C neurones in rabbit nodose ganglia. The BK depolarization was long-lasting and it was dose-dependent (Fig. 3B). BK depolarization was reduced in amplitude as the membrane potential was increased by anodal currents applied to the cell membrane. The BK depolarization was enhanced in a K^+-free Krebs solution (Fig. 3C). These findings indicate that the BK depolarization is brought about mainly by a decrease in K^+ conductance (Higashi, 1980). In the case of a few type C neurones sensitive to BK, the slow depolarization was preceded by a rapid hyperpolarization of 4–10 mV, which was associated with an increased conductance (Higashi et al., 1982b). Moreover, BK at a low concentration (0.1 μM) not only produced membrane depolarization of a few mV, but markedly reduced the CA^{2+}-dependent after-hyperpolarization preceded by the soma spike (Higashi, unpublished observation).

Substance P (SP)

Many of the primary afferent fibres of the vagus have been shown to contain SP (Lundberg et al., 1978). As it was shown that pericellular plexuses of SP-immunoreactive fibres are present in the rabbit nodose ganglia, SP may have a direct action on neuronal cell bodies of the nodose ganglia (Katz and Karten, 1980). However, Wallis et al. (1982), using a sucrose-gap method, demonstrated that bath application of SP to the rabbit nodose ganglion produced no detectable change in resting membrane potential.

SP exists in small dark cells (diameter, 14–30 μm) of rat dorsal root ganglia (Hökfelt et al., 1975) and appears to be involved in pain transmission (see Lembeck and Gamse, 1982). In response to SP (10 μM) applied by superfusion, a certain population of bullfrog dorsal root ganglion cells (presumably type Aβ or C neurones) produced a membrane depolarization accompanied by an increase in input resistance, and reduced a spike after-hyperpolarization which was due to activation of Ca^{2+}-dependent K^+-conductance (Morita et al., 1983b).

Prostaglandins (PGs)

Prostaglandins E_1 and E_2, when injected by the subcutaneous or intramuscular route, elicit pain in man. This effect is generally not as immediate or intense as those caused by BK or Hst, but they outlast and potentiate the pain-producing effects of the other algogenics (see Collier and Schneider, 1972; Zurier, 1974).

Some of the effects of prostaglandins on the rabbit nodose ganglion cells are of interest in the present context. Fowler et al. (1984) demonstrated that pressure-applied soluble extracts prepared from purified human lung mast cells abolished a Ca^{2+}-dependent after-hyperpolarization following the action potentials in type C neurones without affecting membrane potential or input resistance. Similarly, pressure- or bath-applied prostaglandins (PGE_1, $PGF_{2\alpha}$; 1–10 μg/ml) reduced only the amplitude of the after-hyperpolarization, but pressure-applied Hst, on the other hand, did not have significant effects on the after-hyperpolarization (Fowler et al., 1984).

Adenosine phosphates

Erythrocytes after lysis evoke marked pain. This is partly due to their high content of K^+ (>100 mM) and partly to the presence of adenosine phosphates, AMP, ADP and ATP (see Keele et al., 1982). Moreover, it has been demonstrated that electrical activity of rabbit non-myelinated nerve fibres leads to release of adenosine, inosine and hypoxanthine (Maire et al., 1984).

A majority of nodose ganglion cells of the rabbit is sensitive to ATP (Higashi, unpublished observation). In response to ATP (>1 μM) applied by superfusion, type C neurones showed a hyperpolarization of a few mV in amplitude, which was associated with a decrease in input resistance. Since the hyperpolarization was augmented in K^+-free medium, it is probably due to an increase in K^+

conductance. When ATP was applied at high concentrations ($\geqslant 10\ \mu M$), the neurones showed a slowly developing depolarization accompanied by either an increase or a decrease in membrane resistance.

The effects of ATP on nodose ganglion cells are compatible with those on bullfrog dorsal root ganglion cells. Thus, Morita et al. (1983a) reported that ATP (100 nM–1 mM) caused a slow hyperpolarization at relatively low concentrations and produced a slow depolarization at high concentrations by increasing and decreasing K^+-conductance, respectively. Furthermore, ATP at high concentrations ($> 10\ \mu M$) reduced a Ca^{2+}-dependent after-hyperpolarization of the soma spike in dorsal root ganglion cells (Morita et al., 1983b). These results suggest that the ATP-induced depolarization and the reduction of the after-hyperpolarization may result from the depressant effect of ATP on Ca^{2+}-dependent K^+-conductance. On the other hand, Krishtal et al. (1983) investigated the action of adenosine phosphates on the various sensory neurones enzymatically isolated from nodose, vestibular, trigeminal and dorsal root ganglia of the rat and cat, and disclosed that many sensory neurones clamped at a constant holding potential responded with an inward current to the application of either ATP ($K_d = 5\ \mu M$) or ADP ($K_d = 0.5$ mM). The ATP-induced inward current was markedly reduced but did not disappear when external Na^+ was substituted with Tris, choline or tetraethylammonium (TEA). A permeability to divalent cations was not detected when the concentration of Ca^{2+} or Mg^{2+} was increased to 10 mM in the external medium. Substitution of internal fluoride with larger anions, as well as substitution of external NaCl with Na^+-HEPES, did not affect the ATP-activated current. These results may imply that the channels linked to the ATP receptors allow monovalent cations (presumably both Na^+ and K^+) to pass with low selectivity.

Endogenous opiate-like substances

Shefner et al. (1981) found stereospecific binding sites of tritiated dihydromorphine and Leu^5-enkephalin in both the nodose ganglion and the vagus nerve of the rabbit, but they failed to observe any electrophysiological effect of these ligands on the neurone. However, this negative finding may have resulted from a form of desensitization, since much lower concentrations (1–100 nM) both hyperpolarize the resting membrane of type C neurones and also prolong the Ca^{2+}-dependent after-hyperpolarization which follows application of 5-HT, as seen in Fig. 3D (Higashi, unpublished observation).

Higashi et al. (1982a) demonstrated that in approximately 50% of type C neurones, bath application of morphine (1–100 nM) caused a hyperpolarization of a few mV in amplitude. The hyperpolarization was associated with a decreased input resistance and antagonized by a prior exposure of the preparation to naloxone (10 nM). Apparent reversal potential for this morphine-induced hyperpolarization was estimated by employing constant current anelectrotonic pulses; its average value was -86.3 mV, which is similar to the reversal level of the after-hyperpolarization of soma spikes. This suggests that the hyperpolarizing effect of morphine may be due to a selective increase of K^+ conductance. Furthermore, Higashi et al. (1982a) observed that morphine (1–100 nM) initially augmented and then subsequently depressed Ca^{2+}-dependent potentials (the shoulder of the action potential, the slow after-hyperpolarization and the calcium spike in the type C cells), and that this biphasic effect of morphine can be prevented by an equal concentration of naloxone. The enhancement and depression of the Ca^{2+}-dependent potentials are not only concentration dependent but they are also time dependent and can be observed with a given concentration of morphine. It has been reported that opiates inhibit the binding of calcium to brain synaptosomal membrane (Nicholson et al., 1978). Tokimasa et al. (1981) suggested that opiate may prolong Ca^{2+}-dependent after-hyperpolarizations by inhibiting Ca^{2+} binding to an intracellular site normally important in sequestration of Ca^{2+} entering during neuronal activity. In addition, it is well known that an excessive increase in intracellular Ca^{2+} inhibits Ca^{2+} conductance in invertebrate neurones (Kostyuk and Krishtal, 1977). Thus, Higashi et al. (1982a) speculate that the degree of inhibition of Ca^{2+} binding affects the concentration of intracellular free Ca^{2+}, which in turn determines the neuronal response to the opiates. If the extent of opiate-induced inhibition of Ca^{2+} binding is quite small, Ca^{2+}-dependent potentials would be augmented. As the inhibition of Ca^{2+} binding is increased with time or with higher concentrations of morphine, the opiate-induced increase in intracellular free Ca^{2+} would inhibit further Ca^{2+} entry.

Opiate receptors have also been found on the terminal and fibres of dorsal root ganglion cells in adult animals as well as in tissue cultures (Lamotte et al., 1976; Hiler et al., 1978; Fields et al., 1980). Mudge et al. (1979) demonstrated that enkephalin reduced the voltage-dependent calcium current of the action potential in the cultured dorsal root ganglion cells. On the other hand, Williams and Zieglgansberger (1981) failed to observe any electrophysiological effect of the opiates (normorphine, methionine-enkephalin or (D-Ala^2, D-Leu^5)-enkephalin on the dorsal root ganglion cell isolated from adult rats. This negative finding seems to result from a desensitization, since high concentrations (1 μM–1 mM) of the opiates were applied to the bath.

Characterization of the receptors on visceral afferent neurones

Paintal (1964) and Daniel (1968) consider that the excitatory effects of ACh, nicotine, 5-HT and phenyldiguanide on non-ruminant gastric tension receptor afferent discharges are due to the direct action of these substances on the regenerative region of the non-myelinated nerve endings (but also see Cottrell and Iggo, 1984b). The observations described above clearly showed that the cell bodies (type C neurones) of vagal afferent neurones are endowed with algogenic (such as those responding to 5-HT, BK, ACh, Hst, etc.) receptors that may be similar to those located on their axon terminals. The functional roles of these receptors are obscure at the present. Presumably, they could be a remnant of an embryonic stage in which algogenic receptors migrate from cell soma to the axon terminals. A similar receptor distribution has been described for other neuronal elements, such as GABA receptors on the afferent terminals and somata of primary afferent neurones (see Nishi et al., 1974; Gallagher et al., 1978; Curtis, 1979), and the cholinoceptors and adrenoceptors on the somata and axon terminals of the sympathetic nerves to the heart (see Westfall, 1977).

The algesic-induced depolarizations lend themselves to the following classification. The first type concerns 5-HT- and ACh-induced responses concomitant with simultaneously increased Na^+ and K^+ conductance; this depolarization is characterized by rapid onset and short duration. The second type of response is that due to BK, ATP and Hst, in which case K^+ conductance is decreased and the depolarization has a slow onset, and a long-lasting time course. PGs may be classified into the second type since they inhibit Ca^{2+}-dependent K^+ conductance. In several studies (Mense and Schmidt, 1974; Nishi, 1975; Fock and Mense, 1976; Foreman et al., 1979) in which extracellular recordings were obtained with respect to peripheral mammalian afferent nerves, intra-arterial injection of 5-HT or ACh evoked a short burst of repetitive firing followed by a supression of spontaneous firing, while the application of BK and Hst produced long-lasting repetitive firing. These different patterns of the firing evoked by various algesics may be due to different ionic mechanisms underlying their depolarizations.

Since ACh and 5-HT depolarizations are generated by increases in Na^+ and K^+ conductances and are blocked by *d*TC or picrotoxin, there is a possibility that ACh and 5-HT may share the same receptor-ionophore complex. However, in the case of nodose ganglia this possibility is unlikely since in this preparation (1) hexamethonium blocks ACh but not 5-HT depolarization and (2) ACh does not desensitize 5-HT depolarization (Higashi et al.,

1982a). In addition, there appeared to be no interaction between 5-HT and BK receptors, although BK depressed the after-hyperpolarizing phase of 5-HT responses (Higashi et al., 1982b). Similar lack of crossed desensitization between 5-HT, BK and Hst was reported for the endings of muscular group IV afferent units (Hiss and Mense, 1976) and unmyelinated afferents from the skin (Beck and Handwerker, 1974). Krishtal et al. (1983) also reported a lack of crossed desensitization between GABA, proton and ATP receptors in various sensory ganglia. These results suggest that the depolarizing effect of these algogenics on the sensory neurones might be exerted via different receptors.

Not only are visceral sensory type C neurones sensitive to various algogenic substances, but they are also activated by other substances (Cottrell and Iggo, 1984b,c), mechanical stimuli (Falempin et al., 1978; Clerc and Mei, 1983; Cottrell and Iggo, 1984a) and/or thermal variations (Delpierre et al., 1981). On the other hand, visceral afferent type A neurones are less sensitive but not inactive to algogenic substances, as described above. These endings are connected with small myelinated fibres which must belong to type A and possess slowly adapting receptors with a low threshold to mechanical stimuli (see Falempin et al., 1978). Thus, it is likely that the sensory endpoint of type A neurones may be tension receptors, which are less sensitive to algogenics and other irritant chemicals.

Conclusion

The results which we have presented and discussed in this chapter reveal the existence of polymodal receptors in the visceral afferent type C neurones. However, the concept of nociception is difficult to apply to the viscera; cutting, crushing or burning visceral tissue generally produces no pain. Excessive distension of the hollow viscera such as the intestine or bladder can activate mechanoreceptors of C-fibres and evoke pain, but it is not possible to say if such stimuli are tissue-damaging. Furthermore, in many cases of visceral disease pain arises from somatic structures innervated from the same spinal segments as the troubled viscus, and this suggests that the phenomenon has a spinal mechanism (see McMahon, 1984).

Therefore, it is more important to consider the physiological significance of these autocoids and their receptors on the transmission of sensory information. In the case of 5-HT, it is formed and stored locally in the mucosal membrane of rabbit small intestine (Feldberg and Toh, 1953) and is released following a rise in the intraluminal pressure (Bülbring and Lin, 1958). Once released, 5-HT may stimulate non-myelinated afferent fibres of the vagus (Douglas and Richie, 1957) and nerve endings of mesenteric nerves (Niijima, 1980). Douglas and Richie (1957) have proposed that 5-HT may serve a physiological role in the initiation of sensory signals from the gastrointestinal tract. By analogy, it is conceivable that the other algogenics could contribute to modulate sensory input by activating their polymodal receptors at which the centripetal impulses arise (see Cottrell and Iggo, 1984b).

References

Agostoni, E., Chinnock, J. E., Daly, M. De B. and Murray, J. G. (1957) Functional and histological studies of the vagus nerve and its branches to the heart, lungs and abdominal viscera in the cat. J. Physiol. (Lond.), 135: 182–205.

Armett, C. J. and Richie, J. M. (1961) The action of acetylcholine and some related substances on conduction in non-myelinated fibers. J. Physiol. (Lond.), 155: 372–384.

Armstrong, D. (1970) Pain. In E. G. Erdös (Ed.), Handbuch der Experimentalische Pharmakologie, Vol. 25, Springer-Verlag, Berlin, pp. 434–481.

Beck, P. W. and Handwerker, H. O. (1974) Bradykinin and serotonin effects on various types of cutaneous nerve fibres. Pflügers Arch., 347: 207–222.

Bülbring, E. and Lin, R. C. Y. (1958) The effect of intraluminal application of 5-hydroxytryptamine and 5-hydroxytryptophan on peristalsis: the local production of 5-HT and its release in relation to intraluminal pressure and propulsive activity. J. Physiol. (Lond.), 140: 381–407.

Cajal, R. Y. (1909) Histologie du Systeme Nerveux de l'Homme et des Vertebres, A. Maloine, Paris.

Clerc, N. and Mei, N. (1983) Vagal mechanoreceptors located in the lower oesophageal sphincter of the cat. J. Physiol. (Lond.), 36: 487–498.

Collier, H. O. J. and Schneider, C. (1972) Nociceptive response to prostaglandins and analgesic actions of aspirin and morphine. Nature New Biol., 236: 141–143.

Cottrell, D. F. and Iggo, A. (1984a) Tension receptors with vagal afferent fibres in the proximal duodenum and pyloric sphincter of sheep. J. Physiol. (Lond.), 354: 457–475.

Cottrell, D. F. and Iggo, A. (1984b) The responses of duodenal tension receptors in sheep to pentagastrin, cholecystokinin and some other drugs. J. Physiol. (Lond.), 354: 477–495.

Cottrell, D. F. and Iggo, A. (1984c) Mucosal enteroceptors with vagal afferent fibres in the proximal duodenum of sheep. J. Physiol. (Lond.), 354: 497–522.

Curtis, D. R. (1979) Pre- and postsynaptic action of GABA in the mammalian spinal cord. In P. Simon (Ed.), Advances in Pharmacology and Therapeutics, Vol. 2, Neuro-Transmitters, Pergamon Press, Oxford, pp. 281–298.

Daniel, E. E. (1968) Pharmacology of the gastrointestinal tract. In C. F. Code (Ed.), Handbook of Physiology, Section 6, Alimentary Canal, Vol. IV, Motility, American Physiological Society, Washington, D.C., pp. 2267–2324.

De Groat, W. C. and Simonds, W. (1976) Antagonism by picrotoxin of 5-hydroxytryptamine induced depolarization and excitation of the nodose ganglion of the cat. Neurosci. Abstr., 2: 780.

Delpierre, S., Grimaud, C. H., Jammes, Y. and Mei, N. (1981) Changes in activity of vagal bronchopulmonary C fibres by chemical and physical stimuli in the cat. J. Physiol. (Lond.), 316: 61–74.

Dichter, M. A. and Fischback, G. D. (1977) The action potential of chick dorsal root ganglion neurones maintained in cell culture. J. Physiol. (Lond.), 267: 281–298.

Douglas, W. W. and Ritchie, J. M. (1957) On excitation of non-medullated afferent fibres in the vagus and aortic nerves by pharmacological agents. J. Physiol. (Lond.), 138: 31–43.

Douglas, W. W. and Ritchie, J. M. (1960) The excitatory action of acetylcholine on cutaneous non-myelinated fibres. J. Physiol. (Lond.), 150: 501–514.

Evans, D. H. L. and Murray, J. G. (1954) Histological and functional studies on the fibre composition of the vagus nerve of the rabbit. J. Anat. (Lond.), 88: 320–337.

Falempin, M., Mei, N. and Rousseu, J. P. (1978) Vagal mechanoreceptors of the inferior thoracic oesophagus, the lower oesophageal spincter and the stomach in the sheep. Pflügers Arch., 373: 25–30.

Feldberg, W. and Toh, C. C. (1953) Distribution of 5-hydroxytryptamine (serotonin, enteramine) in the wall of the digestive tract. J. Physiol. (Lond.), 119: 352–362.

Fields, H. L., Emson, P. C., Leigh, B. K., Gillbert, R. F. T. and Iversen, L. L. (1980) Multiple opiate sites on primary afferent fibres. Nature, 284: 351–353.

Fjällbrant, N. and Iggo, A. (1961) The effect of histamine, 5-hydroxytryptamine and acetylcholine on cutaneous afferent fibres. J. Physiol. (Lond.), 156: 578–590.

Fock, S. and Mense, S. (1976) Excitatory effect of 5-hydroxytryptamine, histamine and potassium ions on muscular group IV afferent unit: a comparison with bradykinin. Brain Res., 105: 459–469.

Foreman, R. D., Schmidt, R. E. and Willis, W. D. (1979) Effects of mechanical and chemical stimulation of fine muscle afferents upon primate spinothalamic trace cells. J. Physiol. (Lond.), 286: 215–231.

Fowler, D., Weinreich, D. and Gree, R. (1984) A restricted population of vagal neurons have two component spike afterhyperpolarizations. Soc. Neurosci. Abstr., 10: 291.10.

Franz, M. and Mense, S. (1978) Muscle receptors with group IV afferent fibres responding to application of bradykinin. Brain Res., 92: 369–383.

Gallagher, J. P., Higashi, H. and Nishi, S. (1978) Characterization and ionic basis of GABA-induced depolarizations recorded in vitro from cat primary neurons. J. Physiol. (Lond.), 275: 263–282.

Gallego, R. and Eyzaguirre, C. (1978) Membrane and action potential characteristics of A and C nodose ganglion cells studies in whole ganglia and in tissue slices. J. Neurophysiol., 41: 1217–1232.

Harper, A. A. and Lawson, S. N. (1985a) Conduction velocity is related to morphological cell type in rat dorsal root ganglion neurones. J. Physiol. (Lond.), 359: 31–46.

Harper, A. A. and Lawson, S. N. (1985b) Electrical properties of rat dorsal root ganglion neurones with different peripheral nerve conduction velocities. J. Physiol. (Lond.), 359: 47–63.

Higashi, H. (1977) 5-Hydroxytryptamine receptors on visceral primary afferent neurones in the rabbit. Nature, 267: 448–450.

Higashi, H. (1980) Chemoreceptors of visceral primary afferent neurons in the rabbit. Biomedical Res., Suppl. 1: 98–101.

Higashi, H. and Nishi, S. (1982a) 5-Hydroxytryptamine receptors of visceral primary afferent neurones on rabbit nodose ganglion. J. Physiol. (Lond.), 323: 543–567.

Higashi, H. and Nishi, S. (1982b) Effect of barbiturates on the GABA receptor of cat primary afferent neurones. J. Physiol. (Lond.), 332: 299–314.

Higashi, H., Shinnick-Gallagher, P. and Gallagher, J. P. (1982a) Facilitatory and inhibitory effects of morphine on Ca^{++} dependent responses in visceral afferent neurons. Brain Res., 251: 186–191.

Higashi, H., Ueda, N., Nishi, S., Gallagher, J. P. and Shinnick-Gallagher, P. (1982b) Chemoreceptors for serotonin (5-HT), bradykinin (BK), histamine (H) and γ-aminobutyric acid (GABA) on rabbit visceral afferent neurons. Brain Res. Bull., 8: 23–32.

Higashi, H., Morita, K. and North, R. A. (1984) Calcium-dependent after-potentials in visceral afferent neurones of the rabbit. J. Physiol. (Lond.), 355: 479–492.

Hiler, J. M., Simon, E. J., Crain, S. M. and Peterson, E. J. (1978) Opiate receptors in cultures of fetal mouse dorsal root ganglion (DRG) and spinal cord: predominance in DRG neurites. Brain Res., 145: 396–400.

Hiss, E. and Mense, S. (1976) Evidence for existence of different receptor sites for algesic agents at the endings of muscular group IV afferent units. Pflügers Arch., 362: 141–146.

Hökfelt, T., Kewerth, J. O., Nilsson, G. and Pernow, B. (1975) Experimental immunohistochemical studies on the localisation and distribution of substance P in cat primary sensory neurones. Brain Res., 100: 235–252.

Ito, H. (1982) Evidence for initiation of calcium spikes in C-cells of rabbit nodose ganglion. Pflügers Arch., 394: 106–112.

Jaffe, R. A. and Sampson, S. R. (1976) Analysis of passive and active electrophysiologic properties of neurons in mammalian nodose ganglia maintained in vitro. J. Neurophysiol., 39: 802–815.

Juan, H. and Lembeck, F. (1974) Action of peptide and other algesic agents on paravascular pain receptors of the isolated rabbit ear. Naunyn-Schmiedeberg's Arch. Pharmacol., 283: 151–164.

Katz, D. M. and Karten, H. J. (1980) Substance P in the vagal sensory ganglia: location in cell bodies and pericellular arborizations. J. Comp. Neurol., 193: 549–564.

Keele, C. A., Neil, E. and Joels, N. (1982) Samson Wright's Applied Physiology, 13th Edn., Oxford University Press, New York, Toronto, pp. 394–403.

Kostyuk, P. G. and Krishtal, O. A. (1977) Effect of calcium and calcium chelating agents on the inward and outward current in the membrane of mollusc neurones. J. Physiol. (Lond.), 270: 569–580.

Krishtal, O. A., Marchenko, S. M. and Pidoplichko, V. I. (1983) Receptor for ATP in the membrane of mammalian sensory neurones. Neurosci. Lett., 35: 41–45.

Kumazawa, T. and Mizumura, K. (1977) Thin-fibre receptors responding to mechanical, chemical and thermal stimulation in the skeletal muscle of the dog. J. Physiol. (Lond.), 273: 197–199.

Kumazawa, T. and Mizumura, K. (1980) Chemical response of polymodal receptors of the scrotal contents in dogs. J. Physiol. (Lond.), 299: 219–231.

Lamotte, C., Pert, C. B. and Snyder, S. H. (1976) Opiate receptor binding in primate spinal cord: distribution and changes after dorsal root section. Brain Res., 112: 407–412.

Leek, B. F. (1972) Abdominal visceral receptors. In E. Neil (Ed.), Handbook of Sensory Physiology, Vol. 1, IV/1 Enteroceptors, Springer-Verlag, New York, pp. 114–160.

Lembeck, F. and Gamse, R. (1982) Substance P in peripheral sensory processes. In R. Porter and M. O'Connor (Eds.), Substance P in the Nervous System, Pitman, London, pp. 35–48.

Levy, R. A. (1977) The role of GABA in primary afferent depolarization. Prog. Neurobiol., 19: 211–267.

Lundberg, J., Hökfelt, T., Nilsson, G., Terenius, L., Rehfeld, J., Elde, R. and Said, S. (1978) Peptide neurons in the vagus, splanchnic and sciatic nerves. Acta Physiol. Scand., 104: 499–501.

Maire, J. C., Medilanski, J. and Straub, R. W. (1984) Release of adenosine, inosine and hydroxanthine from rabbit non-myelinated nerve fibres at rest and during activity. J. Physiol. (Lond.), 357: 67–77.

McMahon, S. B. (1984) Spinal mechanisms in somatic pain. In A. V. Holden and W. Winlow (Eds.), The Neurobiology of Pain, Manchester University Press, Manchester, pp. 160–178.

Mense, S. (1977) Nervous outflow from skeletal muscle following chemical noxious stimulation. J. Physiol. (Lond.), 267: 75–88.

Mense, S. (1982) Reduction of the bradykinin-induced activation of feline group III and in muscle receptors by acetylsalicylic acid. J. Physiol. (Lond.), 326: 269–283.

Mense, S. and Schmidt, R. F. (1974) Activation of group IV afferent units from muscle by algesic agents. Brain Res., 72: 305–310.

Morita, K. and Katayama, Y. (1984) Two types of acetylcholine receptors on the soma of primary afferent neurons. Brain Res., 290: 348–352.

Morita, K. and Katayama, Y. (1986) 5-Hydroxytryptamine effects on dorsal root ganglion neurones of the bullfrog. Brain Res., in press.

Morita, K., Katayama, Y., Akasu, T. and Koketsu, K. (1983a) Chemosensitivities of bullfrog spinal ganglion cells. J. Physiol. Soc. Jpn., 45(8.9): 423.

Morita, K., Hirai, K. and Katayama, Y. (1983b) Existence of Ca-sensitive K-current regulated by biogenic substances in bullfrog dorsal root ganglion cells. Proc. Int. Union Physiol. Soc., 15: 90.

Mudge, A. W., Leeman, S. E. and Fischback, D. (1979) Enkephalin inhibits release of substance P from sensory neurons in culture and decreases action potential duration. Proc. Natl. Acad. Sci. U.S.A., 76: 526–530.

Neto, F. R. (1978) The depolarizing action for 5-HT on mammalian non-myelinated nerve fibres. Eur. J. Pharmacol., 49: 351–356.

Nicholson, C., Ten Bruggencate, G., Stockle, H. and Steinberg, R. (1978) Calcium and postassium changes in extracellular microenvironment of cat cerebellar cortex. J. Neurophysiol., 41: 1026–1039.

Niijima, A. (1980) Effect of serotonin (5-HT) on the firing rate of afferent discharges recorded from the mesenteric nerves in the rat. Biomed. Res., Suppl. 1: 59–97.

Nishi, K. (1975) The action of 5-hydroxytryptamine on chemoreceptor discharges on the cat's carotid body. Br. J. Pharmacol., 55: 27–40.

Nishi, S., Minota, S. and Karczmar, A. G. (1974) Primary afferent neurons: the ionic mechanism of GABA-mediated depolarization. Neuropharmacology, 13: 215–220.

Paintal, A. S. (1963) Vagal afferent fibres. Ergebn. Physiolog., 52: 74–156.

Paintal, A. S. (1964) Effects of drugs on vertebrate mechanoreceptors. Pharmacol. Rev., 16: 341–380.

Sampson, S. R. and Jaffe, R. A. (1974) Excitatory effect of 5-hydroxytryptamine, veratridine and phenyldiguanide on sensory ganglion cells of the nodose ganglion of the cat. Life Sci., 15: 2157–2165.

Shefner, S. A., North, R. A. and Zukin, R. S. (1981) Opiate effects on rabbit vagus nerve: Electrophysiology and radioligand binding. Brain Res., 221: 109–116.

Simonds, W. F. and De Groat, W. C. (1980) Antagonism by picrotoxin of 5-hydroxytryptamine induced excitation of primary afferent neurons. Brain Res., 192: 592–597.

Stansfeld, C. E. and Wallis, D. I. (1983) Differences in tetrodotoxin (TTX)-sensitivity in group A- and C-cells of the nodose ganglion. J. Physiol. (Lond.), 341: 14–15p.

Stansfeld, C. E. and Wallis, D. I. (1984) Generation of an unusual depolarizing response in rabbit afferent neurones in the absence of divalent cations. J. Physiol. (Lond.), 352: 49–72.

Tokimasa, T., Morita, K. and North, R. A. (1981) Opiates and clonidine prolong Ca^{2+}-dependent after-hyperpolarization. Nature, 294: 162–163.

Wallis, D. I., Stansfeld, C. E. and Nash, H. L. (1982) Depolarizing responses recorded from nodose ganglion cells of the rabbit evoked by 5-hydroxytryptamine and other substances. Neuropharmacology, 21: 31–40.

Westfall, T. C. (1977) Local regulation of adrenergic neurotransmission. Physiol. Rev., 57: 660–728.

Williams, J. and Zieglgansberger (1981) Mature spinal ganglion cells are not sensitive to opiate receptor mediated action. Neurosci. Lett., 21: 211–216.

Yoshida, S., Matsuda, Y. and Samejima, A. (1978) Tetrodotoxin-resistant sodium and calcium components of action potentials in dorsal root ganglion cells of the adult mouse. J. Neurophysiol., 41: 1096–1106.

Zurier, R. B. (1974) Prostaglandins, inflammation and asthma. Arch. Intern. Med., 133: 101–110.

SECTION III

Central Nervous System Mechanisms of Visceral Sensation

F. Cervero and J. F.B. Morrison
Progress in Brain Research, Vol. 67

CHAPTER 11

Spinal cord projections and neuropeptides in visceral afferent neurons

William C. De Groat

Department of Pharmacology and Center for Neuroscience, Medical School, 518 Scaife Hall, University of Pittsburgh, Pittsburgh, PA 15261, U.S.A.

Introduction

During the past few years recently developed neuroanatomical tracing methods have yielded important advances in our knowledge of the organization of visceral afferent pathways at various levels of the spinal cord. Horseradish peroxidase tracing experiments have shown that afferent projections from a number of visceral organs exhibit a similar pattern of termination in the spinal cord and that this pattern is markedly different from that of somatic afferent neurons which innervate the skin. In addition, neurochemical studies in which axonal tracing techniques were combined with immunocytochemistry revealed that a large percentage of visceral afferent neurons exhibit neuropeptide immunoreactivity. These findings raised the possibility that neuropeptides may be important transmitters or neuromodulators in visceral afferent systems.

This chapter will review neuroanatomical experiments which have examined: (1) the segmental distribution and central projections of afferent neurons innervating the urogenital system, large intestine, heart and upper abdominal organs and (2) the identity of peptide neurotransmitters in visceral afferent pathways.

Sacral visceral afferent pathways

Afferent projections from the pelvic viscera to the sacral spinal cord were first studied with horseradish peroxidase (HRP) tracing techniques in the cat (De Groat et al., 1978, 1981; Morgan et al., 1981) and later examined in the rhesus monkey (Nadelhaft et al., 1983) and rat (Nadelhaft and Booth, 1984). In initial experiments the entire population of sacral afferent neurons was labeled by HRP applied to the pelvic nerve, a nerve which carries the afferent and efferent innervation to the urinary bladder, urethra, genital organs and the large intestine. In subsequent studies, afferent pathways to individual organs were also examined.

Pelvic nerve afferent pathways in the cat

In the cat the application of HRP to the pelvic nerve labels a large number of dorsal root ganglion cells (3000–5000) which are usually distributed in all three sacral dorsal root ganglia, with a peak concentration of cells in the S2 ganglion (Table I). The labeled cells are small to medium size (mean, 32 × 23 μm) and are distributed randomly throughout the ganglia ipsilateral to the labeled nerve. Visceral afferent axons in the dorsal roots and the spinal cord also label with HRP. At the dorsal root entry zone of the sacral segments these axons are located among the fine fibers surrounding the bundles of large myelinated axons and are continuous with labeled fibers in Lissauer's tract and the lateral dorsal column (Figs. 1 and 2). Labeled rostrocaudal axons are distributed throughout the mediolateral extent

TABLE I

Visceral afferent pathways in the cat

	Pelvic nerve	Urinary bladder	Large intestine	Renal nerve	Inferior cardiac nerve	Splanchnic nerve	Hypogastric nerve
Number of DRG cells							
Range	2965–5145	800–1330	660–1130	141–880	41–490	1867–2878	167–1204
Mean	3676	1000	900	417	213	2415	692
Segmental distribution of DRG cells							
Range	S1–S3	S1–S3	S1–S3	T12–L4	C8–T9	T3–L1	T12–L5
Peak	S2	S2	S2	L2	T3	T8–T9	L4
Central distribution of afferent projections	L4–C × 7 (Nucleus gracilis)	L7–C × 1	L7–C × 2	T11–L6	C8–T9	T1–T13 (Nucleus gracilis and cuneatus)	T13–L7

See text for references. DRG, dorsal root ganglion.

of Lissauer's tract at the sacral level (Figs. 2 and 3) and extend in the medial half of the tract, several segments rostrally and caudally.

Collaterals from Lissauer's tract enter the sacral gray matter by two routes, which form a thin shell laterally and medially around the dorsal horn (Figs. 1 and 2). At the apex and on the lateral edge of the dorsal horn this shell of labeled afferents (approximately 70 μm wide) is present in lamina I, and a few fibers extend deeper into outer lamina II. Inner laminae II and laminae III–IV are not labeled. The wide band of afferents on the lateral edge of the dorsal horn is termed the lateral collateral pathway (LCP) of Lissauer's tract; whereas the narrower medial band (20 μm wide) is termed the medial collateral pathway (MCP) (Figs. 1 and 2) (Morgan et al., 1981).

Axons in the LCP, which extend ventrally from Lissauer's tract through lamina I into lateral laminae V–VII and X, exhibit four patterns of termination (Fig. 2). In some sections, axons end in lateral lamina V ("a" in Fig. 2A). In other sections, axons extend into medial lamina V and VII and the lower one-third of the dorsal gray commissure ("d" in Fig. 2B). Less frequently, labeled axons extend into dorsomedial lamina V ("c" in Fig. 2B) or ventrally into lateral lamina VII ("e" in Fig. 2B), the region of the sacral parasympathetic nucleus (Nadelhaft et al., 1980).

In serial transverse sections the intensity of labeling in the LCP exhibits considerable variation from section to section. Horizontal sections show that this variability is related to a periodic grouping of collateral bundles along the length of the spinal cord (Fig. 3E,F). The average distance between bundles (center to center) is approximately 215 μm, while the average bundle width is approximately 100 μm. Bundles of axons also extend from lamina I medially through lamina V and VII to the dorsal gray commissure (Fig. 3G).

The MCP consists of a thin band of axons which passes dorsoventrally along the medial edge of the dorsal horn into the region of the dorsal commissure, where the pathway expands into diffuse terminal fields on both sides of the midline (Figs. 1 and 2). Some axons in the MCP extend into lamina V, to overlap with the dorsomedial projections from the LCP (Fig. 2). Horizontal or parasagittal sections reveal that the labeled axons in the dorsal commissure are also organized in a periodic man-

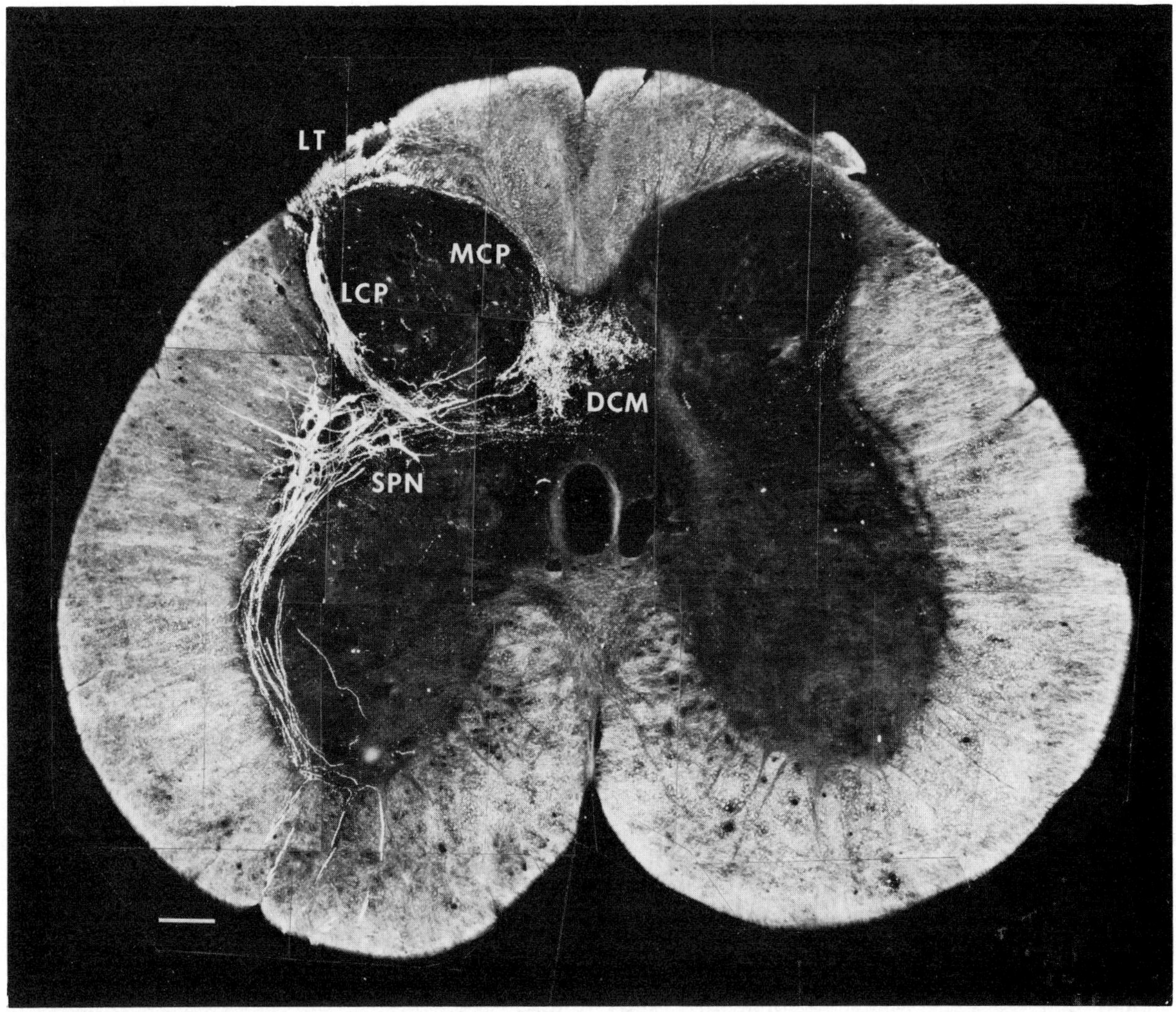

Fig. 1. Transverse section of S2 spinal cord showing labeling of primary afferents and preganglionic neurons after application of HRP to the left pelvic nerve in the cat. Pelvic afferents enter Lissauer's tract (LT). Afferent collaterals enter lamina I and extend laterally in a large bundle, the lateral collateral pathway (LCP), into the area of the sacral parasympathetic nucleus (SPN). Collaterals also extend medially in a smaller group, the medial collateral pathway (MCP), into the dorsal gray commissure (DCM), where they expand into a large terminal field ipsilaterally and contralaterally. Small numbers of afferents are also present in contralateral laminae I and V. This photomicrograph was made using darkfield illumination with polarized light. Bar represents 200 μm. From Morgan et al. (1981).

ner, with clusters of terminals occurring at intervals of approximately 200 μm in the rostrocaudal axis. The clusters are joined by rostrocaudal axons. This general pattern of afferent projections in the ipsilateral LCP and MCP also occurs in the caudal lumbar and coccygeal segments. In the sacral and coccygeal segments afferent projections are also present on the contralateral side of the cord in lateral laminae I and V.

Sacral visceral afferent axons are also present in the ipsilateral dorsal columns, from C × 1 to the nucleus gracilis in the caudal medulla. In the sacral

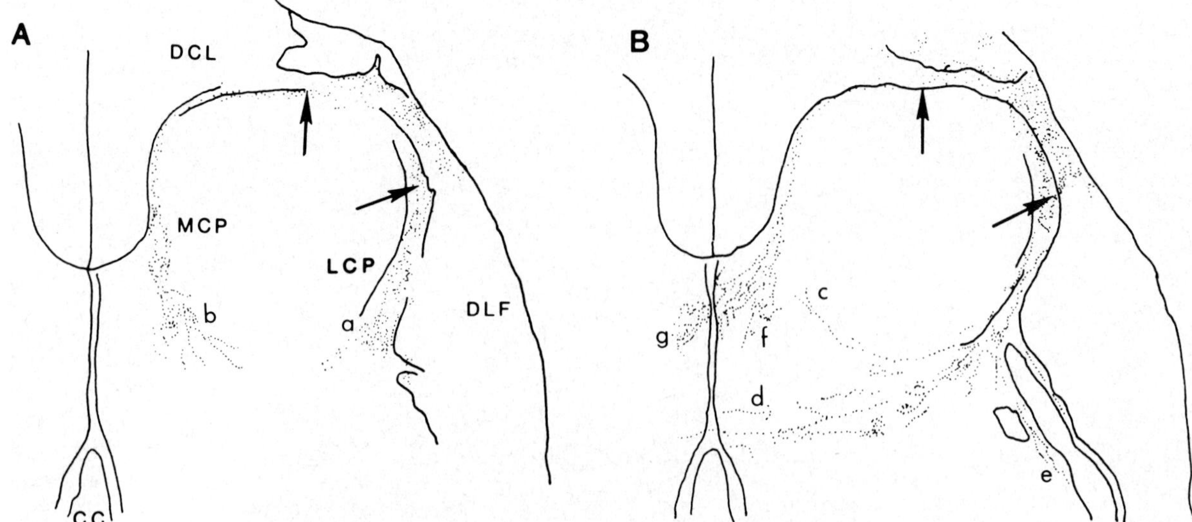

Fig. 2. Different patterns of pelvic nerve afferent collaterals from Lissauer's tract in the S2 segment of the cat. Ventral roots were cut to eliminate efferent labeling. Camera lucida drawings are composed from seven individual sections. These patterns were observed consistently in all experiments in various combinations. They are shown in these configurations only to facilitate their description. The lateral collateral pathway (LCP) exhibited four patterns (a, d, c, e). Many axons ended at the junction of laminae I and V (a), while others continued into lamina V to end in the lower third of the dorsal gray commissure (d). Less frequently, LCP axons ended dorsomedially in medial lamina V (c) or extended into lateral lamina VII (e). The medial collateral pathway (MCP) exhibited three patterns (b, f, g). The most common were the ipsilateral (f) and the contralateral (g) terminal fields in the upper two-thirds of the dorsal gray commissure. Less frequently, axons extended laterally into medial lamina V (b). Arrows show boundaries of Lissauer's tract. DLF, dorsolateral funiculus; DCL, dorsal column, CC, central canal. From Morgan et al. (1981).

segments labeled axons are located throughout the lateral dorsal columns, whereas at more rostral levels (L5–L7) the axons are situated along the posterior and medial borders of the dorsal columns. In lumbar and coccygeal segments collaterals from dorsal column axons extend into the MCP, the dorsal gray commissure and medial lamina V of the dorsal horn.

A small number of labeled axons travel rostrocaudally in the dorsolateral funiculus lateral to Lissauer's tract and the LCP. Fibers extend from these axons into the LCP. Small numbers of labeled ax-

---

→

Fig. 3. The periodic appearance of the lateral collateral pathway from Lissauer's tract (LT) in horizontal sections at various depths of S1 spinal cord. A, B, C, sections near the apex of the dorsal horn through Lissauer's tract. D, E, sections through the middle of the dorsal horn. F, G, sections at the base of the dorsal horn near the junction between laminae I and V. Lateral is toward the top and rostral is to the right of each picture. A, rostrocaudal axons in Lissauer's tract (LT) give off transverse collaterals which form terminal fields (arrows) in lamina I. B, outer lamina I at either end of the section shows terminal fields (arrows) while the center is deeper in lamina I (I) and has fewer terminals. C, Lissauer's tract and lamina I are both densely labeled at this level. D and E, development of discrete bundles of axons in lateral lamina I. Arrow points to a rostrocaudal axon running between groups. F, discrete bundles of axons just dorsal to lamina V. They are spaced at an average distance of 216 μm center to center. Arrow points to a rostrocaudal axon which was traced for 600 μm in tissue beyond that shown in the photomicrograph. G, the bundles of labeled axons have become smaller as they extend medially through lamina V. DLF, dorsolateral funiculus, Bar represents 200 μm. From Morgan et al. (1981).

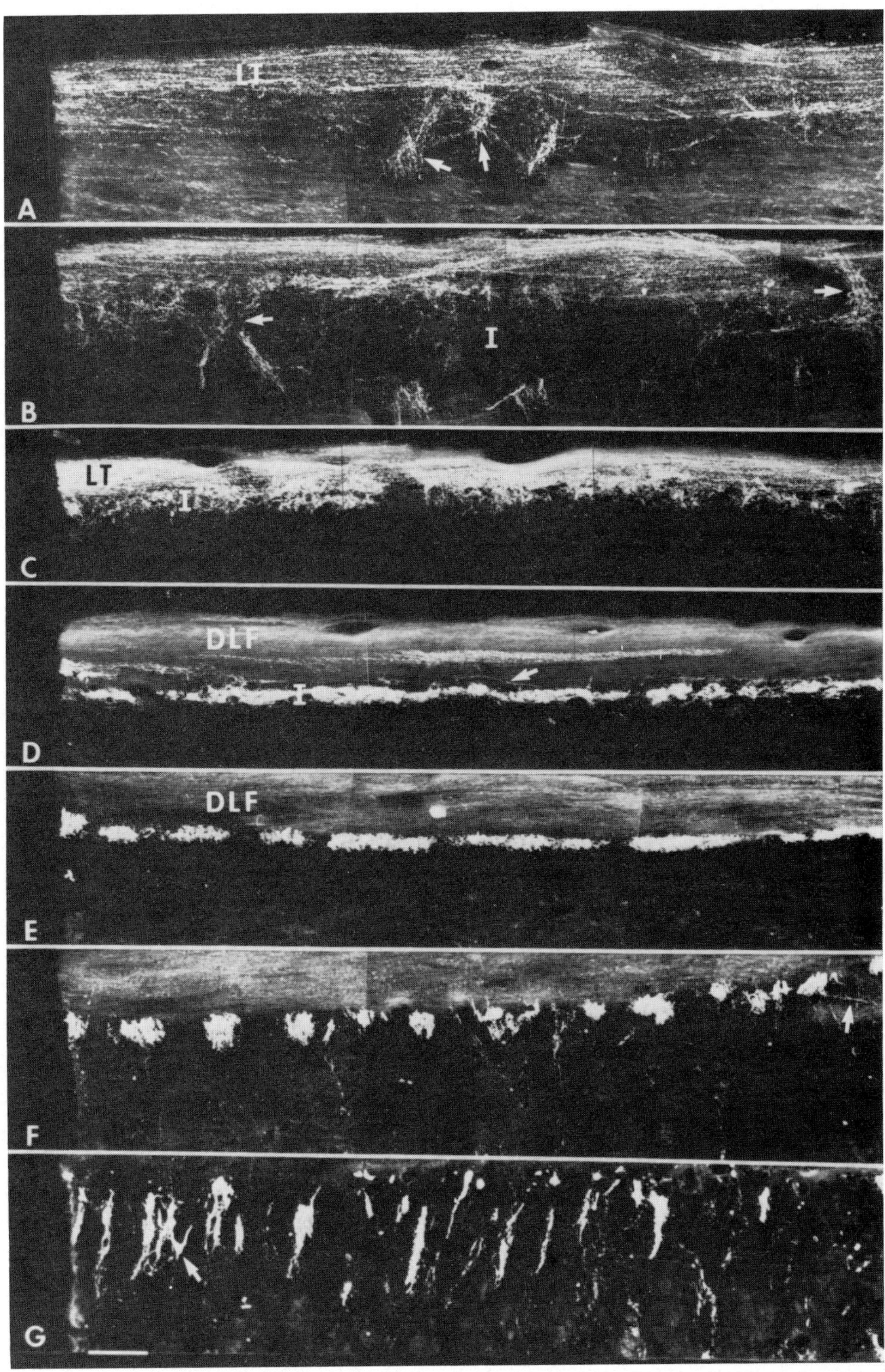

LT
A
B
I
LT
I
C
DLF
I
D
DLF
E
F
G

ons are present in the substantia gelatinosa centralis around the central canal. Some of these axons travel rostrocaudally and send collaterals into other areas of lamina X.

Relatively few axons are present in the ventral horn. However, some of these are of interest since they branch dorsally away from the ventral roots, and therefore have been interpreted as possible ventral root afferents (Morgan et al., 1981).

Afferent projections from the urinary bladder, large intestine and uterine cervix of the cat

The contribution of afferent projections from individual pelvic organs to the LCP and MCP in the sacral spinal cord was also examined with HRP tracing techniques. Preliminary experiments (De Groat et al., 1981, 1986a; C. Morgan, I. Nadelhaft and W. C. De Groat, unpublished data; M. Kawatani and W. C. De Groat, unpublished data) indicate that afferent neurons innervating the urinary bladder (Fig. 4A), large intestine and the uterine cervix project to Lissauer's tract and to lamina I of the sacral dorsal horn in a manner similar to that described above for the general population of afferents in the pelvic nerve. However, the relative density of afferent projections to the LCP and MCP varies according to the organ. Projections to the LCP are prominent for all three afferent pathways, whereas projections to the MCP and dorsal gray commissure are relatively weak for colon afferents in comparison to bladder and uterine afferents and the general population of afferents in the pelvic nerve.

Injections of HRP into the region of the distal urethra-external urethral sphincter also produce central afferent labeling in the LCP and MCP (Fig. 4B) (De Groat et al., 1986a). However, it is not known whether this labeling reflects HRP transported by afferent pathways in the pelvic nerve or the pudendal nerve, which provides an innervation to striated sphincter muscles. Pudendal nerve afferent neurons in the cat (Morgan et al., 1980; Thor et al., 1982, 1986; Ueyama et al., 1984) and monkey (Roppolo et al., 1985; Ueyama et al., 1985) project into the region of the LCP and MCP of the sacral spinal cord but also have a very extensive input into the deeper laminae (II–V) on the medial side of the dorsal horn. The difference between visceral and somatic afferent pathways will be discussed in more detail in a later section.

The relative numbers, segmental distribution and possible overlap of afferent neurons innervating the bladder and large intestine were also analyzed in dye tracing experiments where the afferent innervation to each organ was labeled with a different dye (Fast Blue or Diamidino Yellow). It was shown that similar numbers of dorsal root ganglion cells, the majority of which were localized in the S2 dorsal root ganglion, innervate the bladder (average,

→

Fig. 4. Afferent pathways to the sacral spinal cord. A, camera lucida drawing of the central projections of bladder afferents in the sacral S2 dorsal horn of the cat. Afferent terminals were labeled by transganglionic transport of HRP from nerves on the surface of the bladder. Labeled axons were present in Lissauer's tract (LT), the lateral collateral pathway (LCP), the sacral parasympathetic nucleus (SPN) and the dorsal commissure (DCM). B, afferent projections in the S2 dorsal horn of the cat labeled by HRP injected into the external urethral sphincter. C, two photomicrographs of the same section through the S2 dorsal root ganglion, showing bladder afferent cells (C-1) labeled by Fast Blue injected into the bladder wall and several of these labeled cells containing VIP-immunoreactivity (C-2, arrows). Dye-labeled cells were blue when visualized with light at 340–380 nm excitation wavelength and VIP cells were green when visualized with light at 430–480 nm wavelength. D, the distribution of VIP-immunoreactivity (VIP-IR) in LT and LCP of the S2 segment of the cat spinal cord. E, VIP-IR in the sacral dorsal horn of the S3 segment of the human spinal cord. Large bundles of VIP axons are present in LT and smaller numbers of axons are present in lamina I on the lateral edge of the dorsal horn. F, co-localization of substance P-immunoreactivity and VIP-IR in sacral (S2) dorsal root ganglion cells of the cat. Substance P-immunoreactivity (F-1) stained with TRITC (red color, at 530–560 nm excitation wavelength); in F-2, the same section showing VIP-IR in two of the same ganglion cells (arrows) stained with FITC (green color, at 430–480 nm excitation wavelength). Calibration represents 250 μm in A and B, 50 μm in C, 300 μm in D, 220 μm in E and 60 μm in F. From De Groat et al. (1986a).

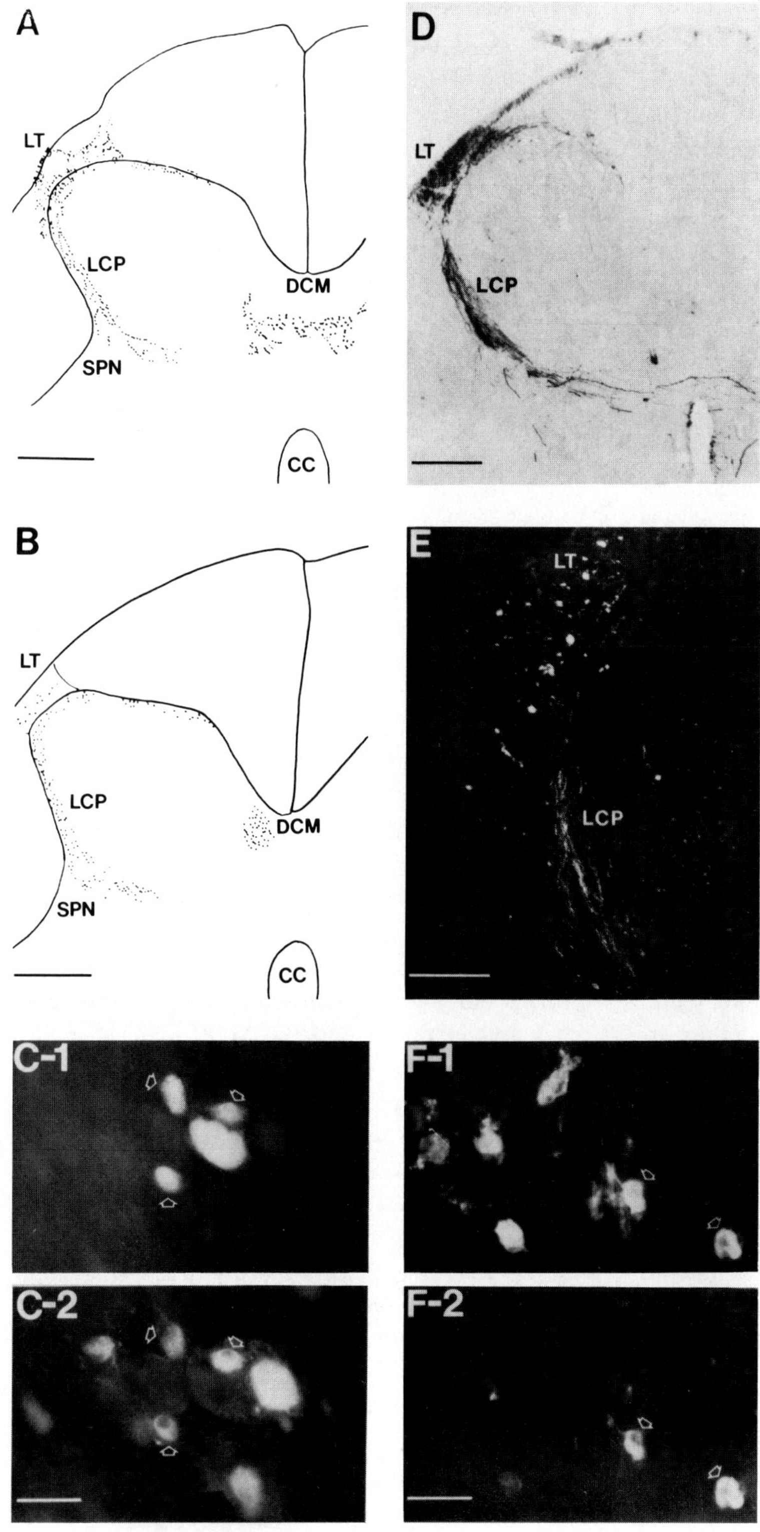
A
LT
LCP
DCM
SPN
CC
B
LT
LCP
DCM
SPN
CC
C-1
C-2
D
LT
LCP
E
LT
LCP
F-1
F-2

1000 cells) and large intestine (average, 900 cells) (Kawatani et al., 1985c). It was also noted that approximately 4–6% of this population of neurons were doubly labeled and presumably provide an innervation to both organs. Other investigators (Taylor and Pierau, 1982; Pierau et al., 1983) have reported that afferent neurons in the L6 dorsal root ganglion of the rat also give rise to dichotomizing fibers that enter separate peripheral nerves. The functional significance of afferent neurons with receptive fields in two adjacent organs is unknown.

Pelvic nerve afferent pathways in the monkey and rat

The central projections of pelvic nerve afferent neurons to the lumbosacral spinal cord of the rhesus monkey (Nadelhaft et al., 1983) and the rat (Nadelhaft and Booth, 1984) are, in general, very similar to those described above for the cat. In both species, visceral afferent axons distribute throughout Lissauer's tract and in thin bands on the lateral and medial edge of the dorsal horn. The LCP is considerably more prominent than the MCP and exhibits a periodic organization, with an average inter-period interval of 260 μm in the monkey and 100 μm in the rat. Axons in the LCP project directly into the sacral parasympathetic nucleus in both species. Deeper laminae (II–IV) of the dorsal horn do not receive afferent projections.

In the monkey, afferent axons from the LCP and MCP form terminal fields at several sites in the dorsal gray commissure: (1) bilaterally at the dorsal border, (2) along the midline and (3) a prominent field in the ventral one-third of the commissure. In the rat, terminal fields occur primarily in the dorsal half of the dorsal gray commissure. Another unusual feature in the rat is a small longitudinal bundle of afferent fibers located immediately ventral to the central canal.

In the rat the number of labeled afferent neurons in the lumbosacral dorsal root ganglia (approximately 1500) agrees well with the number of afferent axons identified in the pelvic nerve (Hulsebosch and Coggeshall, 1982). On the other hand, the number of labeled afferent neurons in the monkey (3000) and cat (3700) is considerably lower than the estimates of the number of afferent axons in the pelvic nerves of these species (monkey, 5,800: Schnitzlein et al., 1954; cat, 14,800: I. Nadelhaft, C. Morgan and W. C. De Groat, unpublished data, see Nadelhaft et al., 1980; Nadelhaft and Booth, 1984). It is possible therefore that visceral afferent neurons in the monkey and cat give rise to multiple axons in the pelvic nerve. The data of Langford and Coggeshall (1981) also suggest that sacral dorsal root ganglion cells in the rat give rise to multiple peripheral axons.

Comparison of visceral and somatic afferent projections to the sacral spinal cord

The functions of the pelvic viscera are closely linked with those of various somatic structures in the perineal region (e.g., urethral and anal sphincter muscles), many of which are innervated by the pudendal nerve (De Groat and Booth, 1984). Since the integration of visceral and somatic mechanisms is essential for the performance of excretory and sexual functions, an overlap of pelvic and pudendal nerve afferent pathways might be expected to occur at certain sites in the sacral spinal cord. This has been demonstrated in both the monkey and the cat (Roppolo et al., 1985; Thor et al., 1986: Ueyama et al., 1985). Pudendal afferent projections overlap with visceral afferents in: (1) the LCP in lateral lamina I and lamina V, (2) the MCP and (3) in the dorsal gray commissure (Fig. 5). Pudendal afferents also project to the intermediate laminae (II–IV) of the dorsal horn, which do not receive significant numbers of visceral afferents. These projections represent input from cutaneous afferents in the perineum (Brown and Fuchs, 1975; Brown, 1982) whereas the projections to the lateral marginal zone and lamina V are likely to represent in part input from deep structures, such as pelvic floor muscles (Craig and Mense, 1983) and urethra. These findings are consistent with electrophysiological studies in cats and monkeys which have revealed prominent convergence of visceral and somatic afferent inputs onto neurons in lamina V and the dorsal

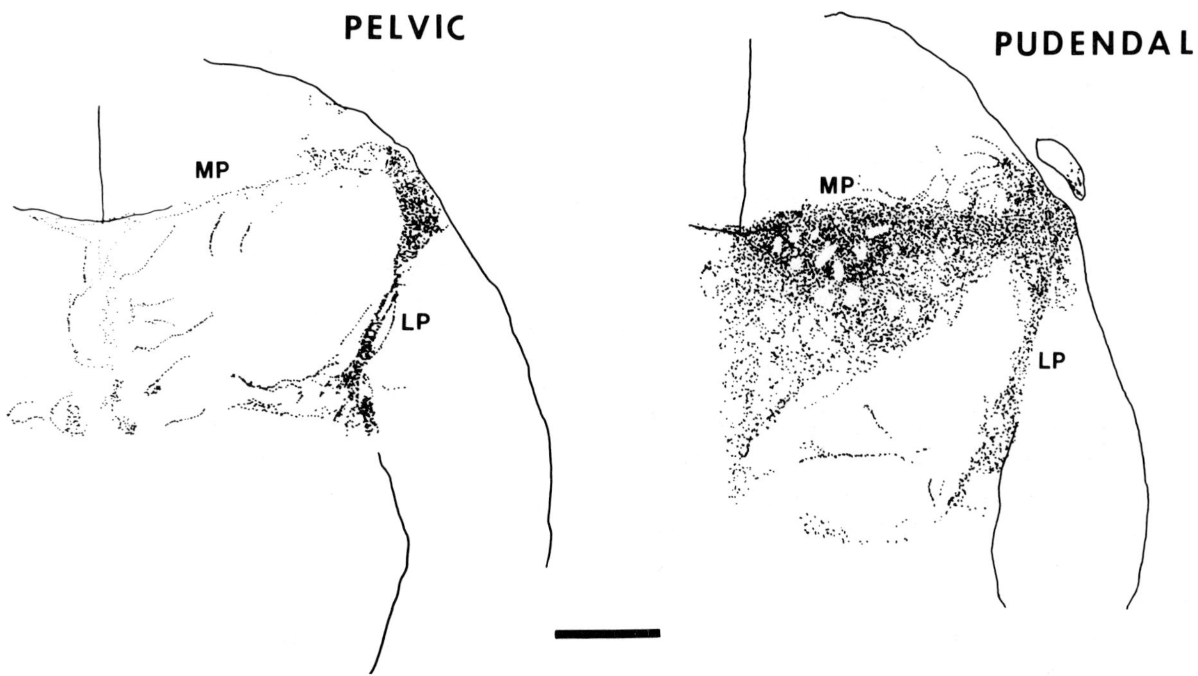

Fig. 5. Distribution of afferent fibers and terminals in the S1 segment of the spinal cord from two different monkeys. In one, HRP was applied to the pelvic nerve and in the other HRP was applied to the pudendal nerve. Note the similarity of the lateral projections (LP) and the difference in the distribution of the medial projections (MP) between the visceral and somatic nerves. Bar represents 400 μm. From Roppolo et al. (1985).

commissure of the lumbosacral spinal cord (De Groat et al., 1981; McMahon and Morrison, 1982; Honda, 1985). The firing patterns of many of these neurons suggest that they may have a role in autonomic reflex mechanisms as well as in sensory pathways (De Groat et al., 1981).

Neuropeptides in sacral visceral afferent pathways

Immunocytochemical studies have revealed a striking similarity between the distribution of visceral afferent projections in the sacral spinal cord and the distribution of certain peptidergic axons and varicosities (De Groat et al., 1983; Kawatani et al., 1983a, 1985b; Basbaum and Glazer, 1983; Honda et al., 1983; Gibson et al., 1984). Vasoactive intestinal polypeptide (VIP) is particularly interesting since it is localized in the cat sacral cord in much higher concentrations than in other spinal segments and since it is present in high densities in Lissauer's tract and the region of the LCP (Figs. 4D and 6). VIP axons are also localized in the lateral marginal zone of the human (Fig. 4E) (Kawatani et al., 1983b; Anand et al., 1983; De Groat et al., 1986a) and the monkey (Roppolo et al., 1983; La Motte and De Lanerolle, 1983; Gibson et al., 1984) sacral spinal cord. In the LCP of the cat, VIP-immunoreactivity is associated wth bundles of axons and varicosities with a similar appearance (Fig. 6) to visceral afferent projections in this region. The bundles are spaced at approximately 210-μm intervals along the length of the spinal cord. VIP axons extend from the LCP to the ventral third of the dorsal gray commissure and cross the midline in a manner similar to the pattern "d" for visceral af-

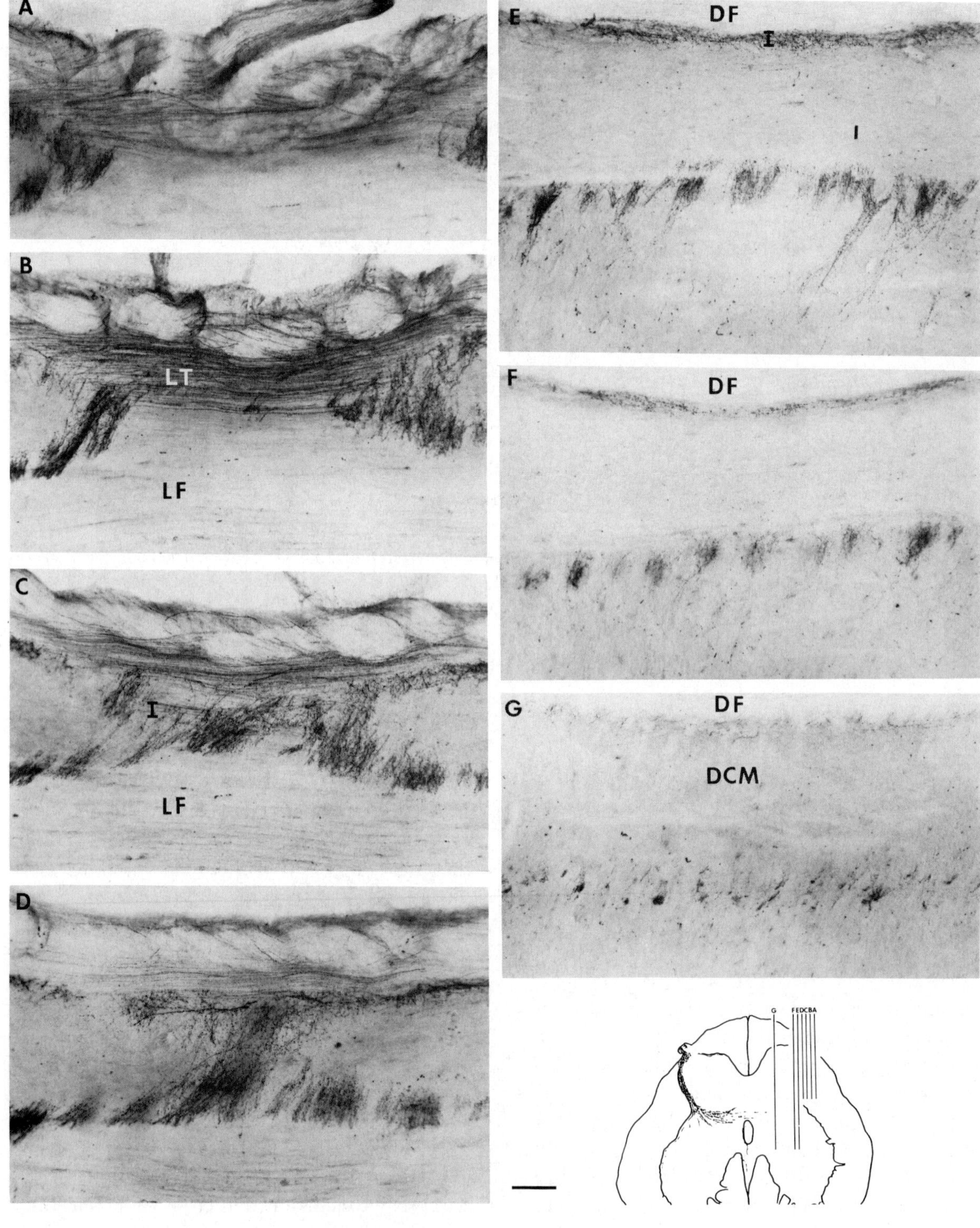
A
B
LT
LF
C
I
LF
D
E
DF
I
I
F
DF
G
DF
DCM
G
FEDCBA

ferents described in Fig. 2B. Rethelyi et al. (1979) and Matsushita and Tanami (1983) identified a similar primary afferent pathway using autoradiographic and HRP techniques, respectively, to label an entire sacral dorsal root.

VIP is present in small dorsal root ganglion cells and VIP varicosities in the sacral spinal cord are eliminated by transection of the sacral dorsal roots in the cat (Kawatani et al., 1983a, 1985b; Honda et al., 1983). These findings coupled with the very localized distribution of VIP axons in the spinal cord prompted the speculation that VIP might be present in sacral visceral afferent neurons (Kawatani et al., 1983a; Basbaum and Glazer, 1983; De Groat et al., 1983; Honda et al., 1983).

This has been confirmed with the use of axonal tracing techniques in combination with immunocytochemistry (De Groat et al., 1983; Kawatani et al., 1983a, 1984, 1985c, 1986). In the cat the entire population of visceral afferent neurons was labeled by applying fluorescent dyes to the pelvic nerve. After sufficient time for axonal transport of the dyes to the sacral dorsal root ganglia, colchicine solution was injected into the ganglia to block axoplasmic transport and to increase the levels of peptides. This technique is considerably more effective than topical or intrathecal administration of colchicine in increasing the immunoreactivity of certain peptides (e.g., VIP, enkephalins and cholecystokinin).

A large percentage of pelvic nerve afferent neurons contain neuropeptides. VIP is the most common peptide (Fig. 4C), occurring in nearly one-half of sacral visceral afferent neurons (mean, 48%; range, 20–60%), followed by leucine enkephalin (30%), substance P (25%), cholecystokinin (29%) and methionine enkephalin (20%) (Kawatani et al., 1984, 1985d). Somatostatin is present in only a small percentage (0.5–2%) of these neurons.

Peptides are present in a considerably higher percentage of sacral visceral neurons than of somatic afferent neurons sending axons into the pudendal nerve (Kawatani et al., 1985d). For example, the sum of the percentages of pelvic nerve afferent neurons containing individual peptides exceeds 100% (approximately 140%), whereas only 72% of pudendal afferent neurons contain peptides. The difference is most striking for VIP, which is present in 42% of visceral afferents compared to only 10% of pudendal afferents. Substance P and leucine enkephalin, on the other hand, are present in similar percentages (21–30%) of these two types of afferent neurons. The significance of the high percentage of visceral afferent neurons containing neuropeptides will be discussed below.

Electron microscopic immunocytochemical studies of the cat sacral spinal cord and dorsal roots indicate that VIP is localized exclusively in unmyelinated afferent axons (Honda et al., 1983; Morgan and O'Hara, 1984). In lateral laminae I and V, VIP-immunoreactivity is associated with large (1–4 μm) vesicle-filled varicosities which sometimes exhibit asymmetrical synaptic specializations in contact with dendrites or somata. The enlargements contained large granular as well as small, agranular, round synaptic vesicles. Thus, VIPergic pathways represent C-fiber afferents which make synaptic connections in the LCP.

Since VIP axons in this region originate exclu-

←

Fig. 6. Sagittal sections showing the VIP distribution in the S1 segment of the spinal cord. Dorsal edge is at the top of each photomicrograph and rostral is to the left. A, VIP-immunoreactivity (VIP-IR) in dorsal rootlets, Lissauer's tract and lamina I. B, rostrocaudal bundles of VIP axons in Lissauer's tract (LT) and lamina I. Dorsoventral VIP fibers in lamina I. C, dorsoventral VIP fibers start to form discrete bundles. Some VIP axons pass dorsoventrally in lamina I(I) from rostrocaudal bundles in Lissauer's tract. D, discrete bundles of VIP axons in the ventral part of lateral lamina I. VIP-IR is not present in inner laminae II and III. E and F, periodic appearance of VIP-IR at the junction between lateral laminae I and V. Ventral projections of VIP axons end abruptly in ventral lamina V. A few VIP fibers extend into lamina VII (bottom) and are present in the medial collateral pathway in lamina I (top of photomicrograph). G, VIP-IR in lateral collateral pathway breaks up into individual fibers or small bundles with a lateromedial orientation (bottom of the photomicrograph), VIP-IR on the medial side of the dorsal horn (medial collateral pathway, top of photomicrograph). DCM, dorsal commissure; DF, dorsal funiculus; LF, lateral funiculus. Calibration bar represents 200 μm. From Kawatani et al. (1985b).

sively in the dorsal root ganglia, VIP-immunoreactivity is a useful marker for unmyelinated afferent projections to the spinal cord. Substance P is also thought to be present, primarily in small-diameter afferents. However, it is noteworthy that the distributions of VIP- and substance P-containing varicosities in the sacral spinal cord are not identical. For example, in the sacral segments of the cat, substance P is distributed more uniformly around the dorsal horn in lamina I, and in deeper laminae, whereas VIP is localized primarily to the region of the LCP. Furthermore, substance P fibers are distributed to the dorsal portion of the dorsal gray commissure, whereas VIP fibers are distributed to the ventral portion of the commissure (Kawatani et al., 1985b). These findings indicate that the two peptides are contained, at least in part, in different populations of neurons, although, as described below, they are co-localized in many dorsal root ganglion cells.

Combined axonal tracing and immunocytochemical experiments revealed that VIP and substance P are also present, as expected, in a considerable percentage of sacral afferent neurons innervating the urinary bladder and large intestine of the cat (Kawatani et al., 1985c; De Groat et al., 1986a). VIP was identified in 25 and 14%, respectively, of sacral dorsal root ganglion cells labeled by dyes injected into the bladder and large intestine, whereas substance P was detected in 22 and 18%, respectively, of bladder and intestinal afferent neurons. Substance P was also identified in lumbosacral afferent neurons innervating the bladder of the rat (Sharkey et al., 1983). Pharmacological studies in the rat (Maggi et al., 1984; Holzer-Petsche and Lembeck, 1985) suggest that substance P is an excitatory transmitter in the afferent limb of the micturition reflex.

The large percentage (140%) of sacral visceral afferent neurons exhibiting neuropeptide-immunoreactivity suggests that more than one peptide may be present in these neurons. This was confirmed using double staining immunocytochemical techniques, where two peptides could be demonstrated on the same tissue section using antisera linked to different fluorochromes (De Groat et al., 1985). Co-localization in unidentified sacral dorsal root ganglion cells was demonstrated for a number of peptides. For example, 59% of VIP-containing neurons also exhibited substance P immunoreactivity (Fig. 4F), whereas approximately 24% of substance P-containing neurons exhibited VIP-immunoreactivity. Leucine-enkephalin neurons exhibited substance P (61%), VIP (48%) and cholecystokinin (14%) but not somatostatin immunoreactivity. Sacral afferent neurons innervating the bladder and large intestine of the cat exhibited similar patterns of peptide co-localization (Kawatani et al., 1985c).

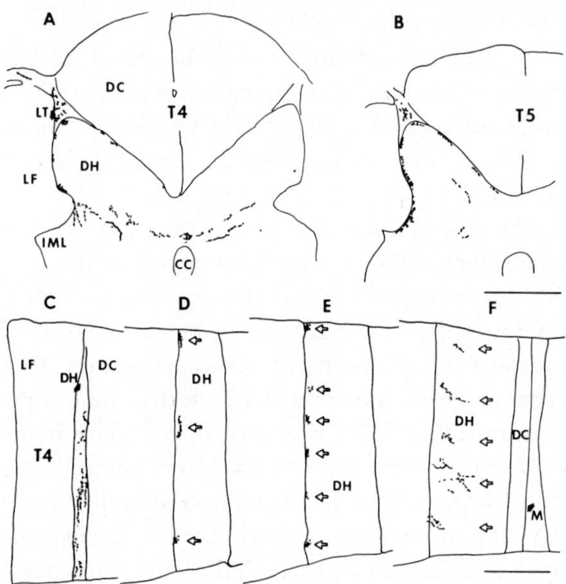

Fig. 7. Camera lucida drawings of projections of cardiac sympathetic afferents to the spinal cord of kitten. In A and B, data are included from five transverse sections of the spinal cord at T4 and T5, respectively. Afferent cardiac sympathetic nerve fibers and collaterals were labeled in Lissauer's tract (LT), along the lateral and medial margins of the dorsal horn (DH), and in laminae I, V, and VII. Some afferent labeling was also observed in laminae V and VII of the contralateral spinal cord. In B, a small group of cardiac afferents could be followed to the vicinity of the sympathetic preganglionic nucleus intermediolateralis (IML). C–F are horizontal serial step sections at T4. Cardiac afferents typically grouped into small bundles (open arrows) along the outer edge of the dorsal horn. These afferents projected across lamina V in a periodic fashion (F). CC, central canal; IML, intermediolateral nucleus; LF, lateral funiculus; M, midline. Calibration is 500 μm. From Kuo et al. (1984a).

Co-localization of peptides has also been reported in lumbosacral dorsal root ganglia of the cat (Snow et al., 1985) and in dorsal root ganglion cells in the rat (Fuxe et al., 1983; Wiesenfeld-Hallin et al., 1984; Dalsgaard et al., 1982a; Tuchscherer and Seybold, 1985) and guinea pig (Gibbins et al., 1985).

Although the significance of peptide co-localization in visceral afferent neurons is uncertain, these observations raise the possibility that several peptides may be released by the same afferent neuron. In this regard, Lowe et al. (1984) and De Groat et al. (1986b) have speculated that enkephalins contained in primary afferent pathways and co-localized with substance P or VIP may be involved in feedback inhibitory mechanisms at primary afferent terminals. In support of this speculation, it has been shown that: (1) opiate receptors are present on afferent terminals (La Motte et al., 1976), (2) exogenous enkephalins or opiate drugs depress the release of substance P from afferent terminals (Jessel and Iversen, 1977; Yaksh et al., 1980) and (3) enkephalins are released from the spinal cord into the cerebrospinal fluid by stimulation of afferent axons in peripheral nerves (Yaksh and Elde, 1981). Thus, it is possible that endogenously released enkephalins may originate in part from primary afferent terminals and act in an autoinhibitory manner at those terminals to depress the release of excitatory transmitters (VIP, substance P) with which they coexist.

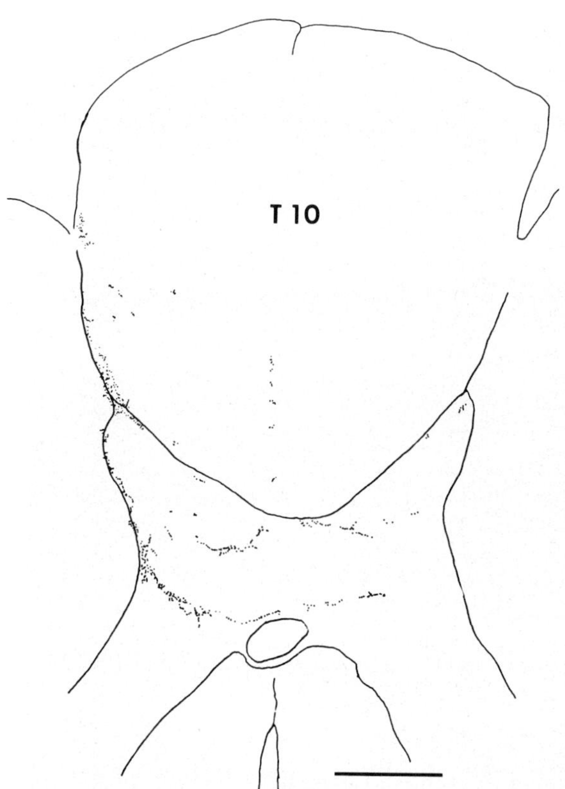

Fig. 8. A camera lucida drawing (from five transverse sections) of the distribution of splanchnic afferent projections to spinal segment T10. The ventral root of this segment was transected in this animal prior to exposing the central cut end of the splanchnic nerve to HRP. The ventral rhizotomy prevented the labeling of splanchnic sympathetic preganglionic neurons and their dendritic arbors, thereby allowing an unobstructed view of the intraspinal distribution of splanchnic afferents. The lateral pathway projected to laminae V and VII and some contralateral fibers were labeled. Calibration is 500 μm. From Kuo and De Groat (1985).

Thoracolumbar visceral afferent pathways

Visceral afferent projections to the thoracolumbar segments of the spinal cord have been studied most extensively in the cat, where pathways to the kidney (Kuo et al., 1983), heart (Kuo et al., 1984a;) splanchnic nerve (Cervero and Connell, 1984; Kuo and De Groat, 1985), hypogastric nerve (Morgan et al., 1986a) and lumbar colonic nerve (Morgan et al., 1986b) were analyzed with HRP tracing techniques. Renal and hypogastric nerve afferent pathways were also examined in the rat (Neuhuber, 1982; Ciriello and Calaresu, 1983).

In general, the pattern of termination of visceral afferent neurons in the thoracolumbar spinal cord is very similar to the termination of pelvic nerve afferent pathways in the sacral spinal cord (Figs. 7 and 8). Afferents are distributed most prominently in: (1) Lissauer's tract, (2) in a thin shell laterally and medially around the dorsal horn and (3) in laminae V–VII and in lamina X around the central canal. Some afferents also project rostrally in the dorsal columns to the dorsal column nuclei (Figs. 9 and 10).

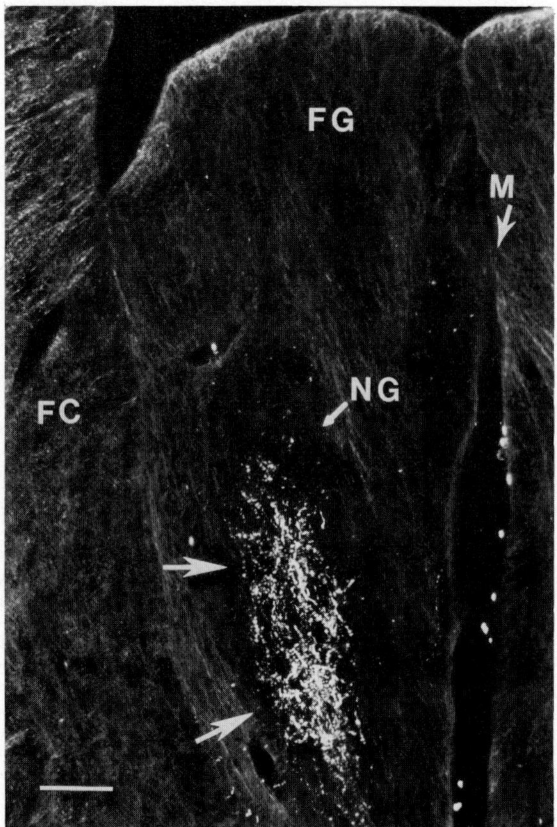

Fig. 9. A high-power, darkfield photomicrograph showing in the coronal plane of the medulla a splanchnic afferent terminal field (large arrows) located in the ipsilateral nucleus gracilis (NG) at a level below the obex. Afferent axons (not shown) were located in a ventrolateral position next to the terminal projection, which occupied the ventral two-thirds of the nucleus. Note that the fasciculus gracilis (FG) dorsal to the gracile nucleus was totally devoid of HRP labeling. FC, fasciculus cuneatus; M, midline. Calibration is 100 μm. From Kuo and De Groat (1985).

Renal and cardiac afferent pathways in the cat

The central projections of renal and cardiac afferent neurons were studied primarily by applying HRP to the renal and inferior cardiac nerves in young kittens (1–10 weeks of age), since in adult cats the central projections do not label or are poorly labeled (Kuo et al., 1983, 1984a). The kidney and heart are innervated by a relatively small number of afferent neurons (i.e., 200–400, Table I) which are distributed across a number of spinal segments: T12–L4 for the kidney (Kuo et al., 1983) and C8–T9 for the heart (Oldfield and McLachlan, 1978; Kuo et al., 1984a; Lee et al., 1984). Labeled dorsal root ganglion cells are detected primarily ipsilateral to the site of HRP application; however, a small percentage (6.8%) of renal afferent neurons are also detected in the contralateral dorsal root ganglia. The density of afferent labeling in the spinal cord generally parallels the segmental distribution of labeled afferent neurons in the dorsal root ganglia. Segments L1–L3 receive the densest input from the kidney, whereas T2–T6 exhibit the most prominent input from the heart (Fig. 7). Labeled axons in Lissauer's tract extend rostral (to T11) and caudal (to L6) from the segments where renal afferent axons enter the spinal cord.

A major projection of labeled afferents from Lissauer's tract to the gray matter occurs along the lateral margin of the dorsal horn (Fig. 7). This projection consists of small bundles of axons ((100–300) × (20–30) μm) passing ventrally through lamina I to lateral lamina V. The distance between

→

Fig. 10. Camera lucida drawings (A–C) of splanchnic afferents and terminals in the lower part of the nucleus gracilis (NG), below the obex. Each drawing was made from a horizontal section of the caudal medulla and its position was depicted in the inset drawing in D. (A–C), the lower edge of these drawings corresponds to the rostral end of C1 and the upper edge to the caudal medulla below the obex. Note that splanchnic afferents were located adjacent to the midline in the fasciculus gracilis (FG) in C1. Upon approaching the nucleus gracilis, these axons shifted ventrolaterally and gave off large nests of collateral terminals to the ventral gracile nucleus (arrows). In addition, some splanchnic afferents sent collaterals across the fasciculus gracilis to the medial edge of the nucleus cuneatus (NC). These collaterals formed small bundles, which presumably terminated in the cuneate nucleus. D, a darkfield photomicrograph showing in a horizontal plane a terminal field of splanchnic afferents (large arrows) in the gracile nucleus below the obex. Splanchnic axons (small arrows) could be seen lateral to the patch of collateral terminals. M, midline. Calibration is 500 μm for A–C and 200 μm in D. From Kuo and De Groat (1985).

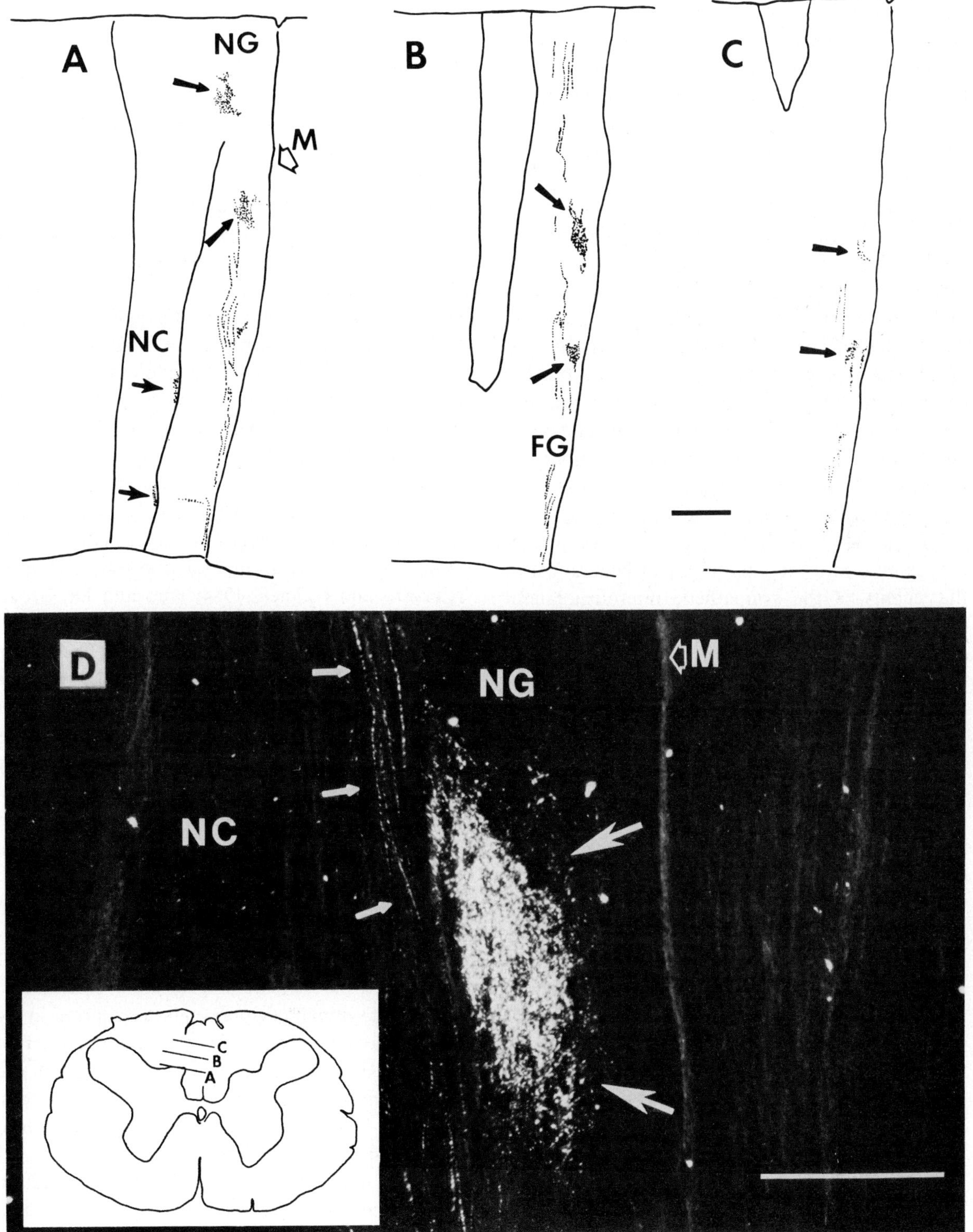
A
NG
M
NC
B
FG
C
D
NG
M
NC
C
B
A

bundles varies between 150 and 700 μm. At the base of the dorsal horn the bundles divide into two groups. One group, consisting of the majority of fibers, turns medially and disperses heavily in the gray matter of the lateral reticulated area. In the lumbar spinal cord this component passes further medially and splits into a dorsal and a ventral projection. The dorsal projection passes over the dorsal border of Clarke's nucleus, reaching the midline just beneath the dorsal columns. The ventral projection passes into laminae VI and VII and extends to the gray matter surrounding the dorsolateral region of the central canal. Clarke's nucleus is devoid of labeling. These two projections extend into the contralateral side of the spinal cord and form a similar pattern of terminal distribution in laminae I and V–VII. The mediolateral projections in lamina V–VII consist of bundles of axons spaced at 200–400 μm along the length of the cord (Fig. 7).

The second group of axons in the lateral projection extends into the lateral part of lamina VII in the vicinity of the sympathetic intermediolateral nucleus and more medially in the area of the nucleus intercalatus.

A medial projection from Lissauer's tract passes through lamina I into the medial region of lamina V. This is more prominent for renal afferents in the lumbar spinal cord. Collaterals from this projection converge at the base of the dorsal column with fibers from the lateral projection. Some afferents then descend along the midline to the dorsal margin of the central canal.

Splanchnic afferent pathways in the cat

The application of HRP to the greater splanchnic nerve of the cat labels on the average 2400 cells in the ipsilateral thoracic dorsal root ganglia. The labeled cells are distributed across eleven ganglia (T3–T13), with a peak distribution between T6–T11 (Kuo et al., 1981; Cervero and Connell, 1984; Cervero et al., 1984; Kuo and De Groat, 1985). Splanchnic afferent neurons represent a relatively small percentage (less than 7%) of the total population of neurons in the thoracic dorsal root ganglia (Cervero et al., 1984). The majority of splanchnic afferent neurons are small to medium size (25–40 μm); however, approximately 13% of the neurons (mean number, 319) have diameters ranging from 45 to 80 μm. These data are consistent with the observation that the splanchnic nerve has considerable numbers of unmyelinated and small myelinated afferent fibers (1500–3000) but relatively few large Aβ-fibers (120–350) (Kuo et al., 1982). The large cells could be afferents connected to pacinian corpuscles (Leek, 1977). Splanchnic afferent neurons are distributed evenly throughout a dorsal root ganglion, although they are sometimes arranged in small clusters of 3–5 neurons. Large splanchnic afferent neurons are preferentially located in the central portion of the ganglion, close to the main bundle of afferent axons (Cervero et al., 1984).

Within the thoracic spinal cord, splanchnic afferent axons project rostrocaudally in Lissauer's tract, from which collaterals pass into lamina I laterally and medially around the dorsal horn (Fig. 8) (Cervero and Connell, 1984; Kuo and De Groat, 1985). The lateral projection is grouped into small bundles of axons [(10–30) × (50–200)μm] occurring at intervals of 300–1000 μm along the length of the spinal cord. Upon reaching laminae V and VII these afferent bundles expand into terminal fields which extend medially as well as rostro-caudally within these laminae. Some of these afferents project to the dorsal gray commissure, to the region around the central canal and to laminae I and V in the contralateral side of the spinal cord (Fig. 8). The intermediate laminae of the dorsal horn (laminae II–IV) and the ventral horn do not receive inputs from the splanchnic nerve. Small groups of afferents from the lateral projection extend into clusters of sympathetic preganglionic neurons in the intermediolateral nucleus at the lateral border of lamina VII. These afferents also pass through the dorsal dendritic arbor of the preganglionic cells. Afferents in these regions of the gray matter also occur in spinal segments where the dorsal and ventral roots were transected prior to HRP application to the splanchnic nerve (Kuo and De Groat, 1985). This demonstrates a strong intersegmental projection of splanchnic afferents from adjacent segments.

Medial projections of splanchnic afferents from the dorsal root entry zone extend into lamina I and also into the ipsilateral dorsal column (Kuo and De Groat, 1985). The labeled fibers in the dorsal column are relatively sparse caudal to T12. However, at midthoracic levels the splanchnic afferents are very prominent and form a vertical column 400–600 μm in height and 80–120 μm in width near the midline. The tract shifts dorsally as it projects from thoracic to cervical levels. At rostral cervical levels the labeled afferents are located in the upper one-third of the dorsal column adjacent to the midline at a depth between 500 and 1000 μm below the surface of the spinal cord. These fibers travel in the fasciculus gracilis, ventral and ventrolateral to the nucleus gracilis in the medulla, where they terminate in four or five clusters distributed along the rostrocaudal axis in the ventral part of the nucleus (Figs. 9 and 10). The location of splanchnic afferent terminals in the ventral portion of the nucleus is consistent with the reports of other investigators who have also identified proprioceptive afferent projections to the ventral part of the dorsal column nuclei (Nyberg and Blomqvist, 1982). The most intense labeling from the splanchnic nerve is located ipsilaterally in the middle and caudal two-thirds of the nucleus, below the level of the obex (Fig. 10). Three terminal clusters are usually present in this region. In horizontal sections the terminal fields range in size from $(400–800) \times (100–300)$ μm and are separated from one another by distances of 400–800 μm (Fig. 10). In transverse sections the length of dorsoventral axis of a terminal field varies from 100 to 600 μm. The volume of a terminal field, which ranges from 0.01 to 0.1 mm^3, is always larger and extends beyond the limits of the cell clusters revealed by Nissl stain in the middle and caudal parts of the nucleus (see Rustioni, 1973; Berkley, 1975). Splanchnic afferents in the dorsal column pathway also form three or four bundles of collaterals on the medial edge of the caudal cuneate nucleus. Weak labeling in the mid portion of the cuneate nucleus and in the dorsal commissural region ventral to the dorsal column nuclei is also present in some animals. Labeled afferents are not detected in the nucleus tractus solitarius or the spinocervical nucleus.

Hypogastric and lumbar colonic nerve afferent pathways in the cat

Afferent neurons sending axons into the hypogastric nerve are located in the dorsal root ganglia bilaterally from T12–L5, with the peak of the distribution in L4 (Oravitz et al., 1982; Baron et al., 1982; Morgan et al., 1986a; Kawatani et al., 1985a). On average, approximately 700 neurons project into the hypogastric nerve. Central projections of hypogastric nerve afferents are distributed most heavily in the medial half of Lissauer's tract, from which axon collaterals enter lamina I to form a thin shell around the dorsal horn. Axons on the lateral edge of the dorsal horn extend: (1) into and medially through lamina V to converge with axons in the medial collateral pathway dorsal to the Clarke's nucleus, (2) through lamina V–VII to the central canal and (3) into lateral lamina VII in the region of the sympathetic intermediolateral cell column. Axons in the lateral pathway occur in bundles, which are spaced on average 235–345 μm center to center.

The hypogastric nerve of the cat contains myelinated and unmyelinated afferent axons which innervate various organs in the pelvic region (Langley and Anderson, 1894; Harris, 1943). Despite the complexity of the nerve, it is interesting to note that the central afferent distribution is very similar to that of the lumbar colonic nerve (Morgan et al., 1986b), which innervates only the large intestine and is composed almost exclusively of unmyelinated afferent and sympathetic postganglionic axons (Harris, 1943). This observation, coupled with earlier studies on renal and cardiac afferent pathways, implies that small myelinated and unmyelinated visceral afferent fibers in the cat terminate in the same regions of the spinal cord and that afferent projections from various organs have similar distributions in the thoracolumbar segments. Other investigators have concluded that myelinated and unmyelinated afferents terminate in different regions of the dorsal horn (Ralston and Ralston, 1979; Gobel and Falls, 1979). The studies of visceral afferents do not support these conclusions.

Renal and hypogastric nerve afferent pathways in the rat

Renal afferent projections to the spinal cord of the rat have been labeled by transganglionic transport of HRP following application of the tracer material to the transected renal nerves or following injection into the kidney (Ciriello and Calaresu, 1983). Renal afferents are present in the ipsilateral dorsal root ganglia from T6–T13 and labeled afferent projections in the spinal cord are present in segments T7–L1. The distribution of afferents from the right kidney is shifted several segments rostral to those from the left kidney.

The central distribution of renal afferents in the rat is markedly different from the distribution of renal afferent projections in the cat or the distribution of other visceral afferent pathways in the rat (Neuhuber, 1982; Nadelhaft and Booth, 1984). Renal afferent axons in the rat are distributed throughout the medial aspect of Lissauer's tract and pass along the medial side of the dorsal horn toward the midline. Collaterals from this pathway terminate in the medial part of lamina I, throughout laminae III and IV and in the ipsilateral dorsal gray commissure. Some axons are also located in medial lamina V. Renal afferents do not project to the contralateral side of the spinal cord.

The central projections of hypogastric nerve and inferior mesenteric plexus afferents in the rat more closely resemble those in the cat (Neuhuber, 1982). Labeled dorsal root ganglion cells are located bilaterally from T11 to L2, with the majority at the L1–L2 level. Central projections of these visceral afferents which are most prominent in caudal T13–L2 segments are distributed throughout Lissauer's tract and in superficial laminae (laminae I and outer II) of the dorsal horn. Axons in inner lamina II are less dense and are more conspicuous on the medial side of the dorsal horn. Longitudinal bundles of afferent axons are also present: (1) in lamina X just ventral to the ependymal layer of the central canal and (2) in lateral extensions from Lissauer's tract into the dorsolateral funiculus and to the nucleus of the dorsolateral funiculus. In the sacral spinal cord of the rat these two areas also receive projections from pelvic nerve afferents (Nadelhaft and Booth, 1984). The longitudinal bundle ventral to the central canal is of particular interest since it includes a variety of peptidergic axons, e.g., VIP, substance P and cholecystokinin (Sasek et al., 1984), some of which appear to be collaterals of primary afferent axons. Labeled hypogastric afferent axons are also present in the ipsilateral nucleus gracilis, slightly rostral to the obex. Only a few labeled axons are present in laminae III, IV and V. In addition, unlike afferents in the cat, the hypogastric afferents in the rat do not project into the sympathetic preganglionic nucleus.

Neuropeptides in thoracolumbar visceral afferent neurons

The distribution of neuropeptides in thoracolumbar visceral afferent neurons of various species (cat, rat, guinea pig) has been studied with axonal tracing in combination with immunocytohemical techniques. In a sample of splanchnic afferent neurons in colchicine-treated T8–T11 dorsal root ganglia of the cat (Kawatani et al., 1985a), substance P and VIP were detected in greater than 60% of the cells, leucine enkephalin in 34%, cholecystokinin in 12% and somatostatin in 2% of the cells. Substance P and VIP were also present in a large percentage (approximately 40%) of hypogastric nerve afferent neurons in L2–L5 dorsal root ganglia of the cat. Leucine enkephalin and cholecystokinin were detected in greater than 20% of the cells, whereas somatostatin was not detected in these cells. In both populations of visceral afferent neurons peptides were associated with small to medium size cells less than 45 μm in diameter, whereas large (45–80 μm) splanchnic afferent neurons did not exhibit peptide immunoreactivity. Approximately 25% of renal afferent neurons in the cat also exhibited substance

P immunoreactivity (Kuo et al., 1984b). Substance P immunoreactivity was detected in afferent neurons projecting to the inferior mesenteric ganglion of the guinea pig (Dalsgaard et al., 1982b) and thoracic neurons innervating the guinea pig pylorus (Lindh et al., 1983) and rat stomach and pancreas (Sharkey et al., 1984).

The distribution of the peptidergic axons in the thoracolumbar dorsal horn of the cat is also suggestive that peptides are present in visceral afferent pathways. Substance P-containing fibers are located in areas of visceral afferent termination in laminae I and V on the lateral edge and at the base of the dorsal horn. The substance P axons at these sites occur in clusters, with a periodic distribution in the longitudinal axis similar to that of visceral afferent fibers (Kawatani et al., 1985b). VIP axons also occur in the marginal zone of the dorsal horn and Lissauer's tract of the thoracolumbar segments (Kawatani et al., 1985b; Kuo et al., 1985); however, the density of VIP fibers is considerably less than in the sacral segments.

Conclusions

HRP tracing studies have revealed that visceral afferent neurons at various levels of the spinal cord and in several species of animals have a similar pattern of central termination (laminae I, V–VII and X) which is markedly different from the central termination of somatic afferent neurons (Brown, 1982; Cervero and Connell, 1984). The anatomical data correlate well with the results of electrophysiological experiments (Pomeranz et al., 1968; De Groat et al., 1981; Milne et al., 1981; McMahon and Morrison, 1982; Cervero, 1982, 1983; Honda et al., 1983; Ammons and Foreman, 1984) in which spinal interneurons and spinal tract neurons receiving visceral sensory inputs have been identified, primarily in laminae I, V–VII and X at the thoracolumbar and sacral segments of the spinal cord.

Visceral afferent projections also overlap with the soma and dendrites of sympathetic and parasympathetic preganglionic neurons in the spinal cord (Nadelhaft et al., 1980, 1983; Morgan et al., 1981, 1986a,b; Kuo and De Groat, 1985). Although evidence for monosynaptic connections between visceral afferent and efferent neurons is sparse (De Groat and Ryall, 1969; Lebedev et al., 1976; Mawe et al., 1984), the proximity of afferent and efferent pathways no doubt has important physiological implications in the organization of autonomic reflex mechanisms.

As noted in other chapters of this volume, viscerosomatic convergence is a prominent characteristic of visceral sensory and visceral reflex pathways in the spinal cord. Electrophysiological and neuroanatomical studies of somatic afferents innervating deep structures related to autonomic function (e.g., perineal muscles and urethra) as well as cutaneous high-threshold afferents have revealed overlap in all visceral afferent terminal fields (laminae I, V–VII and X) (De Groat et al., 1981; Milne et al., 1981; McMahon and Morrison, 1982; Brown, 1982; Cervero, 1983; Foreman and Ohata, 1980; Honda, 1985). This viscerosomatic sensory convergence is likely to provide the anatomical substrate for visceral referred pain as well as for the integration of autonomic and somatic reflex mechanisms.

Immunohistochemical studies suggest that neuropeptides may play an important role in visceral sensory mechanisms at all levels of the spinal cord. A large percentage of sacral and thoracolumbar visceral afferent neurons exhibit peptide immunoreactivity. In addition, in the spinal cord some peptidergic afferent fibers (e.g., substance P and VIP) have a distribution very similar to that of certain components of the visceral afferent pathways.

The co-localization of peptides in visceral afferent neurons raises the possibility that individual neurons may release multiple peptide transmitters at central as well as peripheral afferent terminals. Furthermore, the co-localization in afferent neurons of inhibitory peptides (enkephalins) and excitatory peptides (VIP and substance P) raises the possibility of complex transmitter interactions at visceral afferent synapses.

Acknowledgements

The author would like to thank A. M. Booth, T. Hisamitsu, M. Kawatani, D. Kuo, I. Lowe, C. Morgan, I. Nadelhaft, J. Roppolo, K. Thor, M. Houston, S. Erdman, J. Oravitz and M. Rutigliano for their contributions to these studies, and thanks T. Harvey and T. Smiechowski for typing the manuscript. This work was supported in part by NSF grant, BNS-8507113, NIH grants, AM 317888 and AM 37241 and a Clinical Research Center Grant, MH 30915.

References

Ammons, W. S. and Foreman, R. D. (1984) Responses of T2–T4 spinal neurons to stimulation of the greater splanchnic nerve of the cat. Exp. Neurol., 83: 288–301.

Anand, P., Gibson, S. J., McGregor, G. P., Blank, M. A., Ghatei, M. A., Bacarese-Hamilton, A. J., Polak, J. M. and Bloom, S. R. (1983) A VIP-containing system concentrated in the lumbosacral region of human spinal cord. Nature, 305: 143–145.

Baron, R., Janig, W. and McLachlan, E. M. (1982) Sensory and sympathetic neurons with axons in the hypogastric nerve of the cat. Pflugers Arch., 394: R52.

Basbaum, A. I. and Glazer, E. J. (1983) Immunoreactive vasoactive intestinal polypeptide is concentrated in the sacral spinal cord: A possible marker for pelvic visceral afferent fibers. Somatosensory Res., 1: 69–82.

Berkley, K. J. (1975) Different targets of different neurons in nucleus gracilis of the cat. J. Comp. Neurol., 163: 285–304.

Brown, A. G. (1982) The dorsal horn of the spinal cord. Q. J. Exp. Physiol., 67: 193–212.

Brown, P. B. and Fuchs, J. L. (1975) Somatotopic representation of hindlimb skin in the cat dorsal horn. J. Neurophysiol., 38: 1–9.

Cervero, F. (1982) Noxious intensities of visceral stimulation are required to activate viscero-somatic multireceptive neurones in the thoracic spinal cord of the cat. Brain Res., 240: 350–352.

Cervero, F. (1983) Somatic and visceral inputs to the thoracic spinal cord of the cat: Effects of noxious stimulation of the biliary system. J. Physiol. (Lond.), 337: 51–67.

Cervero, F. and Connell, L. (1984) Distribution of somatic and visceral primary afferent fibres within the thoracic spinal cord of the cat. J. Comp. Neurol., 230: 88–98.

Cervero, F., Connell, L. A. and Lawson, S. N. (1984) Somatic and visceral primary afferents in the lower thoracic dorsal root ganglia of the cat. J. Comp. Neurol., 228: 422–431.

Ciriello, J. and Calaresu, F. R. (1983) Central projections of afferent renal fibres in the rat: An anterograde transport study of horseradish peroxidase. J. Auton. Nerv. System, 8: 273–285.

Craig, A. D. and Mense, S. (1983) The distribution of afferent fibres from the gastrocnemius-soleus muscle in the dorsal horn of the cat, as revealed by transport of HRP. Neurosci. Lett., 41: 233–238.

Dalsgaard, C.-J., Vincent, S. R., Hökfelt, T., Lundberg, J. M., Dahlstrom, A., Schultzberg, M., Dockray, G. J. and Cuello, A. C. (1982a) Co-existence of cholecystokinin- and substance P-like peptides in neurons of the dorsal root ganglia of the rat. Neurosci. Lett., 33: 159–163.

Dalsgaard, C.-J., Hökfelt, T., Elfvin, L. G., Skirboll, L. and Emson, P. (1982b) Substance P containing primary sensory neurons projecting to the inferior mesenteric ganglion: Evidence from combined retrograde tracing and immunohistochemistry. Neuroscience, 7: 647–654.

De Groat, W. C. and Booth, A. M. (1984) Autonomic systems to the urinary bladder and sexual organs. In P. J. Dyck, P. K. Thomas, E. H. Lamber and R. Bunge (Eds.), Peripheral Neuropathy, Vol. I, W. B. Saunders Co., Philadelphia, pp. 285–299.

De Groat, W. C. and Ryall, R. W. (1969) Reflexes to sacral preganglionic parasympathetic neurones concerned with micturition in the cat. J. Physiol. (Lond.), 200: 87–108.

De Groat, W. C., Nadelhaft, I., Morgan, C. and Schauble, T. (1978) Horseradish peroxidase tracing of visceral efferent and primary afferent pathways in the sacral spinal cord of the cat using benzidine processing. Neurosci. Lett., 10: 103–108.

De Groat, W. C., Nadelhaft, I., Milne, R. J., Booth, A. M., Morgan, C. and Thor, K. (1981) Organization of the sacral parasympathetic reflex pathways to the urinary bladder and large intestine. J. Auton. Nerv. System, 3: 135–160.

De Groat, W. C., Kawatani, M., Hisamitsu, T., Lowe, I., Morgan, C., Roppolo, J., Booth, A. M., Nadelhaft, I., Kuo, D. and Thor, K. (1983) The role of neuropeptides in the sacral autonomic reflex pathways of the cat. J. Auton. Nerv. System, 7: 339–350.

De Groat, W. C., Kawatani, M., Houston, M. B. and Erdman, S. L. (1985c) Colocalization of VIP, substance P, CCK, somatostatin and enkephalin immunoreactivity in lumbosacral dorsal root ganglion cells of the cat. Abstract from Vth International Washington Spring Symposium, May 28–31, Washington, DC, p. 48.

De Groat, W. C., Kawatani, M., Hisamitsu, T., Booth, A. M., Roppolo, J. R., Thor, K., Tuttle, P. and Nagel, J. (1986a) Neural control of micturition: The role of neuropeptides. J. Auton. Nerv. System, in press.

De Groat, W. C., Lowe, I. P., Kawatani, M., Morgan, C. W., Kuo, D., Roppolo, J. R., Thor, K. and Nagel, J. (1986b) The identification of enkephalin-like immunoreactivity in sensory ganglion cells. J. Auton. Nerv. System, in press.

Foreman, R. D. and Ohata, C. A. (1980) Effects of coronary

occlusion on thoracic spinal neurones receiving viscerosomatic inputs. Am. J. Physiol., 238: H667–H674.

Fuxe, K., Agnati, L. F., McDonald, T., Locatelli, V., Hökfelt, T., Dalsgaard, C.-J., Battistini, N., Yanaihara, N., Mutt, V. and Cuello, A. C. (1983) Immunohistochemical indications of gastrin releasing peptide-bombesin-like immunoreactivity in the nervous system of the rat. Codistribution with substance P-like immunoreactive nerve terminal systems and coexistence with substance P-like immunoreactivity in dorsal root ganglion cell bodies. Neurosci. Lett., 37: 17–22.

Gibbins, I. L., Furness, J. B., Costa, M., MacIntyre, I., Hillyard, C. J. and Girgis, S. (1985) Colocalization of calcitonin gene-related peptide-like immunoreactivity with substance P in cutaneous, vascular and visceral sensory neurons of guinea pigs. Neurosci. Lett., 57: 125–130.

Gibson, S. J., Polak, J. M., Anand, P., Blank, M. A., Morrison, J. F. B., Kelly, J. S. and Bloom, S. R. (1984) The distribution and origin of VIP in the spinal cord of six mammalian species. Peptides, 5: 201–207.

Gobel, S. and Falls, W. (1979) Anatomical observations of horseradish peroxidase filled terminal primary axonal arborizations in layer II of the substantia gelatinosa of Rolando. Brain Res., 175: 335–340.

Harris, A. J. (1943) An experimental analysis of the inferior mesenteric plexus. J. Comp. Neurol., 79: 1–17.

Holzer-Petsche and Lembeck (1985) Systemic capsaicin treatment impairs the micturition reflex in the rat. Br. J. Pharmacol., 83: 935–941.

Honda, C. N. (1985) Visceral and somatic afferent convergence onto neurons near the central canal in the sacral spinal cord of the cat. J. Neurophysiol., 53: 1059–1078.

Honda, C. N., Rethelyi, M. and Petrusz, P. (1983) Preferential immunohistochemical localization of vasoactive intestinal polypeptide (VIP) in the sacral spinal cord of the cat: Light and electron, microscope observations. J. Neurosci., 5: 2183–2196.

Hulsebosch, C. E. and Coggeshall, R. E. (1982) An analysis of the axon population in the nerves to the pelvic viscera in the rat. J. Comp. Neurol., 211: 1–10.

Jessell, T. M. and Iversen, L. L. (1977) Opiate analgesics inhibit substance P release from rat trigeminal nucleus. Nature, 268: 549–551.

Kawatani, M., Lowe, I., Nadelhaft, I., Morgan, C. and De Groat, W. C. (1983a) Vasoactive intestinal polypeptide in visceral afferent pathways to the sacral spinal cord of the cat. Neurosci. Lett., 42: 311–316.

Kawatani, M., Lowe, I., Moossy, J., Martinez, J., Nadelhaft, I., Eskay, R. and De Groat, W. C. (1983b) Vasoactive intestinal polypeptide (VIP) is localized to the lumbosacral segments of the human spinal cord. Soc. Neurosci. Abstr., 9: 294.

Kawatani, M., Nagel, J., Houston, M. B., Eskay, R., Lowe, I. P. and De Groat, W. C. (1984) Identification of leucine-enkephalin and other neuropeptides in pelvic and pudendal afferent pathways to the spinal cord of the cat. Soc. Neurosci., Abstr., 10: 589.

Kawatani, M., Kuo, D. C. and De Groat, W. C. (1985a) Identification of neuropeptides in visceral afferent neurons in the thoracolumbar dorsal ganglia of the cat. Abstract from Vth International Washington Spring Symposium, May 28–31, Washington, DC, p. 156.

Kawatani, M., Erdman, S. and De Groat, W. C. (1985b) Vasoactive intestinal polypeptide and substance P in afferent pathways to the sacral spinal cord of the cat. J. Comp. Neurol., 241: 327–347.

Kawatani, M., Houston, M. B., Rutigliano, M., Erdman, S. L. and De Groat, W. C. (1985c) Colocalization of neuropeptides in afferent pathways to the urinary bladder and colon: Demonstration with double color immunohistochemistry in combination with axonal tracing techniques. Soc. Neurosci., Abstr., 11: 145.

Kawatani, M., Nagel, J. and De Groat, W. C. (1986d) Identification of neuropeptides in pelvic and pudendal nerve afferent pathways to the sacral spinal cord of the cat. J. Comp. Neurol., in press.

Kuo, D. C. and De Groat, W. C. (1985) Primary afferent projections of the major splanchnic nerve to the spinal cord and gracile nucleus of the cat — an anatomical study using transganglionic transport of horseradish peroxidase. J. Comp. Neurol., 231: 421–434.

Kuo, D. C., Krauthamer, G. M. and Yamasaki, D. S. (1981) The organization of visceral sensory neurons in thoracic dorsal root ganglia (DRG) of the cat studied by horseradish peroxidase (HRP) reaction using the cryostat. Brain Res., 208: 187–191.

Kuo, D. C., Yang, G. C. H., Yamasaki, D. S. and Krauthamer, G. M. (1982) A wide field electron microscopic analysis of the fiber constitutents of the major splanchnic nerve in cat. J. Comp. Neurol., 210: 49–58.

Kuo, D., Nadelhaft, I., Hisamitsu, T. and De Groat, W. C. (1983) Segmental distribution and central projection of renal afferent fibers in the cat studied by transganglionic transport of horseradish peroxidase. J. Comp. Neurol., 216: 162–174.

Kuo, D. C., Oravitz, J. J. and De Groat, W. C. (1984a) Tracing of afferent and efferent pathways in the left inferior cardiac nerve of the cat using retrograde and transganglionic transport of horseradish peroxidase. Brain Res., 321: 111–118.

Kuo, D. C., Oravitz, J. J., Eskay, R. and De Groat, W. C. (1984b) Substance P in renal afferent perikarya identified by retrograde transport of fluorescent dye. Brain Res., 323: 168–171.

Kuo, D. C., Kawatani, M. and De Groat, W. C. (1985) Vasoactive intestinal polypeptide identified in the thoracic dorsal root ganglia of the cat. Brain Res., 330: 178–182.

La Motte, C. C. and De Lanerolle, N. C. (1983) Vasoactive intestinal polypeptide (VIP): Distribution through the length of primate spinal cord. Soc. Neurosci., Abstr., 9: 256.

La Motte, C., Pert, C. B. and Snyder, S. H. (1976) Opiate receptor binding in primate spinal cord: Distribution and changes after dorsal root section. Brain Res., 112: 407–412.

Langford, L. A. and Coggeshall, R. E. (1981) Branching of sensory axons in the peripheral nerve of the rat. J. Comp. Neurol., 203: 745–750.

Langley, J. N. and Anderson, H. K. (1894) The constituents of the hypogastric nerves. J. Physiol. (Lond.), 17: 177–191.

Lebedev, V. P., Rosanov, N. N., Skokelev, V. A. and Smirnov, K. A. (1976) A study of the early somatosympathetic reflex response. Neurosci. Lett., 2: 319–323.

Lee, K. H., Kim, J. and Chung, J. M. (1984) Segmental distribution of dorsal root ganglion cell with axons in the inferior cardiac nerve. Neurosci. Lett., 52: 185–190.

Leek, B. F. (1977) Abdominal and pelvic visceral receptors. Br. Med. Bull., 33: 163–168.

Lindh, B., Dalsgaard, C.-J., Elfvin, L.-G., Hökfelt, T. and Cuello, A. C. (1983) Evidence of substance P immunoreactive neurons in dorsal root ganglia and vagal ganglia projecting to the guinea pig pylorus. Brain Res., 269: 365–369.

Lowe, I. P., Kawatani, M., Thor, K. and De Groat, W. C. (1984) Identification of leucine-enkephalin in primary afferent pathways to the spinal cord of the cat. Abstracts of the 29th International Congress of Neurovegetative Research, Berlin, Germany, March 19–24.

Maggi, C. A., Santicioli, P. and Meli, A. (1984) The effects of topical capsaicin on rat urinary bladder motility in vivo. Eur. J. Pharmacol., 103: 41–50.

Matsushita, M. and Tanami, T. (1983) Contralateral termination of primary afferent axons in the sacral and caudal segments of the cat, as studied by anterograde transport of horseradish peroxidase. J. Comp. Neurol., 220: 206–218.

Mawe, G. M., Bresnahan, J. C. and Beattie, M. S. (1984) Primary afferent projections from dorsal and ventral roots to autonomic preganglionic neurons in the cat sacral spinal cord: Light and electron microscopic observations. Brain Res., 290: 152–157.

McMahon, S. B. and Morrison, J. F. B. (1982) Spinal neurones with long projections activated from the abdominal visceral of the cat. J. Physiol. (Lond.), 322: 1–20.

Milne, R. J., Foreman, R. D., Giesler, G. J. Jr. and Willis, W. C. (1981) Convergence of cutaneous and pelvic visceral nociceptive inputs onto primate spinothalamic neurons. Pain, 11: 163–183.

Morgan, C. and O'Hara, P. (1984) Electron microscopic identification of vasoactive intestinal polypeptide (VIP) in visceral primary afferent axons in the sacral spinal cord of the cat. Anat. Rec., 208: 121.

Morgan, C., De Groat, W. C. and Nadelhaft, I. (1980) The central distribution within Lissauer's tract and the spinal gray matter of primary afferents from the pelvic nerve and pudendal nerve of the cat demonstrated by transganglionic transport of HRP. Soc. Neurosci., Abstr., 6: 116.

Morgan, C., Nadelhaft, I. and De Groat, W. C. (1981) The distribution of visceral primary afferents from the pelvic nerve within Lissauer's tract and the spinal gray matter and its relationship to the sacral parasympathetic nucleus. J. Comp. Neurol., 201: 415–440.

Morgan, C., De Groat, W. C. and Nadelhaft, I. (1986a) The spinal distribution of sympathetic preganglionic and visceral primary afferent neurons which send axons into the hypogastric nerves of the cat. J. Comp. Neurol., 243: 23–40.

Morgan, C., Nadelhaft, I. and De Groat, W. C. (1986b) The spinal distribution of visceral primary afferent neurons which send axons into the lumbar colonic nerves of the cat. Soc. Neurosci., Abstr., in press.

Nadelhaft, I. and Booth, A. M. (1984) The location and morphology of preganglionic neurons and the distribution of visceral afferents from the rat pelvic nerve: A horseradish peroxidase study. J. Comp. Neurol., 226: 238–245.

Nadelhaft, I., Morgan, C. W. and De Groat, W. C. (1980) Localization of the sacral autonomic nucleus in the spinal cord of the cat by the horseradish peroxidase technique. J. Comp. Neurol., 193: 265–281.

Nadelhaft, I., Roppolo, J., Morgan, C. and De Groat, W. C. (1983) Parasympathetic preganglionic neurons and visceral primary afferents in monkey sacral spinal cord revealed following the application of horseradish peroxidase to pelvic nerve. J. Comp. Neurol., 216: 36–52.

Neuhuber, W. (1982) The central projections of visceral primary afferent neurons of the inferior mesenteric plexus and hypogastric nerve and the location of the related sensory and preganglionic sympathetic cell bodies in the rat. Anat. Embryol., 164: 413–425.

Nyberg, G. and Blomqvist, A. (1982) The termination of forelimb nerves in the feline cuneate nucleus demonstrated by the transganglionic transport method. Brain Res., 248: 209–222.

Oldfield, B. J. and McLachlan, E. M. (1978) Localization of sensory neurons traversing the stellate ganglion of the cat. J. Comp. Neurol., 182: 915–922.

Oravitz, J. J., Morgan, C., Nadlehaft, I. and De Groat, W. C. (1982) Sympathetic preganglionic neurons and visceral primary afferents supplying the pelvic viscera in the cat. Soc. Neurosci., Abstr., 8: 269.

Pierau, F. K., Taylor, D. C. M. and Fellmer, G. (1983) Convergence of somatic and visceral inputs in the peripheral nerves of cat and rat. Neurosci. Lett. (Suppl.), 24: S285.

Pomeranz, B., Wall, P. D. and Weber, W. V. (1968) Cord cells responding to fine myelineated afferents from viscera, muscle and skin. J. Physiol. (Lond.), 199: 511–532.

Ralston, H. J. and Ralston, D. D. (1979) The distribution of dorsal root axons in laminae I, II and III of the macaque spinal cord: A quantitative electron microscopic study. J. Comp. Neurol., 184: 643–684.

Rethelyi, M., Trevino, D. L. and Perl, E. R. (1979) Distribution of primary afferent fibers within the sacrococcygeal dorsal horn: An autoradiographic study. J. Comp. Neurol., 185: 603–622.

Roppolo, J. R., Nadelhaft, I. and De Groat, W. C. (1983) The preferential distribution of vasoactive intestinal polypeptide (VIP) in the sacral spinal cord of the rhesus monkey. Soc. Neurosci., Abstr., 9: 293.

Roppolo, J. R., Nadelhaft, I. and De Groat, W. C. (1985) The organization of pudendal motoneurons and primary afferent projections in the spinal cord of the rhesus monkey revealed by horseradish peroxidase. J. Comp. Neurol., 234: 475–488.

Rustioni, A. (1973) Non-primary afferents to the nucleus gracilis from the lumbar cord of the cat. Brain Res., 51: 81–95.

Sasek, C. A., Seybold, V. S. and Elde, R. P. (1984) The immunohistochemical localization of nine peptides in the sacral parasympathetic nucleus and the dorsal gray commissure in rat spinal cord. Neuroscience, 12: 855–873.

Schnitzlein, H. N., Hoffman, H. H., Tucker, C. C. and Quigley, M. B. (1954) The pelvic splanchnic nerves of the male rhesus monkey. J. Comp. Neurol., 100: 57–65.

Sharkey, K. A., Williams, R. G., Schultzberg, M. and Dockray, G. J. (1983) Sensory substance P-innervation of the urinary bladder: Possible site of action of capsaicin in causing urine retention in rats. Neuroscience, 10: 861–868.

Sharkey, K. A., Williams, R. G. and Dockray, G. J. (1984) Sensory substance P innervation of the stomach and pancreas. Gastroenterology, 87: 914–920.

Snow, P. J., Cameron, A. A. and Leah, J. D. (1985) Pain transmission in identified pathways. Neurosci. Lett. (Suppl.), 19: S17.

Taylor, D. C. M. and Pierau, F. K. (1982) Double fluorescence labelling supports electrophysiological evidence for dichotomizing peripheral sensory nerve fibers in rat. Neurosci. Lett., 33: 1–6.

Thor, K. B., Kuo, D. C., De Groat, W. C., Blais, D. and Backes, M. (1982) Alterations of HRP-labelled pudendal nerve afferent projections in the sacral spinal cord of the cat during neonatal development and after spinal cord transection: Correlation with physiological plasticity of a spinal somatovesical reflex. Soc. Neurosci., Abstr., 8: 305.

Thor, K. B., Kawatani, M. and De Groat, W. C. (1986) Plasticity in the reflex pathways to the lower urinary tract of the cat during postnatal development and following spinal cord injury. In M. Goldberger, A. Gorio and M. Murray (Eds.), Development and Plasticity of the Mammalian Spinal Cord, Fidia Research Series, Vol. III, Livana Press, Padova, Italy, pp. 105–121.

Tuchscherer, M. M. and Seybold, V. S. (1985) Immunohistochemical studies of substance P, cholecystokinin-octapeptide and somatostatin in dorsal root ganglia of the rat. Neuroscience, 14: 593–605.

Ueyama, T., Mizuno, N., Nomura, S., Konishi, A., Itoh, K. and Arakawa, H. (1984) Central distribution of afferent and efferent components of the pudendal nerve in cat. J. Comp. Neurol., 222: 38–46.

Ueyama, T., Mizuno, N., Takahashi, O., Nomura, S., Arakawa, H. and Matsushima, R. (1985) Central distribution of efferent and afferent components of the pudendal nerve in macaque monkeys. J. Comp. Neurol., 232: 548–556.

Wiesenfeld-Hallin, Z., Hökfelt, T., Lundberg, J. M., Forssmann, W. G., Reinecke, M., Tschopp, F. A. and Fischer, J. A. (1984) Immunoreactive calcitonin gene-related peptide and substance P coexist in sensory neurons to the spinal cord and interact in spinal behavioral responses of the rat. Neurosci. Lett., 52: 199–204.

Yaksh, T. L. and Elde, R. P. (1981) Factors governing the release of methionine-enkephalin-like immunoreactivity from the mesencephalon and spinal cord of the cat in vivo. J. Neurophysiol., 46: 1056–1075.

Yaksh, T. L., Jessell, T. M., Gamse, R., Mudge, A. W. and Leeman, S. E. (1980) Intrathecal morphine inhibits substance P release from mammalian spinal cord in vivo. Nature, 286: 155–157.

F. Cervero and J. F.B. Morrison
Progress in Brain Research, Vol. 67

CHAPTER 12

Somatic and visceral sensory integration in the thoracic spinal cord

F. Cervero and J. E. H. Tattersall

Department of Physiology, University of Bristol Medical School, University Walk, Bristol BS8 1TD, U.K.

Introduction

Sympathetic and parasympathetic nerves contain not only autonomic efferent axons but also the afferent fibres that carry visceral sensory signals. The existence of visceral afferent fibres in the splanchnic nerves was first recognised by Langley and Anderson (1894), who estimated a ratio of efferent to afferent fibres in these nerves of approximately 10:1. The cell bodies of these afferent fibres were believed to be in the thoracic spinal ganglia. Subsequent histological and physiological examinations of sympathetic and parasympathetic nerves (Ranson, 1921) confirmed the existence of afferent fibres in these nerves and the involvement of visceral afferent fibres in the signalling of visceral pain.

During the course of these early studies it became apparent that most internal organs have a dual afferent innervation. Some visceral afferent fibres join sympathetic nerves, such as the splanchnic nerves, whereas other afferent fibres from the same viscera course in parasympathetic nerves, such as the vagus and pelvic nerves. Therefore, it was thought that visceral afferents in sympathetic and in parasympathetic nerves carried fundamentally different kinds of visceral afferent signals. A parallel was established between the dual afferent innervation of many viscera and the dual effects that can be evoked by the stimulation of internal organs, i.e., unconscious reflex activity and conscious sensory experiences. It was finally concluded that visceral sensation (and especially visceral pain) is mediated by afferent fibres in sympathetic nerves and that the activation of afferent fibres running in parasympathetic nerves does not evoke visceral sensations and is concerned only with the reflex regulation of visceral function. This view became standard opinion in textbooks and reference monographs (Ruch, 1946) and has survived, almost untouched, until present times.

Although most forms of visceral pain from abdominal organs are mediated by afferent fibres in sympathetic nerves, it is possible to evoke non-painful visceral sensations by stimulation of vagal and pelvic afferent fibres. These non-painful sensory experiences include some of the sensations known as "organic" or "general" sensations (such as hunger, satiety and nausea) and some of the sensory perceptions evoked by the distension of the urinary bladder. The pathways that mediate non-painful sensory signals from viscera and the involvement of the vagus nerve in visceral sensation are discussed at length in other chapters of this book.

The notion that visceral pain from abdominal organs can be mediated by afferent activity in sympathetic nerves is supported by experimental evidence from studies that have correlated the stimulation of abdominal viscera with the patterns of behaviour evoked by such stimulation. Once a relationship is established between a particular form of visceral stimulation and a behavioural response it is then possible to examine the afferent pathway for the response by repeating the test stimulus after sectioning or blocking sympathetic and parasympathetic nerves. Schrager and Ivy (1928) described the patterns of behaviour elicited in conscious dogs when the gallbladder or the cystic duct was distended with a chronically implanted balloon. The motor reactions interpreted as signs of distress and the inhibition of respiration that followed distension of the biliary system were completely abolished in animals which had their right splanchnic nerves sectioned. However, other consequences of biliary distension, such as increased salivation (nausea ?) and vomiting, persisted after splanchnic nerve section and were only abolished by section of the vagi nerves. Similar results were reported by Davis et al. (1929) using conscious dogs with chronically implanted cannulae in their biliary systems. In their experiments, pain reactions to distension of the gallbladder were abolished by section of the splanchnic nerve or by lesions of the spinal cord, but not by section of the vagi. In a study by Cannon (1933), using cats with chronically implanted electrodes around their splanchnic and vagi nerves, no signs of pain were observed following electrical stimulation of the vagus nerve below the recurrent branch. In contrast, motor behaviour indicative of pain was readily elicited by electrical stimulation of the splanchnic nerve. More recently, Stulrajter et al. (1978) have repeated these experiments using cats and dogs with chronically implanted balloons in the biliary systems and have confirmed the earlier reports. Pain reactions produced by stimulation of the gallbladder could only be evoked if the splanchnic nerves of the experimental animals were intact.

Neurophysiological studies have also given support to the notion that afferent fibres in sympathetic nerves mediate visceral pain. The reflexes produced by noxious stimulation of viscera were used by Sherrington (1906) to illustrate his argument for a close relationship between adequate stimuli and nociceptive responses. Among the reflexes described by Sherrington as being always associated with nociceptive reactions was the transient increase in blood pressure elicited by noxious stimulation of somatic or visceral structures. This blood pressure change could be evoked in conscious as well as in anaesthetized or decerebrate animals, and therefore could be used as an index of nociception even when consciousness was prevented by experimental interference. Sherrington (1906) and Davis et al. (1932) then showed that nociceptive reactions evoked by noxious stimulation of the gallbladder were still present after section of both vagi, and therefore were mediated by afferent fibres in sympathetic nerves. A similar conclusion was reached by Moore and Singleton (1933) and Moore (1938), who studied nociceptive reactions evoked in anaesthetized cats by the injection of irritants in mesenteric arteries. They showed that the flexor reflexes elicited in their animals by such noxious visceral stimulation were abolished by section of the splanchnic nerves and the thoracic sympathetic chain, but not by section of the vagi. More recently, similar conclusions were reached by Cervero (1982), who studied blood pressure increases evoked by noxious stimulation of the ferret's biliary system, and by Stulrajter et al. (1978), Ordway and Longhurst (1983) and Ammons and Foreman (1984), who analysed cardiovascular responses to noxious biliary stimulation in the cat.

A considerable body of clinical evidence gives additional support to the idea that abdominal visceral pain is mediated by afferent fibres in sympathetic nerves. It has been known for some time that stimulation of the splanchnic nerves in conscious humans under local anaesthesia elicits severe pain (Leriche, 1939). Clinical studies using a combination of stimulation and blocking techniques have repeatedly shown that abdominal pain is elicited by stimulation of sympathetic but not of parasympathetic nerves, and is relieved by section or blockade of sympathetic but not of parasympathetic nerve trunks (White, 1943).

Thus, it is possible to conclude from the behavioural, neurophysiological and clinical evidence that most forms of pain from abdominal viscera are mediated by afferent fibres in sympathetic nerves and that the parasympathetic afferent innervation of these organs is not immediately concerned with visceral sensation. While this generalisation applies, with few exceptions, to visceral pain from upper abdominal viscera, it is important to point out that non-painful visceral sensations or visceral pain from other internal organs may be elicited by the stimulation of afferent fibres in somatic or in parasympathetic nerves. However, since visceral pain from the upper abdomen is almost exclusively mediated by afferent fibres in sympathetic nerves, the analysis of viscero-somatic integration in the lower thoracic spinal cord should provide some insight into the mechanisms used by the nervous system to integrate visceral sensory information at the level of the first synaptic relay. In another chapter of this book, Foreman and colleagues discuss the role of the upper thoracic spinal cord in the integration of nociceptive signals from the heart. In this chapter we will review the processing by the lower thoracic cord of sensory signals from abdominal viscera.

Visceral pain and referred pain

Discomfort and pain are the sensory experiences most commonly evoked from abdominal viscera. In contrast with the bright and well-localised pain evoked by noxious stimulation of the skin, pain of internal origin is often dull, aching and ill-localized. These well-known peculiarities of visceral pain have formed the basis for an argument on the localisation of visceral sensation in general, and of visceral pain in particular. In 1888, Ross described visceral pain as being of two sorts: "splanchnic" pain, derived directly from a viscus and felt in the same viscus, and "somatic" pain, a form of visceral pain felt in a part of the body away from the originating viscus. Ross's "splanchnic" pain was later termed "true" visceral pain, implying the direct localization of its source in the originating viscus. On the other hand, the wrongly localised "somatic" pain of Ross was subsequently renamed "referred" visceral pain by Head (1893), who wished to emphasize the referral to the skin and other superficial structures of sensations originating from internal organs.

The argument on the localisation of deep and visceral pain was thoroughly reviewed by Lewis (1942). He concluded that visceral pain is always poorly localised and referred to somatic structures adjacent to or remote from the viscus of origin. To Lewis, the imprecise localization of visceral pain is due to the lack of a detailed central representation of visceral structures within the central nervous system. Therefore, the better localised and so-called "true" visceral pain must be due to the spread of the visceral lesion and the activation of somatic nerves close to the injured or diseased organ. If the stimulation of an internal organ leads to a circumscribed and well-localized sensation of pain, this is probably due to the internal stimulus affecting adjacent structures innervated by somatic nerves (i.e., peritoneum, muscle, ligaments). The lack of evidence for a sensory channel specifically concerned with the transmission of visceral sensory impulses and the considerable amount of experimental data on viscero-somatic convergence in the central nervous system are powerful arguments against the existence of a specific visceral mechanism for the so-called "true" visceral pain.

Models of viscero-somatic integration

Unpleasant sensory experiences triggered by the activation of visceral afferent fibres are referred to somatic structures, and hence wrongly localized. A number of different mechanisms have been suggested in order to explain the somatic localization of the sensory experiences evoked from viscera. All these models take into account the clinical observation that visceral pain is usually referred to a somatic area innervated by the same spinal cord segments that receive the input from the originating viscus (Mackenzie, 1909). Therefore, all neurophysiological interpretations of visceral pain are based on viscero-somatic integration, that is, the convergence of inputs from viscera and from somatic structures onto sensory neurones whose activation leads to the experience of somatic pain.

The simplest form of viscero-somatic convergence occurs in primary afferent fibres with multiple peripheral branches that innervate sensory receptors in skin, muscle and viscera. Several authors have described dorsal root ganglion neurones with dual or multiple peripheral branches, including neurones with branches in somatic and visceral nerves (Adrian et al., 1931; Langford and Coggeshall, 1981; Bahr et al., 1981; Pierau et al., 1984). This arrangement has been claimed as evidence for the pre-spinal convergence hypothesis of referred visceral sensation (Lewis, 1942; Pierau et al., 1984). However, Pierau et al. (1984) have reported that such "dichotomizing" primary afferent neurones constitute less than 1% of the total number of cells in the lower thoracic dorsal root ganglia of the cat, which shows that only a small minority of afferent fibres have two or more peripheral branches. In addition, there is no functional evidence that the different branches of the dichotomising afferent neurones are connected to physiologically active receptor endings in skin and viscera. Therefore, prespinal convergence cannot totally account for all manifestations of referred visceral sensation. Before general statements are made about the role of dichotomising primary afferent fibres in referred pain, it is necessary to establish the precise function of the somatic and visceral branches of such primary afferent neurones.

Most of the hypotheses put forward to explain the referral of visceral pain are based on models of viscero-somatic integration within the central nervous system. Ross (1888) and Head (1893) suggested that the excitation of visceral nerves projecting to the spinal cord would result in the subsequent spread of this activation to somatic cells within the same spinal cord segments. Mackenzie (1909) provided a comprehensive model of viscero-somatic convergence by suggesting that visceral impulses arriving to the spinal cord could produce an "irritable focus" within the grey matter (Fig. 1). Such an area of "irritation" would be responsible for the activation of somatic sensory neurones (and hence the referred sensation) and for the triggering of somatic and visceral reflexes. All these initial attempts to explain referred visceral pain on the basis of viscero-somatic convergence within the spinal cord were finally put together by Ruch (1946) in his "convergence-projection" theory of referred pain. According to Ruch: "some visceral afferents converge with cutaneous pain afferents to end upon the same neuron at some point in the sensory pathway. The first opportunity for this is in the spinothalamic tract. The resulting impulses, upon reaching the brain, are interpreted as having come from

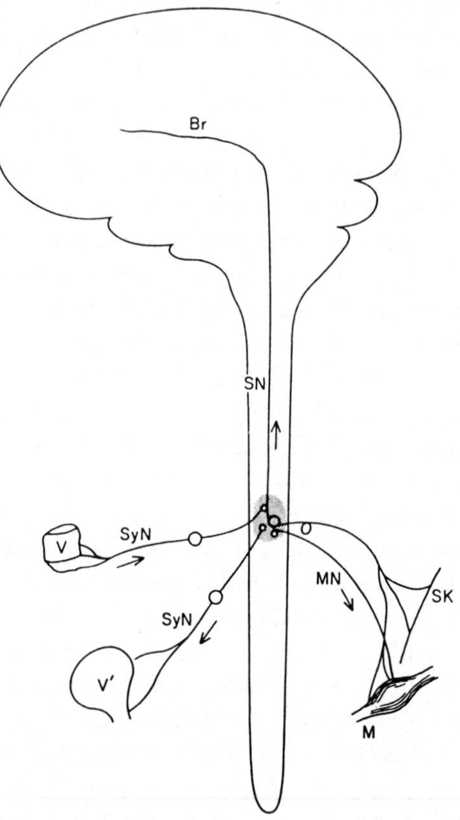

Fig. 1. Mackenzie's interpretation of the mechanisms of visceral pain and related reflexes. An adequate stimulus from a viscus (V) is conveyed to the spinal cord by sympathetic nerves (SyN) and stimulates spinal cord cells. If the stimulus activates a sensory pathway (SN) projecting to the brain (Br) it results in pain being referred to the peripheral distribution of the somatic nerve from the skin (SK). The visceral stimulus also activates other neurones which cause contractions of muscles (M), supplied by motor nerves (MN) and viscero-visceral reflexes (V'). If the visceral stimulus is of sufficient strength it may leave an "irritable focus" in the spinal cord (shaded area), resulting in cutaneous hyperalgesia and persistent muscle spasm. Diagram from Mackenzie (1909).

the skin, an interpretation which has been learned from previous experiences in which the same tract fiber was stimulated by cutaneous afferents". Ruch's hypothesis has been at the centre of modern neurophysiological studies on referred visceral sensation and has received considerable experimental support, particularly those aspects of the theory that predicted the existence of viscero-somatic convergence in the spinal cord. What remains to be tackled experimentally is the second part of Ruch's proposal; i.e., that convergent signals evoked by visceral impulses are wrongly localized to somatic structures because of previously learned experiences.

Visceral input to the lower thoracic spinal cord

Visceral afferent fibres reach the lower thoracic spinal cord via the thoraco-lumbar sympathetic chain and the "rami communicanti". These visceral afferent fibres have their cell bodies in the thoracic spinal ganglia and their central branches enter the spinal cord through the dorsal roots (Fig. 2). Some primary afferent fibres join the thoracic ventral roots (Coggeshall, 1980), but it is not clear whether these fibres actually reach the spinal cord by this route (Risling et al., 1984).

All visceral afferent fibres that enter the lower thoracic spinal cord join the sympathetic chain by way of the splanchnic nerves (Bain et al., 1935; Gernandt and Zottermann, 1946). These nerves consist of a larger "greater splanchnic nerve" and one or more smaller "lesser splanchnic nerves". The presence of visceral afferent fibres in the splanchnic nerves has long been recognised (Langley and Anderson, 1894), and early estimates indicated a ratio of efferent to afferent fibres in these nerves of about 10:1. Recently, Kuo et al. (1982) have published a comprehensive report on the composition and fibre spectrum of the greater splanchnic nerve of the cat. According to these authors, the greater splanchnic nerve contains no more than 3,000–3,500 afferent fibres, a figure of less than 20% of the total number of fibres in this nerve. The vast majority of these afferents (2,000–3,000) are unmyelinated fibres (C-fibres); 250–400 are $A\delta$-fibres and 120–350 are $A\beta$-fibres. Thus, the visceral afferent input to the lower thoracic spinal cord is entirely mediated by a small number of visceral afferent fibres, 90% of which are unmyelinated. This visceral input includes all afferent fibres involved in the signalling

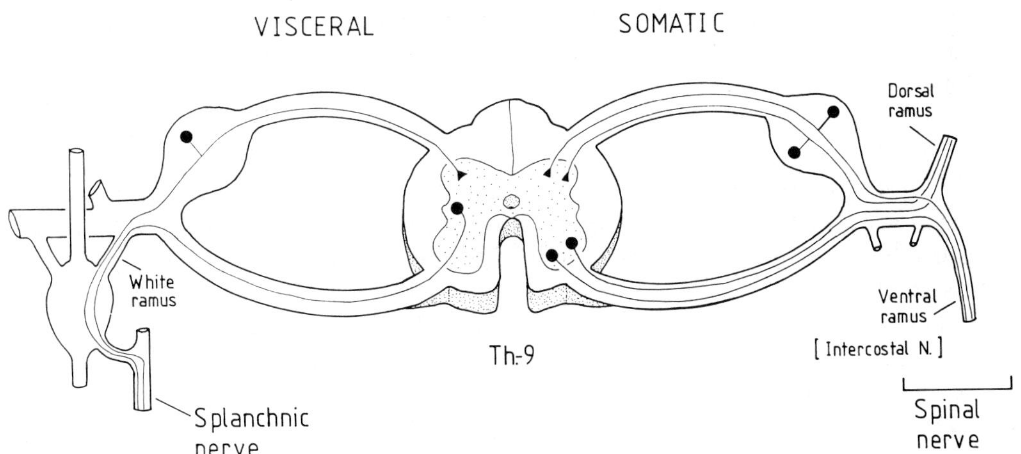

Fig. 2. Afferent pathways to the lower thoracic spinal cord. Primary afferent fibres have their cell bodies in the dorsal root ganglia. The visceral afferent fibres (left) reach the cord via the thoraco-lumbar sympathetic chain and the "rami communicanti", and the somatic fibres (right) via the dorsal and ventral rami of the spinal nerves. Their central branches enter the cord through the dorsal roots. Also shown are the efferent pathways which leave the cord through the ventral roots: on the left, preganglionic sympathetic neurones; and on the right, somatic motoneurones. Adapted from Cervero and Connell (1984b).

of visceral pain from upper abdominal viscera, i.e., the stomach, duodenum, upper jejunum, biliary system, liver and pancreas. These few visceral afferent fibres pass to the sympathetic chain from the splanchnic nerves and enter the spinal cord between the T2 and L2 segments (McSwiney and Suffolk, 1938; Hazarika et al., 1964; Mei et al., 1970; Kuo et al., 1981; Torigoe et al., 1985). Although there are some discrepancies between different reports as to the exact upper and lower limits of the spinal cord entry of splanchnic afferent fibres, it is quite clear that these afferents enter the cord through more than ten different segments.

The majority of the splanchnic afferent fibres project to the lower thoracic segments (T6–T11), and therefore these segments contain the main area of projection of visceral afferent fibres from the upper abdomen. Using transganglionic transport of horseradish peroxidase (HRP) through the splanchnic nerves, it has been possible to estimate the proportion of visceral primary afferent fibres in the lower thoracic spinal ganglia (Cervero et al., 1984). Fewer than 7% of all dorsal root ganglion cells in the T8 and T9 ganglia were found to be labelled with HRP via the ipsilateral splanchnic nerves. Thus, even in the main area of projection of the splanchnic nerve, the actual number of afferent fibres that reach the spinal cord is very small. Since many of these fibres are involved in the signalling of visceral pain from the upper abdomen, it follows that this form of visceral sensation is mediated by the activation of very few visceral afferent fibres. Such a low density of sensory innervation leaves little scope for fine discrimination and precise localization, and it is probably one of the reasons for the diffuse nature of visceral pain.

Although splanchnic afferent fibres enter the thoracic spinal cord over many segments, there is a certain degree of "viscero-topic" organization in the rostro-caudal distribution of visceral afferent from different internal organs. The upper segments (T3–T6) receive afferent fibres from the oesophagus, stomach and duodenum whereas the lower segments (T6–L1) receive fibres from the pyloric region of the stomach, the biliary system, the liver and portal vein and the kidneys (Hazarika et al., 1964; Ciriello and Calaresu, 1983; Kuo et al., 1983; Magni and Carobi, 1983; Barja and Mathison, 1984; Iwamoto et al., 1984).

The mode of termination of visceral afferent fibres within the spinal cord is described in detail by De Groat in another chapter of this book. Visceral afferent fibres that enter the lower thoracic segments of the cord project, as in the lumbar and sacral regions, to laminae I and V of the dorsal horn, sparing the intermediate laminae. The functional significance of this mode of termination of visceral afferent fibres within the spinal cord will be discussed in the following paragraphs.

Somatic input to the lower thoracic spinal cord

The thoracic spinal cord receives somatic primary afferent fibres via the dorsal and ventral rami of the thoracic spinal nerves (Fig. 2). The skin area innervated by afferent fibres in a single spinal nerve constitutes one dermatome. Dermatomes in the cat were first delineated by Sherrington (1893, 1898), using the technique of "remaining sensibility". This involves sectioning at least two dorsal roots rostral and two caudal to the one under study, to produce an insensitive area on either side of the isolated dermatome, and then testing for sensitivity by observing reflex responses to pinching of the skin. Dermatomes have since been defined using electrical recording methods in the lumbo-sacral cord by Kuhn (1953) and in the thoracic cord by Hekmatpanah (1961). Dermatomes T4–L2 were found by Hekmatpanah (1961) to be bands of skin extending in uniform width from the middorsal to the midventral line. There is considerable overlap between adjacent dermatomes and the degree of this varies according to the method used to map the dermatomes (Hekmatpanah, 1961; Kirk and Denny-Brown, 1970; Denny-Brown et al., 1973). The results of Denny-Brown et al. (1973) suggest that each point on the body is innervated by axons from at least five different dorsal roots, and that the size of a dermatome is determined by interactions between primary afferent fibres and dorsal horn neurones with axons in Lissauer's tract.

The dorsal ramus of each thoracic spinal nerve carries afferent fibres which innervate the dorsal one-third of the corresponding dermatome and the ventral ramus (intercostal nerve) supplies the ventral two-thirds of the dermatome (Ygge, 1984). Studies using HRP to label somatic and visceral nerves have shown that the vast majority (over 90%) of cell bodies in the lower thoracic dorsal root ganglia (T7–T11) are connected with afferent fibres in somatic nerves (Cervero et al., 1984).

The total rostro-caudal extent of the somatic projection to the thoracic cord through a single spinal nerve in cats and rats is two and two-thirds segments, including the segment of entry, the entire segment rostral to it and two-thirds of the segment caudal to it (Smith, 1983; Ygge and Grant, 1983;

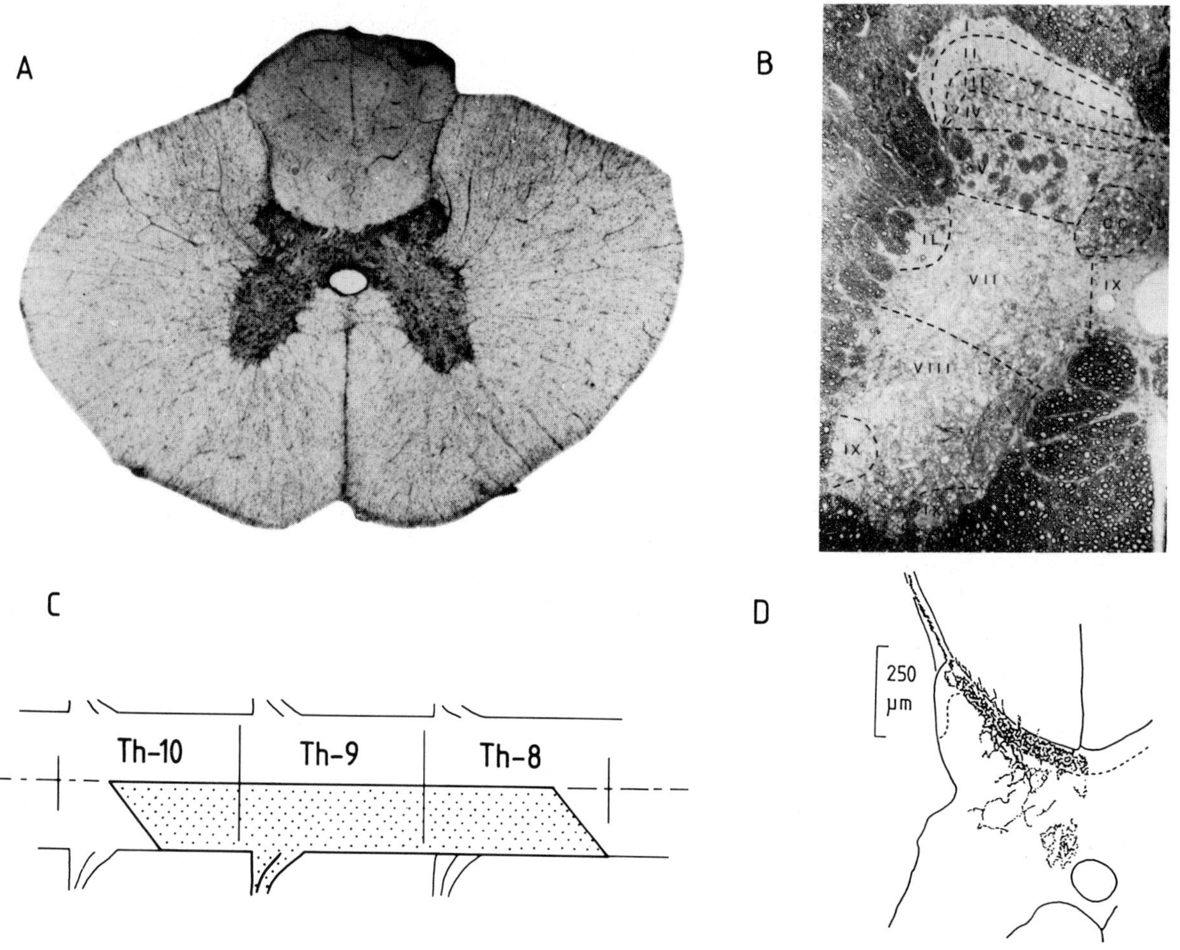

Fig. 3. Somatic primary afferent projection to the thoracic spinal cord. A, transverse section of the 9th thoracic segment, showing the extent of the grey matter. B, semithin transverse section of the T9 grey matter, stained with Toluidine Blue. Rexed's laminae are indicated by the broken lines. C, diagrammatic representation of the rostro-caudal extent of the projection through the 9th thoracic spinal nerve. The projection is ipsilateral, and includes the entire T8 segment and two-thirds of the T10 segment. Note the lateral to medial shift in the rostro-caudal axis of the cord. D, reconstruction from three 80-μm transverse serial sections of HRP-labelled fibres and terminals in the T9 segment following application of HRP to the ventral ramus of the T9 spinal nerve. The projection of this ramus is confined to the medial two-thirds of the dorsal horn. From Cervero and Connell (1984b).

Cervero and Connell, 1984b). There is a lateral to medial shift in the position of the somatic projection in the rostro-caudal axis of the cord (Smith, 1983; Ygge and Grant, 1983; Cervero and Connell, 1984b): the projection through the T9 nerve reaches more medial areas of the T10 segment in its caudal end, and more lateral areas of the T8 segment in its rostral end (Fig. 3C).

The pattern of termination of somatic afferent fibres within the spinal cord is different from that of the visceral afferent fibres. There are areas of heavy termination in laminae I and II and more scattered fibres and terminals in laminae III, IV and V and in Clarke's column (Fig. 3D), probably reflecting a lower density of neurones in these areas of the grey matter (Ygge and Grant, 1983; Cervero and Connell, 1984a,b).

Application of HRP to the dorsal and ventral rami of a spinal nerve has revealed a somatotopic arrangement of the somatic projection to the thoracic dorsal horn (Ygge and Grant, 1983; Cervero and Connell, 1984b). Afferents from the dorsal one-third of the dermatome project to the lateral one-third of the dorsal horn, whereas those from the ventral two-thirds of the dermatome project to the medial two-thirds of the dorsal horn (Fig. 3D). In addition, the projection of each ramus shows the lateral to medial shift described above in the rostro-caudal axis of the cord, at least in the rat (Smith, 1983; Ygge and Grant, 1983). Intracellular staining of single primary afferent fibres with HRP has confirmed this somatotopic organisation (Cervero and Tattersall, 1985a,b).

Viscero-somatic integration

Convergence of visceral and somatic inputs onto neurones in the thoracic spinal cord is well documented (Pomeranz et al., 1968; Gokin, 1970; Hancock et al., 1975; Foreman, 1977; Gokin et al., 1977; Guilbaud et al., 1977; Foreman and Ohata, 1980; Blair et al., 1981; Foreman et al., 1981). Two types of thoracic spinal neurone can be distinguished, on the basis of their responses to electrical stimulation of the greater splanchnic nerve (Fig. 4): (a) "somatic" neurones, which can be excited by stimulation of cutaneous or subcutaneous receptive fields, but do not receive inputs from visceral afferent fibres in the splanchnic nerve; and (b) "viscero-somatic" cells, which respond also to stimulation of somatic structures, but in addition can be driven from the splanchnic nerve or by natural stimulation of viscera such as the gallbladder (Cervero, 1982, 1983a,b; Cervero and Tattersall, 1985a,b). No evidence has been reported for the existence of significant numbers of spinal cord neurones which receive only visceral inputs.

Facilitatory and inhibitory interactions have been demonstrated between somatic and visceral

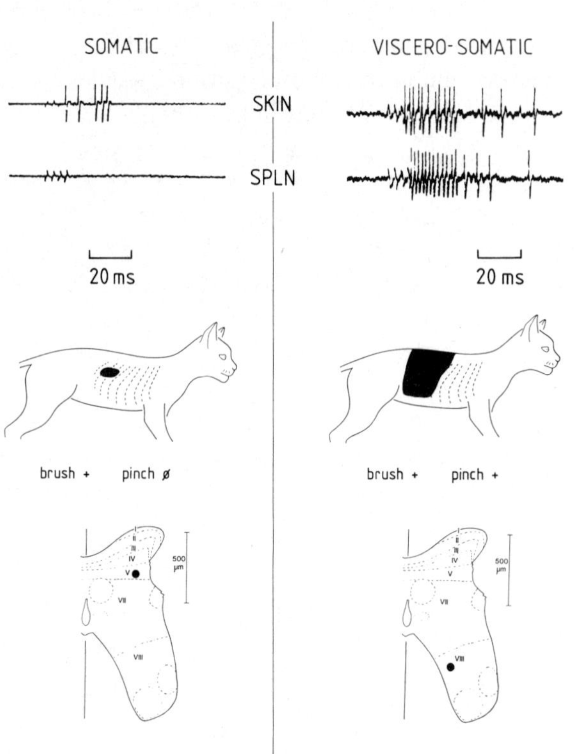

Fig. 4. Responses of a somatic (left) and a viscero-somatic neurone (right) to electrical stimulation of their cutaneous receptive fields (top traces) and of the splanchnic nerve (lower traces). The cutaneous receptive fields of the two neurones are shown: the somatic neurone was excited by brush but not by pinch, whereas the viscero-somatic cell responded to both types of stimulation. At the bottom are shown the locations of the recording sites.

inputs onto viscero-somatic neurones in the thoracic cord. Simultaneous cutaneous and visceral stimuli evoke a larger response than either stimulus would evoke on its own (Pomeranz et al., 1968; Gokin et al., 1977). If a volley in the splanchnic nerve precedes a cutaneous stimulus, then the response to the cutaneous input is reduced: estimates for the duration of the inhibition vary between 150 and 400 mseconds (Pomeranz et al., 1968; Gokin et al., 1977; Foreman et al., 1981). Conversely, the response of a cell to a splanchnic volley can be inhibited by a preceding cutaneous stimulus. Gokin et al. (1977) found variations in the degree of inhibition following cutaneous or visceral stimulation, according to the location of the neurone. The inhibition produced by a cutaneous input was greatest in viscero-somatic neurones in the dorsal horn, and had a duration of 600–900 mseconds; the greatest inhibition following a splanchnic volley was found in the neurones of lamina VIII. A conditioning volley in the splanchnic nerve inhibits the response of a neurone to a second volley in the same nerve. Similarly, an electrical stimulus in the cutaneous receptive field of a neurone inhibits the response to a second cutaneous stimulus. The duration of the inhibition is around 600 mseconds in both cases (Cervero and Tattersall, unpublished observations).

Although the number of visceral afferent fibres entering the thoracic cord is small in relation to the number of somatic afferents, a large proportion (56–75%) of thoracic spinal neurones respond to stimulation of the splanchnic nerve (Cervero, 1983a,b; Cervero and Tattersall, 1985a,b). This indicates extensive divergence of visceral inputs to the thoracic cord. Most spinothalamic tract cells are excited by activity in splanchnic Aδ-fibres (Hancock et al., 1975; Foreman et al., 1981), which in turn constitute a relatively small proportion of afferents in the nerve (Kuo et al., 1982). Some have also been shown to respond to C-fibre stimulation, but no effect of visceral Aβ afferent fibres upon spinal neurones has been found (Hancock et al., 1975; Foreman et al., 1981; Cervero, 1983a). Aβ-fibres, of which there are 120–350 in each splanchnic nerve, are known to innervate mesenteric Pacinian corpuscles (Sheehan, 1933). Kuo and De Groat (1985) have reported a direct projection of Aβ visceral afferent fibres through the dorsal columns to the gracile nucleus, but the available evidence suggests that these large visceral fibres do not contribute to neuronal integration at the level of the spinal cord. If this is the case, then they are the only primary afferent fibres which do not have a projection to the dorsal horn. The functional significance of such an input to the central nervous system remains to be analysed in more detail.

The majority of somatic neurones are located in laminae II, III, IV and V of the dorsal horn (Fig. 5). In contrast, viscero-somatic cells are concentrated in laminae I, V, VII and VIII, and are almost completely absent from laminae II, III and IV (Fig. 5) (Pomeranz et al., 1968; Gokin, 1970; Hancock et al., 1975; Gokin et al., 1977; Blair et al., 1981; Cervero, 1983a,b; Cervero and Tattersall, 1985a,b). This follows the pattern of termination of visceral afferents, whose endings are absent from laminae II–IV of the dorsal horn. The absence of viscero-somatic neurones from lamina II (the substantia gelatinosa)

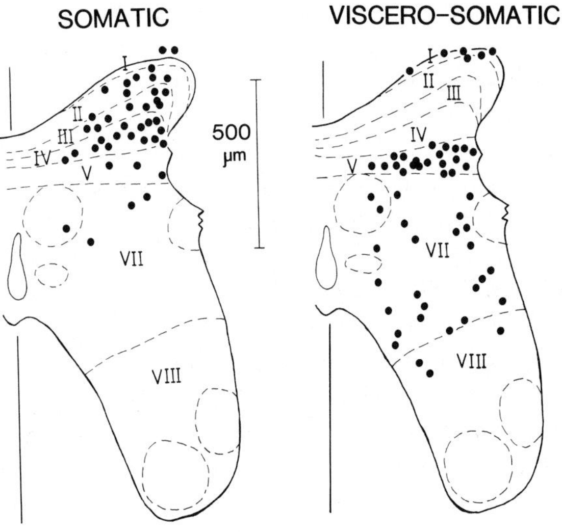

Fig. 5. Locations of the recording sites of 41 somatic neurones and 55 viscero-somatic neurones. Recording sites have been superimposed on a standard section of the T11 spinal cord segment. Lamination of the grey matter has been indicated. From Cervero (1983b).

is further evidence that there is no direct projection of visceral afferent fibres, which are predominantly unmyelinated, to this part of the dorsal horn, even though it receives the major projection of somatic afferent C-fibres. Gokin et al. (1977) have reported monosynaptic or disynaptic visceral inputs onto neurones in lamina V, whereas neurones in deeper laminae receive inputs mediated by at least two or three synapses. De Groat and his colleagues (see De Groat's chapter in this volume) have demonstrated a rostro-caudal periodicity of 300–1000 μm in the distribution of visceral primary afferents in the "lateral bundle", the projection which courses down the lateral border of the dorsal horn. It has been our impression when making electrode tracks through the thoracic spinal cord that viscero-somatic cells are concentrated in clusters along the length of the cord. If this is so, then the periodicity of visceral afferent termination may be reflected in the clustering of viscero-somatic neurones.

All somatic and viscero-somatic neurones can be excited by natural stimulation of somatic receptive fields, but the nature of the effective stimulus differs between the two groups. The majority of somatic cells are driven exclusively by low-intensity stimulation, such as touch or hair movement ("class 1" or "mechanoreceptive"). In contrast, most viscero-somatic neurones receive nociceptive inputs, such as pinch or noxious heat, either exclusively ("class 3" or "nocireceptive") or together with low-threshold inputs ("class 2" or "multireceptive"). On the basis of their recordings from neurones in laminae IV and V, Guilbaud et al. (1977) concluded that only cells which respond to noxious cutaneous stimulation receive visceral inputs. However, other studies have revealed a significant proportion of viscero-somatic neurones which receive only non-nociceptive cutaneous inputs (Hancock et al., 1975; Milne et al., 1981; Cervero, 1983a; Cervero and Tattersall, 1985a,b). Many of the viscero-somatic neurones in laminae V, VII and VIII are excited more strongly by stimulation of subcutaneous tissues, particularly muscle, than by stimulation of the skin. This is in line with the clinical signs of referred visceral sensation, which usually takes the form of pain in subcutaneous structures, especially muscle cramp, rather than cutaneous pain.

Neurones in the thoracic cord are not clearly segregated according to the types of cutaneous input they receive. Nocireceptive cells, although present in significant numbers in lamina I, are found throughout the rest of the grey matter. Similarly, mechanoreceptive and multireceptive neurones are present in or around the marginal zone (Cervero, 1983a; Cervero and Tattersall, 1985a,b). This suggests that the separation of neurones according to their cutaneous inputs is less marked than in the lumbo-sacral cord. The exception to this is found in the somatic cells of lamina I, which seem to be almost exclusively of the class 3 (nocireceptive) type (Cervero and Tattersall, unpublished observations).

The sizes of somatic receptive fields differ between the somatic and viscero-somatic groups of neurones. In a recent study in the cat, Cervero and Tattersall (1985a,b) classified receptive field sizes as small (<4 cm^2), medium (4–10 cm^2) or large (>10 cm^2). 80% of all neurones had receptive fields larger than 4 cm^2 in area, which is comparable with neurones in the lumbo-sacral cord having receptive fields on the upper hindlimb and pelvic regions. This suggests that the level of spatial discrimination in the thoracic area is similar to that in the upper hindlimb, a conclusion which is consistent with the results of psychophysical studies. Neurones with small or medium receptive fields were equally distributed between the somatic and viscero-somatic groups, but 80% of those neurones with large receptive fields had visceral inputs. 64% of all cells had receptive fields which included three or more dermatomes. Most of these could be driven from the splanchnic nerve, whereas neurones with receptive fields which included less than three dermatomes were equally divided between the somatic and viscero-somatic groups. Thus, viscero-somatic neurones tend to have larger receptive fields than do somatic cells. In terms of the "convergence-projection" theory of referred pain, it would be expected that noxious visceral stimuli would result in poorly localised referred sensations. Additionally, since most neurones receiving somatic nociceptive inputs are viscero-somatic, it could be predicted that noxious stimulation of somatic structures would be less well localised than would non-noxious stimuli.

All somatic, and most viscero-somatic, neurones have receptive fields which include the dermatome corresponding to the spinal cord segment in which recordings are made (T11). A few viscero-somatic cells (6%), however, have receptive fields which do not include the corresponding dermatome (Cervero and Tattersall, 1985a,b). This might result in the referral of visceral sensation to more distant cutaneous areas.

As described earlier, afferent fibres from the dorsal one-third of the dermatome terminate in the lateral one-third of the dorsal horn, whereas those from the ventral two-thirds project to the medial two-thirds of the dorsal horn. If dorsal horn neurones in the thoracic cord are classified according to their locations within the grey matter and to the dorso-ventral positions of their cutaneous receptive fields, a clear tendency can be observed for those neurones with dorsal receptive fields to be located in the lateral one-third of the grey matter (Cervero and Tattersall, 1985a,b). Neurones with ventral receptive fields, however, do not appear to be differentially distributed within the dorsal horn (Cervero and Tattersall, 1985a,b). Thus, the somatotopic arrangement of thoracic neurones seems to be less well-defined than that of the primary afferents. Preliminary studies using intracellular injections of HRP have revealed extensive branching of primary afferent collaterals in the grey matter, and large dendritic fields of dorsal horn neurones. Furthermore, the cell density in the thoracic grey matter seems to be rather low, and the cross-sectional area of the dorsal horn is considerably smaller than in the lumbar segments (see Fig. 3). All these morphological characteristics do not seem well suited to a clear somatotopic organisation. In view of the relatively featureless nature of the costal region, compared with limbs and paws for example, it is perhaps not surprising that the somatotopic arrangement of the thoracic spinal cord is less distinct than that in the lumbo-sacral cord.

Natural stimulation of viscera

Most of the studies on visceral inputs to the thoracic spinal cord have employed electrical stimulation of visceral afferent fibres in the splanchnic nerve. Natural stimulation of viscera can be achieved by using techniques such as controlled distension of the gallbladder and biliary ducts. These techniques permit the distinction between noxious and innocuous intensities of visceral stimulation (Cervero, 1982, 1983a).

Cervero (1983a) examined the responses to biliary distension of neurones in the thoracic spinal cord to biliary distension. About 30% of all viscero-somatic neurones were excited by changes in biliary pressure. With the exception of one recording site in lamina III, all biliary-driven units were found in or ventral to lamina V and none was located in lamina I. All these neurones were excited only at noxious levels of distension, that is, levels of biliary pressure which evoked pseudo-affective reflexes, including transient changes in blood pressure.

In a study of biliary afferent fibres in the ferret, Cervero (1982) described two types of primary afferent fibres: low threshold, which responded to innocuous stimuli, and high threshold, which required noxious levels of biliary pressure for excitation. The low-threshold afferents clearly included a variety of functional types of receptor, and probably subserve local motor-secretory reflexes or systemic reflexes related to gastrointestinal function (Cervero, 1982). It is apparent that spinal cord neurones receive inputs only from the high-threshold biliary afferents. The observation that noxious intensities of biliary stimulation are necessary to excite thoracic spinal neurones (Fig. 6) is in line with studies showing that only noxious stimulation of the heart is effective in exciting thoracic spinal neurones driven by cardiac afferent fibres (Foreman, 1977; Foreman and Ohata, 1980). Similarly, spinothalamic tract cells in the sacral cord of the monkey can be excited by noxious stimulation of the testicles (Milne et al., 1981). Thus, it would appear that for those internal organs from which clear patterns of visceral pain can be elicited, noxious in-

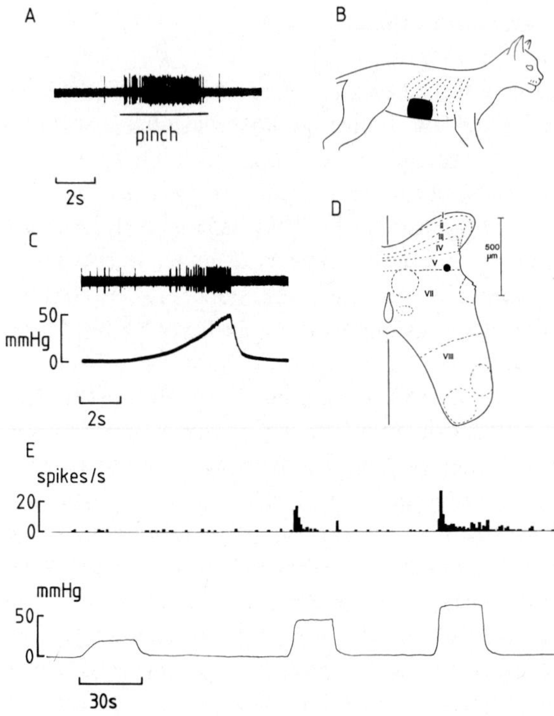

Fig. 6. Responses of a viscero-somatic neurone excited by distension of the gallbladder. A, response to pinching of the somatic receptive field. The response was greatest if subcutaneous structures were stimulated in addition to the skin. This cell did not respond to brushing of the skin. B, the somatic receptive field. C, response of the neurone (upper trace) to a steady increase in biliary pressure (lower trace). D, location of the recording site in lamina V. E, ratemeter record (upper trace) of responses to various levels of biliary pressure (lower trace). The neurone was not excited by pressures below about 25 mmHg.

tensities of stimulation are necessary to excite viscero-somatic neurones in the spinal cord. However, this is not the case in other viscera with more complex patterns of innervation and/or giving rise to a variety of sensations, for example, the urinary bladder (McMahon and Morrison, 1982).

Supraspinal linkage of thoracic viscero-somatic neurones

Ascending pathways

A major requirement of the "convergence-projection" theory of referred pain is that visceral inputs to the spinal cord should excite neurones which project through pathways that carry cutaneous nociceptive information (Ruch, 1946). Traditionally, the most important ascending pathways for the transmission of somatic pain are thought to be those in the ventrolateral quadrant, namely, the spinothalamic and spinoreticular tracts (Nathan, 1977; Webster, 1977; Willis and Coggeshall, 1978). The distribution of the cells of origin of these tracts closely follows that of viscero-somatic neurones. Spinothalamic tract (STT) cells are located mainly in laminae I, V, VII and VIII of the spinal cord and project through contralateral pathways (Carstens and Trevino, 1978; Blair et al., 1981). Spinoreticular tract (SRT) neurones are concentrated in laminae VII and VIII, although there are some in the dorsal horn (Fields et al., 1975; Maunz et al., 1978). They project ipsi- and contralaterally in the cat, but mainly ipsilaterally in primates (Fields et al., 1975).

The great majority of STT neurones in the thoracic cord receive viscero-somatic convergence, and all receive somatic nociceptive inputs (Foreman and Weber, 1980; Blair et al., 1981; Foreman et al., 1981). In this respect, they are similar to STT neurones in the lumbo-sacral cord (Giesler et al., 1981; Milne et al., 1981).

Gokin et al. (1977) recorded viscero-somatic neurones in laminae V, VII and VIII of the thoracic cord which could be excited antidromically from either the ipsilateral or contralateral ventrolateral quadrant of the cord at the C2 level, and from the reticular formation. They found also that almost all neurones in the reticular formation responded to stimulation of both visceral and high-threshold somatic afferents (Gokin et al., 1977; Pavlasek et al., 1977). Many of the axons recorded in the ventrolateral white matter by Fields et al. (1970) received viscero-somatic convergence. Although the identity of the tracts to which these axons belonged was not determined, the authors suggested that they were probably spinoreticular.

Cervero (1983b) found that most viscero-somatic neurones projecting through the cervical cord did so via a crossed ventrolateral pathway, supporting the view that the spinothalamic and spinoreticular tracts carry most of the viscero-somatic convergent information (Fields and Winter, 1970; Fields et al., 1970; Gokin et al., 1977). Viscero-somatic neurones with axons projecting in the contralateral ventrolateral quadrant were located in laminae I and VII. None of the postsynaptic dorsal column neurones recorded was viscero-somatic. Spinocervical tract neurones were found to be very infrequent in the thoracic cord, and it is of interest to note that spinocervical neurones in the lumbar cord do not respond to excitation of urinary bladder afferents (Cervero and Iggo, 1978; McMahon and Morrison, 1982). Thus, it appears that the spinothalamic and spinoreticular tracts are the main pathways of projection for viscero-somatic neurones.

Descending control

As described earlier, visceral sensory information is carried by ascending pathways which also transmit cutaneous nociceptive signals. It would thus be expected that descending controls which affect transmission of cutaneous nociceptive information would also modify the transmission of visceral signals. Indeed, STT and SRT neurones, which receive visceral inputs, have been shown to be under inhibitory control from the brain stem (Grillner et al., 1968; Beall et al., 1976; McCreery and Bloedel, 1975; Willis et al., 1977; Ammons et al., 1984).

Using the technique of reversible spinalisation by means of a cold block, two categories of viscero-somatic neurones in the thoracic cord can be distinguished (Cervero et al., 1985). The first type exhibit increased responses to splanchnic nerve stimulation in the spinal state, indicating that they receive tonic descending inhibition in the intact animal. These neurones can also be phasically inhibited by electrical stimulation in the nucleus raphe magnus (NRM) and adjacent reticular formation, and by stimulation of the ipsilateral dorsolateral funiculus (Cervero, 1983b; Cervero et al., 1985). Approximately half of these neurones are located in the dorsal horn.

The second type of neurone shows a reduction or complete abolition of the splanchnic-evoked response in the spinal state. Since the background activity and responses to cutaneous stimulation are not affected in the same manner, and indeed are often increased during spinalisation, this indicates that the visceral input to these neurones is predominantly or exclusively mediated through supraspinal pathways. The majority of these cells are located in the ventral horn and most of them are phasically excited by electrical stimulation in the NRM and reticular formation (Cervero et al., 1985). This type of descending excitation is very similar to that described by Cervero and Wolstencroft (1984) on neurones in laminae VII and VIII of the lumbar spinal cord. A parallel could be established between these laminae VII/VIII neurones of the lumbar cord and the second type of viscero-somatic neurone. The latter cells are also located in the ventral horn, have excitatory visceral inputs mediated by long polysynaptic pathways, can be driven by stimulation of the NRM and reticular formation and some of them have long axons projecting to these brain stem areas. Like their counterparts in the lumbar cord, they could be elements in a long spinal-bulbo-spinal loop, which in this case can mediate excitation to thoracic spinal cord neurones after visceral stimulation. Stimulation of viscera is known to activate neurones in the NRM and reticular formation (Lumb, this volume), thus closing a spinal-bulbo-spinal loop and providing an anatomical and functional substrate for the type of general response that can include motor and autonomic reflexes as well as a diffuse visceral sensation. This kind of response is typical of the reaction of the central nervous system to a noxious visceral stimulus.

Conclusions

The lower thoracic spinal cord receives the bulk of the visceral sensory input mediated by the sympathetic splanchnic nerves. These afferent fibres transmit nociceptive signals from many abdominal viscera to the spinal cord, where visceral and somatic sensory information are jointly processed. All the available experimental evidence supports the main postulates of the "convergence-projection" theory of referred visceral pain (Ruch, 1946). In spite of extensive electrophysiological investigations of the thoracic spinal cord, no pathway has been found carrying exclusively visceral sensory information. This indicates that "true" visceral pain is not due to the activation of specific visceral sensory channels but, more likely, is the consequence of the spread of the visceral lesion to regions innervated by somatic nerves, whose stimulation leads to restricted and well-localised experiences of deep pain. Therefore, excitation of visceral sensory receptors always evokes sensory experiences that are ill-localized, poorly discriminated and referred to somatic structures.

Viscero-somatic convergent neurones in the thoracic spinal cord fulfil all the requirements of the "convergence-projection" theory: (i) they are driven by convergent somatic and visceral inputs, (ii) their somatic inputs include afferent drives from deep somatic structures such as muscle, ligaments and tendons, (iii) most have inputs from cutaneous nociceptors, (iv) their visceral drives are active only at noxious intensities of visceral stimulation, and (v) some of them have axons projecting to the thalamus and to the reticular formation via crossed ventro-lateral pathways.

Recent studies of the thoracic spinal cord have provided considerable experimental support for traditional models of viscero-somatic convergence, but have also revealed new neurophysiological mechanisms that could explain some of the clinical characteristics of referred visceral sensation. Visceral pain from upper abdominal viscera is mediated by the very few visceral afferent fibres contained in the splanchnic nerves. These primary afferents excite second-order neurones in the spinal cord, which in turn generate extensive divergence within the spinal cord and brain stem, sometimes involving long supraspinal loops. Such a divergent input can activate many different systems, motor and autonomic as well as sensory, and thus trigger the general reactions that are characteristic of visceral nociception: a diffuse and ill-localized pain referred to somatic areas, viscero-visceral reflexes that alter autonomic control of viscera and viscero-somatic reflexes that result in prolonged muscle spasms.

We conclude that the organization of viscero-somatic convergence in the thoracic spinal cord can be compared to that of a trip-wire alarm mechanism. Such a system requires a few peripheral sensors capable of triggering extensive sensory-motor reactions when excited by visceral nociceptive stimulation. The low density of visceral sensory innervation and the extensive divergence of the visceral input within the central nervous system are probably responsible for the diffuse localization and poor discrimination of the sensations evoked by visceral nociceptive stimulation.

References

Adrian, E. D., Cattell, McK. and Hoagland, H. (1931) Sensory discharges in single cutaneous nerve fibres. J. Physiol. (Lond.), 72: 377–391.

Ammons, W. S. and Foreman, R. D. (1984) Cardiovascular and T_2–T_4 dorsal horn cell responses to gallbladder distension in the cat. Brain res., 321: 267–277.

Ammons, W. S., Blair, R. W. and Foreman, R. D. (1984) Raphe Magnus inhibition of primate T_1–T_4 spinothalamic cells with cardiopulmonary visceral input. Pain, 20: 247–260.

Bahr, R., Blumberg, H. and Jänig, W. (1981) Do dichotomizing afferent fibres exist which supply visceral organs as well as somatic structures? A contribution to the problem of referred pain. Neurosci. Lett., 24: 25–28.

Bain, W. A., Irving, J. T. and McSwiney, B. A. (1935) The afferent fibers from the abdomen in the splanchnic nerve. J. Physiol. (Lond.), 84: 323–333.

Barja, F. and Mathison, R. (1984) Sensory innervation of the rat portal vein and the hepatic artery. J. Auton. Nerv. System, 10: 117–125.

Beall, J. E., Martin, R. F., Applebaum, A. E. and Willis, W. D. (1976) Inhibition of primate spinothalamic tract neurons by stimulation in the region of the nucleus raphe magnus. Brain Res., 114: 328–333.

Blair, R. W., Weber, R. N. and Foreman, R. D. (1981) Characteristics of primate spinothalamic tract neurons receiving viscero-somatic convergent inputs in the T3–T5 segments. J. Neurophysiol., 46: 797–811.

Cannon, B. (1933) A method of stimulating autonomic nerves in the unanaesthetized cat with observations on the motor and sensory effects. Am. J. Physiol., 105: 366–372.

Carstens, E. and Trevino, D. L. (1978) Laminar origins of spinothalamic projections in the cat as determined by the retrograde transport of horseradish peroxidase. J. Comp. Neurol., 182: 151–166.

Cervero, F. (1982) Afferent activity evoked by natural stimulation of the biliary system in the ferret. Pain, 13: 137–151.

Cervero, F. (1983a) Somatic and visceral inputs to the thoracic spinal cord of the cat: effects of noxious stimulation of the biliary system. J. Physiol. (Lond.), 337: 51–67.

Cervero, F. (1983b) Supraspinal connections of neurones in the thoracic spinal cord of the cat: ascending projections and effects of descending impulses. Brain Res., 275: 251–261.

Cervero, F. and Connell, L. A. (1984a) Fine afferent fibres from viscera do not terminate in the substantia gelatinosa of the thoracic spinal cord. Brain Res., 294: 370–374.

Cervero, F. and Connell, L. A. (1984b) Distribution of somatic and visceral primary afferent fibres within the thoracic spinal cord of the cat. J. Comp. Neurol., 230: 88–98.

Cervero, F. and Iggo, A. (1978) Natural stimulation of urinary bladder afferents does not affect transmission through lumbosacral spinocervical tract neurones in the cat. Brain Res., 156: 375–379.

Cervero, F. and Tattersall, J. E. H. (1985a) Somatotopic organisation in the thoracic spinal cord of the cat. J. Physiol. (Lond.), 361: 45P.

Cervero, F. and Tattersall, J. E. H. (1985b) Cutaneous receptive fields of somatic and viscero-somatic neurones in the thoracic spinal cord of the cat. J. Comp. Neurol., 237: 325–332.

Cervero, F. and Wolstencroft, J. H. (1984) A positive feedback loop between spinal cord nociceptive pathways and antinociceptive areas of the cat's brain stem. Pain, 20: 125–138.

Cervero, F., Connell, L. A. and Lawson, S. N. (1984) Somatic and visceral primary afferents in the lower thoracic dorsal root ganglia of the cat. J. Comp. Neurol., 228: 422–431.

Cervero, F., Lumb, B. M. and Tattersall, J. E. H. (1985) Supraspinal loops that mediate visceral inputs to thoracic spinal cord neurones in the cat: involvement of descending pathways from raphe and reticular formation. Neurosci. Lett., 56: 189–194.

Ciriello, J. and Calaresu, F. R. (1983) Central projections of afferent renal fibres in the rat: an anterograde transport study of horseradish peroxidase. J. Auton. Nerv. System, 8: 273–285.

Coggeshall, R. E. (1980) Law of separation of function of the spinal roots. Physiol. Rev., 60: 716–755.

Davis, L., Hart, J. T. and Crain, R. C. (1929) The pathway for visceral afferent impulses within the spinal cord. Surg. Gynecol. Obst., 48: 647–651.

Davis, L., Pollock, L. J. and Stone, T. T. (1932) Visceral pain. Surg. Gynecol. J. Obstet., 55: 418–427.

Denny-Brown, D., Kirk, E. J. and Yanagisawa, N. (1973) The tract of Lissauer in relation to sensory transmission in the dorsal horn of spinal cord in the macaque monkey. J. Comp. Neurol., 151: 175–200.

Fields, H. L. and Winter, D. L. (1970) Somatovisceral pathway: rapidly conducting fibres in the spinal cord. Science, 167: 1729–1730.

Fields, H. L., Partridge, L. D., Jr. and Winter, D. L. (1970) Somatic and visceral field properties of fibres in ventral quadrant white matter of the cat spinal cord. J. Neurophysiol., 33: 827–837.

Fields, H. L., Wagner, G. M. and Anderson, S. D. (1975) Some properties of spinal neurons projecting to the medial brainstem formation. Exp. Neurol., 47: 118–134.

Foreman, R. D. (1977) Viscero-somatic convergence onto spinal neurones responding to afferent fibres located in the inferior cardiac nerve. Brain Res., 137: 164–168.

Foreman, R. D. and Ohata, C. A. (1980) Effects of coronary artery occlusion on thoracic spinal neurones receiving viscerosomatic inputs. Am. J. Physiol., 238: H667–H674.

Foreman, R. D. and Weber, R. N. (1980) Responses from neurones of the primate spinothalamic tract to electrical stimulation of afferents from the cardiopulmonary region and somatic structures. Brain Res., 186: 463–468.

Foreman, R. D., Hancock, M. B. and Willis, W. D. (1981) Responses of spinothalamic tract cells in the thoracic spinal cord of the monkey to cutaneous and visceral inputs. Pain, 11: 149–162.

Gernandt, B. and Zotterman, Y. (1946) Intestinal pain: an electrophysiological investigation on mesenteric nerves. Acta Physiol. Scand., 12: 56–72.

Giesler, G. J., Yezierski, R. P., Gerhart, K. D. and Willis, W. D. (1981) Spinothalamic tract neurones that project to medial and/or lateral thalamic nuclei: evidence for a physiologically novel population of spinal cord neurones. J. Neurophysiol., 46: 1285–1308.

Gokin, A. P. (1970) Synaptic activation of interneurones in the thoracic spinal cord by cutaneous muscle and visceral afferents. Neirofiziologiya, 2: 563–572.

Gokin, A. P., Kostyuk, P. G. and Preobrazhensky, N. N. (1977) Neuronal mechanisms of interactions of high-threshold visceral and somatic afferent influences in spinal cord and medulla. J. Physiol. (Paris), 73: 319–333.

Grillner, S., Hongo, T. and Lund, S. (1968) The origin of descending fibres monosynaptically activating spinoreticular neurones. Brain Res., 10: 259–262.

Guilbaud, G., Benelli, G. and Besson, J. M. (1977) Responses of thoracic dorsal horn interneurones to cutaneous stimulation and to the administration of algogenic substances into the mesenteric artery in the spinal cat. Brain Res., 124: 437–448.

Hancock, M. B., Foreman, R. D. and Willis, W. D. (1975) Convergence of visceral and cutaneous input onto spinothalamic tract cells in the thoracic spinal cord of the cat. Exp. Neurol., 47: 240–248.

Hazarika, N. H., Coote, J. and Downman, C. B. B. (1964) Gastrointestinal dorsal root viscerotomes in the cat. J. Neurophysiol., 27: 107–116.

Head, H. (1893) On disturbances of sensation with special reference to the pain of visceral disease. Brain, 16: 1–133.

Hekmatpanah, J. (1961) Organization of tactile dermatomes, C_1 through L_4, in cat. J. Neurophysiol., 24: 129–140.

Iwamoto, G. A., Waldrop, T. G., Longhurst, J. C. and Ordway, G. A. (1984) Localization of the cells of origin for primary afferent fibres supplying the gall bladder of the cat. Exp. Neurol., 84: 709–714.

Kirk, E. J. and Denny-Brown, D. (1970) Functional variation in dermatomes in the macaque monkey following dorsal root lesions. J. Comp. Neurol., 139: 307–320.

Kuhn, R. A. (1953) Organization of tactile dermatomes in cat and monkey. J. Neurophysiol., 16: 169–182.

Kuo, D. C. and De Groat, W. C. (1985) Primary afferent projections of the major splanchnic nerve to the spinal cord and gracile nucleus of the cat. J. Comp. Neurol., 231: 421–434.

Kuo, D. C., Krauthamer, G. M. and Yamasaki, D. S. (1981) The organization of visceral sensory neurones in the thoracic dorsal root ganglia (DRG) of the cat studied by horseradish peroxidase reaction using the cryostat. Brain Res., 208: 187–191.

Kuo, D. C., Yang, G. C. H., Yamaskai, D. S. and Krauthamer, G. M. (1982) A wide field electron microscopic analysis of the fiber constituents of the major splanchnic nerve in the cat. J. Comp. Neurol., 210: 49–58.

Kuo, D. C., Nadelhaft, I., Hisamitsu, T. and De Groat, W. C. (1983) Segmental distribution and central projections of renal afferent fibres in the cat studied by transganglionic transport of horseradish peroxidase. J. Comp. Neurol., 216: 162–174.

Langford, L. A. and Coggeshall, R. E. (1981) Branching of sensory axons in the peripheral nerve of the rat. J. Comp. Neurol., 203: 745–750.

Langley, J. N. and Anderson, H. K. (1894) The constituents of the hypogastric nerves. J. Physiol. (Lond.), 17: 177–191.

Leriche, R. (1939) The Surgery of Pain, Bailliere, Tindal and Cox, London, pp. 472.

Lewis, T. (1942) Pain, The MacMillan Company, New York, pp. 192.

Mackenzie, J. (1909) Symptoms and Their Interpretation, Shaw and Sons, London, pp. 297.

Magni, F. and Carobi, C. (1983) The afferent and preganglionic parasympathetic innervation of the rat liver, demonstrated by the retrograde transport of horseradish peroxidase. J. Auton. Nerv. System, 8: 237–260.

Maunz, R. A., Pitts, N. G. and Peterson, B. W. (1978) Cat spinoreticular neurones: locations, responses and changes in responses during repetitive stimulation. Brain Res., 148: 365–379.

McCreery, D. B. and Bloedel, J. R. (1975) Reduction of the response of cat spinothalamic neurons to graded mechanical stimuli by electrical stimulation of the lower brain stem. Brain Res., 97: 151–156.

McMahon, S. B. and Morrison, J. F. B. (1982) Spinal neurones with long projections activated from the abdominal viscera of the cat. J. Physiol. (Lond.), 322: 1–20.

McSwiney, B. A. and Suffolk, S. F. (1938) Segmental distribution of certain visceral afferent neurones of the pupillodilator reflex in the cat. J. Physiol. (Lond.), 93: 104–116.

Mei, N., Ranieri, F. and Crousillat, J. (1970) Limites et distribution des afferences splanchniques au niveau des ganglions spinaux chez le chat. C.R. Soc. Biol., 164: 1058.

Milne, R. J., Foreman, R. D., Giesler, G. J., Jr. and Willis, W. D. (1981) Convergence of cutaneous and pelvic visceral nociceptive inputs onto primate spinothalamic neurones. Pain, 11: 163–183.

Moore, R. M. (1938) Some experimental observations relating to visceral pain. Surgery, 3: 534–555.

Moore, R. M. and Singleton, A. O. (1933) Studies on the painsensibility of arteries: II: peripheral paths of afferent neurones from the arteries of the extremities and of the abdominal viscera. Am. J. Physiol., 104: 267–275.

Nathan, P. W. (1977) Pain. Br. Med. Bull., 33: 149–156.

Ordway, G. A. and Longhurst, J. C. (1983) Cardiovascular reflexes arising from the gall bladder of the cat. Circ. Res., 52: 26–35.

Pavlasek, J., Gokin, A. P. and Duda, P. (1977) Visceral pain: responses of the reticular formation neurons to gallbladder distension. J. Physiol. (Paris), 73: 335–346.

Pierau, F.-K., Fellmer, G. and Taylor, D. C. M. (1984) Somato-visceral convergence in cat dorsal root ganglion neurones demonstrated by double-labelling with fluorescent tracers. Brain Res., 321: 63–70.

Pomeranz, B., Wall, P. D. and Weber, W. V. (1968) Cord cells responding to fine myelinated afferents from viscera, muscle and skin. J. Physiol. (Lond.), 199: 511–532.

Ranson, S. W. (1921) Afferent paths for visceral reflexes. Physiol. Rev., 1: 477–522.

Risling, M., Dalsgaard, C. J., Cukierman, A. and Cuello, A. C. (1984) Electron microscopic and immunohistochemical evidence that unmyelinated ventral root axons make U-turns or enter the spinal pia mater. J. Comp. Neurol., 225: 53–63.

Ross, J. (1888) On the segmental distribution of sensory disorders. Brain, 10: 333–361.

Ruch, T. C. (1946) Visceral sensation and referred pain. In J. F. Fulton (Ed.), Howell's Textbook of Physiology, 15th Edn., Saunders, Philadelphia, pp. 385–401.

Schrager, V. L. and Ivy, A. C. (1928) Symptoms produced by distension of the gallbladder and biliary ducts. Surg. Gynecol. J. Obstet., 47: 1–13.

Sheehan, D. (1933) The afferent nerve supply of the mesentery and its significance in the causation of abdominal pain. J. Anat., 67: 233–249.

Sherrington, C. S. (1893) Experiments in the examination of the peripheral distribution of the posterior roots of some spinal nerves. Phil. Trans. Roy. Soc. Lond. B., 184: 641–763.

Sherrington, C. S. (1898) Experiments in the examination of the peripheral distribution of the posterior roots of some spinal nerves. Part II. Phil. Trans. Roy. Soc. Lond. B, 190: 45–186.

Sherrington, C. S. (1906) The Integrative Action of the Nervous System, Yale University Press, New Haven, pp. 344.

Smith, C. L. (1983) The development and post-natal organisation of primary afferent projections to the rat thoracic spinal cord. J. Comp. Neurol., 220: 29–43.

Stularajter, V., Pavlasek, J., Strauss, P., Duda, P. and Gokin, A. P. (1978) Some neuronal, autonomic, and behavioural correlates to visceral pain elicited by gall-bladder stimulation. Activ. Nerv. Sup. (Praha), 20: 203–209.

Torigoe, Y., Cernucan, R. D., Nishimoto, J. A. S. and Blanks, R. H. J. (1985) Sympathetic preganglionic efferent and afferent neurones mediated by the greater splanchnic nerve in rabbit. Exp. Neurol., 87: 334–348.

Webster, K. E. (1977) Somaesthetic pathways. Br. Med. Bull., 33: 113–120.

White, J. C. (1943) Sensory innervation of the viscera. Studies on visceral afferent neurones in man based on neurosurgical procedures for the relief of intractable pain. Res. Pub. Assoc. Res. Nerv. Mental Dis., 23: 373–390.

Willis, W. D. and Coggeshall, R. E. (1978) Sensory Mechanisms of the Spinal Cord, Plenum Press, New York, pp. 382–397.

Willis, W. D., Haber, L. H. and Martin, R. F. (1977) Inhibition of spinothalamic tract cells and interneurones by brain stem stimulation in the monkey. J. Neurophysiol., 40: 968–981.

Ygge, J. (1984) On the organisation of the thoracic spinal ganglion and nerve in the rat. Exp. Brain Res., 55: 395–401.

Ygge, J. and Grant, G. (1983) The organisation of the thoracic spinal nerve projection in the rat dorsal horn demonstrated with transganglionic transport of horseradish peroxidase. J. Comp. Neurol., 216: 1–9.

F. Cervero and J. F.B. Morrison
Progress in Brain Research, Vol. 67

CHAPTER 13

Visceral inputs to sensory pathways in the spinal cord

W. D. Willis Jr.

Marine Biomedical Institute and Departments of Anatomy and of Physiology and Biophysics, University of Texas Medical Branch, 200 University Boulevard, Galveston, TX 77550-2772, U.S.A.

Introduction

Although visceral afferent information does not reach consciousness to any appreciable extent under ordinary circumstances, there are occasions when visceral sensations predominate, as during nausea or visceral pain. Thus, there must be ascending pathways that can transmit visceral sensory information to the brain when required, and there are interpretive mechanisms for processing this information. However, the neural apparatus for visceral sensation need not be nearly as elaborate as that involved in somatic sensation, since it is not called upon to encode a finely grained viscerotopic map and stimulus intensity and quality need not be defined precisely (see review by Cervero, 1983a). In fact, a hallmark of visceral pain is its tendency to be confused with somatic sensation and to be referred to somatic structures (Head, 1893; Mackenzie, 1893, 1909; Lewis, 1942; Ruch, 1946). Another facet of visceral pain is that it may be associated with a region of cutaneous hyperalgesia ("referred" tenderness; Head, 1893; Mackenzie, 1893). Autonomic and somatic reflexes may accompany visceral pain (Ruch, 1946).

Some investigators have expressed the opinion that there is no true visceral sensation (e.g., Mackenzie, 1893). This view would seem to be supported by the observation that abdominal viscera can be handled, cut, crushed or burned without a concomitant sensation (Moore, 1938; White and Smithwick, 1941; Lewis, 1942). On the other hand, if adequate stimuli are used, there is good evidence favoring the occurrence of visceral sensation. For example, a sense of distension is produced when the stomach is inflated with a balloon (Nathan, 1981). Similarly, the application of mechanical stimuli exceeding 30 g/cm^2 to the stomach wall in a patient with a gastric fistula produced a pressure sensation (Wolf, 1965). In the same patient, pinching the gastric mucosa, electrical stimulation of the mucosa, or application of chemical stimuli did not cause pain when the stomach lining was normal, but the same stimuli did provoke pain when the gastric mucosa was inflamed (Wolf, 1965).

These observations suggest that sensation can arise from the abdominal viscera, provided that an adequate stimulus is used. One class of sensation is interpreted as distension or pressure and another as pain. Pain is most prominent when inflammation is present. Given the abundance of Pacinian corpuscles in the abdomen of at least several species, including the cat and man, it seems likely that there should be another class of mechanically evoked sensation dependent upon the detection of mechanical transients. Alternatively, the input from abdominal Pacinian corpuscles may play a role in cardiovascular reflexes (Ruch, 1946), since these receptors can often be shown to discharge in synchrony with the pulse (Gammon and Bronk, 1935).

This chapter will be concerned chiefly with a review of what is known about the ascending sensory pathways that convey visceral sensory information. First, however, a brief overview will be given of the pattern of visceral afferent input to the spinal cord.

Visceral afferent input to the spinal cord

Organization of visceral afferent fibers

Afferent fibers supplying sensory receptors in the viscera generally reach the central nervous system by way of components of the autonomic nervous system. Some of these visceral afferent fibers enter the brain stem by way of cranial nerves, to synapse in nuclei there, whereas other visceral afferent fibers pass through the sympathetic chain or the sacral parasympathetic nerves to reach the spinal cord (White and Smithwick, 1941).

At least some primary afferent fibers may have peripheral terminations in both visceral and somatic structures, since some individual dorsal root ganglion cells can be activated by electrical stimulation of both the sympathetic chain and a cutaneous nerve (Bahr et al., 1981; see also Taylor and Pierau, 1982). Thus, one basis for convergence of visceral and somatic sensory information onto central neurons may be by way of shared primary afferent fibers, as originally suggested on theoretical grounds by Sinclair et al. (1948). However, another basis of viscerosomatic convergence would be at the level of neurons in the central nervous system that are activated independently by visceral and somatic primary afferent fibers (see below). The latter mechanism would be most consistent with the "convergence-projection theory" of referred pain (Ruch, 1946). Referred tenderness (Head, 1893; Mackenzie, 1893) could be produced by central facilitation of transmission from somatic afferents by tonic nociceptive input from a visceral structure, a mechanism similar to that proposed to explain secondary hyperalgesia of the area of skin outside of a region of damage (Hardy et al., 1952; Kenshalo et al., 1982). The possible occurrence of primary afferent fibers with both cutaneous and visceral receptive fields would provide an alternative explanation for referred tenderness on the basis of axon reflexes and the release of substances, such as peptides, in the skin that might sensitize adjacent nerve endings (cf. Sinclair et al., 1948; Fitzgerald, 1979).

Most of the visceral afferent fibers that enter the spinal cord do so through the dorsal roots. However, some may traverse ventral roots (Fig. 1; Coggeshall et al., 1974; Clifton et al., 1976; Floyd et al., 1976). The ventral root afferent fibers include both myelinated and unmyelinated axons, but most of these fibers are unmyelinated. There is controversy about the proportion of unmyelinated ventral root afferent fibers that actually penetrate the spinal cord from the ventral root, since the number of ven-

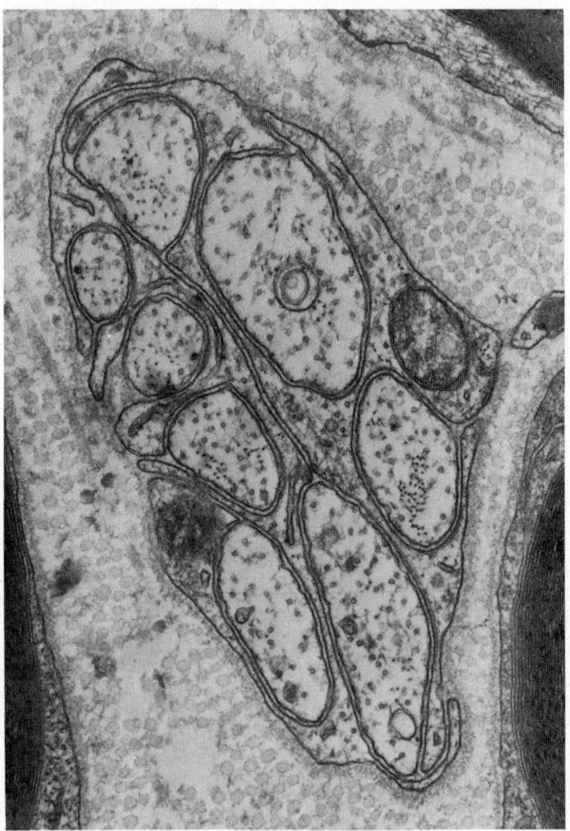

Fig. 1. The electron micrograph shows a group of unmyelinated fibers in a ventral root of the human. These are likely to be ventral root afferent fibers, since most such fibers in the cat are removed by dorsal root ganglionectomy. From Coggeshall et al. (1975).

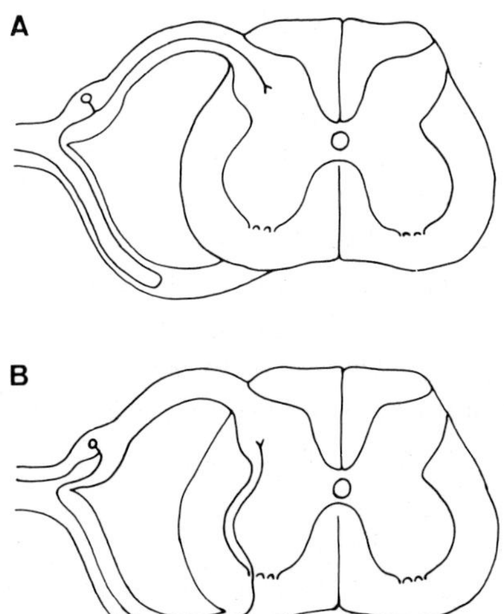

Fig. 2. A and B show two different routes that may be followed by ventral root afferent fibers in gaining entrance to the spinal cord. From Coggeshall (1979).

tral root afferent fibers is diminished when the ventral root is sectioned progressively nearer the spinal cord (Risling et al., 1984). Many of the ventral root afferent fibers may loop and enter the cord over the dorsal root (Fig. 2A). There is electrophysiological, behavioral and clinical evidence for such looping fibers (Magendie, 1822; Frykholm et al., 1953; White and Sweet, 1955; Chung et al., 1983). However, at least some ventral afferent fibers must penetrate the cord directly from the ventral root (Fig. 2B), since horseradish peroxidase has been shown to be conveyed both retrogradely and anterogradely between the spinal cord and ventral root afferent fibers (Maynard et al., 1977; Yamamoto et al., 1977; Light and Metz, 1978; Mawe et al., 1984). There is also some electrophysiological evidence for such directly projecting fibers (Longhurst et al., 1980; Voorhoeve and Nauta, 1983). These fibers may be more common in the sacral spinal cord than at other levels.

Immunocytochemical studies suggest that many visceral afferent fibers contain a neuroactive peptide, such as substance P, somatostatin or vasoactive intestinal polypeptide (VIP) (Hökfelt et al., 1976; Alm et al., 1977; Kawatani et al., 1983). However, a large number of different candidate neurotransmitters/neuromodulators are found in dorsal root ganglion cells (Dodd et al., 1984), and it seems likely that several of these, in addition to substance P, somatostatin and VIP, may be utilized by visceral afferent fibers. It will be of considerable interest if it can be shown that a given neurotransmitter is consistently associated with a given class of visceral primary afferent fiber.

Terminations of visceral afferent fibers in the spinal cord

The projections of visceral afferent fibers have been traced to their termination zone in the spinal cord by several techniques. One approach has been to utilize the transganglionic transport of horseradish peroxidase (HRP) applied to a visceral nerve. Another is to map the distribution of chemical components of visceral afferent fibers, such as substance P or VIP (recognizing the fact that substance P, for instance, is also found in some somatic afferent fibers).

A surprising finding in these mapping studies is that visceral afferent fibers have a somewhat different terminal distribution in the dorsal horn than do somatic afferent fibers. Small myelinated somatic afferent fibers have been found to end largely in laminae I and V and to some extent in lamina X, at least in the sacral spinal cord (Light and Perl, 1979), whereas unmyelinated somatic afferent fibers terminate in laminae I and II (LaMotte, 1977; Gobel 1979; Réthelyi et al., 1979). The distribution of somatic afferent fibers to the thoracic spinal cord is illustrated in Fig. 3A, right. By contrast, few visceral afferent fibers end in the substantia gelatinosa (lamina II), but most instead prefer laminae I and V (Fig. 3A, left, and 3B; Morgan et al., 1981; Kawatani et al., 1983; Cervero and Connell, 1984a,b; see also Neuhuber, 1982). This observation is of particular interest with respect to the transmission of visceral sensory information to the brain, since many of the neurons in laminae I (Christensen and Perl, 1970; Price and Mayer, 1974; Cervero et al., 1976; Menetrey et al., 1977; Woolf and Fitzgerald,

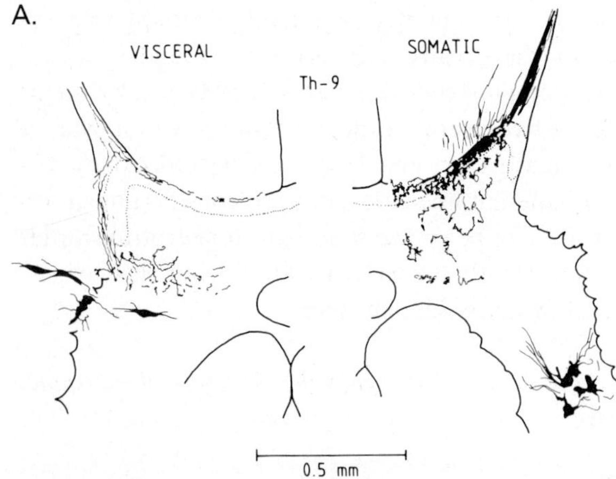

1983) and V (Hillman and Wall, 1969; Price and Mayer, 1974; Handwerker et al., 1975; Menetrey et al., 1977) are nociceptive, and several nociceptive ascending tracts originate in part from neurons in these laminae (see below). By contrast, most of the neurons of lamina II are thought to be interneurons (see review by Cervero and Iggo, 1980), although a few are ascending tract cells (Giesler et al., 1978; Willis et al., 1978). The lack of a prominent visceral primary afferent input to the substantia gelatinosa implies a different kind of processing for visceral and cutaneous information.

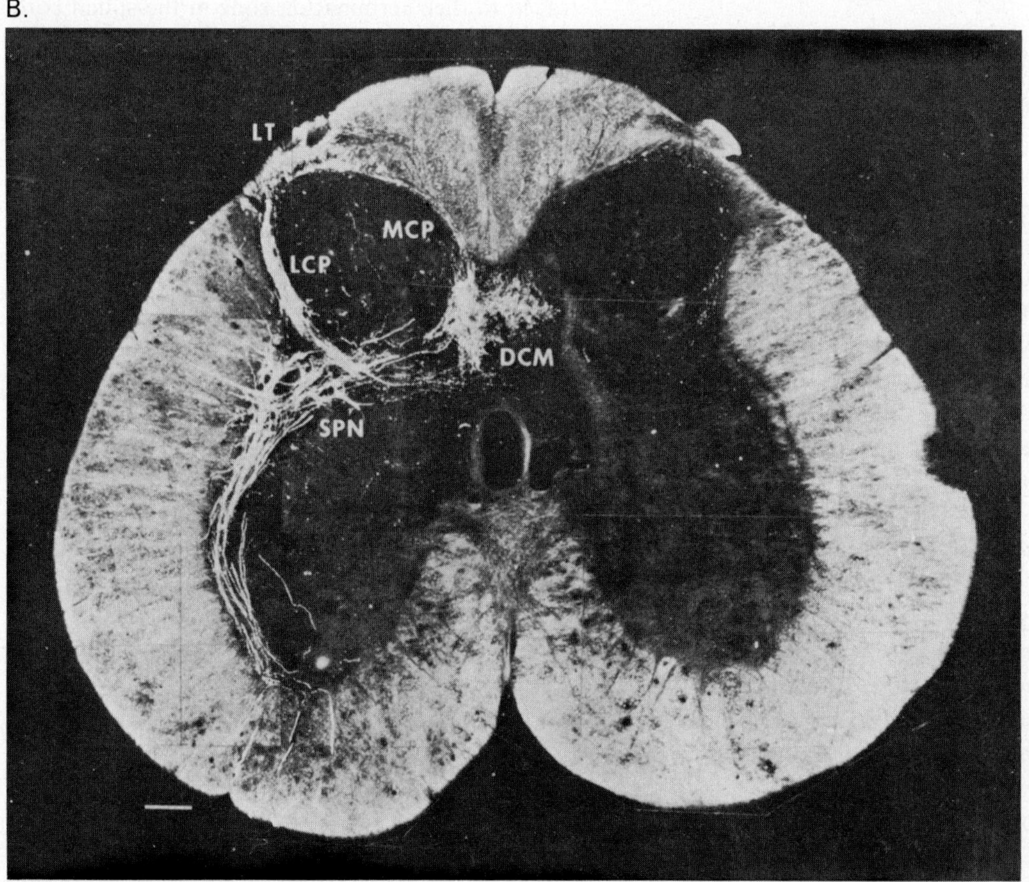

Fig. 3. A shows the pattern of termination of visceral afferent fibers (left) and of somatic afferent fibers (right) in the thoracic spinal cord, as demonstrated by the transganglionic transport of HRP from the splanchnic nerve. From Cervero and Connell (1984a). B shows the distribution of visceral afferent fibers and of parasympathetic preganglionic neurons in the sacral cord following transport of HRP from the pelvic nerve. LT, Lissauer's tract; LCP, lateral collateral pathway; MCP, medial collateral pathway; SPN, sacral parasympathetic nucleus; DCM, dorsal gray commissure. From Morgan et al. (1981).

Responses of spinal interneurons to visceral input

A detailed consideration of the responses of spinal cord interneurons to visceral inputs will be found in the chapters by Cervero and Tattersall and by Foreman et al. in this volume (see also Pomeranz et al., 1968; Selzer and Spencer, 1969; Fields et al., 1970a; Hancock et al., 1973; Foreman, 1977; Gokin et al., 1977; Guilbaud et al., 1977; Foreman and Ohata, 1980; Cervero, 1982, 1983b; McMahon and Morrison, 1982b; Takahashi and Yokota, 1983; Ammons and Foreman, 1984; Honda, 1985). The activity of such interneurons is undoubtedly of crucial importance both for the modulation of the transmission of sensory information along the long ascending tracts to the brain and for the organization of reflex responses to visceral stimulation. A major challenge for future investigations will be the determination of the patterns of connectivity of spinal cord interneurons receiving visceral input. For instance, it will be a significant step to learn how to recognize which interneurons belong to sensory or to motor pathways or to determine if a given interneuron contributes to both sensory and reflex responses.

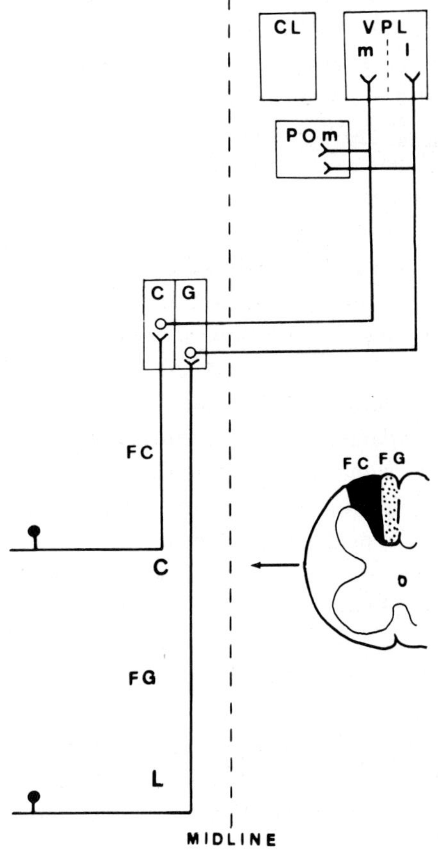

Fig. 4. The organization of the dorsal column-medial lemniscus pathway. C (below), cervical; C (above), nucleus cuneatus; CL, central lateral nucleus; FC, FG, fasciculus cuneatus and gracilis; G, nucleus gracilis; POm, medial part of the posterior nucleus, VPLm and VPLl, medial and lateral parts of the ventral posterior lateral nucleus. From Willis and Coggeshall (1978).

The studies of spinal interneurons that respond to visceral inputs cited above establish a number of points that apply also to ascending tract cells: (1) there may be some spinal cord neurons that have a purely visceral input (see Gokin et al., 1977; McMahon and Morrison, 1982a; Cervero, 1983b; Honda, 1985), (2) many spinal cord neurons show a convergent input from visceral and cutaneous primary afferent fibers, and the cutaneous receptive fields of these neurons reflect the pattern of pain referral in human visceral disease, (3) there are inhibitory interactions between visceral and cutaneous inputs, suggesting a mechanism by which inputs from either source may modulate the responses of central neurons to inputs from the other source (cf. Fields et al., 1970a).

The transmission of visceral information by sensory tracts ascending in the dorsal part of the spinal cord

Visceral information is conveyed to the brain by way of several of the tracts that ascend from the spinal cord. Although visceral information does reach the cerebellum and other components of the motor system, emphasis here will be primarily upon pathways likely to play an important role in sensation.

Visceral sensation appears to depend upon sensory pathways that ascend in both the dorsal and the ventral parts of the spinal cord. This is demonstrated by the results of cordotomies in human patients (Hyndman and Wolkin, 1943; Nathan,

1963). Dorsal pathways appear to mediate the sensations of bladder and rectal distension, the passage of urine and feces, and the completion of urination and defecation, since these sensations remain after visceral pain is eliminated by anterolateral cordotomies (White, 1943; Nathan, 1963). Non-painful sensations of gastric distension also persist after commissural myelotomy (Nathan, 1981).

Dorsal column-medial lemniscus pathway

One of the major somatosensory pathways is the dorsal column-medial lemniscus path (Fig. 4; see review by Willis and Coggeshall, 1978). This system includes collaterals of primary afferent fibers that ascend in the fasciculus gracilis or fasciculus cuneatus of the dorsal funiculus, to end synaptically in the nucleus gracilis or nucleus cuneatus of the caudal medulla oblongata. Second-order projections from the dorsal column nuclei cross the midline and ascend to the ventral posterior lateral nucleus and the medial part of the posterior nucleus of the thalamus, and third-order projections from the thalamus terminate in somatosensory areas of the cerebral cortex.

The dorsal column-medial lemniscus pathway has been studied primarily with respect to its capability for transmitting information concerning tactile and proprioceptive sensibilities (see Willis and Coggeshall, 1978). However, at least some visceral sensory information is also carried by axons in the dorsal column (Amassian, 1951; Aidar et al., 1952; Gardner et al., 1955; Rigamonti and Hancock, 1974). There is evidence that Pacinian corpuscles in the abdomen of the cat can excite neurons of the dorsal column nuclei (Perl et al., 1962; Gordon and Jukes, 1964). Presumably, the processing of the responses to stimulation of these receptors would be done by neurons at higher levels of the somatovisceral sensory system in much the same manner as for the Pacinian corpuscles in subcutaneous tissue.

Other kinds of visceral responses have also been recorded from axons of the dorsal column. For example, Yamamoto and his colleagues (Yamamoto et al., 1956) describe the activation of dorsal column fibers in the cat during distension of the urinary bladder. This observation is consistent with the finding that patients upon whom a cordotomy has been performed for the relief of pain in the pelvic region can still sense urinary tract distension (Hyndman and Wolkin, 1943; White, 1943). Perhaps primary afferent fibers mediating the sensation of innocuous distension of certain viscera ascend in the dorsal column.

Evidently, the dorsal column-medial lemniscus pathway should not be considered strictly a somatic sensory system, but rather a somatovisceral system. Furthermore, the visceral representation in this pathway appears to be topographically organized, since the collaterals of visceral afferent fibers from pelvic viscera are found in the fasciculus gracilis and not cuneatus (Yamamoto et al., 1956) and since the ascending collaterals of visceral Aβ-fibers in the greater splanchnic nerve terminate in the trunk representation of the dorsal column nuclei (Rigamonti and Hancock, 1974, 1978).

The most likely role for the dorsal column-medial lemniscus pathway in visceral sensation would seem to be in mediating such sensations as the feelings of distension of the bladder and rectum and the expulsion of urine and feces. Presumably, this pathway also participates in the recognition of mechanical transients signalled by Pacinian corpuscles in the abdominal viscera. However, this is only a supposition based on evidence for the function of Pacinian corpuscles in somatic sensation (see Willis and Coggeshall, 1978).

Postsynaptic dorsal column pathway

The dorsal column nuclei receive input from the spinal cord not only from collaterals of primary afferent fibers that ascend without synaptic interruption in the dorsal column but also from spinal cord neurons that project rostrally through the dorsal column (and also the dorsolateral funiculus). This latter pathway is often called the postsynaptic dorsal column path or second-order dorsal column path (see Willis and Coggeshall, 1978; Willis, 1985), since the neurons are postsynaptic to sensory input from primary afferent fibers.

There have been only a few studies of the response characteristics of the neurons belonging to the postsynaptic dorsal column pathway, and most of these do not address the question of whether or not these neurons respond to visceral stimuli (Uddenberg, 1968; Angaut-Petit, 1975; Brown et al., 1983; Lu et al., 1983; Giesler and Cliffer, 1985). In one recent study, recordings were made from six neurons identified as belonging to the postsynaptic dorsal column pathway by antidromic activation from the dorsal column and not from the dorsolateral funiculus (Cervero, 1983c). Although all of the cells had cutaneous receptive fields on the trunk, none could be activated by stimulating the splanchnic nerve. Thus, there is no evidence at present for a role of the postsynaptic dorsal column pathway in visceral sensation.

Spinocervicothalamic pathway

Another major somatosensory pathway that ascends in the dorsolateral funiculus is the spinocervical tract (see reviews by Willis and Coggeshall, 1978; Brown, 1981; Willis, 1985). This path originates from neurons that are located chiefly in laminae III and IV, and it synapses in the lateral cervical nucleus, which is found in the first two cervical segments. The lateral cervical nucleus projects, among other places, through the contralateral medial lemniscus to the contralateral ventral posterior lateral nucleus.

Evidence concerning a possible role in visceral sensation for the spinocervicothalamic pathway is mixed. Most studies have not addressed this question (see Brown, 1981). Two reports indicate that spinocervical tract cells in the lumbar spinal cord are not affected by visceral input (Cervero and Iggo, 1978; McMahon and Morrison, 1982a). However, one of two spinocervical tract cells recorded in the thoracic spinal cord was excited by both somatic and visceral inputs (Cervero, 1983c). The positive results came from a highly unusual spinocervical tract cell that was located in lamina VIII. There is also a report that there are neurons in the lateral cervical nucleus that can be activated by stimulation of the greater splanchnic nerve (Rigamonti and De Michelle, 1977).

The spinocervicothalamic pathway cannot be ruled out as making some contribution to visceral sensation. However, it seems unlikely that its contribution would be substantial.

The transmission of visceral information by sensory pathways ascending in the ventral part of the spinal cord

Cordotomies interrupting the anterolateral white matter of the human spinal cord can be used for the relief of visceral pain (Hyndman and Wolkin, 1943; White and Sweet, 1955; Nathan, 1963). Thus, visceral pain is conveyed by pathways ascending in this part of the cord. Sexual sensations may also be eliminated by bilateral cordotomies (Hyndman and Wolkin, 1943; White and Sweet, 1955).

Spinal neurons with axons ascending in the ventrolateral funiculus

Several studies have demonstrated that spinal cord neurons with axons in the ventrolateral funiculus frequently respond to both somatic and visceral inputs (Fields et al., 1970b; Cervero, 1983c). It is likely that many of the neurons belonged to the spinoreticular, spinomesencephalic or spinothalamic tracts (Fig. 5; see Willis and Coggeshall, 1978; Willis, 1985). An important observation made by Cervero (1983c) is that these neurons are often under descending excitatory control.

Spinoreticular tract

The spinoreticular tract originates from neurons located in several laminae, including I and V–VIII (Willis and Coggeshall, 1978; Willis, 1985). However, the largest proportion of spinoreticular neurons appear to be in laminae VII and VIII (Kevetter

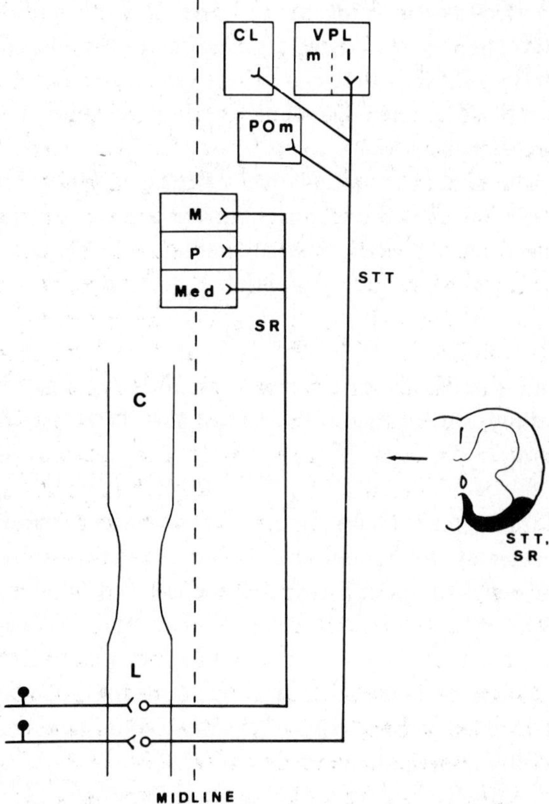

Fig. 5. Sensory pathways of the ventral lateral quadrant. C, cervical; CL, central lateral nucleus; L, lumbar; M, midbrain; Med, medulla oblongata; P, pons; POm, medial part of posterior nucleus; SR, spinoreticular tract; STT, spinothalamic tract; VPL-l and VPL-m; lateral and medial parts of the ventral posterior lateral nucleus.

et al., 1982). The axons of spinoreticular neurons may ascend in the ventrolateral white matter on either side of the spinal cord, and they terminate in several of the reticular formation nuclei of the medulla and pons (Mehler et al., 1960).

Most electrophysiological investigations of neurons identified as belonging to the spinoreticular tract have employed somatic stimuli to activate these cells (Fields et al., 1975, 1977; Maunz et al., 1978; Haber et al., 1982). A recent study by Cervero and Wolstencroft (1984) demonstrated that spinoreticular neurons located chiefly in lamina VIII could often be excited by stimulation in the nucleus raphe magnus and the medullary reticular formation. This observation is consistent with the finding of Giesler et al. (1981) that primate spinothalamic tract neurons projecting to the medial thalamus have large receptive fields, due to a spinobulbospinal loop, and that stimulation in the reticular formation can excite these neurons. At least some of these spinothalamic tract cells gave off collaterals at the level of the reticular formation, and so were likely to have been spinoreticular as well as spinothalamic projections (cf. Kevetter and Willis, 1982). Thus, spinoreticular neurons and some of the spinothalamic tract neurons that project to the medial thalamus may be part of a positive feedback loop involving the spinal cord and the reticular formation. As mentioned above, Cervero (1983c) recorded from neurons with axons that ascended the ventrolateral funiculus that were activated by descending pathways and that received a visceral afferent input. It seems reasonable to suppose that many of these neurons were spinoreticular cells with a visceral input. However, it will be necessary to substantiate this with recordings of responses from identified spinoreticular neurons following visceral afferent stimulation.

Foreman and his colleagues (1984) have shown that spinoreticular neurons identified by antidromic activation from the medullary reticular formation are commonly excited by inputs from both somatic and visceral afferent fibers. The neurons studied were at the T2–T4 segmental level and about half of those tested could be activated by electrical stimulation of the ansa subclavia or the sympathetic chain. Somatic receptive fields were most commonly of the high-threshold type and could be either simple (often on the left forelimb and upper trunk) or complex (sometimes bilateral). Some of the cells projected to both the reticular formation and the thalamus.

Spinomesencephalic tract

The spinomesencephalic tract projects from the spinal cord to various nuclei in the midbrain (Fig. 5). It could be regarded as a component of the spinoreticular pathway, but there are sufficient differences in its organization to warrant a separate nomenclature.

The cells of origin of the spinomesencephalic tract appear to be concentrated in laminae I and V of the side of the spinal cord contralateral to their midbrain targets (Willis et al., 1979; Menetrey et al., 1982; Liu, 1983). This is a major point of difference in the spinomesencephalic and spinoreticular tracts, since, as mentioned above, most spinoreticular neurons projecting to the pontomedullary reticular formation are in laminae VII and VIII and many have ipsilateral axons.

The spinomesencephalic tract terminates in a number of midbrain structures, including the lateral periaqueductal gray and the nucleus cuneiformis (see review by Willis, 1985).

There have so far been only a few investigations of the response properties of spinomesencephalic tract cells (e.g., Price et al., 1978; Menetrey et al., 1980). These do not address the question of visceral input to these neurons. However, from the facts that at least some spinomesencephalic tract cells are also spinothalamic tract cells, as shown by antidromic activation from both sites (Price et al., 1978), and that spinothalamic tract cells often have a visceral input (see below), it seems highly likely that the spinomesencephalic tract will be found to play an important role in the transmission of nociceptive information from the viscera.

Spinothalamic tract

The spinothalamic tract is generally regarded as a major pathway for the transmission of pain and temperature sensations and a minor pathway for tactile sensation (Foerster and Gagel, 1932; Noordenbos and Wall, 1979). The pathway originates from neurons in the spinal cord, projects largely up the contralateral ventrolateral funiculus and terminates in the thalamus, on the side opposite the sensory input (Fig. 5). A small proportion of spinothalamic axons project to the ipsilateral thalamus (Willis et al., 1979).

The spinothalamic tract in the monkey originates from neurons located in all laminae of the spinal cord gray matter (Trevino and Carstens, 1975; Willis et al., 1979). However, these neurons are most concentrated in laminae I and V. Distributions similar to those in the monkey have been reported for the rat (Giesler et al., 1979) and for the cervical spinal cord of the cat (Carstens and Trevino, 1978). However, in the lumbosacral enlargement of the cat spinal cord, spinothalamic tract neurons appear to be concentrated in laminae I, VII and VIII (Trevino and Carstens, 1975; Carstens and Trevino, 1978). In primates, spinothalamic tract cells projecting to lateral parts of the thalamus are found chiefly in laminae I and V, whereas spinothalamic tract cells projecting to the medial thalamus are more likely to be found in laminae VII and VIII (Willis et al., 1979).

The spinothalamic tract projects to a number of thalamic nuclei, incuding the ventral posterior lateral nucleus (in the monkey and rat, but minimally or not at all in the cat), the medial part of the posterior nucleus, the central lateral nucleus, the nucleus submedius, and several others (see review by Willis, 1985).

Neurons belonging to the spinothalamic tract both in the cat (Hancock et al., 1975; Rucker and Holloway, 1982; Foreman et al., 1984; Rucker et al., 1984) and in the monkey (Foreman et al., 1981; Milne et al., 1981; Ammons et al., 1984a) have been shown to respond to visceral input. Although some of the visceral input may have been from mechanoreceptors (Milne et al., 1981), most appeared to have been from nociceptors. Both excitatory and inhibitory actions have been described (Foreman et al., 1981; Milne et al., 1981). Most of the spinothalamic tract cells receiving visceral input have also received a convergent input from a somatic receptive field, although Rucker et al. (1984) did not find a somatic receptive field for three of the spinothalamic tract cells in their sample.

In several of the studies of spinothalamic tract cells with viscerosomatic convergence, visceral input was produced by electrical stimulation of a visceral nerve, such as the greater splanchnic nerve (Hancock et al., 1975; Foreman et al., 1981; Rucker and Holloway, 1982; Ammons et al., 1984a; Rucker et al., 1984) or the sympathetic chain (Foreman and Weber, 1980; Blair et al., 1981; Foreman et al., 1984). In these cases, it could not be detemined if the visceral input was nociceptive. However, the effective afferent volleys were generally conducted in Aδ- and C-fibers, and so there is a strong possibility that the excitatory effects were due to activity conveyed by nociceptive afferent fibers. By contrast, volleys in Aβ-fibers of a visceral nerve were usually ineffective in exciting spinothalamic tract cells. For example, none of the cells examined by Foreman et al. (1981) or by Rucker et al. (1984) appeared to respond to volleys in Aβ-fibers in the splanchnic nerve; furthermore, five of seven neurons tested by Hancock et al. (1975) did not respond to Aβ volleys. However, one of the remaining cells did, and another may have been excited by Aβ volleys.

An intriguing recent finding is that spinothalamic tract cells can be inhibited by afferent volleys evoked by electrical stimulation of the vagus nerve (Ammons et al., 1983a,b). The responses of spinothalamic tract cells with visceral input can also be inhibited by stimulation of the nucleus raphe magnus in the medulla oblongata (Ammons et al., 1984b).

The somatic receptive field properties of spinothalamic tract cells that could be activated by electrically evoked volleys in visceral nerves have been

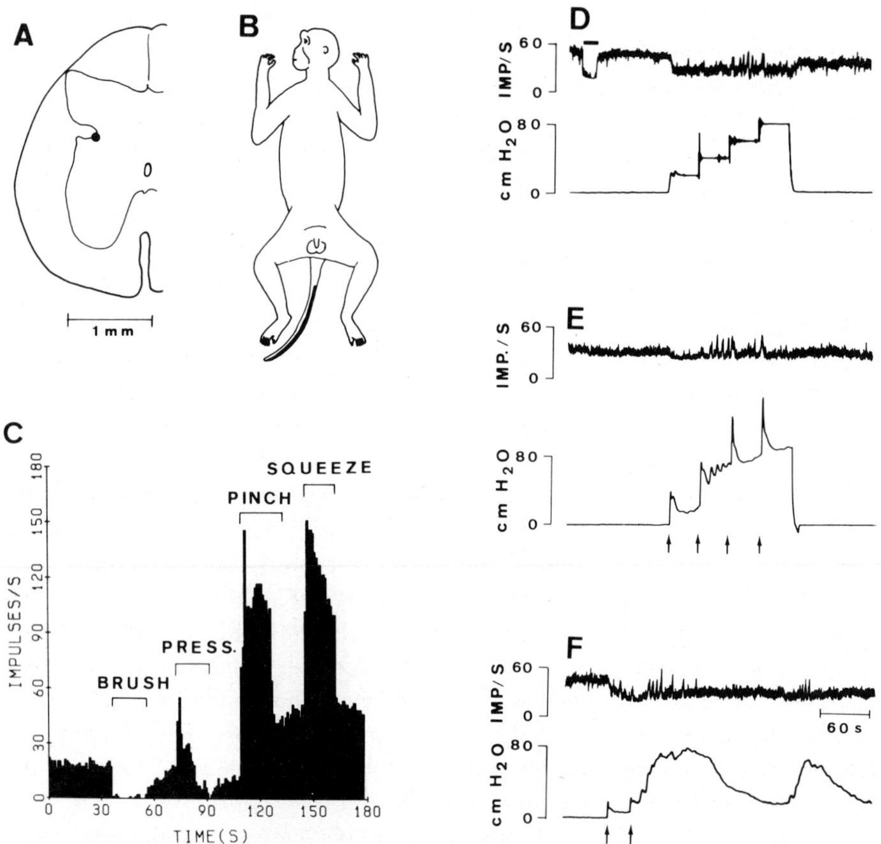

Fig. 6. Responses of a high-threshold primate spinothalamic tract cell to cutaneous and visceral stimuli. See text. In D–F, the upper traces are ratemeter records of the discharges of the neuron and the lower traces show bladder pressure. The reduced firing rate in D (horizontal bar) was produced by brushing the hair on the tail. In E, 10 ml of fluid were injected into the bladder at each time indicated by an arrow. In F, 5 ml were injected at each arrow. From Milne et al. (1981).

diverse (Hancock et al., 1975; Foreman et al., 1981; Rucker et al., 1984). Some of the spinothalamic tract cells with viscerosomatic convergence have been classified on the basis of their responses to somatic stimulation as low threshold (excited just by innocuous mechanical stimulation of the skin); others have been nociceptive, including both high-threshold (nociceptive-specific) cells (excited just by noxious intensities of cutaneous stimuli) and wide dynamic range (multireceptive) neurons (excited by innocuous mechanical stimuli but more by noxious intensities of stimulation).

Several studies of spinothalamic tract cells have utilized mechanical or chemical stimulation of visceral afferent fibers, rather than electrical stimulation of visceral nerves, to modulate the activity of these neurons (Milne et al., 1981; Blair et al., 1982, 1984). The results of the studies by Foreman's group on the responses of primate spinothalamic tract cells in the upper thoracic spinal cord to stimulation of cardiopulmonary afferent fibers have been reviewed in the chapter by Foreman et al. in this volume. The findings of Milne et al. (1981) will be emphasized here.

An example of the responses of a primate spinothalamic neuron with a convergent input from afferents supplying the urinary bladder and the skin of the tail is shown in Fig. 6. The neuron was activated antidromically from the contralateral ventral posterior lateral thalamic nucleus (not shown). The cell was located in the lateral part of lamina V in the sacral spinal cord (Fig. 6A), and it had a somatic receptive field along the ipsilateral side of the tail (Fig. 6B). Brushing the hairy skin in the receptive field on the tail caused inhibition of the background activity of the cell (Fig. 6C, BRUSH). Pressure produced by application of an arterial clip to the skin caused an initial excitation followed by an inhibition (Fig. 6C, PRESS.). Stronger and clearly noxious stimuli, such as the application of an arterial clip with a very firm grip (Fig. 6C, PINCH) or squeezing the skin with serrated forceps (Fig. 6C, SQUEEZE), caused a potent excitation of the cell. When the bladder was distended by the introduction of saline through a cannula, the cell was inhibited at low pressures, but excited in phasic bursts when pressure was high, especially during bladder contractions (Fig. 6D–F).

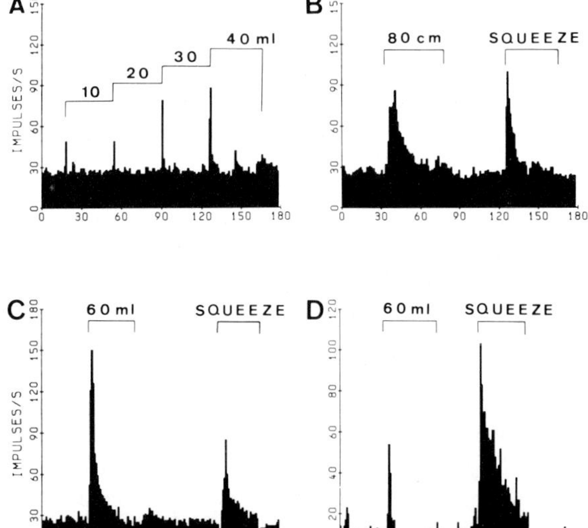

Fig. 7. Responses of two high-threshold primate spinothalamic tract neurons to distension of the urinary bladder. In A, fluid was injected into the bladder rapidly in 10-ml increments. In B, the bladder pressure was raised to 80 cm of water. The same histogram shows the response to squeezing the skin with forceps. In C, the response of the same neuron is shown to rapid injection of 60 ml of fluid. Note that the response was greater than that produced by squeezing the skin, either in this histogram or in that of B. The responses in D were from another high-threshold spinothalamic neuron (located in lamina I) and indicate that cutaneous stimulation could be more effective than visceral stimulation, depending upon the unit. From Milne et al. (1981).

Some spinothalamic tract cells were mainly excited by bladder distension. For example, in Fig. 7 are shown the responses of two different spinothalamic tract cells. Each was activated by the introduction of fluid into the bladder and also by noxious mechanical stimulation of the cutaneous receptive field (but not by innocuous mechanical stimulation). It is interesting that under the appropriate conditions the response to bladder distension could exceed the response to squeezing the skin with forceps (Fig. 7C).

Another type of visceral afferent input used to

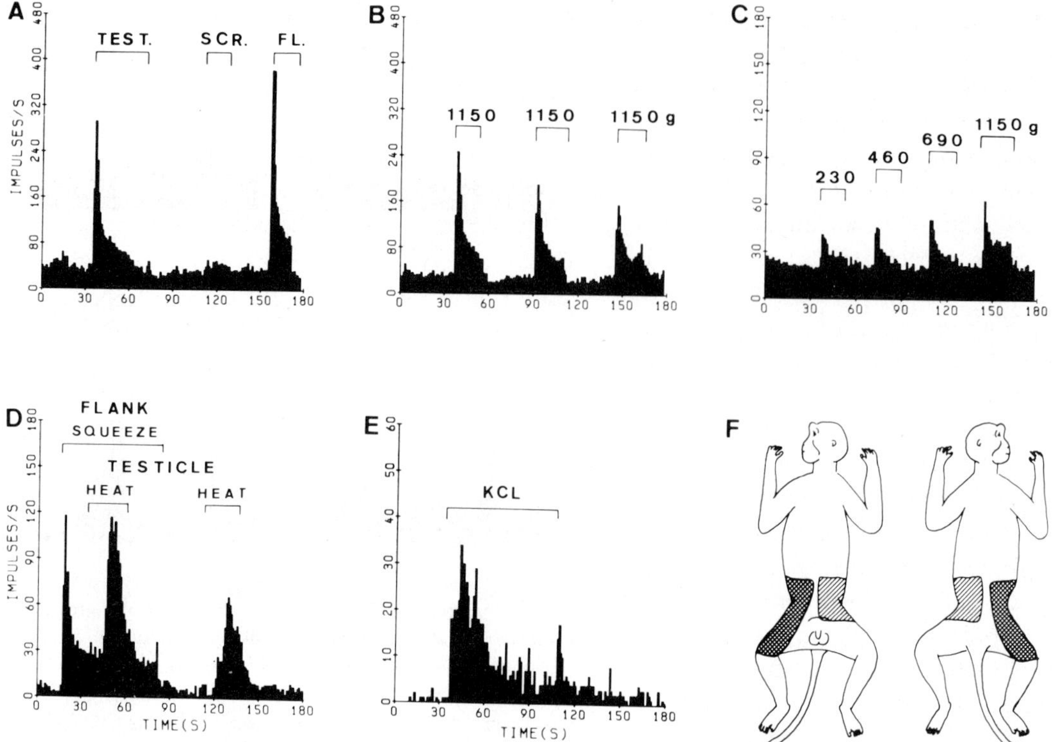

Fig. 8. Responses of three different wide dynamic range primate spinothalamic tract cells to noxious stimulation of the testicle or of the skin. See text. The receptive fields in F are for two of the cells. Note that the receptive fields extend over both the dorsal and ventral surfaces of the trunk (and in one case proximal hindlimb). From Milne et al. (1981).

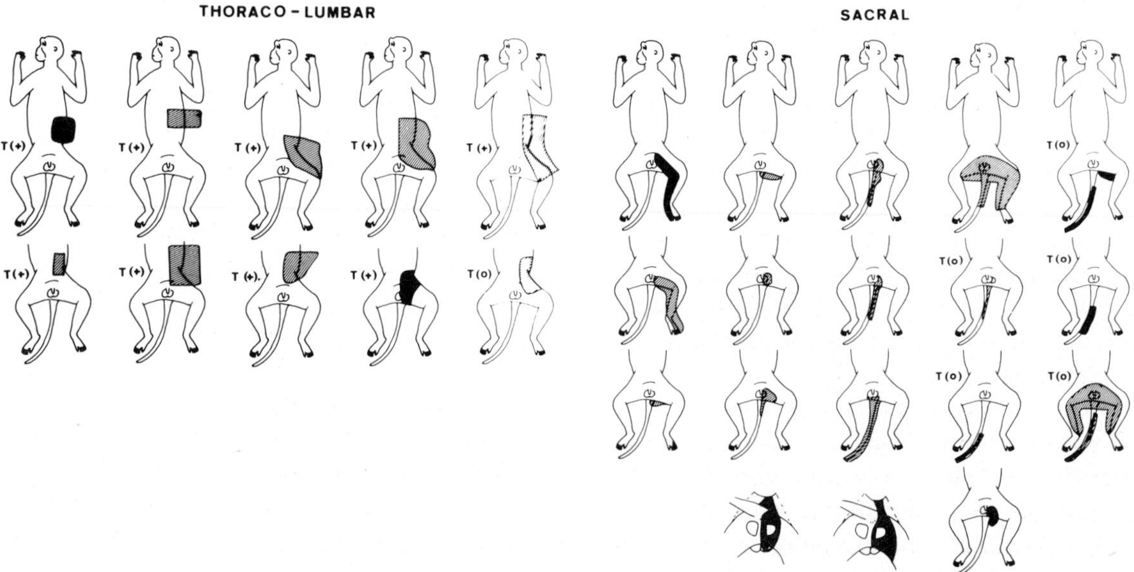

Fig. 9. Receptive fields of primate spinothalamic neurons located either near the thoracolumbar junction or at the sacral level. T(+) means that testicular input was present; T(O) means that it was tested but was not present. The apparent skin flaps indicate that the receptive fields extended onto the dorsal surface. From Milne et al. (1981).

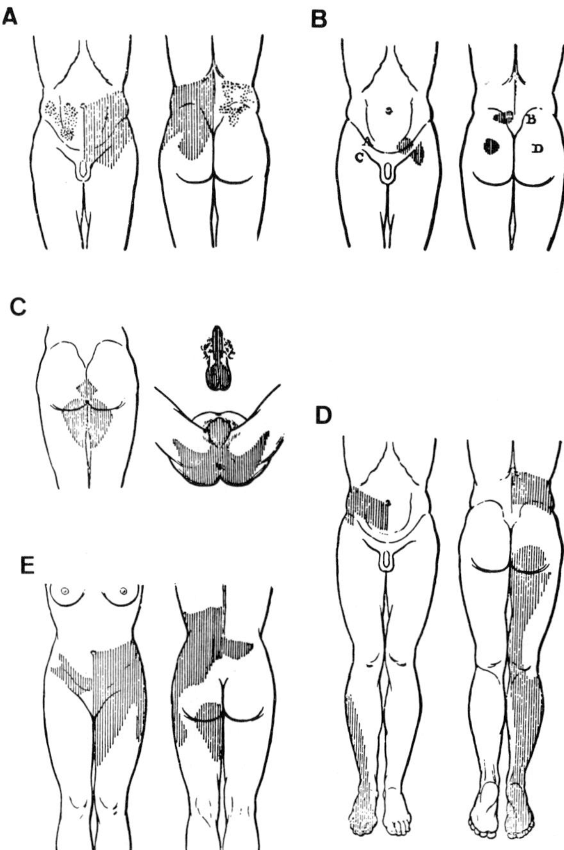

Fig. 10. Distribution of referred tenderness in: A, severe renal colic; B, gonorrheal epididymitis; C, bladder pain; D, acute inflammation of right lobe of prostate; E, second stage of labor. From Head (1893).

activate primate spinothalamic tract neurons was noxious stimulation of the testicle. Examples of such responses are shown in Fig. 8. Compression of the testicle, but not squeezing the skin of the scrotum, activated a spinothalamic tract cell, as did squeezing the skin over the ipsilateral flank (Fig. 8A). Repeated compression of the testicle caused adaptation of the responses (Fig. 8B), perhaps because of receptor fatigue, but it was still possible in such cells to demonstrate a graded increment in the response as the force of compression was increased (Fig. 8C). The input produced by heating the testicle summed with that produced by noxious stimulation of the skin (Fig. 8D). Noxious chemical stimulation of testicular nociceptive afferent fibers was also effective (Fig. 8E). The cells responding to testicular inputs were located in the lower thoracic and upper lumbar segments (and not the sacral spinal cord), and they had receptive fields that were largely on the flanks (Fig. 8F).

The patterns of viscero-somatic convergence onto spinothalamic tract cells in the thoraco-lumbar and sacral spinal cords are shown in Fig. 9. The former cells generally had somatic receptive fields on the flank, whereas the latter had receptive fields over the perineum, along the tail, or on the medial aspects of one or both hindlimbs. It is instructive to compare these somatic receptive fields with the distribution of referred pain in cases of renal, testicular or pelvic pathology (Fig. 10).

Responses to visceral afferent stimulation at higher levels of the viscerosomatic sensory transmission system

Only a few studies have been done that demonstrate activity in the thalamus or cerebral cortex in response to visceral afferent stimulation. However, responses can be recorded in response to volleys in visceral nerves as the result of electrical stimulation (e.g., Amassian, 1951; Aidar et al., 1952; Gardner et al., 1955; McLeod, 1958; Tyner, 1979) and, in at least one study, of intestinal distension (Carstens and Yokota, 1980). Clearly, more work is needed in this direction to define better the means by which visceral sensory information is processed in the brain.

Conclusions

Experimental studies of the visceral afferent system at the spinal cord level reveal several similarities and differences between this system and the somatic afferent system. Conclusions that can be drawn from this review include the following.

(1) Some visceral afferent fibers may branch peripherally to supply receptors in different tissues.

The visceral afferent fibers that do this may supply both visceral and somatic receptors. Such afferents could serve as part of the mechanism for referred pain and tenderness. (Somatic afferent fibers that supply receptors in more than one somatic tissue have also been found.)

(2) It is likely that some visceral afferent fibers, particularly in the sacral spinal cord, enter the cord by way of the ventral root. This possibility needs further investigation.

(3) Some visceral afferent fibers may utilize a peptide, such as substance P or vasoactive intestinal polypeptide, as a neurotransmitter or neuromodulator. Somatic afferent fibers may contain the same peptide, as in the case of substance P, but there may be cases in which a peptide is unique to visceral afferent fibers (possibly vasoactive intestinal polypeptide).

(4) Fine somatic afferent fibers terminate in laminae I, II and V of the spinal cord dorsal horn, whereas fine visceral afferent fibers end largely in laminae I and V. This avoidance of the substantia gelatinosa by unmyelinated visceral afferent fibers suggests that the processing of information from somatic and visceral structures in the dorsal horn is quite different.

(5) Spinal cord interneurons frequently receive a convergent input from somatic and visceral afferent fibers. Although some interneurons have a peripheral input that appears to be restricted to visceral afferents, most interneurons with visceral input have a convergent input from somatic tissue. The convergent inputs may reflect the neural processing responsible for pain referral. Besides excitatory interactions between somatic and visceral inputs, there are also inhibitory interactions.

(6) The ascending sensory pathways from the spinal cord that convey visceral information to the brain include pathways in both the dorsal and the ventral parts of the cord. In man, the dorsal pathways appear to be responsible for such sensations as bladder and rectal fullness and the passage of urine and feces, whereas the ventral pathways are concerned with pain (and also sexual sensations).

(7) Dorsal spinal cord pathways that may transmit visceral sensations include the dorsal column-medial lemniscus path and perhaps the spinocervical tract. The latter does not appear to be very important in this respect, and the postsynaptic dorsal column path has not been shown to participate in visceral activity.

(8) The responses that have been recorded in the dorsal column-medial lemniscus pathway due to the activation of visceral afferent fibers are consistent with the visceral sensory functions of the dorsally situated spinal cord pathway mentioned in conclusion 6.

(9) Ventral pathways that convey visceral information include the spinoreticular and spinothalamic tracts. It seems very likely that the spinomesencephalic tract will also be found to contribute to visceral sensation.

(10) The spinothalamic tract is the visceral sensory path that has been the most studied. Cells of this pathway commonly receive a convergent input from both somatic and visceral afferent fibers. Most of the visceral input can be attributed to $A\delta$- and C-fibers, although some spinothalamic neurons may receive an input from $A\beta$-fibers in visceral nerves.

(11) Several classes of spinothalamic tract cells, based on responses to somatic stimuli, can also be activated by visceral afferents. These classes of cells include low-threshold, wide dynamic range and high-threshold neurons.

(12) Some spinothalamic tract cells can be excited or inhibited by innocuous visceral stimuli, for instance by small amounts of bladder distension. However, more prominent excitatory responses are produced by noxious stimuli, such as the production of high bladder pressures or the activation of testicular nociceptors.

(13) Spinothalamic tract cells with viscerosomatic convergent inputs typically have somatic receptive fields in areas that resemble the patterns of pain referral in humans. Thus, they may contribute to the phenomenon of referred pain and tenderness, consistent with the convergence-projection theory of Ruch (1946).

(14) Although a few studies have demonstrated

responses of neurons in the thalamus and cerebral cortex to visceral afferent stimulation, much more work is required to determine the mechanisms by which visceral sensory processing is accomplished at the level of the brain.

Acknowledgements

The author thanks Helen Willcockson for her assistance in preparing the figures and Phyllis Waldrop for typing the manuscript. He is indebted to his colleagues with whom some of the work described was done in collaborative experiments. The work in the author's laboratory was supported by NIH grants NS 09743 and NS 11255.

References

Aidar, O., Geohegan, W. A. and Ungewitter, L. H. (1952) Splanchnic afferent pathways in the central nervous system. J. Neurophysiol., 15: 131–138.

Alm, P., Alumets, J., Hakanson, R. and Sundler, F. (1977) Peptidergic (vasoactive intestinal peptide) nerves in the genitourinary tract. Neuroscience, 2: 751–754.

Amassian, V. E. (1951) Fiber groups and spinal pathways of cortically represented visceral afferents. J. Neurophysiol., 14: 445–460.

Ammons, W. S. and Foreman, R. D. (1984) Responses of T2–T4 spinal neurons to stimulation of the greater splanchnic nerves of the cat. Exp. Neurol., 83: 288–301.

Ammons, W. S., Blair, R. W. and Foreman, R. D. (1983a) Vagal afferent inhibition of primate thoracic spinothalamic neurons. J. Neurophysiol., 50: 926–940.

Ammons, W. S., Blair, R. W. and Foreman, R. D. (1983b) Vagal afferent inhibition of spinothalamic cell responses to sympathetic afferents and bradykinin in the monkey. Circ. Res., 53: 603–612.

Ammons, W. S., Blair, R. W. and Foreman, R. D. (1984a) Greater splanchnic excitation of primate T1–T4 spinothalamic neurons. J. Neurophysiol., 51: 592–603.

Ammons, W. S., Blair, R. W. and Foreman, R. D. (1984b) Raphe magnus inhibition of primate T1–T4 spinothalamic cells with cardiopulmonary visceral input. Pain, 20: 247–260.

Angaut-Petit, D. (1975) The dorsal column system: II. Functional properties and bulbar relay of the postsynaptic fibres of the cat's fasciculus gracilis. Exp. Brain Res., 22: 471–493.

Bahr, R., Blumberg, H. and Jänig, W. (1981) Do dichotomizing afferent fibers exist which supply visceral organs as well as somatic structures? A contribution to the problem of referred pain. Neurosci. Lett., 24: 25–28.

Blair, R. W., Weber, R. N. and Foreman, R. D. (1981) Characteristics of primate spinothalamic tract neurons receiving viscerosomatic convergent inputs in T3–T5 segments. J. Neurophysiol., 46: 797–811.

Blair, R. W., Weber, R. N. and Foreman, R. D. (1982) Responses of thoracic spinothalamic neurons to intracardiac injections of bradykinin in the monkey. Circ. Res., 51: 83–94.

Blair, R. W., Ammons, W. S. and Foreman, R. D. (1984) Responses of thoracic spinothalamic and spinoreticular cells to coronary artery occlusion. J. Neurophysiol., 51: 636–648.

Brown, A. G. (1981) Organization in the Spinal Cord. The Anatomy and Physiology of Identified Neurones, Springer-Verlag, Berlin, 238 pp.

Brown, A. G., Brown, P. B., Fyffe, R. E. W. and Pubols, L. M. (1983) Receptive field organization and response properties of spinal neurones with axons ascending the dorsal columns in the cat. J. Physiol., 337: 575–588.

Carstens, E. and Trevino, D. L. (1978) Laminar origins of spinothalamic projections in the cat as determined by the retrograde transport of horseradish peroxidase. J. Comp. Neurol., 182: 151–166.

Carstens, E. and Yokota, T. (1980) Viscerosomatic convergence and responses to intestinal distension of neurons at the junction of midbrain and posterior thalamus in the cat. Exp. Neurol., 70: 392–402.

Cervero, F. (1982) Noxious intensities of visceral stimulation are required to activate viscerosomatic multireceptive neurons in the thoracic spinal cord of the cat. Brain Res., 240: 350–352.

Cervero, F. (1983a) Mechanisms of visceral pain. In S. Lipton and J. Miles (Eds.), Persistent Pain, Vol. 4, Grune and Stratton, New York, pp. 1–19.

Cervero, F. (1983b) Somatic and visceral inputs to the thoracic spinal cord of the cat: effects of noxious stimulation of the biliary system. J. Physiol., 337: 51–67.

Cervero, F. (1983c) Supraspinal connections of neurones in the thoracic spinal cord of the cat: ascending projections and effects of descending impulses. Brain Res., 275: 251–261.

Cervero, F. and Connell, L. A. (1984a) Fine afferent fibers from viscera do not terminate in the substantia gelatinosa of the thoracic spinal cord. Brain Res., 294: 370–374

Cervero, F. and Connell, L. A. (1984b) Distribution of somatic and visceral primary afferent fibres within the thoracic spinal cord of the cat. J. Comp. Neurol., 230: 88–98.

Cervero, F. and Iggo, A. (1978) Natural stimulation of urinary bladder afferents does not affect transmission through lumbosacral spinocervical tract neurones in the cat. Brain Res., 156: 375–379.

Cervero, F. and Iggo, A. (1980) The substantia gelatinosa of the spinal cord. A critical review. Brain, 103: 717–772.

Cervero, F. and Wolstencroft, J. H. (1984) A positive feedback loop between spinal cord nociceptive pathways and antinociceptive areas of the cat's brain stem. Pain, 20: 125–138.

Cervero, F. Iggo, A. and Ogawa, H. (1976) Nociceptor-driven dorsal horn neurones in the lumbar spinal cord of the cat. Pain, 2: 5–24.

Christensen, B. N. and Perl, E. R. (1970) Spinal neurons specifically excited by noxious or thermal stimuli: marginal zone of the dorsal horn. J. Neurophysiol., 33: 293–307.

Chung, J. M., Lee, K. H., Endo, K. and Coggeshall, R. E. (1983) Activation of central neurons by ventral root afferents. Science, 222: 934–935.

Clifton, G. L., Coggeshall, R. E., Vance, W. H. and Willis, W. D. (1976) Receptive fields of unmyelinated ventral root afferent fibres in the cat. J. Physiol., 256: 573–600.

Coggeshall, R. E. (1979) Afferent fibers in the ventral root. Neurosurgery, 4: 443–448.

Coggeshall, R. E., Coulter, J. D. and Willis, W. D. (1974) Unmyelinated axons in the ventral roots of the cat lumbosacral enlargment. J. Comp. Neurol., 153: 39–58.

Coggeshall, R. E., Applebaum, M. L., Fazen, M., Stubbs, T. B. and Sykes, M. T. (1975) Unmyelinated axons in human ventral roots, a possible explanation for the failure of dorsal rhizotomy to relieve pain. Brain, 98: 157–166.

Dodd, J., Jahr, C. E. and Jessell, T. M. (1984) Neurotransmitters and neuronal markers at sensory synapses in the dorsal horn. Adv. Pain Res. Therap., 6: 105–121.

Fields, H. L., Meyer, G. A. and Partridge, L. D. (1970a) Convergence of visceral and somatic input onto spinal neurons. Exp. Neurol., 26: 36–52.

Fields, H. L., Partridge, L. D. and Winter, D. L. (1970b) Somatic and visceral receptive field properties of fibers in ventral quadrant white matter of the cat spinal cord. J. Neurophysiol., 33: 827–837.

Fields, H. L., Wagner, G. M. and Anderson, S. D. (1975) Some properties of spinal neurons projecting to the medial brainstem reticular formation. Exp. Neurol., 47: 118–134.

Fields, H. L., Clanton, C. H. and Anderson, S. D. (1977) Somatosensory properties of spinoreticular neurons in the cat. Brain Res., 120: 49–66.

Fitzgerald, M. (1979) The spread of sensitization of polymodal nociceptors in the rabbit from nearby injury and by antidromic nerve stimulation. J. Physiol., 297: 207–216.

Floyd, K., Koley, J. and Morrison, J. F. B. (1976) Afferent discharge in the sacral ventral roots of cat. J. Physiol., 259: 37P–38P.

Foerster, O. and Gagel, O. (1932) Die Vorderseitenstrangdurchschneidung beim Menschen. Eine klinisch-patho-physiologisch-anatomische Studie. Z. Ges. Neurol. Psychiat., 138: 1–92.

Foreman, R. D. (1977) Viscerosomatic convergence onto spinal neurons responding to afferent fibers located in the inferior cardiac nerve. Brain Res., 137: 164–168.

Foreman, R. D. and Ohata, C. A. (1980) Effects of coronary artery occlusion on thoracic spinal neurons receiving viscerosomatic inputs. Am. J. Physiol., 238: H667–674.

Foreman, R. D. and Weber, R. N. (1980) Responses from neurons of the primate spinothalamic tract to electrical stimulation of afferents from the cardiopulmonary region and somatic structures. Brain Res., 186: 463–468.

Foreman, R. D., Hancock, M. B. and Willis, W. D. (1981) Responses of spinothalamic tract cells in the thoracic spinal cord of the monkey to cutaneous and visceral inputs. Pain, 11: 149–162.

Foreman, R. B., Blair, R. W. and Weber, R. N., (1984) Viscerosomatic convergence onto T2–T4 spinoreticular, spinoreticular-spinothalamic, and spinothalamic tract neurons in the cat. Exp. Neurol., 85: 597–619.

Frykholm, R., Hyde, J., Norlen, G. and Skoglund, C. R. (1953) On pain sensations produced by stimulation of ventral roots in man. Acta Physiol. Scand., 29 (suppl. 106): 455–469.

Gammon, G. D. and Bronk, D. M. (1935) The discharge of impulses from Pacinian corpuscles in the mesentery and its relation to vascular changes. Am. J. Physiol., 114: 77–84.

Gardner, E., Thomas, L. M. and Morin, F. (1955) Cortical projections of fast visceral afferents in the cat and monkey. Am. J. Physiol., 183: 438–444.

Giesler, G. J. and Cliffer, K. D. (1985) Postsynaptic dorsal column pathway of the rat. II. Evidence against an important role in nociception. Brain Res., 326: 347–356.

Giesler, G. J., Cannon, J. T., Urca, G. and Liebeskind, J. C. (1978) Long ascending projections from substantia gelatinosa Rolandi and the subjacent dorsal horn in the rat. Science, 202: 984–986.

Giesler, G. J., Menetrey, D. and Basbaum, A. I. (1979) Differential origins of spinothalamic tract projections to medial and lateral thalamus in the rat. J. Comp. Neurol., 184: 107–126.

Giesler, G. J., Yezierski, R. P., Gerhart, K. D. and Willis, W. D. (1981) Spinothalamic tract neurons that project to medial and/or lateral thalamic nuclei: evidence for a physiologically novel population of spinal cord neurons. J. Neurophysiol., 46: 1285–1308.

Gobel, S. (1979) Neural circuitry in the substantia gelatinosa of Rolando: anatomical insights. Adv. Pain Res. Therap., 3: 175–195.

Gokin, A. P., Kostyuk, P. G. and Preobrazhensky, N. N. (1977) Neuronal mechanisms of interactions of high-threshold visceral and somatic afferent influences in spinal cord and medulla. J. Physiol. (Paris). 73: 319–333.

Gordon, G. and Jukes, M. G. M. (1964) Dual organization of the exteroceptive components of the cat's gracile nucleus. J. Physiol., 173: 263–290.

Guilbaud, G., Benelli, G. and Besson, J. M. (1977) Responses of thoracic dorsal horn interneurons to cutaneous stimulation and to the administration of algogenic substances into the mesenteric artery in the spinal cat. Brain Res., 124: 437–448.

Haber, L. H., Moore, B. D. and Willis, W. D. (1982) Electrophysiological response properties of spinoreticular neurons in the monkey. J. Comp. Neurol., 207: 75–84.

Hancock, M. B., Rigamonti, D. D. and Bryan, R. N. (1973) Convergence in the lumbar spinal cord of pathways activated by splanchnic nerve and hind limb cutaneous nerve stimulation. Exp. Neurol., 38: 337–348.

Hancock, M. B., Foreman, R. D. and Willis, W. D. (1975) Convergence of visceral and cutaneous input onto spinothalamic tract cells in the thoracic spinal cord of the cat. Exp. Neurol., 47: 240–248.

Handwerker, H. O., Iggo, A. and Zimmermann, M. (1975) Segmental and supraspinal actions on dorsal horn neurons responding to noxious and non-noxious skin stimuli. Pain, 1: 147–165.

Hardy, J. D., Wolff, H. G. and Goodell, H. (1952) Pain Sensations and Reactions, Williams and Wilkins, New York (reprinted (1967) by Hafner, New York), 435 pp.

Head, H. (1893) On disturbances of sensation with especial reference to the pain of visceral disease. Brain, 16: 1–132.

Hillman, P. and Wall, P. D. (1969) Inhibitory and excitatory factors influencing the receptive fields of lamina 5 spinal cord cells. Exp. Brain Res., 9: 284–306.

Hökfelt, T., Elde, R., Johansson, O., Luft, R., Nilsson, G. and Arimura A. (1976) Immunohistochemical evidence for separate populations of somatostatin-containing and substance P-containing primary afferent neurons in the rat. Neuroscience, 1: 131–136.

Honda, C. N. (1985) Visceral and somatic afferent convergence onto neurons near the central canal in the sacral spinal cord of the cat. J. Neurophysiol., 53: 1059–1078.

Hyndman, O. R. and Wolkin, J. (1943) Anterior chordotomy. Further observations on physiological results and optimum manner of performance. Arch. Neurol. Psychiat., 50: 129–148.

Kawatani, M., Loew, I. P., Nadelhaft, I., Morgan, C. and De Groat, W. C. (1983) Vasoactive intestinal polypeptide in visceral afferent pathways to the sacral spinal cord of the cat. Neurosci. Lett., 42: 311–316.

Kenshalo, D. R., Jr., Leonard, R. B., Chung, J. M. and Willis, W. D. (1982) Facilitation of the responses of primate spinothalamic cells to cold and to tactile stimuli by noxious heating of the skin. Pain, 12: 141–152.

Kevetter, G. A. and Willis, W. D. (1982) Spinothalamic cells in the rat lumbar cord with collaterals to the medullary reticular formation. Brain Res., 238: 181–185.

Kevetter, G. A., Haber, L. H., Yezierski, R. P., Chung, J. M., Martin, R. F. and Willis, W. D. (1982) Cells of origin of the spinoreticular tract in the monkey. J. Comp. Neurol., 207: 61–74.

LaMotte, C. (1977) Distribution of the tract of Lissauer and the dorsal root fibers in the primate spinal cord. J. Comp. Neurol., 172: 529–562.

Lewis, T. (1942) Pain, Macmillan, London, 192 pp.

Light, A. R. and Metz, C. B. (1978) The morphology of the spinal cord efferent and afferent neurons contributing to the ventral roots of the cat. J. Comp. Neurol., 179: 501–516.

Light, A. R. and Perl, E. R. (1979) Spinal termination of functionally identified primary afferent neurons with slowly conducting myelinated fibers. J. Comp. Neurol., 186: 133–150.

Liu, R. P. C. (1983) Laminar origins of spinal projection neurons to the periaqueductal gray of the rat. Brain Res., 264: 118–122.

Longhurst, J. C., Mitchell, J. H. and Moore, M. B. (1980) The spinal cord ventral root: an afferent pathway of the hind-limb pressor reflex in cats. J. Physiol., 301: 467–476.

Lu, G. W., Bennett, G. J., Nishikawa, N., Hoffert, M. J. and Dubner, R. (1983) Extra- and intracellular recordings from dorsal column postsynaptic spinomedullary neurons in the cat. Exp. Neurol., 82: 456–477.

Mackenzie, J. (1893) Some points bearing on the association of sensory disorders and visceral disease. Brain, 16: 321–354.

Mackenzie, J. (1909) Symptoms and Their Interpretation, Shaw and Sons, London, 304 pp.

Magendie, F. (1822) Expériences sur les fonctions des racines des nerfs qui naissent de la moelle épiniere. J. Physiol. Exp. Pathol., 2: 366–371. (Reprinted (1974) in Cranefield, P. F. The Way In and The Way Out, Futura, Mount Kisco, NY), 660 pp.

Maunz, R. A., Pitts, N. G. and Peterson, B. W. (1978) Cat spinoreticular neurons: locations, responses and changes in responses during repetitive stimulation. Brain Res., 148: 365–379.

Mawe, G. M., Bresnahan, J. C. and Beattie, M. S. (1984) Primary afferent projections from dorsal and ventral roots to autonomic preganglionic neurons in the cat sacral spinal cord: light and electron microscopic observations. Brain Res., 290: 152–157.

Maynard, C. W., Leonard, R. B., Coulter, J. D. and Coggeshall, R. E. (1977) Central connections of ventral root afferents as demonstrated by the HRP method. J. Comp. Neurol., 172: 601–608.

McLeod, J. G. (1958) The representation of the splanchnic afferent pathways in the thalamus of the cat. J. Physiol., 140: 462–478.

McMahon, S. B. and Morrison, J. F. B. (1982a) Spinal neurones with long projections activated from the abdominal viscera of the cat. J. Physiol., 322: 1–20.

McMahon, S. B. and Morrison, J. F. B. (1982b) Two groups of spinal interneurones that respond to stimulation of the abdominal viscera of the cat. J. Physiol., 322: 21–34.

Mehler, W. R., Feferman, M. E. and Nauta, W. J. H. (1960) Ascending axon degeneration following anterolateral cordotomy. An experimental study in the monkey. Brain, 83: 718–751.

Menetrey, D., Giesler, G. J. and Besson, J. M. (1977) An analysis of response properties of spinal cord dorsal horn neurones to nonnoxious and noxious stimuli in the spinal rat. Exp. Brain Res., 27: 15–33.

Menetrey, D., Chaouch, A. and Besson, J. M. (1980) Location and properties of dorsal horn neurons at origin of spinoreticular tract in lumbar enlargement of the rat. J. Neurophysiol., 44: 862–877.

Menetrey, D., Chaouch, A., Binder, D. and Besson, J. M. (1982)

The origin of the spinomesencephalic tract in the rat: an anatomical study using the retrograde transport of horseradish peroxidase. J. Comp. Neurol., 206: 193–207.

Milne, R. J., Foreman, R. D., Giesler, G. J. and Willis, W. D. (1981) Convergence of cutaneous and pelvic visceral nociceptive inputs onto primate spinothalamic neurons. Pain, 11: 163–183.

Moore, R. M. (1938) Some experimental observations relating to visceral pain. Surgery, 3: 534–555.

Morgan, C., Nadelhaft, I. and De Groat, W. C. (1981) The distribution of visceral primary afferents from the pelvic nerve to Lissauer's tract and the spinal gray matter and its relationship to the sacral parasympathetic nucleus. J. Comp. Neurol., 201: 415–440.

Nathan, P. W. (1963) Results of antero-lateral cordotomy for pain in cancer. J. Neurol. Neurosurg. Psychiat., 26: 353–362.

Nathan, P. W. (1981) Gastric sensation: report of a case. Pain, 10: 259–262.

Neuhuber, W. (1982) The central projections of visceral primary afferent neurons of the inferior mesenteric plexus and hypogastric nerve and the location of the related sensory and preganglionic sympathetic cell bodies in the rat. Anat. Embryol., 164: 413–425.

Noordenbos, W. and Wall, P. D. (1976) Diverse sensory functions with an almost totally divided spinal cord. A case of spinal cord transection with preservation of part of one anterolateral quadrant. Pain, 2: 185–195.

Perl, E. R., Whitlock, D. G. and Gentry, J. R. (1962) Cutaneous projection to second-order neurons of the dorsal column system. J. Neurophysiol., 25: 337–358.

Pomeranz, B., Wall, P. D. and Weber, W. V. (1968) Cord cells responding to fine myelinated afferents from viscera, muscle and skin. J. Physiol., 199: 511–532.

Price, D. D. and Mayer, D. J. (1974) Physiological laminar organization of the dorsal horn of *M. mulatta*. Brain Res., 79: 321–325.

Price, D. D., Hayes, R. L., Ruda, M. A. and Dubner, R. (1978) Spatial and temporal transformations of input to spinothalamic tract neurons and their relation to somatic sensations. J. Neurophysiol., 41: 933–947.

Réthelyi, M., Trevino, D. L. and Perl, E. R. (1979) Distribution of primary afferent fibers within the sacrococcygeal dorsal horn: an autoradiographic study. J. Comp. Neurol., 185: 603–622.

Rigamonti, D. D. and De Michelle, D. (1977) Visceral afferent projection to the lateral cervical nucleus. In F. P. Brooks and P. W. Evans (Eds.), Nerves and the Gut, Charles B. Slack, Inc., Thorofare, NJ, pp. 327–333.

Rigamonti, D. D. and Hancock, M. B. (1974) Analysis of field potentials elicited in the dorsal column nuclei by splanchnic nerve A-beta afferents. Brain Res., 77: 326–329.

Rigamonti, D. D. and Hancock, M. B. (1978) Viscerosomatic convergence in the dorsal column nuclei of the cat. Exp. Neurol., 61: 337–348.

Risling, M., Dalsgaard, C. J., Cukierman, A. and Cuello, A. C. (1984) Electron microscopic and immunohistochemical evidence that unmyelinated ventral root axons make U-turns or enter the spinal pia mater. J. Comp. Neurol., 225: 53–63.

Ruch, T. C. (1946) Visceral sensation and referred pain. In J. F. Fulton (Ed.), Fulton and Howell's Textbook of Physiology, 15th Edn., Saunders, Philadelphia, pp. 385–401.

Rucker, H. K. and Holloway, J. A. (1982) Viscerosomatic convergence onto spinothalamic tract neurons in the cat. Brain Res., 243: 155–157.

Rucker, H. K., Holloway, J. A. and Keyser, F. G. (1984) Response characteristics of cat spinothalamic tract neurons to splanchnic nerve stimulation. Brain Res., 291: 383–387.

Selzer, M. and Spencer, W. A. (1969) Convergence of visceral and cutaneous afferent pathways in the lumbar spinal cord. Brain Res., 14: 331–348.

Sinclair, D. C., Weddell, G. and Feindel, W. H. (1948) Referred pain and associated phenomena. Brain, 71: 184–211.

Takahashi, M. and Yokota, T. (1983) Convergence of cardiac and cutaneous afferents onto neurons in the dorsal horn of the spinal cord in the cat. Neurosci. Lett., 38: 251–256.

Taylor, D. C. M. and Pierau, F. K. (1982) Double fluorescence labelling supports electrophysiological evidence for dichotomizing peripheral sensory nerve fibres in rats. Neurosci. Lett., 33: 1–6.

Trevino, D. L. and Carstens, E. (1975) Confirmation of the location of spinothalamic neurons in the cat and monkey by the retrograde transport of horseradish peroxidase. Brain Res., 98: 177–182.

Tyner, C. F. (1979) Splanchnic nerve activation of single cells in the cat's postcruciate motorsensory cortex. Exp. Neurol., 63: 76–93.

Uddenberg, N. (1968) Functional organization of long, second-order afferents in the dorsal funiculus. Exp. Brain Res., 4: 377–382.

Voorhoeve, P. E. and Nauta, J. (1983) Do nociceptive ventral root afferents exert central somatic effects? Adv. Pain Res. Ther., 5: 105–110.

White, J. C. (1943) Sensory innervation of the viscera: Studies on visceral afferent neurones in man based on neurosurgical procedures for the relief of intractable pain. Res. Publ. Ass. Nerv. Mental Dis., 23: 373–390.

White, J. C. and Smithwick, R. H. (1941) The Autonomic Nervous System. Anatomy, Physiology, and Surgical Application, 2nd Edn., The Macmillan Co., New York, 469 pp.

White, J. C. and Sweet, W. H. (1955) Pain. Its Mechanisms and Neurosurgical Control, Thomas, Springfield, 136 pp.

Willis, W. D. (1985) The Pain System. The Neural Basis of Nociceptive Transmission in The Mammalian Nervous System, Karger, Basel, 346 pp.

Willis, W. D. and Coggeshall, R. E. (1978) Sensory Mechanisms of The Spinal Cord, Plenum Press, New York, 485 pp.

Willis, W. D., Leonard, R. B. and Kenshalo, D. R., Jr. (1978) Spinothalamic tract neurons in the substantia gelatinosa. Science, 202: 986–988.

Willis, W. D., Kenshalo, D. R., Jr. and Leonard, R. B. (1979)

The cells of origin of the primate spinothalamic tract. J. Comp. Neurol., 188: 543–574.

Wolf, S. (1965) The Stomach, Oxford University Press, New York, 321 pp.

Woolf, C. J. and Fitzgerald, M. (1983) The properties of neurones recorded in the superficial dorsal horn of the rat spinal cord. J. Comp. Neurol., 221: 313–328.

Yamamoto, S., Sugihara, S. and Kuru, M. (1956) Microelectrode studies on sensory afferents in the posterior funiculus of cat. Jpn. J. Physiol., 6: 68–85.

Yamamoto, T., Takahashi, K., Satomi, H. and Ise, H. (1977) Origins of primary afferent fibers in the spinal ventral roots in the cat as demonstrated by the horseradish peroxidase method. Brain Res., 126: 350–354.

F. Cervero and J. F.B. Morrison
Progress in Brain Research, Vol. 67

CHAPTER 14

Neural mechanisms of cardiac pain

Robert D. Foreman, Robert W. Blair and W. Steve Ammons

University of Oklahoma Health Sciences Center, Department of Physiology and Biophysics, P.O. Box 26901, Oklahoma City, OK 73190, U.S.A.

Introduction

Cardiac pain often manifests itself as deep, diffuse, aching, somatic sensations arising from the chest, left arm and sometimes the right arm and jaw (Harrison and Reeves, 1968). This form of visceral pain can originate during ischemia of the heart but can also be associated with diseases of the esophagus, lungs and even the gallbladder (Christie and Conti, 1981). The purpose of this chapter is to describe the underlying neural mechanisms that can be used to explain pain associated with heart disease and gallbladder disease. An assessment of the stimuli that can be used to generate activity of the system transmitting noxious information will be discussed. Finally, neural mechanisms to explain the similarity in cardiac pain and in some cases of gallbladder disease will be addressed.

Spinothalamic tract system

The classical pain pathway, the lateral spinothalamic tract, has been studied to determine how this system responds to noxious stimuli applied to the heart and the gallbladder. The spinothalamic tract was chosen because primate (Yoss, 1953; Kennard, 1954; Poirier and Bertrand, 1955; Vierck and Luck, 1979) and human (Brown-Sequard, 1860; Spiller, 1905; Head and Thompson, 1906; Foerster and Gagel, 1932; White and Sweet, 1955, 1959) studies have shown that disruption of this system in the anterolateral spinal cord causes analgesia. Furthermore, a large proportion of primate spinothalamic tract cells respond to noxious stimuli (Willis et al., 1974; Price et al., 1978; Chung et al., 1979a; Kenshalo et al., 1979; Blair et al., 1982). Since anesthetized animals were used in the studies discussed in this chapter, identification of the activity of cells in the classical pain pathway provided a more accurate basis for studying the neural mechanisms of cardiac pain. Thus, for these studies electrical activity of the cells of origin of the spinothalamic tract was recorded during perturbations applied to the somatic structures, heart, and the gallbladder.

Somatic receptive fields

Mechanical stimuli applied to the skin and muscle at different intensities are used to classify spinothalamic tract cells according to their responsiveness to somatic inputs. Innocuous stimuli selectively activate a few spinothalamic tract cells; however, a much larger population of cells also responds more vigorously to noxious stimuli (Giesler et al., 1976; Price et al., 1978; Chung et al., 1979a; Craig and Kniffki, 1982; Willis, 1985). The three general classes of these cells are low-threshold, wide dynamic range (or multireceptive) and high-threshold (or nociceptive specific) (Willis, 1985). There is a small population of cells which are classified as high-threshold inhibitory because hair movement inhibits the spontaneous cell activity, but a noxious stimulus markedly increases the discharge rate (Blair et al., 1981).

Noxious stimuli applied to muscle also activate spinothalamic tract cells. Algesic chemicals, such as bradykinin and serotonin, injected into the arterial circulation of muscle can excite spinothalamic tract cells having receptive fields that encompass the muscle (Foreman et al., 1977, 1979).

A common feature of visceral pain is referral of pain to the overlying somatic structures. Angina pectoris in humans is sometimes reflected to the left chest and often the left forearm (Fig. 1). Somatic boundaries for the spinothalamic tract cells in primates that received sympathetic input from the cardiopulmonary region often extended from the left chest and down the forelimb, including the inner aspect of the arm (Fig. 2). The receptive fields for the spinothalamic tract cells with high-threshold input tended to have smaller receptive fields than for cells classified as wide dynamic range (Blair et al., 1981).

Another important characteristic of the receptive fields was that many of the high-threshold cells received skin and muscle input. The sensation associated with muscle pain is usually described as a dull, aching, poorly located sensation (Lewis, 1942). This sensation may be due to many of the spinothalamic tract cells receiving muscle input.

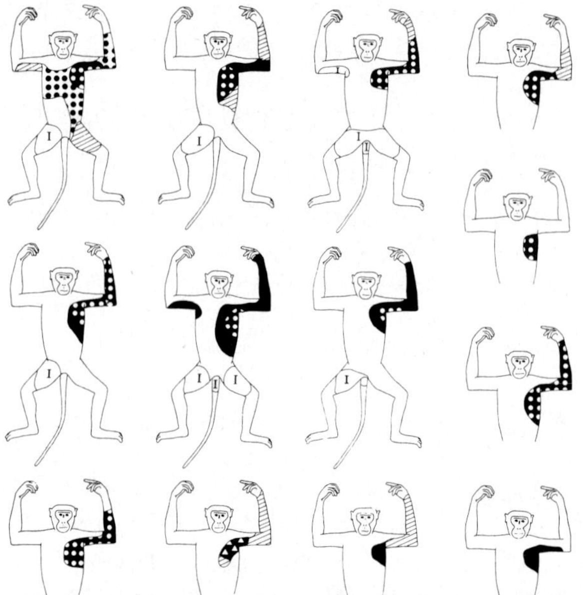

Fig. 2. Somatic receptive fields of primate spinothalamic tract cells found in the T2–T5 segments. Black areas, input from skin and muscle; white dots, excitatory hair field overlaying skin and muscle field; black dots, excitatory hair input only; hatching, area eliciting response only from muscle; white triangles, inhibitory input from hair movement; I, inhibitory receptive field from skin or muscle. From Ammons et al. (1985b).

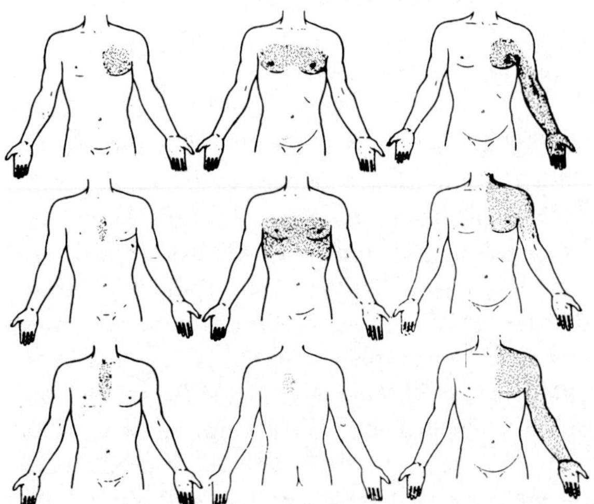

Fig. 1. Somatic fields where deep referred pain was perceived in myocardial infarction and during angina pectoris in humans. From Teodori and Galletti (1985).

Sympathetic afferent fibers

A common feature of spinothalamic tract cells in these studies is the convergence of visceral input onto the same cells receiving somatic input. Receptors located in the cardiopulmonary region have axons travelling in sympathetic nerves that are sensitive to mechanical deformation and to chemicals. Receptors are found in the ventricles and atria (Ueda et al., 1969; Malliani et al., 1972; Malliani, 1982), superior and inferior vena cava (Ueda et al., 1969), aorta (Uchida, 1975b; Malliani and Pagani,

1976), pulmonary vessels (Nishi et al., 1974; Kostreva et al., 1975; Lombardi et al., 1976), and in or near the coronary arteries (Brown, 1967, 1979; Uchida and Murao, 1974). Pressure changes within the different chambers of the heart and blood vessels (Ueda et al., 1969; Malliani et al., 1973; Uchida and Murao, 1974; Uchida, 1975a) and strain changes occurring during diastole increase activity of sympathetic afferent fibers. In addition to mechanical stimuli, receptors respond to noxious stimuli such as coronary artery occlusion and injections of algesic chemicals, particularly bradykinin (Baker et al., 1980; Lombardi et al., 1981). Currently, at least two views exist about the type of receptor that is responsive to noxious stimuli. Baker et al. (1980) suggest that a specific nociceptor exists that is responsive primarily to noxious cardiac stimuli. In contrast, Malliani et al. (1985) suggest that the same receptor may be sensitive to innocous and noxious stimuli. They argue that low discharge rates are interpreted as innocuous, and high discharge rates provide the information to allow the central nervous system to perceive pain. This disagreement about the role of receptors and their input may be misleading because integration of noxious input within the central nervous system, particularly in the classical pain transmission pathways, has not been involved in the arguments about the mechanisms underlying cardiac pain. An analysis of cell activity during mechanical deformation and the application of noxious chemicals may indicate whether mechanoreceptors, chemosensitive endings, or both, provide important inputs for cells of the central nervous system.

Axons attached to receptors in cardiopulmonary structures, particularly the heart, are composed of myelinated and unmyelinated fibers (Emery et al., 1978; Seagard et al., 1978). These afferent fibers course in the inferior cardiac nerve and ansa subclavia through the stellate ganglion to the rami communicantes. Cell bodies for these afferent fibers are located in the dorsal root ganglia from C8 to T9, with the greatest concentration in the T2–T6 ganglia (Oldfield and McLachlan, 1978; Chung et al., 1979b; Kuo et al., 1984).

Spinothalamic tract cells respond to both Aδ- and C-fiber input from cardiopulmonary afferents (Blair et al., 1981). At low intensities of electrical stimulation a volley of activity appeared which was correlated with Aδ-fiber activity. When the intensity and the duration of the stimulus was increased, a later volley of activity with conduction velocities in the range for C-fibers occurred. The minimum afferent conduction velocity for the Aδ peak was approximately 9 m/second and for the C-fiber peak was about 1.0 m/second. Approximately 50% of the cells received only Aδ-fiber input, 40% received both Aδ- and C-fiber input and 10% received only C-fiber input (Blair et al., 1981). The exact reason for these different categories is not understood at the present time; however, theories of cardiac pain based only upon results of peripheral studies should be questioned until these peripheral studies can be combined with more studies of the central nervous system.

Sympathetic afferent fibers of the inferior cardiac nerve terminate in the gray matter of the thoracic spinal cord (Kuo et al., 1984). Once afferent fibers reach the spinal cord a prominent lateral projection travels in Lissauer's tract. Axons then extend ventrally through lamina I into lamina V and the dorsolateral region of lamina VII. These axons terminate in regions of the gray matter containing spinothalamic tract neurons and neurons involved with autonomic mechanisms.

Spinothalamic tract cells with viscerosomatic convergence were found in laminae I, IV, V, and VII (Fig. 3). Since the gray matter is so small in the T2–T5 segments, fine discrimination between laminae IV and V may be difficult. However, electrophysiological locations correlate well with anatomical studies (Willis et al., 1974; Trevino and Carstens, 1975). Kuo et al. (1984) noted that small bundles of axons penetrated the gray matter every 200–420 μm in a rostrocaudal direction. We found that spinothalamic neurons often seemed to occur in clusters. These clusters extended approximately 200 μm in the rostral-caudal direction (Blair et al., 1982). Our anecdotal observations combined with the anatomical evidence indicate that a close

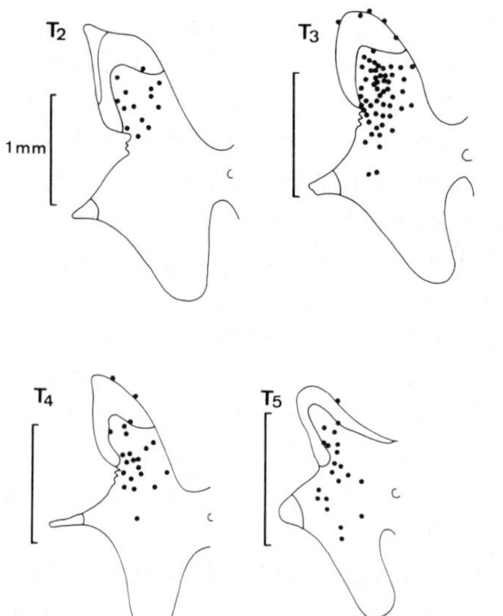

Fig. 3. Locations of spinothalamic tract cells in the gray matter segments T2–T5. The filled circles represent the locations of the lesions made after cell analyses were completed.

relationship between spinothalamic tract cell location and axonal termination exists.

"Natural" stimulation of sympathetic afferents

Aviado and Schmidt (1955) presented the hypothesis that several forms of stimuli might produce the onset of pain and reflexes in the heart. These forms of stimuli are the following: (1) reduced coronary arterial pressure distal to an occlusion acting on coronary artery pressoreceptors, (2) ischemia stimulating myocardial pressoreceptors, (3) liberation of chemical substances formed by tissue breakdown or platelet disintegration, and (4) myocardial ischemia stimulating visceral nociceptors.

Electrical stimulation of afferent fibers from the cardiopulmonary region activates spinothalamic tract cells. Since afferent fibers can arise from various structures in the thorax, electrical stimulation provides no evidence for fibers originating from the heart. In addition, electrical stimulation elicits a volley of information that does not occur under normal circumstances, whereas natural stimuli provide a temporal dispersion of the afferent activity onto cells. The stimuli used to study cardiac pain were either bradykinin injections into the left atrium or coronary artery occlusion. The use of these techniques may provide stimulation of receptors similar to that described by Aviado and Schmidt (1955).

Bradykinin

Bradykinin was chosen because it is an endogenous algesic chemical that is released following a traumatic injury. Injections of bradykinin into the heart also produced pseudoaffective responses, indicative of pain (Guzman et al., 1962). Increased amounts of bradykinin are found in the effluent of the coronary sinus following coronary artery occlusion (Kimura et al., 1973; Hashimoto et al., 1977). Sympathetic afferent fibers are excited when bradykinin is injected into the heart or dripped on the epicardium (Nishi et al., 1974; Baker et al., 1980; Lombardi et al., 1981).

For tests on spinothalamic tract cells, bradykinin (2 μg/kg) was injected through a catheter placed in the left atrial appendage. By this route bradykinin can stimulate endocardial receptors of the left atrium and left ventricle directly or other receptors after entering the coronary circulation. Bradykinin excited approximately 75% of the spinothalamic tract cells tested (Blair et al., 1982). After a delay of approximately 15 seconds, spinothalamic tract cells markedly increased their discharge rate (Fig. 5A). The response was sustained for variable periods of time and then activity gradually decreased. In addition, pinching the skin (Fig. 4B) demonstrated that cells were responsive to both visceral and somatic input. Infusion of 2% lidocaine into the paracardial sac anesthetized fibers that leave the heart. Spinothalamic tract cells were not activated after the lidocaine infusion (Fig. 4C), yet excitability of the cell had not changed because it still responded to the skin input (Fig. 4D). This evidence showed that spinothalamic tract cells are activated from receptors located in the heart. Other control tests, such as bradykinin injections into the aorta near the aortic arch and near the brachiocephalic artery, had very little effect on cell activity (Blair et al., 1982). Nitroglycerin injections to lower blood pressure did not activate the cells; therefore, the fall in blood pressure following bradykinin injections was not responsible for cell activation.

An important characteristic of the responses of spinothalamic tract cells to bradykinin is the long latency between the injection of bradykinin and the increased discharge rate of the cells. This long latency may originate at the receptor, because approximately the same latency existed when single-unit recordings were made from sympathetic afferent fibers and injections were made in the coronary circulation (Malliani et al., 1969; Brown and Mal-

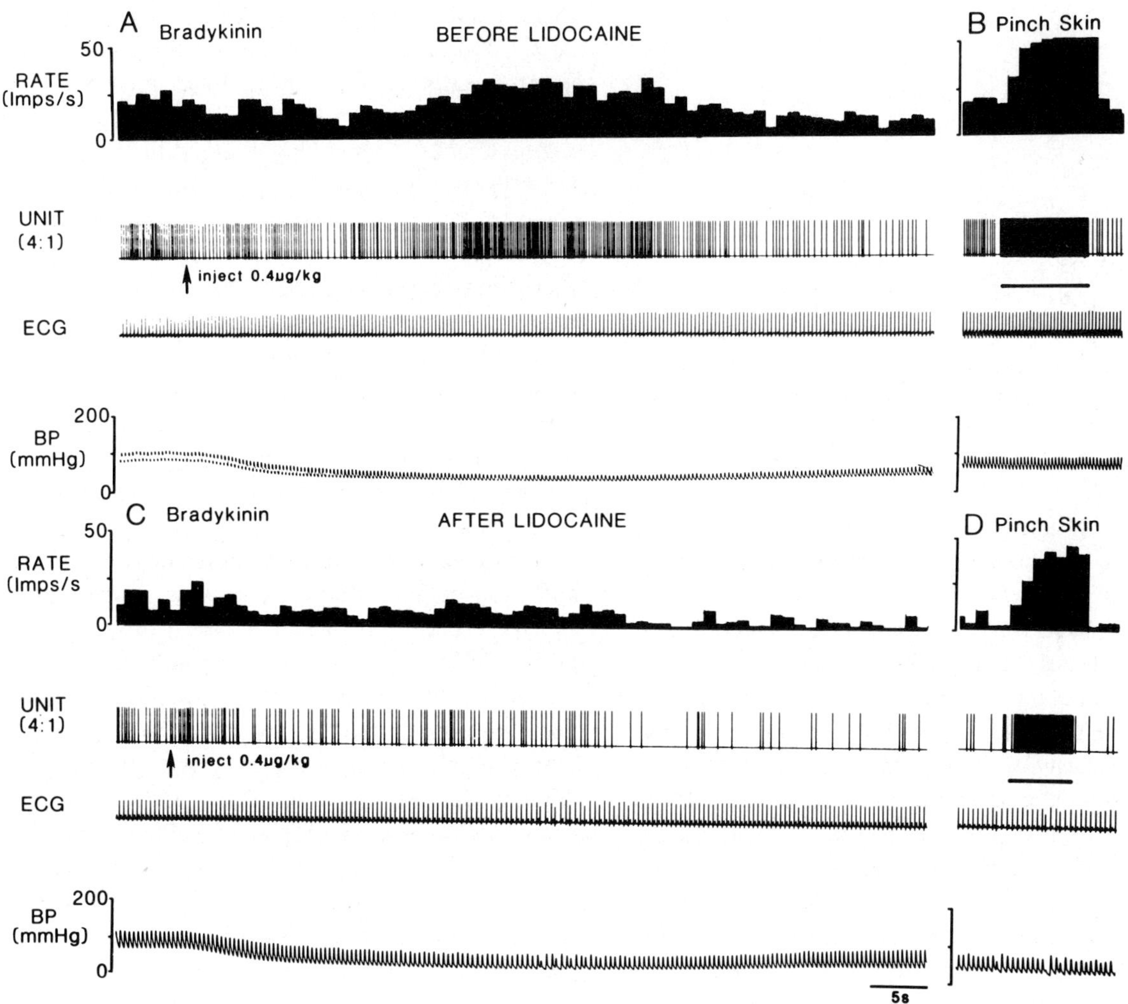

Fig. 4. Responses of a cell to intracardiac bradykinin (2 μg/kg) and somatic pinch before and after lidocaine perfusion over the surface of the heart. In the unit trace, one deflection represents four action potentials. A and C show responses to left atrial injection of bradykinin before and after lidocaine is administered. B and D show cell responses to pinching of the skin overlying the left triceps muscle before and after lidocaine perfusion. The arrow is the time bradykinin was injected. The line under the unit traces indicates the duration of the pinch. BP, blood pressure. From Blair et al. (1982).

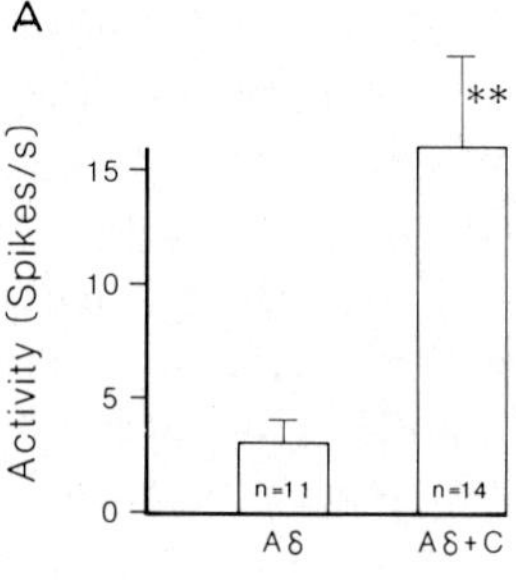

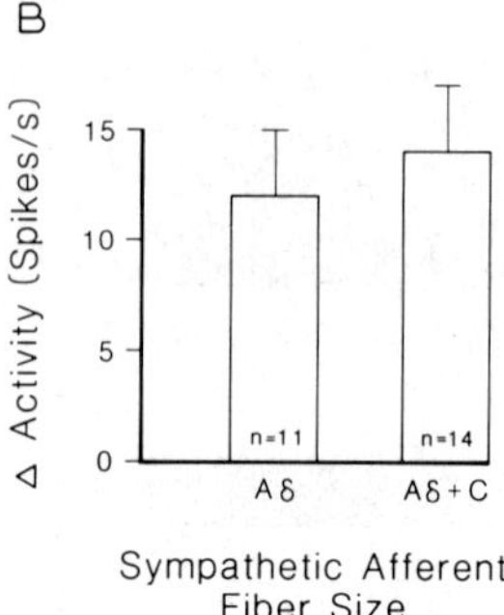

Fig. 5. Relationship between the type of visceral afferent fiber input on spontaneous activity (A) and change in activity of spinothalamic cells to intracardiac bradykinin (B). ** $P < 0.01$. From Blair et al. (1982).

liani, 1971). Needleman (1976) suggested that there might be a cascading phenomenon before the receptor is activated.

Combined results of electrical stimulation and of cell responses to bradykinin injections provide some ideas about the effects of activity transmitted in Aδ- and C-fibers. Spinothalamic tract cells that responded only to Aδ- but not C-fiber input had a very low level of spontaneous activity (Fig. 5A). In contrast, cells responsive to both Aδ- and C-fiber volleys had a significantly higher spontaneous activity than cells responding to Aδ input alone (Blair et al., 1982; Fig. 5A). These results suggest a difference in the processing of information depending upon the fibers synapsing on spinothalamic tract cells. The difference between these two populations of cells could result from a greater degree of tonic descending suppression of cells with Aδ input. This seems unlikely, because Cervero (1983c) has shown that the amplitude of the Aδ volley of spinal neurons does not increase when the descending pathways are blocked during spinal cord cooling. An alternative is that cells with both Aδ- and C-fiber inputs receive more synaptic input from sympathetic afferent fibers than cells with only Aδ input.

Bradykinin injections activated both the cells receiving only Aδ input as well as cells receiving Aδ- and C-fiber input (Fig. 5B). Based on recordings from sympathetic afferent fibers, Baker et al. (1980) suggested that the cardiac nociceptors were C-fibers. Data supporting this theory of nociception from C-fibers were also presented for somatic afferents (Guilbaud et al., 1976). Since spinothalamic tract cells transmit noxious information, cells receiving C-fiber input should respond to bradykinin and cells with no C-fiber input should not respond. However, 68% of the cells receiving only Aδ input responded to bradykinin, but three cells with C-fiber input only did not respond. In addition, cell activity for the population receiving only Aδ input increased by 400%, whereas the cell population receiving Aδ- and C-fiber input increased by 88% (Blair et al., 1982). Thus, the larger percentage change resulting from Aδ input may be an important signal for transmitting noxious cardiac input to the thalamus.

Entrainment of spinothalamic tract cell activity with each cardiac cycle may provide insights into the type of receptors being activated following bradykinin injections. Approximately 40% of the spinothalamic tract cells increased their cell activity after bradykinin injections, and several seconds later cell activity was entrained to the cardiac cycle (Blair et al., 1982; Ammons et al., 1983, 1985a,b). The initial random increase in cell activity is likely due to activation of mechanosensitive and chemosensitive afferents, and the later entrained activity may be due to sensitization of mechanosensitive afferent fibers. Bradykinin excites afferent fibers sensitive to mechanical as well as chemical events in the heart (Baker et al., 1980; Lombardi et al., 1981). In summary, most of the spinothalamic tract cells seem to be sensitive primarily to chemical stimulation of the heart, although a population of cells also become active with mechanical events of the heart.

Bradykinin has been used as a noxious cardiac stimulus in many studies. However, Pagani and his colleagues (1985) have shown recently that bradykinin produces pressor reflexes without eliciting pseudoaffective pain response in conscious dogs. Our interpretation of the effects of bradykinin differs from the conclusions of Pagani et al. (1985), because we have shown that spinothalamic tract cells responding to cardiac injections of bradykinin vigorously excited 75% of the cells we studied. Since the spinothalamic tract is the classical pain pathway, we assume that animals would have perceived pain in the conscious state. This assumption is supported by the work of Hoffman et al. (1981), who showed that response characteristics of trigeminothalamic tract cells to noxious stimuli were similar in the conscious and the anesthetized preparations. Therefore, the anesthetized state does not seem to provide a logical explanation for the difference. There may be some problem with effects of noxious stimuli on laboratory-conditioned dogs. There is a possibility that these animals may be conditioned so that they are able to suppress responses to pain. Conditioning may activate the descending control system that effectively suppresses noxious information. An animal in a novel situation might express pseudoaffective responses more readily, because the animals are not conditioned to the investigators or their environment. Furthermore, earlier reports in the literature showed that bradykinin does cause pain in animals (Guzman et al., 1962; Besson et al., 1974) and in humans (Armstrong et al., 1953, 1957; Elliot et al., 1960; Lim and Guzman, 1968; Keele and Armstrong, 1969; Bleehen and Keele, 1977; Chahl, 1979; Chahl and Kirk, 1975). Thus, bradykinin certainly is a noxious stimulus, but may be one of several substances that are released and contribute to the pain felt during myocardial ischemia.

Animals used by Pagani et al. (1985) should have been trained to avoid an aversive noxious stimulus. If this psychological tool had been used, then the assessment of pain could have been valid. Unfortunately, their studies do not conclusively demonstrate that the animals did not experience an aversive behavior to bradykinin.

Coronary artery occlusion

Coronary artery occlusion is a technique used for simulating ischemia that is often associated with cardiac pain, and particularly angina pectoris. Experimental coronary artery occlusions differ from the clinical manifestations of coronary heart disease, because in the clinical situation there is usually a gradual occluding of diseased vessels and angina pectoris is often experienced only during increased exertion. However, there is a population of patients who experience angina pectoris, because the coronary arteries seem to close suddenly when coronary vasospasm occurs.

Experimental coronary artery occlusion usually excites sympathetic afferent fibers approximately 10–20 seconds after the onset (Brown, 1967; Brown and Malliani, 1971; Uchida and Murao, 1974; Bosnjak et al., 1979; Casati et al., 1979) and often initiates cardiac reflexes (Malliani et al., 1969; Brown and Malliani, 1971; Malliani and Lombardi, 1978; Brown, 1979; Felder and Thames, 1981). To determine if spinothalamic tract cells responded to experimental coronary artery occlusion, the effects on cell activity of occluding either left circumflex artery or left anterior descending artery were examined (Blair et al., 1984b). The activity of 19 spinothalamic tract cells, as well as spinoreticular tract cells, was recorded during occlusion of one coronary artery, and 14 cells were tested for responses to left anterior descending and left circumflex occlusion, making a total of 47 responses (Blair et al., 1984b). Four different patterns of responses were observed. These patterns were: (1) cell activity generally increased during myocardial ischemia produced by the experimental occlusion (IS response), (2) cell activity increased at the onset of the occlusion, adapted, and then increased again as ischemia developed (ON-IS response), (3) cell activity increased at the onset or release of occlusion and rapidly adapted or remained elevated throughout the

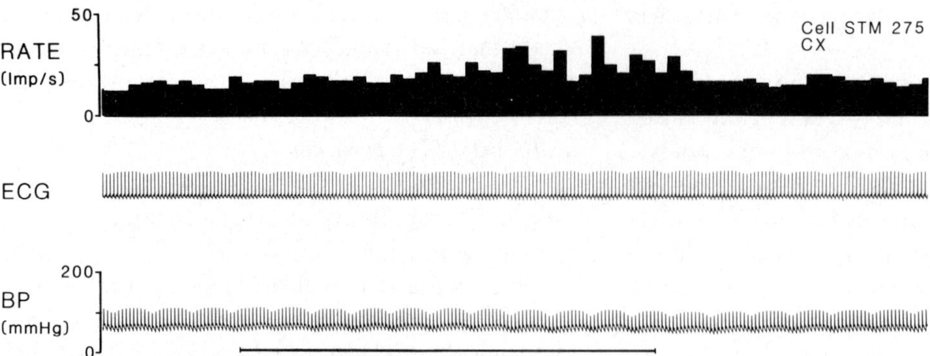

Fig. 6. Responses of a primate spinothalamic tract cell to occlusion of the left circumflex (CX) coronary artery. The top trace is cell discharge rate in impulses per second (imp/s), second trace is electrocardiogram (ECG), and third trace is blood pressure (BP). Duration of occlusion is indicated by black line under blood pressure trace. This record shows a response classified as ischemic (IS). From Blair et al. (1984b).

occlusion (ON response), and (4) no response to occlusion (NR). For cells responsive during ischemia the average latency following onset of the occlusion to onset of increased activity was 13 seconds, and cell activity increased from 12 to 20 spikes/second (Fig. 6) ($P < 0.001$). Although the ECG does not show much change in this figure, systolic bulging was observed, and the heart in the area supplied by the coronary artery markedly changed its color. Thus, these cells were most likely responding to ischemia produced during the experimental occlusion. In contrast, cells that responded immediately to the occlusion might be caused by deformation of receptors within or near the coronary artery.

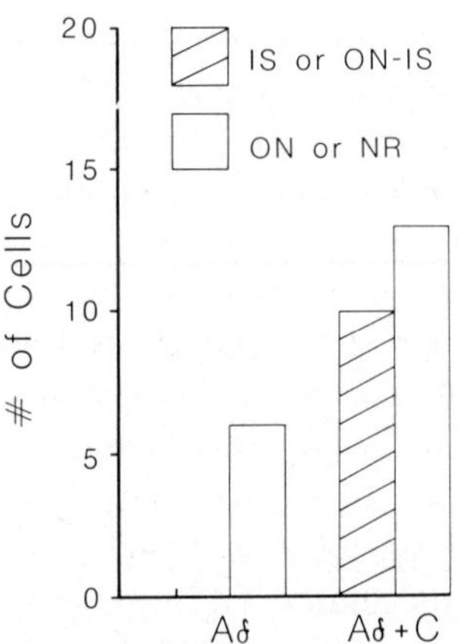

Fig. 7. Relationship between the response of cell to occlusion and the type of visceral afferent fiber input onto the cell. Responses are divided according to the response to ischemia. Note that C-fiber input was significantly related ($P < 0.05$) to the response to ischemia. Modified from Blair et al. (1984b).

All spinothalamic tract cells responsive to coronary artery occlusion received sympathetic afferent input from Aδ-fibers. In addition, 23 cells received input from C-fibers. To determine whether the type of input was related to class of response, cells were grouped according to their response to ischemia (Fig. 7). A cell was classified as responsive to ischemia if it had an ischemic (IS) or on-ischemic (ON-IS) response to occlusion of any single coronary artery. No cells with only Aδ input responded to ischemia, but ten cells with both Aδ- and C-fiber inputs did respond. Thus, sympathetic afferent activity from C-fibers seemed to be necessary for eliciting an ischemic response, but not all cells with C-fiber input responded to ischemia.

The role of the C-fibers in signaling nociceptive information for visceral (Baker et al., 1980) as well as somatic (Guilbaud et al., 1976) afferent fibers has been emphasized. The effectiveness of the C-fiber input appears to differ, depending on the type of noxious cardiac stimulus. C-fibers were not necessary for the spinothalamic tract cell responses to bradykinin, but they were necessary for the responses to ischemia. There is a possibility that the bradykinin stimulus activates both chemosensitive and mechanosensitive fibers whereas the experimental occlusion stimulus activates primarily the chemosensitive fibers. The chemosensitive fibers appear to be primarily comprised of C-fibers (Baker et al., 1980). Further support for this distinction comes from the observation that about half of the cells responsive to bradykinin exhibited cell activity associated with the cardiac cycle, leading to the suggestion that mechanoreceptors were sensitized. In addition, the type of input was not related to whether a cell would exhibit an IS or ON response to occlusion. These results demonstrate that any model for cardiac pain must take into consideration the complexities of the interactions occurring in the spinal cord and not depend entirely on the studies of peripheral fibers.

Mechanisms of cardiac pain

Ischemic heart disease often elicits pain. The symptoms are complex and often without any definite pattern. This pain, which seems to be without rules, was addressed by Procacci and Zoppi (1985). They suggest that very careful observation of symptoms associated with angina pectoris may be diagnosed even if laboratory signs are initially negative. To diagnose cardiac pain appropriately, a physician must not only investigate where the pain is felt, but also distinguish between true visceral pain and referred pain and, in addition, determine if the pain is referred to deep or superficial structures. According to Procacci and Zoppi (1985), as described initially by Ross (1887), visceral pain is dull, aching or boring, not well-localized and described differently by patients. This pain is always accompanied by a sense of malaise and a sense of being ill. In addition, strong autonomic reflexes and an intense alarm reaction are associated with visceral pain. Referred pain occurs when an algogenic process recurs frequently or becomes more intense and prolonged within a visceral organ. The location is more exact and the painful sensation is gradually felt in more superficial structures, sometimes far from the site of origin.

Patients experiencing angina pectoris often sense pain that is generally referred, often deep, and lasts for 30 seconds to 30 minutes. Pain is not associated with a feeling of impending death, nausea and vomiting, but it is related to exertion, cold, abundant meals, and strong emotions (Procacci and Zoppi, 1985).

Neurophysiological mechanisms described in this chapter provide a partial explanation for the clinical presentations of patients experiencing angina pectoris. The "convergence-projection" theory of Ruch (1961) provides the best explanation for describing the neural mechanisms associated with referred pain. Ruch (1961) stated that "some visceral afferents converge with cutaneous pain afferents to end upon the same neuron at some point in the sensory pathway — spinal, thalamic or cortical — and that the system of fibers is sufficiently organized topographically to provide the dermatomal reference". The first synapse where the viscerosomatic convergence occurs is the spinothalamic tract. All thoracic spinothalamic tract cells receive visceral and somatic convergence. Both cutaneous and muscle afferent fibers usually originating from the chest and/or left arm excite these spinothalamic tract cells. Noxious cardiac stimuli such as coronary artery occlusion and algesic chemical injections excite these spinothalamic tract cells terminating in the ventral posterior lateral nucleus. The neospinothalamic tract is primarily responsible for relaying information from a specific part of the body surface to a specific region of the ventral posterior lateral nucleus of the thalamus. The somatotopic organization of this system may subserve sensory discriminative aspects of pain (Mehler et al., 1960; Melzack and Casey, 1968; Price and Dubner, 1977). The receptive fields shown in Fig. 2 support this concept of neospinothalamic tract cells with discrete, localized somatic receptive fields. The neospinothalamic tract system provides information about sensory-discriminitive responses, but not about autonomic and behavioral changes. The paleospinothalamic tract system projects to the medial thalamus and may provide the neural substrate for motivational-affective aspects of pain (Mehler et al., 1960; Melzack and Casey, 1968). Motivational-affective components associated with ischemic heart disease may be produced, because the paleo-(medial) spinothalamic tract is activated. Our work has shown that this pathway receives visceral and somatic inputs (Ammons et al., 1985b) and transmits information about noxious cardiac stimuli (Ammons et al., 1985a).

Ischemic heart disease also produces autonomic responses which likely involve the brainstem and bulbospinal pathways. Autonomic adjustments during angina pectoris may occur because sympathetic afferent fibers activate spinal pathways, such as the spinoreticular and spinoreticular-spinothalamic tracts that are excited by somatic manipulation and noxious cardiac stimuli (Foreman et al., 1984; Blair et al., 1984a,b), that project to medullary regions involved with cardiovascular adjustments (Wang and Ranson, 1939; Alexander, 1946; Gebber, 1980; Barman and Gebber, 1983; Blair, 1985).

In summary, neural mechanisms underlying clinical symptoms associated with angina pectoris have been described. We have not explained the distinction that Procacci and Zoppi (1985) make between visceral pain and referred pain. Their description of visceral pain implies a separate pathway being responsible only for visceral pain. All spinal cord studies using identified projecting neurons to the brainstem have not demonstrated a separate ascending pathway specific for visceral information. Perhaps visceral pain and referred pain use the same pathway but central processing is different at different times in the disease process. This should be examined in future studies.

Anginal-like pain

Chest pain can occur with a variety of disorders that originate from both somatic and visceral structures (Cohn and Brunwald, 1980). Angina pectoris, a common chest pain originating from the visceral structures, was discussed in the previous section. Since a significant number of patients may exhibit anginal-like pain but have normal cardiac function, another level of complexity needs to be addressed. Many of these patients may have gastrointestinal disorders, particularly hiatal hernia, gastritis, gallbladder disease, splenic flexure syndrome, esophageal spasm or peptic ulcer (Miller, 1942; Ravdin et al., 1955; Palmer, 1958; Hampton et al., 1959; Wehrmacher, 1964; Henderson et al., 1978). This next section will provide an explanation for the referral of gastrointestinal pain to somatic structures that are normally associated with heart disease. This work was designed to determine the central organization of spinothalamic tract cells in relation to their role as a pathway for integration of anginal-like pain associated with heart disease, gallbladder disease and other abdominal pain.

Splanchnic stimulation

Previous investigators have shown that dorsal horn cells of the T7–T11 segments respond to electrical stimulation of the splanchnic nerve (Pomeranz et al., 1968; Fields et al., 1970; Gokin et al., 1977; Cervero, 1983a,b,c), gallbladder distension (Cervero, 1983a) or injections of algesic substances into the mesenteric artery (Guilbaud et al., 1977). Spinothalamic tract cells of the T7–T11 segments having viscerosomatic input respond to electrical stimulation of the Aδ- and C-fibers of the splanchnic nerve (Foreman et al., 1981; Hancock et al., 1975). Anatomical studies have also demonstrated that the splanchnic afferent fibers enter the spinal cord in the T3–T13 segments, with the major concentration found in the T5–T11 segments (Kuo et al., 1981; Cervero et al., 1984). These afferents penetrate the lateral aspect of the dorsal horn and terminate in laminae I and V and the intermediolateral cell column (Kuo and De Groat, 1983; Cervero and Connell, 1984).

Do spinothalamic tract cells found in the T1–T5 segments receive visceral input from both the abdominal region and the cardiopulmonary region? The answer to this question is yes, since electrical stimulation of the splanchnic nerve in primates excited 63 of 85 spinothalamic tract cells that also responded to electrical stimulation of cardiopulmonary afferent fibers and activation of somatic fields (Fig. 9; Ammons et al., 1984b). All cells with splanchnic input exhibited an early volley of activity in response to both the splanchnic and cardiopulmonary sympathetic afferent stimulation. Average latency for the early volley was about 11 mseconds and for the cardiopulmonary sympathetic afferent fibers was approximately 5 mseconds. Excitation of splanchnic-responsive spinothalamic tract cells differs from approximately 25% of the dorsal horn cells of the cat that were inhibited by

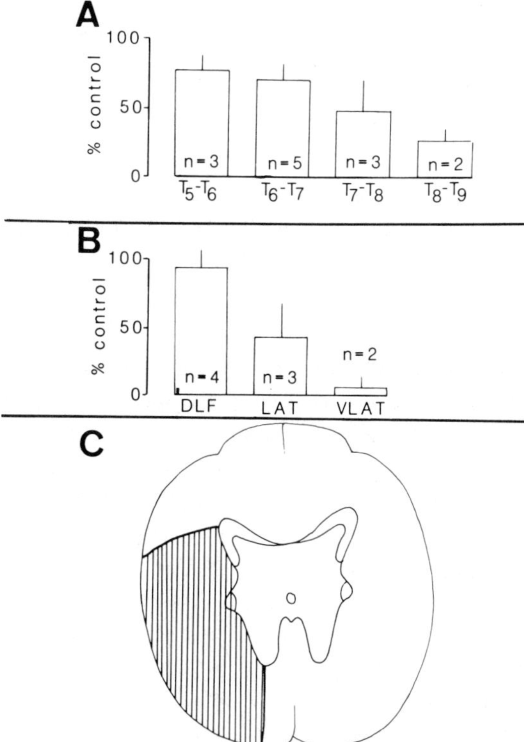

Fig. 8. A, effects of cutting the left sympathetic chain on responses of seven spinothalamic tract cells to splanchnic nerve stimulation. The number of cell discharges in response to splanchnic nerve stimulation with all nerves intact was designated 100%. After the chain was interrupted, the number of spikes evoked by splanchnic nerve stimulation was expressed as a percentage of intact response. B, effects of cutting different areas of the spinal cord. DLF, dorsolateral funiculus; LAT, lateral column; VLAT, ventrolateral column. C, the striped area represents a summation of all lesions that reduced the cell response to splanchnic nerve stimulation. From Ammons et al. (1984b).

splanchnic stimulation and gallbladder distension (Ammons and Foreman, 1984). Inhibition by splanchnic stimulation may be unique for these segments since all the dorsal horn cells studies in the T9–T11 segments were excited following splanchnic stimulation (Cervero, 1983a,b). Suppression of dorsal horn cell activity in the T1–T5 segments could be due to a species difference. Alternatively, dorsal horn cells having no ascending projections may provide a mechanism for controlling information as it is transmitted from the splanchnic nerve to these segments, whereas spinothalamic tract cells are excited in order to ensure that noxious information reaches higher brain structures.

Splanchnic afferent information is transmitted to the T1–T5 segments via the sympathetic chain and propriospinal pathways (Bain et al., 1935; Downman, 1955; Downman and Evans, 1957). Approximately 20% of the responses to splanchnic stimulation were lost after the sympathetic chain between the T5 and T6 white rami communicantes was cut (Fig. 8). This indicates that afferent input may reach spinothalamic tract cells by direct input of splanchnic afferent fibers via the sympathetic chain. Most of the splanchnic input that entered the spinal cord in segments caudal to T5 was disrupted when the lateral and ventrolateral funiculi were interrupted. Most likely, this ipsilateral projection represents propriospinal connections between the upper and lower thoracic segments. However, we have not eliminated the possibility that this pathway is part of an ascending limb of a supraspinal loop.

Gallbladder distension

Electrical stimulation of the splanchnic nerve demonstrated that connections existed between this nerve and the T1–T5 spinothalamic tract cells, but this did not provide evidence that the gallbladder was involved in activation of these neurons. Therefore, we studied gallbladder distension while recording from spinothalamic tract cells (Ammons et al., 1984a). Gallbladder distension excited 36% of the cells that were also responsive to electrical stimulation of the cardiopulmonary afferent fibers.

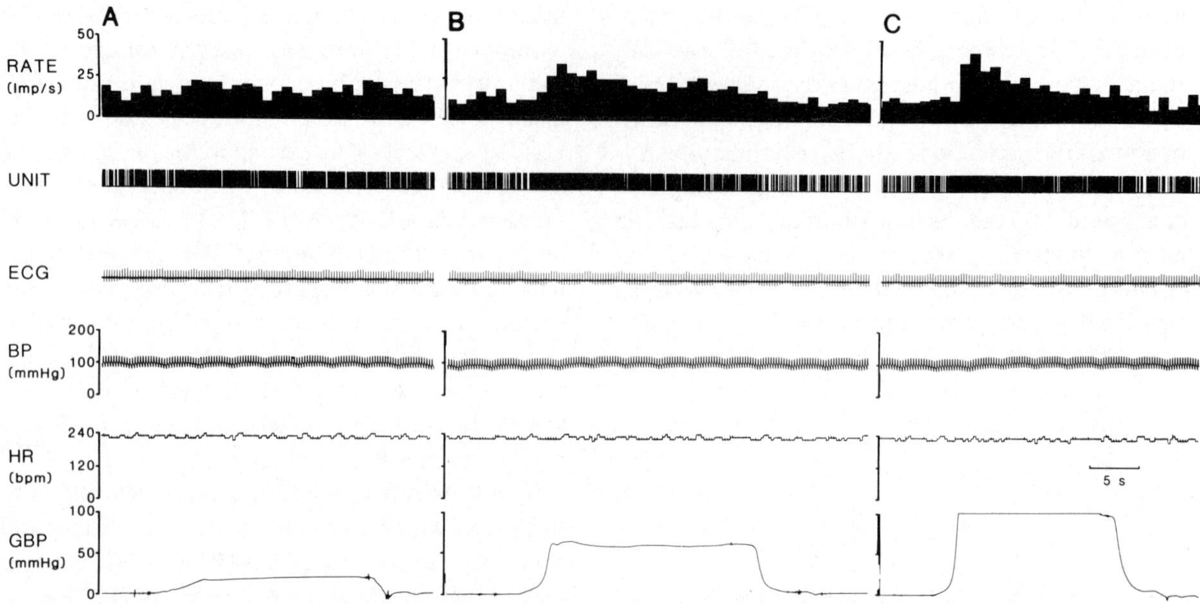

Fig. 9. Responses of a wide dynamic range spinothalamic tract neuron to gallbladder distension of 20 (A), 60 (B) and 100 (C) mmHg. RATE, discharge frequency in impulses/second; UNIT, output of window discriminator; ECG, electrocardiogram; BP, blood pressure; HR, heart rate; GBP, gallbladder pressure. From Ammons et al. (1984a).

The gallbladder was inflated to pressures between 10 and 100 mmHg in order to elicit responses in spinothalamic tract cells. The first bladder distension was set between 40 and 60 mmHg. If cell activity changed, then a series of tests of gallbladder pressure versus cell response was performed.

Gallbladder responsive cells were particularly sensitive to the phasic component of distension. Most cells rapidly increased their discharge rate during this phase and then adapted to a lower rate of discharge for the duration of the distension (Fig. 9). This early phasic component was comparable to the responses obtained in spinothalamic tract cells responding to distension of the urinary bladder (Milne et al., 1981). The magnitude of the phasic component was related to the intensity of the stimulus (Fig. 10). This type of signal may be best suited for informing the thalamus about sudden changes in gallbladder pressure.

Another population of spinothalamic tract cells was characterized as tonic responsive cells because their activity was sustained for the duration of the stimulus. Some of the cells included in this population had both a phasic and a tonic component. These cells differed from the phasic responsive cells,

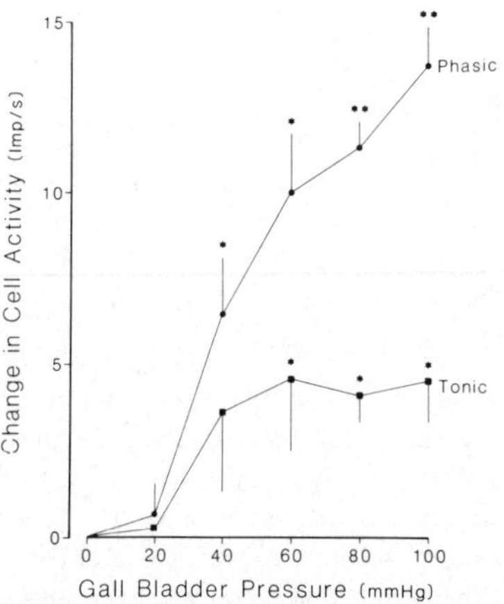

Fig. 10. Relationship between gallbladder pressure on the abscissa and change in spinothalamic tract cell activity on the ordinate. The data represent 13 phasic responses (filled circles) and 12 tonic responses (filled squares). * $P < 0.05$ compared to the control value (no distension); ** $P < 0.01$. From Ammons et al. (1984a).

because the magnitude of cell activity was not related to the intensity of the distension (Fig. 10). Tonic responsive cells may be most effective for signalling an abnormally high pressure in the gallbladder. The phasic and tonic responding cells may be the neurophysiological correlates of sudden colic-type gallbladder pain and chronic gallbladder pain, respectively.

The threshold gallbladder pressure for activating spinothalamic tract cells was 50 mmHg. No apparent relation existed between threshold and cell class, sympathetic input, or cell location, but thresholds for phasic responses (40 mmHg) were lower than for tonic responses (60 mmHg, $P < 0.05$). During acute cholecystitis gallbladder pressures may rise to levels approaching 60 mmHg (Csendes and Sepulveda, 1980); therefore, the high thresholds necessary for activating spinothalamic tract cells fit their function of signalling pain.

Gallbladder responsive cells displayed some other unique properties which may contribute to our understanding of the similarities between angina pectoris and the anginal-like pain associated with gallbladder disease. These cells were more likely to respond to intracardiac bradykinin (Fig. 11A) and to respond with a greater frequency (Fig. 11B). 90% of the gallbladder responsive cells responded to bradykinin, while only 55% of the non-responsive cells did so ($P < 0.05$). The group of cells with both gallbladder input and bradykinin responses included a greater number of cells that responded to Aδ- and C-fiber inputs. This does not mean that C-fibers are necessary for responses, since cells with only Aδ input responded to bradykinin. More likely, the presence of C-fiber input increases the probability of responsiveness to these stimuli. Thus, there is a subpopulation of spinothalamic tract cells that appear to be more responsive to inputs from both the gallbladder and the heart. This subpopulation could provide a mechanism for pain referral to the same somatic structures for either gallbladder distension or myocardial ischemia. This may explain why patients who have both heart and gallbladder disease are likely to experience anginal-like pain during their gallbladder attacks (Ravdin et al., 1942). However, why is pain of gallbladder disease referred to the abdomen in some patients and to the chest and arm in other patients? No evidence exists yet to explain this difference, but it is likely that the processing of information is different in these two groups of patients.

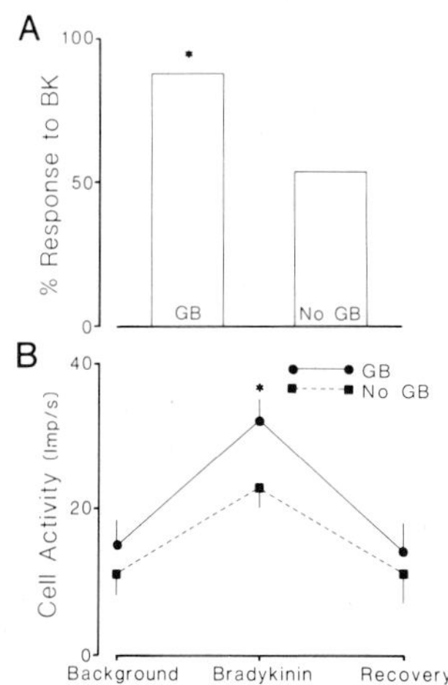

Fig. 11. Responses of gallbladder responsive cells and nonresponsive cells to injection of bradykinin (BK) into left atrium. A, percentage of cells with gallbladder input (GB) or no gallbladder input (No GB) responding to bradykinin. B, change in cell activity elicited by bradykinin injection. Bradykinin values represent peak activity during responses. * $P < 0.05$ compared with cells without gallbladder input. From Ammons et al. (1984a).

Conclusions

This chapter has described not only somatic and visceral inputs onto spinothalamic neurons, but also input from two different visceral organs. The demonstrated input from two organs provides an explanation for anginal-like pain that is sometimes associated with severe gallbladder disease, but raises a further crucial question. Since viscerosomatic convergence involves more than one organ, why is visceral pain often restricted to somatic structures overlying the diseased organ? This type of widespread convergence seems to provide a mechanism whereby the sensation of referred pain should be much more diffuse. What mechanisms provide for the selective input of pain sensation? The following selectivity hypothesis is proposed to provide ideas for future directions.

Selectivity for sympathetic afferent inputs from different organs and for somatic structures exists, even though convergence onto spinal neurons and tract neurons has been demonstrated. Selectivity may occur because input from one organ determines the response of a cell or cells to the input from another organ. The type of interaction that occurs may depend upon the ascending tract or interneurons utilized. At least two mechanisms may be important for the selectivity hypothesis. Interneurons, spinal neurons that do not project to supraspinal areas, may determine what information can activate ascending tract neurons. Descending control activated by the vagal afferent fibers, for example, may differentially modulate the input from two different visceral organs and/or somatic structures. Alternatively, visceral afferent input from a distant visceral organ, such as the urinary bladder, may inhibit rather than facilitate the activity of the thoracic neurons. In a preliminary study we have shown that urinary bladder distension most commonly inhibits the activity of T2–T5 spinal neurons. This response contrasts with the excitatory response that was obtained by distending the gallbladder. Such differential response may contribute to the integration of information that contributes to the selectivity of inputs and to the localization of referred pain to structures overlying the diseased visceral organ.

References

Alexander, R. S. (1946) Tonic and reflex functions of medullary sympathetic cardiovascular centers. J. Neurophysiol., 9: 205–207.

Ammons, W. S. and Foreman, R. D. (1984) Cardiovascular and T_2–T_4 dorsal horn cell responses to gallbladder distension in the cat. Brain Res., 321: 267–277.

Ammons, W. S., Blair, R. W. and Foreman, R. D. (1983) Vagal afferent inhibition of spinothalamic cell responses to sympathetic afferents and bradykinin in the monkey. Circ. Res., 53: 603–612.

Ammons, W. S., Blair, R. W. and Foreman, R. D. (1984a) Responses of primate T_1–T_5 spinothalamic neurons to gallbladder distension. Am. J. Physiol., 247: R995–R1001.

Ammons, W. S., Blair, R. W. and Foreman, R. D. (1984b) Greater splanchnic excitation of primate T_1–T_5 spinothalamic neurons. J. Neurophysiol., 51: 592–603.

Ammons, W. S., Girardot, M.-N. and Foreman, R. D. (1985a) Effects of intracardiac bradykinin on T_2–T_5 spinothalamic cells projecting to medial thalamus. Am. J. Physiol., 249: R147–R152.

Ammons, W. S., Girardot, M.-N. and Foreman, R. D. (1985b) Characteristics of T_2–T_5 spinothalamic neurons with viscerosomatic convergent inputs projecting to medial thalamus. J. Neurophysiol., 54: 73–89.

Armstrong, D., Dry, R. M. L., Keele, C. A. and Markham, J. W. (1953) Observations on chemical excitation of cutaneous pain in man. J. Physiol., 326–351.

Armstrong, D., Jepson, J. B., Keele, C. A. and Stewart, J. W. (1957) Pain producing substance in human inflammatory exudates and plasma. J. Physiol., 135: 350–370.

Aviado, D. M. and Schmidt, C. F. (1955) Reflexes from stretch receptors in blood vessels, heart and lungs. Physiol. Rev., 35: 247–300.

Bain, W. A., Irving, J. T. and McSwiney, B. A. (1935) The afferent fibres from the abdomen in the splanchnic nerves. J. Physiol. (Lond.), 84: 323–333.

Baker, D. G., Coleridge, H. M., Coleridge, J. C. G. and Nerdrum, T. (1980) Search for a cardiac nociceptor: stimulation by bradykinin of sympathetic afferent nerve endings in the heart of the cat. J. Physiol. (Lond.), 306: 519–536.

Barman, S. M. and Gebber, G. L. (1983) Sequence of activation of ventrolateral and dorsal medullary sympathetic neurons. Am. J. Physiol., 245: R438–R447.

Besson, J. M., Guilbaud, G. and Lombard, M. C. (1974) Effects of bradykinin intra-arterial injection into the limbs upon bulbar and mesencephalic reticular unit activity. Adv. Neurol., 4: 207–215.

Blair, R. W. (1985) Noxious cardiac input onto neurons in medullary reticular formation. Brain Res., 326: 335–346.

Blair, R. W., Weber, R. N. and Foreman, R. D. (1981) Characteristics of primate spinothalamic tract neurons receiving viscerosomatic convergent inputs in T_3–T_5 segments. J. Neurophysiol., 46: 797–811.

Blair, R. W., Weber, R. N. and Foreman, R. D. (1982) Responses of thoracic spinothalamic neurons to intracardiac injection of bradykinin in the monkey. Circ. Res., 51: 83–94.

Blair, R. W., Weber, R. N. and Foreman, R. D. (1984a) Responses of spinoreticular and spinothalamic cells to intracardiac bradykinin. Am. J. Physiol., 246: H500–H507.

Blair, R. W., Ammons, W. S. and Foreman, R. D. (1984b) Responses of thoracic spinothalamic and spinoreticular cells to coronary artery occlusion. J. Neurophysiol., 51: 636–648.

Bleehen, T. and Keele, C. A. (1977) Observations on the algogenic actions of adenosine compounds on the human blister base preparation. Pain, 3: 367–377.

Bosnjak, Z. K., Zuperku, E. J., Coon, R. L. and Kampine, J. P. (1979) Acute coronary artery occlusion and cardiac sympathetic afferent activity. Proc. Soc. Exp. Biol. Med., 161: 142–148.

Brown, A. M. (1967) Excitation of afferent cardiac sympathetic nerve fibres during myocardial ischaemia. J. Physiol. (Lond.), 190: 35–53.

Brown, A. M. (1979) Cardiac reflexes. In R. M. Berne (Ed.), Handbook of Physiology, The Cardiovascular System, The Heart, Vol. 1, American Physiological Society, Bethesda, pp. 677–689.

Brown, A. M. and Malliani, A. (1971) Spinal sympathetic reflexes initiated by coronary receptors. J. Physiol. (Lond.), 212: 685–705.

Brown-Sequard, C. E. (1860) Course of Lectures on the Physiology and Pathology of the Central Nervous System, Lippincott, Philadelphia.

Casati, R., Lombardi, F. and Malliani, A. (1979) Afferent sympathetic unmyelinated fibres with left ventricular endings in cats. J. Physiol. (Lond.), 292: 135–148.

Cervero, F. (1983a) Somatic and visceral inputs in to the thoracic spinal cord of the cat: effects of noxious stimulation of the biliary system. J. Physiol., 337: 51–67.

Cervero, F. (1983b) Mechanisms of visceral pain. In S. Lipton and J. Miles (Eds.), Persistent Pain: Modern Methods of Treatment, Vol. 4, Grune and Stratton Ltd., London, pp. 1–19.

Cervero, F. (1983c) Supraspinal connections of neurones in the thoracic spinal cord of the cat: ascending projections and effects of descending impulses. Brain Res., 275: 251–261.

Cervero, F. and Connell, L. A. (1984) Distribution of somatic and visceral primary afferent fibres within the thoracic spinal cord of the cat. J. Comp. Neurol., 230: 88–98.

Cervero, F., Connell, L. A. and Lawson, S. N. (1984) Somatic and visceral primary afferents in the lower thoracic dorsal root ganglia of the cat. J. Comp. Neurol., 228: 422–431.

Chahl, L. A. (1979) Pain induced by inflammatory meditors. In R. F. Beers and E. G. Bennett (Eds.), Mechanisms of Pain and Analgesic Compounds, Raven Press, New York, pp. 273–284.

Chahl, L. A. and Kirk, E. J. (1975) Toxins which produce pain. Pain, 1: 3–49.

Christie, L. G. and Conti, C. R. (1981) Systematic approach to evaluation of angina-like chest pain: Pathophysiology and clinical testing with emphasis on objective documentation of myocardial ischaemia. Am. Heart J., 102: 897–912.

Chung, J. M., Kenshalo, D. R. Jr., Gerhart, K. D. and Willis, W. D. (1979a) Excitation of primate spinothalamic neurons by cutaneous C-fiber volleys. J. Neurophysiol., 42: 1354–1369.

Chung, K., Chung, J. M., LaVelle, F. W. and Wurster, R. D. (1979b) Sympathetic neurons in the cat spinal cord projecting to the stellate ganglion. J. Comp. Neurol., 185: 23–30.

Cohn, P. F. and Braunwald, E. (1980) Chronic coronary artery disease. In E. Braunwald (Ed.), Heart Disease, Saunders, Philadelphia, pp. 1387–1486.

Craig, A. D. and Kniffki, K. D. (1982) Lumbosacral lamina I cells projecting to medial and/or lateral thalamus in the cat. Soc. Neurosci. Abstr., 8: 95.

Csendes, A. and Sepulveda, A. (1980) Intraluminal gallbladder pressure measurements in patients with chronic or acute cholecystites. Am. J. Surg., 13: 383–385.

Downman, C. B. B. (1955) Skeletal muscle reflexes of splanchnic and intercostal nerve origin in acute spinal and decerebrate cats. J. Neurophysiol., 18: 217–235.

Downman, C. B. B. and Evans, M. H. (1957) The distribution of splanchnic afferents in the spinal cord of cat. J. Physiol. (Lond.), 137: 66–79.

Elliott, D. F., Horton, E. W. and Lewis, G. P. (1960) Actions of pure bradykinin. J. Physiol. (Lond.), 153: 473–480.

Emery, D. G., Foreman, R. D. and Coggeshall, R. E. (1978) Categories of axons in the inferior cardiac nerve of the cat. J. Comp. Neurol., 177: 301–310.

Felder, R. B. and Thames, M. D. (1981) The cardiocardiac sympathetic reflex during coronary occlusion in anesthetized dogs. Circ. Res., 48: 685–692.

Fields, H. L., Meyer, G. A. and Partridge, L. D. Jr. (1970) Convergence of visceral and somatic inputs onto spinal neurons. Expt. Neurol., 26: 36–52.

Foerster, O. and Gagel, O. (1932) Die Vorderseitenstrangdurchschneidung beim Menschen. Eineklinisch-pathophysiologisch-anatomische Studie. Z. Ges. Neuro. Psychiat., 138: 1–92.

Foreman, R. D., Schmidt, R. F. and Willis, W. D. (1977) Convergence of muscle and cutaneous input onto primate spinothalamic tract neurons. Brain Res., 124: 555–560.

Foreman, R. D., Schmidt, R. F. and Willis, W. D. (1979) Effects of mechanical and chemical stimulation of fine muscle afferents upon primate spinothalamic tract cells. J. Physiol., 286: 215–231.

Foreman, R. D., Hancock, M. B. and Willis, W. D. (1981) Responses of spinothalamic tract cells in the thoracic spinal cord of the monkey to cutaneous and visceral inputs. Pain, 11: 149–162.

Foreman, R. D., Blair, R. W. and Weber, R. N. (1984) Viscerosomatic convergence onto T_2–T_4 spinoreticular, spinoreticular-spinothalamic and spinothalamic tract neurons in the cat. Expt. Neurol., 85: 597–619.

Gebber, G. L. (1980) Central oscillators responsible for sympathetic nerve discharge. Am. J. Physiol., 239: H143–H155.

Giesler, G. J., Menetrey, D., Guilbaud, G. and Besson, J. M. (1976) Lumbar cord neurons at the origin of the spinothalamic tract in the rat. Brain Res., 118: 320–324.

Gokin, A. P., Kostyuk, P. G. and Preobrazhensky, N. N. (1977) Neuronal mechanisms of interactions of high-threshold visceral and somatic afferent influences in spinal cord and medulla. J. Physiol. (Paris), 73: 319–333.

Guilbaud, G., LeBars, D. and Besson, J. M. (1976) Bradykinin as a tool in neurophysiological studies of pain mechanisms. In J. J. Bonica and D. AlbeFessard (Eds.), Advances in Pain Research and Therapy, Vol. I, Raven Press, New York, pp. 67–73.

Guilbaud, G., Benelli, G. and Besson, J. M. (1977) Response of thoracic dorsal horn interneurones to cutaneous stimulation and to the administration of algogenic substances into the mesenteric artery in the spinal cat. Brain Res., 124: 437–448.

Guzman, F., Braun, C. and Lim, R. K. S. (1962) Visceral pain and the pseudaffective response to intra-arterial injection of bradykinin and other algesic agents. Arch. Int. Pharmacodyn. Ther., 136: 353–383.

Hampton, A. G., Beckwith, J. R. and Wood, J. E. Jr. (1959) The relationship between heart disease and gall bladder disease. Ann. Int. Med., 50: 1135–1148.

Hancock, M. B., Foreman, R. D. and Willis, W. D. (1975) Convergence of visceral and cutaneous input onto spinothalamic tract cells in the thoracic spinal cord of the cat. Expt. Neurol., 47: 240–248.

Harrison, T. R. and Reeves, T. J. (1968) Patterns and causes of chest pain. In Principles and Problems of Ischemic Heart Disease, Year Book Medical Publishers, Inc., Chicago, pp. 197–204.

Hashimoto, K., Hirose, M., Furukawa, S., Haykawa, H. and Kimura, E. (1977) Changes in hemodynamics and bradykinin concentration in coronary sinus blood in experimental coronary artery occlusion. Jpn. Heart J., 18: 679–689.

Head, H. and Thompson, T. (1906) The grouping of afferent impulses within the spinal cord. Brain, 29: 537–741.

Henderson, R. D., Wigle, H. D., Sample, K. and Manyat, G. (1978) Atypical chest pain of cardiac and esophageal origin. Chest, 73: 24–41.

Hoffman, D. S., Dubner, R., Hayes, R. L. and Medlin, T. P. (1981) Neuronal activity in medullary dorsal horn of awake monkeys trained in a thermal discrimination task. I. Responses to innocuous and noxious thermal stimuli. J. Neurophysiol., 46: 409–427.

Keele, C. A. and Armstrong, D. (1969) Substances Producing Pain and Itch, Edward Arnold, London.

Kennard, M. A. (1954) The course of ascending fibers in the spinal cord of the cat essential to the recognition of painful stimuli. J. Comp. Neurol., 100: 511–524.

Kenshalo, D. R. Jr., Leonard, R. B., Chung, J. M. and Willis, W. D. (1979) Responses of primate spinothalamic neurons to graded and to repeated noxious heat stimuli. J. Neurophysiol., 42: 1370–1389.

Kimura, E., Hashimoto, K., Furukawa, S. and Hayakawa, H. (1973) Changes in bradykinin level in coronary sinus blood after the experimental occlusion of coronary artery. Am. Heart J., 85: 635–647.

Kostreva, D. R., Zuperku, E. J., Hess, R. L., Coon, R. L. and Kampine, J. P. (1975) Pulmonary afferent activity recorded from sympathetic nerves. J. Applied Physiol., 39: 37–40.

Kuo, D. C. and De Groat, W. C. (1983) Central projection of afferent fibers of the major splanchnic nerve (MSPLN) in the cat. Anat. Rec., 205: 104A.

Kuo, D. C., Krauthomer, G. M. and Yamasaki, D. S. (1981) The organization of visceral sensory neurones in the thoracic dorsal root ganglia (DRG) of the cat studied by horseradish peroxidase (HRP) reaction using the cryostat. Brain Res., 208: 187–191.

Kuo, D. C., Oravitz, J. J. and De Groat, W. C. (1984) Tracing of afferent and efferent pathways in the left inferior cardiac nerve of the cat using retrograde and transport of horseradish peroxidase. Brain Res., 321: 111–118.

Lewis, T. (1942) Pain, The MacMillan Press Ltd., London, p. 192.

Lim, K. S. and Guzman, F. (1968) Manifestations of pain in analgesic evaluation in animals and man. In A. Soulairac, J. Cohn and J. Charpentier (Eds.), Pain, Academic Press, London, pp. 119–152.

Lombardi, F., Malliani, A. and Pagani, M. (1976) Nervous activity of afferent sympathetic fibers innervating the pulmonary veins. Brain Res., 113: 197–200.

Lombardi, F., Della Bella, P., Casati, R. and Malliani, A. (1981) Effects of intracoronary administration of bradykinin on the impulse activity of afferent sympathetic unmyelinated fibers with left ventricular endings in the cat. Circ. Res., 48: 69–75.

Malliani, A. (1982) Cardiovascular sympathetic afferent fibers. Rev. Physiol. Biochem. Pharmacol., 94: 11–74.

Malliani, A. and Lombardi, F. (1978) Neural reflexes associated with myocardial ischemia. In P. J. Schwartz, A. M. Brown, A. Malliani and A. Zanchetti (Eds.), Neural Mechanisms in Cardiac Arrhythmias, Raven Press, New York, pp. 209–219.

Malliani, A. and Pagani, M. (1976) Afferent sympathetic nerve fibres with aortic endings. J. Physiol. (Lond.), 263: 157–169.

Malliani, A., Schwartz, P. J. and Zanchetti, A. (1969) A sympathetic reflex elicited by experimental coronary occlusion. Am. J. Physiol., 217: 703–709.

Malliani, A., Peterson, D. F., Bishop, V. S. and Brown, A. M. (1972) Spinal sympathetic cardiocardiac reflexes. Circ. Res., 30: 158–166.

Malliani, A., Recordati, G. and Schwartz, P. J. (1973) Nervous activity of afferent cardiac sympathetic fibres with atrial and ventricular endings. J. Physiol. (Lond.), 229: 457–469.

Malliani, A., Pagani, M. and Lombardi, F. (1985) Visceral versus somatic mechanisms. In P. D. Wall and R. Melzack (Eds.), Pain, Churchill Livingstone, Edinburgh, pp. 100–109.

Mehler, W. R., Feferman, M. E. and Nauta, W. J. H. (1960) Ascending axon degeneration following anterolateral cordotomy. An experimental study in the monkey. Brain, 83: 718–751.

Melzack, R. and Casey, K. L. (1968) Sensory, motivational and central control determinants of pain. In D. Kenshalo (Ed.), The Skin Senses, Thomas, Springfield, IL, pp. 423–443.

Miller, H. R. (1942) The interrelationship of disease of coronary arteries and gallbladder. Am. Heart J., 24: 579–587.

Milne, R. J., Foreman, R. D., Giesler, G. J. and Willis, W. D. (1981) Convergence of cutaneous and pelvic visceral nociceptive inputs onto primate spinothalamic neurons. Pain, 11: 163–183.

Needleman, P. (1976) The synthesis and function of prostaglandins in the heart. Fed. Proc., 35: 2376–2381.

Nishi, K., Sakanashi, M. and Takenaka, F. (1974) Afferent fibres from pulmonary arterial baroreceptors in the left cardiac sympathetic nerve of the cat. J. Physiol. (Lond.), 240: 53–66.

Oldfield, B. J. and McLachlan, E. M. (1978) Localization of sensory neurons traversing the stellate ganglion of the cat. J. Comp. Neurol., 182: 915–922.

Pagani, M., Furlan, R., Guzzetti, S., Rimoldi, O., Sandrone, G. and Malliani, A. (1985) Analysis of the pressor sympathetic reflex produced by intracoronary injections of bradykinin in conscious dogs. Circ. Res., 56: 175–183.

Palmer, E. D. (1958) Chest pain of colon origin. Gastroenterologia, 90: 15–21.

Poirier, L. J. and Bertrand, C. (1955) Experimental and anatomical investigation of the lateral spinothalamic and spinotectal tracts. J. Comp. Neurol., 102: 745–757.

Pomeranz, B., Wall, P. D. and Weber, W. V. (1968) Cord cells responding to fine myelinated afferents from viscera, muscle and skin. J. Physiol. (Lond.), 199: 511–532.

Price, D. D. and Dubner, R. (1977) Neurons that subserve the sensory-discriminative aspects of pain. Pain, 3: 307–338.

Price, D. D., Hayes, R. L., Ruda, M. A. and Dubner, R. (1978) Spatial and temporal transformations of input to spinothalamic tract neurons and their relation to somatic sensations. J. Neurophysiol., 41: 933–947.

Procacci, P. and Zoppi, M. (1985) Heart pain. In P. D. Wall and R. Melzack (Eds.), Pain, Churchill Livingstone, Edinburgh, pp. 309–318.

Ravdin, I. S., Royster, H. P. and Sanders, G. B. (1942) Reflexes originating in the common duct giving rise to pain simulating angina pectoris. Ann. Surg., 115: 1055–1062.

Ravdin, I. S., Fitz-Hugh, T. Jr., Wolferth, C. C., Barbieri, E. A. and Ravdin, R. G. (1955) Relation of gallstone disease to angina pectoris. Arch. Surg., 70: 333–342.

Ross, J. (1887) On the segemental distribution of sensory disorders. Brain, 10: 333–361.

Ruch, T. C. (1961) Pathophysiology of pain. In T. C. Ruch, H. D. Patton, J. W. Woodbury and A. L. Towe (Eds.), Neurophysiology, Saunders, Philadelphia, pp. 350–368.

Seagard, J. L., Pederson, H. J., Kostreva, D. R., Van Horn, D. L., Cusik, J. F. and Kampine, J. P. (1978) Ultrastructural identification of afferent fibers of cardiac origin in thoracic sympathetic nerves in the dog. Am. J. Anat., 153: 217–232.

Spiller, W. G. (1905) The occasional clinical resemblance between caries of the vertebrae and lumbothoracic syringomyelia, and the location within the spinal cord of the fibres for the sensations of pain and temperature. Univ. PA. Med. Bull., 18: 147–154.

Teodori and Galletti (1985) In P. D. Wall and R. Melzac (Eds.), Textbook of Pain, Churchill Livingstone, Edinburgh, 315 pp.

Trevino, D. L. and Carstens, E. (1975) Confirmation of the location of spinothalamic neurons in the cat and monkey by the retrograde transport of horseradish peroxidase. Brain Res., 98: 177–182.

Uchida, Y. (1975a) Afferent sympathetic nerve fibers with mechanoreceptors in the right heart. Am. J. Physiol., 228: 223–230.

Uchida, Y. (1975b) Afferent aortic nerve fibers with their pathways in cardiac sympathetic nerves. Am. J. Physiol., 228: 990–995.

Uchida, Y. and Murao, S. (1974) Excitation of afferent cardiac sympathetic nerve fibers during coronary occlusion. Am. J. Physiol., 226: 1094–1099.

Ueda, H., Uchida, Y. and Kamisaka, K. (1969) Distribution and responses of the cardiac sympathetic receptors to mechanically induced circulatory changes. Jpn. Heart J., 10: 70–81.

Vierck, C. J. and Luck, M. M. (1979) Loss and recovery of reactivity to noxious stimuli in monkeys with primary spinothalamic cordotomies, followed by secondary and tertiary lesions of other cord sectors. Brain, 102: 233–248.

Wang, S. C. and Ranson, S. W. (1939) Autonomic responses to electrical stimulation of the lower brain stem. J. Comp. Neurol., 71: 437–455.

Wehrmacher, E. H. (1964) Pains in the Chest, Thomas, Springfield, IL, pp. 342–361.

White, J. C. and Sweet, W. H. (1955) Pain, Its Mechanisms and Neurosurgical Control, Thomas, Springfield, IL.

White, J. C. and Sweet, W. H. (1969) Pain and the Neurosurgeon, Thomas, Springfield, IL.

Willis, W. D. (1985) The Pain System: The Neural Basis of Nociceptive Transmission in the Mammalian Nervous System, S. Karger, Basel, pp. 145–212.

Willis, W. D., Trevino, D. L., Coulter, J. D. and Maunz, R. A. (1974) Responses of primate spinothalamic tract neurons to natural stimulation of hindlimb. J. Neurophysiol., 37: 358–372.

Yoss, R. D. (1953) Studies of the spinal cord. 3. Pathways for deep pain within the spinal cord and brain. Neurology, 3: 163–175.

F. Cervero and J. F.B. Morrison
Progress in Brain Research, Vol. 67

CHAPTER 15

Sensory-motor integration in urinary bladder function

Stephen B. McMahon

Sherrington School of Physiology, St. Thomas' Hospital Medical School, London SE1 7EH, U.K.

Introduction

The sophistication of the neural pathways controlling bladder function can be appreciated if one considers the dual function of this viscus. For prolonged periods the organ maintains a reservoir function, relaxing to accommodate relatively large volumes of fluid — up to 5% or so of total body weight. Then, at intermittent intervals an exact opposite function is required; that is, a brief coordinated and strong contraction of the musculature of the bladder accompanied by relaxation of sphincter tone to permit micturition. In man, voiding of a large proportion of bladder contents is normal, at the end of which the bladder reverts to its reservoir function.

The importance of afferent information in controlling these processes is clear: micturition is normally heralded by a sensation of urinary fullness, which gives way to urgency and finally pain if unheeded (Denny-Brown and Robertson, 1933a; Nathan, 1956). Conversely, deafferentation of the bladder abolishes normal micturition (Barrington, 1914), and the bladder volume remains high and an "overflow" incontinence persists. Afferent information arising from other visceral structures can also exert an action on the bladder in man. Chronic constipation is often associated with urinary retention, and micturition is inhibited during copulation.

This chapter will consider the neuronal mechanisms that operate in the normal filling and emptying phases of bladder function. The experimental evidence derives mostly from animal studies, but there are no reasons to believe that human bladder reflexes have a fundamentally different organisation. It is beyond the scope of this chapter to consider in detail the changes in bladder reflexes that are known to occur after spinal injury — conditions in which alternative pathways are revealed and in which dyssynergia of vesical smooth muscle and sphincter is a common occurrence (Denny-Brown and Robertson, 1933b; Yalla et al., 1976).

Normal bladder motility

The cystometrogram represents one approach to the experimental study of bladder function. To construct such a cystometrogram, quantities of saline are repeatedly injected into an animal or human bladder, through an indwelling catheter, and the motility of the organ is recorded. The steady level of pressure attained at each volume is recorded and plotted graphically. An example of a cystometrogram is shown in Fig. 1a, the data for which were obtained from a conscious dog trained to accept a urethral catheter. The initial injections produce a small rise in intravesical pressure to a few mmHg, but there is then a plateau phase where a considerable volume increase is associated with very little change in pressure. Finally, an "elbow" is reached in this curve, and pressure henceforth rises rapidly. In this experiment micturition with emptying of bladder contents occurred when volumes reached this steep part of the curve. What is not apparent from the cystometrogram is that the plateau phase

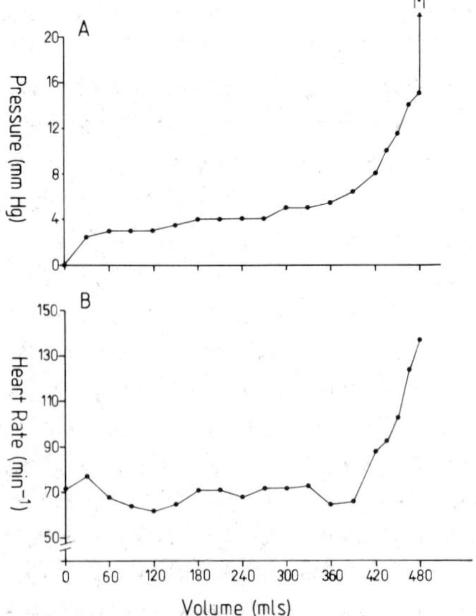

Fig. 1. A, cystometrogram obtained from a conscious bitch trained to accept a urethral catheter. The bladder volume was slowly increased and the steady level of pressure associated with different volumes is plotted here. Note the three phases of the cystometrogram — the initial rise in pressure at small volumes followed by a prolonged plateau phase before the curve finally steepens. At M, micturition with a large rise in bladder pressure occurred and the bladder emptied. B, the average heart rate of the dog during the filling shown in A. Note the tachycardia at volumes greater than 400 ml and pressures above 6 mmHg. Courtesy of Dr. R. A. Summerhill.

is associated with a quiescent bladder, whilst beyond the elbow of the curve waves of vesical contraction are often seen which do not produce any voiding. Denny-Brown and Robertson (1933a) in their classical studies reported that such waves, in man, were associated with an urgent desire to micturate. Animal studies (Ruch, 1960; Gjone, 1965; Edvardsen, 1968b) suggest that this steep portion of the curve results from an increase in detrussor tone following activation of pelvic nerve afferents, since the curve is considerably flattened (and the contractions are lost) by pelvic nerve afferent or efferent section. In Fig. 1b it can be seen that higher bladder volumes can trigger other autonomic reflexes, in this case an increase in heart rate, presumably also by activation of vesical afferents. This observation is also of interest since tachycardia and pressor responses in anaesthetised animals have been used by some workers as criteria to label a stimulus as noxious: in the current experiments, on conscious dogs, the animals never showed signs of distress at bladder volumes initiating tachycardia.

Cystometrographic techniques show that in conscious animals and man, the contractility of detrussor muscle is sensed, and "tone" is only pronounced at relatively high volumes that cause a large input from bladder afferents. In decerebrate animals the excitability of bladder reflexes is higher (Barrington, 1914; Tang and Ruch, 1956). For example, Fig. 2 shows the motility pattern recorded from a decerebrate rat when bladder volume was increased by 0.5 ml, and intravesical pressure rose to 6 mmHg. In this case, the urethra was closed and no voiding occurred, yet a series of large contractions occurred regularly. These large contractions are known as micturition reflexes and the volume necessary to elicit them is the micturition threshold. In this isovolumic state, with a bladder volume greater than the micturition threshold, the rate of occurrence of "spontaneous" micturition reflexes varies between about 0.3 and 6 per minute (De Groat and Ryall, 1969), faster rates being associated with higher volumes (McPherson, 1966). The contractions are not as such spontaneous, since they are reflex in nature and are abolished by deafferentation of the bladder, but their timing is unpredictable and long quescient periods occur be-

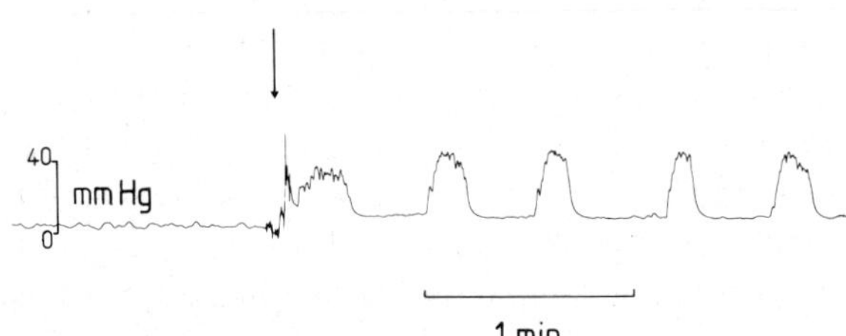

Fig. 2. Motility pattern seen in the bladder of a decerebrate rat. The initial volume of the bladder was 0.2 ml and this was increased by 0.5 ml at the arrow. A series of large active micturition contractions ensues, separated by quiescent periods, when intravesical pressure achieved about 6 mmHg. The urethral outlet was closed.

tween contractions, even though the bladder volume does not change.

The remainder of this chapter will consider in detail how visceral sensory information is processed in order to produce these two phases of bladder motility.

Expulsion phase (micturition reflex)

The urinary bladder, like many viscera, receives an efferent innervation from both parasympathetic and sympathetic arms of the autonomic nervous system. The former is carried by pelvic nerves originating in sacral spinal segments, and the latter by the hypogastric nerves originating in the inferior mesenteric ganglion (in turn supplied by the upper lumbar segments) and also by fine strands from the lumbosacral sympathetic chain (Langley and Anderson, 1896a).

The early experiments of Langley and Anderson (1894, 1896a,b) showed that the smooth muscle of the body of the bladder (the fundus) contracted under parasympathetic influence, whilst sympathetic firing relaxed all but the trigone and neck region. Afferents from bladder travel with both parasympathetic and sympathetic nerves, and as discussed by Jänig and Morrison (this volume), apart from a small proportion of Pacinian-like afferents, they form an apparently homogeneous population of fibres, all activated by intravesical pressures in the normal physiological range.

Section of sacral dorsal roots, eliminating pelvic afferent input, was shown by Barrington (1914) to abolish micturition reflexes. However, they persist after hypogastric nerve section. Bladder contractions were also abolished by thoracic spinal cord transections, but were still present in cats decerebrated at an intercollicular level (Barrington, 1921, 1941). Barrington concluded that the micturition reflex utilised long ascending, spino-bulbar, and descending, bulbo-spinal, pathways with a controlling "centre" in the pons. Wang and Ranson (1939), and later Ruch (1960), suggested that the centre was at or near the locus coeruleus, a view supported from more recent stimulation experiments (Sato et al., 1978). It was thus proposed that micturition occurred because filling of the bladder led to excitation of mechanoreceptive afferents travelling in the pelvic nerve, which activated a spino-bulbo-spinal pathway onto pelvic nerve efferents, causing contraction and emptying of the bladder.

In the 1960s electrophysiological techniques were applied in the study of micturition. Recordings from pelvic nerve branches to the bladder or from single preganglionic cell bodies in cat spinal cord segments S1–S3 showed that these became active during micturition contractions and that electrical stimulation of pelvic nerve afferents could induce long latency firing (typically 80–120 mseconds) which was abolished by spinalisation (Bradley and Teague, 1968, 1972; De Groat and Ryall, 1968, 1969). Indeed, intracellular recordings from preganglionic cells showed that in acutely spinal animals only inhibitory postsynaptic potentials (IPSPs) could be elicited at short latency (De Groat and Ryall, 1969).

To complete this picture, it was then shown that stimulation in the brainstem, near the site of Barrington's micturition centre, could elicit firing in pelvic efferents with approximately half of the total latency found for pelvic afferent to efferent reflexes (Lalley et al., 1972). Conversely, recordings from the same brainstem area showed evoked potentials following pelvic nerve stimulation, again at about half the latency for the whole loop reflex (De Groat, 1975). Therefore, this electrically induced reflex has been considered the electrophysiological substrate of micturition contractions.

The slowly adapting mechanoreceptors in the bladder wall are connected to finely myelinated (Aδ) or unmyelinated (C) afferent fibres (see Jänig and Morrison, this volume). Excitation of the Aδ-fibres has been found sufficient to activate the spino-bulbo-spinal pathway of the micturition reflex (De Groat et al., 1982). The reflex activation of pelvic nerve efferents to the bladder does not produce a simple increase in firing frequency. Rather, the efferents fire in bursts, with the average firing within a burst relatively constant under a variety of conditions (De Groat et al., 1981). Thus, gradual distension of the bladder, and therefore gradual increase in afferent firing, does not initially evoke efferent firing. Once the micturition threshold is reached the efferent pathway is apparently "switched-on" maximally for short periods of time. Interneuronal networks, not the efferents themselves, appear to be responsible for this bursting, since direct activation of the cells by ionophoretic application of excitatory amino acids causes tonic firing (De Groat et al., 1981). This maximally-on/maximally-off pattern of firing in pelvic efferents, whilst uncharacteristic of autonomic efferents in general, is perhaps appropriate for micturition where an all or none retention/expulsion control is required.

The role of pelvic nerve afferent C-fibres in micturition is unclear. Capsaicin, the pungent ingredient of chilli peppers, can impair C-fibre function if administered systemically to an animal or locally to a nerve (Fitzgerald, 1983). Neonatal destruction of C-fibres by capsaicin can induce urinary retention in rats (Sharkey et al., 1983), suggesting that C-fibre firing summates with that from Aδ-fibres. In acutely spinalized animals, as mentioned above, no short-latency reflex firing can be elicited. However, in a proportion of animals a weak spinal reflex can be elicited in the pelvic nerve at high intensities of stimulation of pelvic afferents, with a latency consistent with the slow conduction velocities of C-fibres (De Groat et al., 1982). This weak reflex is not sufficient for normal micturition contractions to occur.

The mechanisms described do not operate in chronically spinalized animals, where so-called automatic micturition occurs. In these animals, an entirely spinal mechanism is responsible for coordinated micturition (Barrington, 1931; De Groat et al., 1982). This appears to be a modified and greatly strengthened form of the small reflex sometimes seen electrophysiologically in acute spinal preparations. It too is mediated by pelvic nerve afferent C-fibres (De Groat et al., 1982). However, the fact that stimulation at C-fibre strength is necessary to elicit the reflex does not mean that only C-fibres are important. It is very likely that summation from Aδ-fibres, which are also activated by high-intensity stimulation, contributes to, or perhaps is essential for, operation of the reflex.

The changes seen in chronic spinal animals are not simply small shifts in excitability since there are fundamental differences in the properties of this reflex, such as a change in the effect of cutaneous perineal stimulation from inhibition to excitation. In many ways, the reflexes that emerge in chronic spinal animals resemble those present in neonates (De Groat et al., 1982); they may emerge because of the loss of influences from the brainstem.

Normal adult animals apparently have a highly specific micturition reflex, activated only by pelvic nerve afferents from the bladder and travelling by a spino-bulbo-spinal pathway. Therefore, we might expect especial response properties in the spinal neurones mediating these reflexes. Several studies have reported recordings from cells receiving input from the urinary bladder (Kamikawa et al., 1962; Fields et al., 1970; Cervero and Iggo, 1978; Milne et al., 1981) and recently from spinal cord cells with ascending axons that terminate in supraspinal structures, and likely mediators of the spino-bulbar limb of the reflex (McMahon and Morrison, 1982a). Recordings from such cells show that they can be either excited or inhibited by small rises in bladder pressure, with thresholds close to normal micturition thresholds. Interestingly, the response thresholds of all the spinal neurones that were activated by vesical pressure changes were within the physiological range. The same neurones increased their levels of firing at vesical pressures that might be considered noxious. Thus, these observations support the notion of an intensity rather than specificity code for noxious visceral events from the bladder (Malliani et al., 1984). Fig. 3 illustrates one such response of a cat dorsal horn cell to a series of distensions of the bladder. These cells were also tested for their response specificity. Firstly, all cells were found to possess a somatic receptive field — a general finding in studies of viscero-sensory mechanisms. Secondly, although this type of cell had a visceral receptive field in only one viscus, electrical

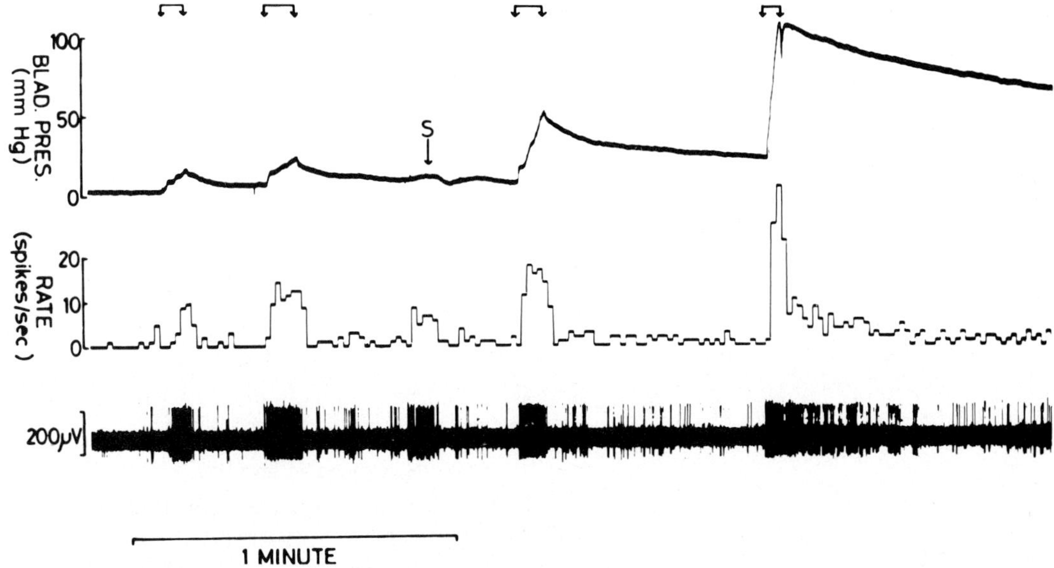

Fig. 3. Responses of a cat dorsal horn cell to a series of bladder distensions. The upper trace is a record of intravesical pressure. The lower trace shows the spike train and the middle trace the derived spike rate (in 1-second bins). Each set of double arrows indicates the injection of 10 ml of saline into the bladder. Initial bladder volume was 5 ml. S indicates a small spontaneous bladder contraction. Note the large increases in rate associated with this small increase in intravesical pressure. From McMahon and Morrison (1982a), with permission.

stimulation of afferents in both sympathetic and parasympathetic nerves activated them in a similar way in the great majority of cases (Table I).

This seems paradoxical since these other inputs cannot substitute for the pelvic afferents in producing micturition. Of course, other possible sources of convergence were not tested in these studies and it could be that many of these would also have been effective. It is of interest that the properties of interneurones confined to the sacral cord (i.e., without ascending axons) showed markedly different properties (Table I). In these cells, convergence from different visceral nerves was not common (McMahon and Morrison, 1982b).

These findings led to a reexamination of the stimuli which could elicit reflex firing in parasympathetic nerves to the bladder (McMahon and Morrison, 1982c). Surprisingly, it was found that a number of sources were effective at evoking this reflex — all those in fact which had been found to converge onto ascending spino-bulbar neurones — but not when the bladder was empty and intravesical pressure very low. This means that there was some facilitatory effect of afferent input from the bladder on these reflex pathways. It could be that this convergence had been overlooked previously because, whilst repetitive pelvic nerve stimulation would raise bladder pressure and hence permit the reflex to occur, stimulation of other nerves would not do

TABLE I

Percentages of cat dorsal horn cells responding to stimulation of only pelvic parasympathetic nerve or showing convergence from both parasympathetic and sympathetic nerves

	Parasympathetic only	Parasympathetic and sympathetic
Cells with ascending axons	20%	80%
Sacral interneurones	71%	29%

Modified from McMahon and Morrison (1982a,b).

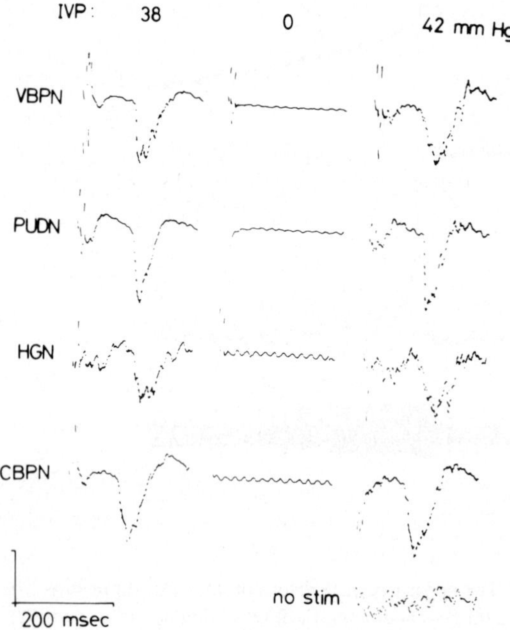

Fig. 4. The average of 16 responses in vesical parasympathetic efferents following electrical stimulation (at start of sweep) of vesical branches of the pelvic nerve (VBPN, top row), pudendal nerve (PUDN, second row), hypogastric nerve (HGN, third row) and colonic branches of the pelvic nerve (CBPN, fourth row). An averaged control response using no electrical stimulation is shown on the bottom right. Responses were recorded at different intravesical pressures: 38 mmHg (first column), 0 mmHg (second column) and 43 mmHg (third column). Vertical calibration: 60 μV for responses in first row and 30 μV for all others. All responses obtained from one animal. From McMahon and Morrison (1982c), with permission.

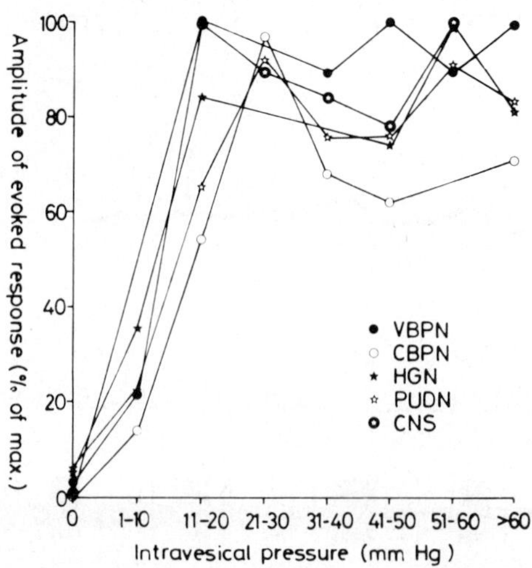

Fig. 5. The relationship between the amplitude of 16 averaged evoked responses in the vesical parasympathetic efferents following electrical stimulation of the vesical (VBPN) or colonic (CBPN) branches of the pelvic nerve, the hypogastric nerve (HGN), the pudendal nerve (PUDN) or below a hemitransection of the spinal cord at the second cervical segment (CNS), at different intravesical pressures and low intracolonic pressure. The responses in all experiments have been pooled into bins of intravesical pressure, as indicated on the abscissa. From McMahon and Morrison (1982c), with permission.

so. This facilitatory or gating influence proved to be mediated by pelvic nerve afferents from the bladder and not by hypogastric afferents (McMahon and Morrison, 1982c). It appeared to act at a spinal level since its activation allowed descending volleys in bulbo-spinal pathways to evoke pelvic nerve discharges. Fig. 4 shows examples of evoked reflex responses obtained from one animal, where it can be seen that many afferent sources produce reflexes at similar latencies, and Fig. 5 shows that each of these reflexes has a similar dependence on the level of intravisical pressure, suggesting they were all regulated by the same mechanism.

Thus, there appear to be two separate pathways regulating micturition; a spino-bulbo-spinal pathway activated from a variety of sources, and a sacral cord pathway which itself cannot activate pelvic efferents, but which can facilitate or gate the effects of the spino-bulbo-spinal path. It is the specificity in the sacral pathway which confers specificity on the micturition reflex. The ascending systems carry information from a variety of sources, and this may simply represent neuronal economy since the pathway might subserve several unrelated functions. As we have shown (McMahon and Morrison, 1982b), the majority of sacral cord interneurones possess appropriate specificity in terms of visceral nerve inputs. However, it was found that many of these interneurones exhibited reciprocal inputs from bladder and bowel (i.e., one excitatory receptive field and one inhibitory one), both of which were mediated by pelvic nerve affer-

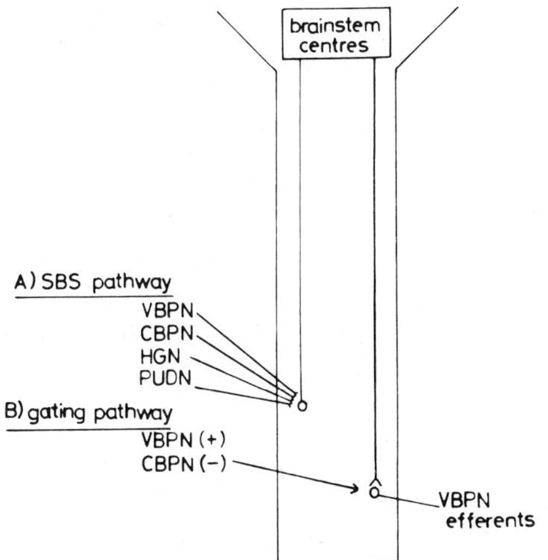

Fig. 6. Summary of the neuronal pathways controlling firing in pelvic efferents to the bladder (VBPN efferents). A long spino-bulbo-spinal reflex actually activates the efferents. This pathway shows extensive convergence from afferents in a number of nerves (VBPN, vesical branches of the pelvic nerve; CBPN, colonic branches of the pelvic nerve; HGN, hypogastric nerve; PUDN, pudendal nerve). However, the ability of discharges in the descending limb of this path to activate the efferents is regulated or gated by a second, sacral pathway. This cannot itself normally drive the efferents. It is switched on by activity in pelvic afferents from the bladder, and off by activity in pelvic afferents from the colon. It does not show the convergence seen in the spino-bulbo-spinal pathway, and it is this property which confers specificity on micturition.

ents. This too is consistent with the properties of micturition. Denny-Brown and Robertson (1933a) noted that defaecation and micturition usually alternated, and several experimental studies have shown the inhibitory action of bowel distension on micturition (Kock and Pompeius, 1963; De Groat, 1971; Floyd et al., 1982b).

Fig. 6 summarises this scheme of the nervous control of vesical emptying. The presence of a sacral cord pathway could be the anatomical basis for the emergence of automatic micturition in chronic spinal animals.

Filling phase

The ability of the bladder to relax and accommodate a variable, sometimes large, volume of urine is for man as important as its ability to contract and expel its contents. In numerical terms urinary incontinence is a far greater problem than retention. There are two distinct schools of thought as to how the accommodatory function is achieved. The first maintains that the mechanism is intrinsic to the organ and has no neural component whilst the second holds that the activation of sympathetic efferents that relax the bladder underlies the phenomenon.

In the former theory the physical properties of smooth muscle are considered sufficient for relaxation (Tang and Ruch, 1956; Klevmark, 1974, 1977). In the work of Klevmark, the motility of the bladder in cats was examined when they were filled at slow, physiological rates, i.e., one to fifteen times the normal urinary diuretic rate. At the lowest of these rates there was no significant increase in intravesical pressure up to a volume sufficient to elicit a micturition contraction. At the higher of the diuretic rates there was only a modest increase in intravesical pressure and, most importantly, this rate of rise was indistinguishable from that seen in denervated preparations. These results would suggest that any active neuronal control of the smooth muscle would operate only at high volumes and high filling rates. It is possible to criticise such essentially negative results on the grounds that the observations were made under barbiturate anaesthesia (Klevmark, 1974, 1977), which might abolish or reduce reflexes (Bradley and Teague, 1972).

The alternative theory of active relaxation is based on the observations that hypogastric nerve section can increase motility (Gjone, 1965; Edvardsen, 1968a) and that the slope of the cystometrogram (obtained at non-physiological filling rates) is greater in sympathectomised preparations. Since thoracic spinalization did not abolish this difference, an entirely spinal reflex has been proposed.

Electrophysiological investigations on the firing of hypogastric efferents have been performed (De Groat and Lalley, 1972; Floyd et al., 1982a), but in all these cases the exact destination and the actions of the recorded fibres has been unknown. Nevertheless, the gross effects of hypogastric nerve stimulation indicate that many efferents can relax the bladder. De Groat and Lalley (1972) have demonstrated that hypogastric activity can be elicited by pelvic nerve stimulation and increases as bladder pressure rises. It has also been shown that similar firing can be evoked from hypogastric afferents to the bladder (Floyd et al., 1982a), and a high degree of convergence onto this reflex pathway has been directly demonstrated (Spillane et al., 1980). These electrophysiological reflexes can be seen in animals spinalised at thoracic levels. The main problem in associating such reflexes with relaxation in bladder filling is that the reflex is most readily seen at higher intravesical pressure levels, with relatively small actions at pressures below the micturition threshold. High bladder pressures are of course seen in micturition but this is the one time that bladder relaxation is not required! It has been proposed that during micturition contractions a supraspinal influence inhibits the sympathetic firing (De Groat and Lalley, 1972).

It is possible that these reflexes have no functional role in normal micturition, but are utilised perhaps in unusual circumstances, such as to counter rapid increases in intravesical pressure that occur with changes in posture, for example. It is also possible that these efferents have vasomotor or gastrointestinal actions, since bladder distension is known to exert such actions (Mukherjee, 1957; Taylor, 1965; Garret et al., 1974).

Conclusions

The study of an autonomic or vegetative event such as micturition has shown that it is inappropriate to consider these functions as "simple" reflexes. In the periphery, a high level of co-ordinated activity between different structures is necessary for the successful operation of this system. It is clear that even apparently simple reflexes, such as the pelvic nerve efferent firing that is seen on pelvic afferent stimulation, do not represent simple central circuity. Rather, multiple pathways exhibiting complex interactions and with high levels of convergence are seen. This makes the "simple" reflex all the more remarkable: it is apparent in spite of complex central processes and not because of simple ones.

It is also clear that afferent information from the viscera, although perhaps not conveyed over as many paths as is the case with other tissues nor producing the same fine gradation of sensory experience, is nevertheless carefully discriminated and utilised in physiological processes.

References

Barrington, F. J. F. (1914) The nervous control of micturition. Q. J. Expt. Physiol., 8: 33–71.

Barrington, F. J. F. (1921) The relation of the hindbrain to micturition. Brain, 44: 23–53.

Barrington, F. J. F. (1931) The component reflexes of micturition in the cat. Parts I and II. Brain, 54: 177–188.

Barrington, F. J. F. (1941) The component reflexes of micturition in the cat. Part III. Brain, 64: 239–243.

Bradley, W. E. and Teague, C. T. (1968) Spinal cord organisation of micturition reflex afferents. Expt. Neurol., 22: 504–516.

Bradley, W. E. and Teague, C. T. (1972) Electrophysiology of pelvic and pudendal nerves in the cat. Expt. Neurol., 35: 378–393.

Cervero, F. and Iggo, A. (1978) Natural stimulation of urinary bladder afferents does not affect transmission through lumbrosacral spinocervical tract neurones in the cat. Brain Res., 156: 375–379.

De Groat, W. C. (1971) Inhibition and excitation of sacral parasympathetic neurones by visceral and cutaneous stimuli in the cat. Brain Res., 33: 499–503.

De Groat, W. C. (1975) Nervous control of the urinary bladder of the cat. Brain Res., 87: 201–211.

De Groat, W. C. and Lalley, P. M. (1972) Reflex firing in the lumbar sympathetic outflow to activation of vesical afferent fibres. J. Physiol., 226: 289–309.

De Groat, W. C. and Ryall, R. W. (1968) The identification and characteristics of sacral parasympathetic preganglionic neurones. J. Physiol., 196: 563–577.

De Groat, W. C. and Ryall, R. W. (1969) Reflexes to sacral parasympathetic neurones concerned with micturition in the cat. J. Physiol., 200: 87–108.

De Groat, W. C., Nadelhaft, I., Milne, R. J., Booth, A., Morgan, A. M. and Thor, K. (1981) Organisation of the sacral parasympathetic reflex pathways to the urinary bladder and large intestine. J. Auton. Nerv. System, 3: 135–160.

De Groat, W. C., Booth, A. M., Milne, R. J. and Roppolo, J.

R. (1982) Parasympathetic preganglionic neurones in the sacral spinal cord. J. Auton. Nerv. System, 5: 23–43.

Denny-Brown, D. and Robertson, E. G. (1933a) On the physiology of micturition. Brain, 56: 149–190.

Denny-Brown, D. and Robertson, E. G. (1933b) The state of the bladder and its sphincters in complete transverse lesions of the spinal cord and cavda equina. Brain, 56: 397–463.

Edvardsen, P. (1968a) Nervous control of the urinary bladder in cats. I. The collecting phase. Acta Physiol. Scand., 72: 157–171.

Edvardsen, P. (1968b) Nervous control of the urinary bladder in cats. II. The expulsion phase. Acta Physiol. Scand., 72: 172–182.

Fields, H. L., Partridge, L. D. and Winter, D. L. (1970) Somatic and visceral receptive field properties of fibres in ventral quadrant white matter of the cat spinal cord. J. Neurophysiol., 33: 827–837.

Fitzgerald, M. (1983) Capsaicin and sensory neurones: a review. Pain, 15: 109–130.

Floyd, K., Hick, V. E. and Morrison, J. F. B. (1982a) The influence of visceral mechanoreceptors on sympathetic efferent discharge in the cat. J. Physiol., 323: 65–76.

Floyd, K., McMahon, S. B. and Morrison, J. F. B. (1982b) Inhibitory interactions between colonic and vesical afferents in the micturition reflex of the cat. J. Physiol., 323: 45–52.

Garrett, J. R., Howard, E. R. and Jones, W. (1974) The internal anal sphincter of the cat: A study of nervous mechanisms affecting tone and reflex activity. J. Physiol., 243: 153–166.

Gjone, R. (1965) Peripheral autonomic influences on the motility of the urinary bladder in the cat. I. Rhythmic contractions. Acta Physiol. Scand., 65: 370–377.

Kamikawa, K., Tatsua, S., Koshino, K. and Kuru, M. (1962) Analysis of lateral column units related to vesical reflexes. Exp. Neurol., 6: 271–284.

Klevmark, B. (1974) Motility of the urinary bladder in cats during filling at physiological rates. I. Intravesical pressure patterns studied by a new method of cystometry. Acta Physiol. Scand., 90: 565–577.

Klevmark, B. (1977) Motility of the urinary bladder in cats during filling at physiological rates. II. Effects of extrinsic bladder denervation on intramural tension and on intravesical pressure patterns. Acta Physiol. Scand., 101: 176–184.

Kock, N. G. and Pompeius, R. (1963) Inhibition of vesical motor activity induced by anal stimulation. Acta Chir. Scand., 126: 244–250.

Lalley, P. M., De Groat, W. C. and McLain, P. L. (1972) Activation of the sacral parasympathetic pathway to the urinary bladder by brain stem stimulation. Fed. Proc., 31: 386.

Langley, J. N. and Anderson, H. K. (1894) The constituents of the hypogastric nerves. J. Physiol., 17: 177–191.

Langley, J. N. and Anderson, H. K. (1896a) The innervation of the pelvic and adjoining viscera. Part. II. The bladder. J. Physiol., 19: 71–84.

Langley, J. N. and Anderson, H. K. (1896b) The innervation of the pelvic and adjoining viscera. Part VI. Histological and physiological effects of section of the sacral nerves. J. Physiol., 19: 372–384.

Malliani, A., Pagani, M. and Lombardi, F. (1984) Visceral versus somatic mechanisms. In P. D. Wall and R. Melzack (Eds.), Textbook of Pain, Churchill Livingstone, London, pp. 100–110.

McMahon, S. B. and Morrison, J. B. F. (1982a) Spinal neurones with long projections activated from the abdominal viscera. J. Physiol., 322: 1–20.

McMahon, S. B. and Morrison, J. F. B. (1982b) Two groups of spinal interneurones that respond to stimulation of the abdominal viscera. J. Physiol., 322: 21–34.

McMahon, S. B. and Morrison, J. F. B. (1982c) Factors that determine the excitability of parasympathetic reflexes to the bladder. J. Physiol., 322: 35–44.

McPherson, A. (1966) The effect of somatic stimuli on the bladder in the cat. J. Physiol., 185: 185–196.

Milne, R. J., Foreman, R. D., Ghesler, G. J. and Willis, W. D. (1981) Convergence of cutaneous and pelvic visceral nociceptive inputs onto primate spinothalamic neurons. Pain, 11: 163–183.

Mukherjee, S. R. (1957) Effect of bladder distension on arterial blood pressure and renal circulation in acute spinal cats. J. Physiol., 138: 300–306.

Nathan, P. W. (1956) Sensations associated with micturition. Br. J. Urol., 28: 126–131.

Ruch, T. C. (1960) Central control of the bladder. In J. Field and H. W. Magoun (Eds.), Handbook of Physiology, Section I, Vol. 2, American Physiological Society, Washington, pp. 1207–1224.

Sato, K., Shimizo, N., Toyama, M. and Maeda, T. (1978) Localisation of the micturition reflex centre at dorsolateral pontine tegmentum of the rat. Neurosci. Lett., 8: 27–33.

Sharkey, K. A., Williams, R. G., Shulz, M. and Dockray, G. J. (1983) Sensory substance P innervation of the urinary bladder: Possible site of action of capsaicin in causing urine retention in rats. Neurosurgery, 10: 861–868.

Spillane, K., McMahon, S. B. and Morrison, J. F. B. (1980) Peripheral and central pathways influencing activity of sympathetic efferents in the hypogastric nerve. Proc. I.U.P.S., 14: 715.

Tang, P. C. and Ruch, T. C. (1956) Localisation of brain stem and diencephalic areas controlling the micturition reflex. J. Comp. Neurol., 106: 213–245.

Taylor, D. E. M. (1965) Reflex effects of slow bladder filling on the blood pressure in cats. Q. J. Exp. Physiol., 50: 263–270.

Wang, S. C. and Ranson, W. S. (1939) Autonomic responses to electrical stimulation of the lower brain stem. J. Comp. Neurol., 71: 437–455.

Yalla, S. V., Rossier, A. B. and Fam, B. (1976) Dyssynergic vesicourethral responses during bladder rehabilitation in spinal cord injury patients: Effects of suprapubic percussion, crede method and bethanecol chloride. J. Urol., 115: 575–579.

F. Cervero and J. F.B. Morrison
Progress in Brain Research, Vol. 67

CHAPTER 16

Spinal cord integration of visceral sensory systems and sympathetic nervous system reflexes

W. Jänig

Physiologisches Institut, Christian-Albrechts-Universität, Olshausenstrasse 40, D-2300 Kiel, F.R.G.

Introduction

The activity in the sympathetic preganglionic neurones is a result of integrative processes in the spinal cord, brain stem, hypothalamus and suprahypothalamic brain structures. In the peripheral autonomic ganglia, this product of integration is transmitted synaptically to the postganglionic neurones and from here to the target organs. The spinal cord is an integrative organ in its own right and a major highway of liaison between the brain and the inner world (Lloyd, 1960).

Very little is known about the neuronal elements, synaptic processes, transmitters and temporospatial excitatory and inhibitory processes of the spinal integration of neuronal autonomic processes. A systematic analysis of the activity of single sympathetic neurones recorded intra- and extracellularly in vivo has recently been started, giving an insight into the differentiation of spinal sympathetic systems and the integrative properties of the spinal cord (Jänig, 1985; Dembowsky et al., 1985a).

This review focusses on the discharge patterns of sympathetic pre- and postganglionic neurones. The discharge patterns are composed of reflexes which can be elicited in the neurones under standardized experimental conditions. Many of these reflexes and discharge patterns probably cannot be seen during the neuronal ongoing regulations of the target organs in unanaesthetized animals. They are artificial entities which are used by the experimenter in his analysis and, so to speak, are the language of the neurones, by which they reveal some properties of the central organization of the systems, provided the experimenter asks reasonable questions, i.e., uses meaningful, adequate stimuli. The analysis of the discharge patterns of sympathetic neurones is an important step towards, first, the description of the different types of "final common sympathetic paths" to the target organs, second, the recognition of functionally different types of preganglionic neurones in the spinal cord and, third, the development of general ideas about the central organization of the sympathetic systems.

This review is restricted to the description of lumbar pre- and postganglionic sympathetic neurones which supply target organs in skin and skeletal muscle of the cat hindlimb, and in the lower abdominal and pelvic cavity. Details of the functional and other properties of the neurones have been given extensively in the literature (Jänig, 1985; Baron et al., 1985c,d; Bahr et al., 1986a–c; Bartel et al., 1986; Jänig and McLachlan, 1986a,b). Special emphasis has been placed on the spinal cord and on the role of the visceral afferent inputs.

The methods employed in the neurophysiological and histological studies on cats have been described extensively in the literature referred to in this review. Necessary details of procedures have been given either in the text or in the legends.

The pre- and postganglionic channels to the target organs

Spinal motoneurones integrate activity in spinal afferents, spinal interneurones and in supra-spinal motor centres and relay the product of the integration in their activity to the skeletal muscle. In this way, the motoneurones are interpreted as the "final common motor paths"; cutting these paths leads to complete paralysis and, finally, to degeneration of the skeletal muscle fibres.

For the autonomic target organs the above situation is more complex. The activity of the sympathetic preganglionic neurones is the result of the integration of activity in spinal primary afferents, spinal descending systems from supraspinal brain centres and activity in spinal interneurones. In this way, the preganglionic sympathetic neurones could be named — in analogy to the motoneurones to skeletal muscle — "final common sympathetic motor paths". However, this notion is not necessarily valid and needs some modification and restrictions when seen from the sympathetic target organs.

First, the activity of the preganglionic neurones is synaptically transmitted to postganglionic neurones in the sympathetic para- and prevertebral ganglia. Considerable convergence and divergence of preganglionic axons and non-nicotinic (muscarinic, cholinergic and peptidergic) synaptic processes may occur in the ganglia; furthermore, spinal visceral afferent neurones and afferent neurones with cell bodies in the periphery may establish synapses on postganglionic neurones in prevertebral ganglia. Thus, there is strong evidence showing that integration occurs in sympathetic ganglia, and this may particularly apply to the prevertebral ganglia (Szurszewski, 1981; Simmons, 1985). However, our knowledge about the physiological role of this integration of neuronal activity in sympathetic ganglia during ongoing regulations of sympathetic target organs is very limited.

Experiments conducted recently on guinea-pig sympathetic ganglia show that the synaptic input to most postganglionic neurones in the lumbar sympathetic chain is dominated by one (or, rarely, two) preganglionic fibres; thus, these postganglionic neurones discharge impulses only when the "dominant" preganglionic axons are stimulated. Most postganglionic neurones in the inferior mesenteric ganglion require summation of synaptic inputs from several preganglionic axons in order to discharge (McLachlan et al., 1984; see also Skok and Ivanov, 1983). These results are consistent with our own measurements showing that postganglionic neurones supplying skeletal muscle and skin of the cat hindlimb exhibit only small scatterings of latency and well-defined thresholds upon electrical stimulation of the preganglionic axons in the lumbar sympathetic trunk and the lumbar white rami with single pulses (U. Halsband, W. Jänig, M. Michaelis and K. Sternberg, unpublished observation); most postganglionic neurones in the inferior mesenteric ganglia supplying pelvic organs exhibit considerably larger scatterings of latency in their responses to electrical stimulation of the preganglionic axons with single pulses, some of them showing latency differences of up to 50 ms between the responses (W. Jänig, M. Schmidt, A. Schnitzler and U. Wesselmann, unpublished observation). Also, these results may mean that integration is important in pre- but not in paravertebral sympathetic ganglia (but see Hoffmeister et al., 1978; Jänig et al., 1982, 1983a; Blumberg and Jänig, 1983). Support for the notion that the pre- and postganglionic sympathetic channels are — cum grano salis — functionally the "final common sympathetic motor paths", and separate, with respect to the target organs, has been given by extensive neurophysiological analysis of the respective post- and preganglionic neurones which supply skeletal muscle and skin (Jänig, 1985; see Fig. 2 and below). The same may even be true for the lumbar sympathetic supply to pelvic organs and viscera: visceral vasoconstrictor neurones and different types of motility-regulating neurones could recently be classified by way of their distinct reflex patterns, preganglionically (Bahr et al., 1986a–c; Bartel et al., 1986) as well as postganglionically (see below).

Second, the responses of most autonomic effector organs are dependent not only on the activity

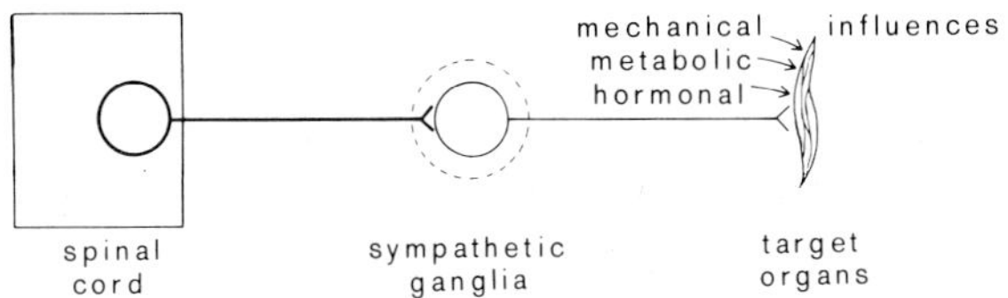

Fig. 1. The final common sympathetic motor path as a neuronal link between spinal cord and sympathetic target organ.

in the postganglionic neurones but also on other, non-neural factors (Fig. 1). Hormonal, local metabolic, mechanical (myogenic), environmental (temperature) and neural influences may be integrated by the autonomic target organs to the autonomic effector responses. In the visceral domain, postganglionic sympathetic neurones may not influence effector organs directly but only indirectly, by controlling the transmitter released from preganglionic parasympathetic axons or by ending synaptically on postganglionic parasympathetic neurones or on enteric neurones.

Both levels of integration, that in the sympathetic ganglia and that at the target organs, probably vary in importance between different sympathetic systems. For example, integration in the ganglia and at the target organ may be of minor importance, or not important at all, for the pre-/postganglionic pilomotor, sudomotor and vasodilator channels, of some importance for the pre-/postganglionic vasoconstrictor channels (Jänig et al., 1982, 1983a; Blumberg and Jänig, 1983) and of great importance for the pre-/postganglionic motility-regulating channels to the viscera. This entails that target organ activity is highly correlated with the neural activity in certain sympathetic systems, such as the pilomotor and sudomotor systems (see Grosse and Jänig, 1976; Jänig and Kümmel, 1977), but less in other sympathetic systems, such as the vasoconstrictor systems.

Keeping the limitations outlined above in mind, it appears justified to us to denote the sympathetic pre-/postganglionic channels to skeletal muscle and skin as "final common sympathetic motor paths" for the integrated central activity (Fig. 2). Substantial neurophysiological evidence exists which shows

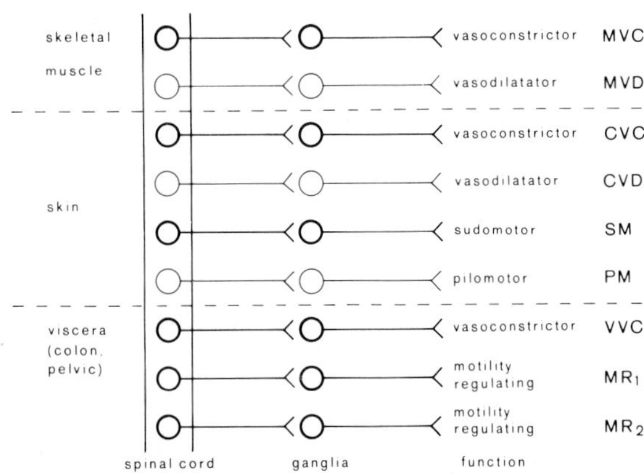

Fig. 2. Sympathetic systems supplying the skeletal muscle, skin (of the hindlimb and tail) and viscera (colon and pelvic organs) in the cat. The systems drawn heavily have ongoing activity in the anaesthetized cat. The properties of the CVD neurones are not as well established as those of the other systems (see Bell et al., 1985). SM neurones supply only sweat glands of the hairless skin of the paws (see Jänig and Kümmel, 1977, 1981). PM neurones supply only erector pili muscles on the tail and back (see Grosse and Jänig, 1976). The MR neurones consist probably of more than two types (see Bahr et al., 1986a). Modified from Jänig (1984).

that the different types of neurones exhibit characteristic discharge patterns and that there is probably no or only very little cross-talk between different sympathetic channels in the sympathetic ganglia (see Jänig, 1985). Experiments conducted recently show that this may even be true for the lumbar sympathetic supply to the distal colon and the pelvic organs (see below).

Some functional quantitative morphological aspects of the sympathetic lumbar outflow in the cat

Most sympathetic preganglionic neurones which are involved in regulation of target organs in skeletal muscle and skin of the cat hindlimb and tail are situated in the segments T13–L5. A few may be found further rostral. As we know from Langley's work (Langley, 1891a,b, 1894, 1894/95; Langley and Sherrington, 1891) and from experiments conducted recently (Sonnenschein and Weissman,

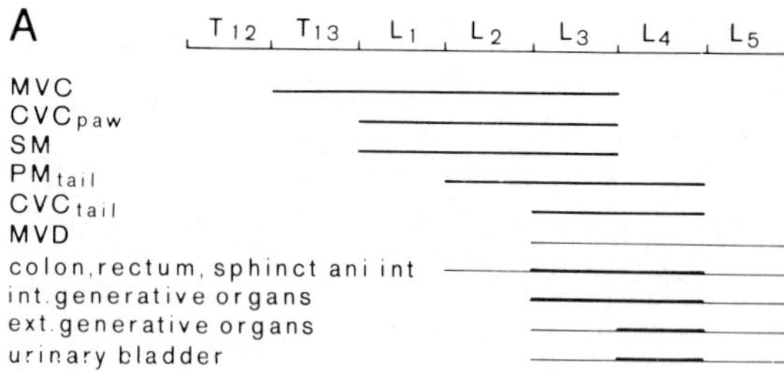

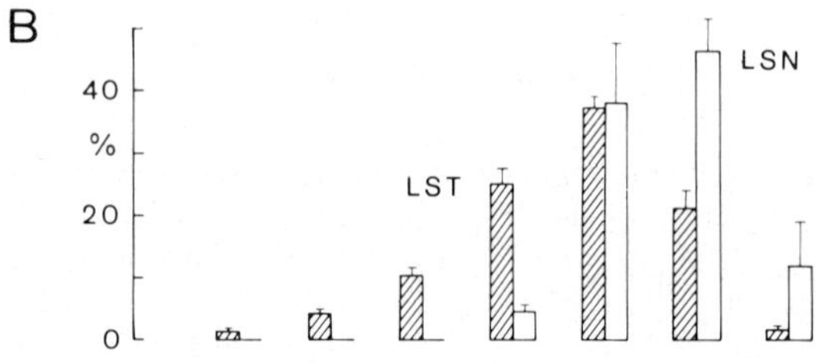

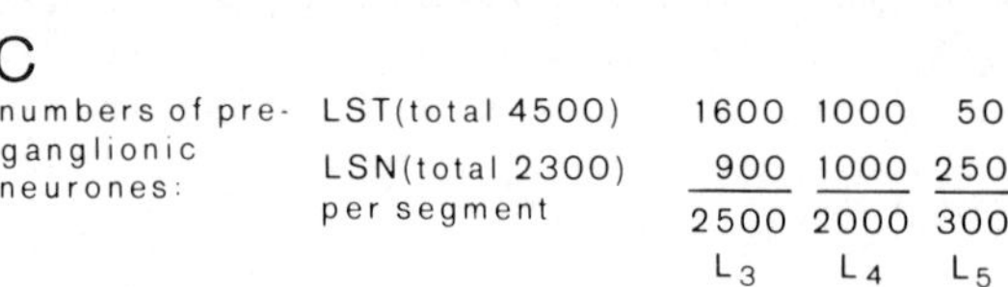

C

numbers of preganglionic neurones:		L3	L4	L5
	LST (total 4500)	1600	1000	50
	LSN (total 2300)	900	1000	250
	per segment	2500	2000	300

Fig. 3. A, autonomic effects elicited by electrical ventral root stimulation in the cat. MVC, MVD: vasoconstriction, vasodilation in skeletal muscle of the hindlimb (Sonnenschein and Weissman, 1978). CVC: vasoconstriction in paw skin and tail skin (Langley, 1891a,b, 1894/5). SM: sweat secretion on foot pads (Langley, 1894, 1894/5). PM: piloerection on the tail (Langley and Sherrington, 1891). Colon, rectum, sphincter ani internus: decrease of motility, contraction, pallor (Langley and Anderson, 1895a). Internal generative organs: contraction, pallor (Langley and Anderson, 1895d). Urinary bladder: short contraction (Langley and Anderson, 1895b). External generative organs: pallor, contraction, retractor, penis and smooth cutaneous muscles (Langley and Anderson, 1895c). B, segmental distribution of preganglionic neurones which project in the lumbar sympathetic trunk (LST) distal to ganglion L_5 (distal to the most caudal lumbar splanchnic nerve, hatched columns) and in the lumbar splanchnic nerves (LSN, open columns) of the cat. These segmental distributions were determined from experiments in which horseradish peroxidase (HRP) solution was applied to the freshly cut LST or LSN nerves. HRP-labelled preganglionic neurones were counted in the respective spinal segments. Mean ± 1 S.E.M. LST, n = 9, from Jänig and McLachlan (1986a); LSN, n = 4, from Baron et al. (1985b). C, numbers of preganglionic neurones. The total numbers of neurones were evaluated from the animals with the best HRP labelling (LST, n = 6; LSN, n = 3). From Baron et al. (1985b) and Jänig and McLachlan (1986a,b).

1978), preganglionic outflow for each target organ has its characteristic, though widely overlapping, segmental distribution (upper part of Fig. 3A). This may be due to the location of the observed target organ, but is probably also characteristic for the functional types of preganglionic neurones (compare the segmental distribution of the vasoconstriction in skeletal muscle (MVC) with that of the active vasodilation in skeletal muscle (MVD) in Fig. 3A). The segmental distribution of the different effector responses in skeletal muscle and skin corresponds reasonably well to the segmental distribution of the preganglionic neurones which project in the lumbar sympathetic trunk distal to the ganglion L5 (distal to the most caudal lumbar splanchnic nerve; see hatched columns in Fig. 3B; Jänig and McLachlan, 1986a). The corresponding postganglionic somata lie in the paravertebral ganglia L5–L7 for the hindlimb (McLachlan and Jänig, 1983) and in the ganglia S2 and S3 for the tail (Langley, 1894; Langley and Sherrington, 1891), a few being found more caudally or rostrally. It should be kept in mind that the ganglia of the lumbar sympathetic trunk have been named according to the origin of the white rami they receive and not according to the destination of their grey rami. Thus, ganglion L4 receives its white ramus (rami) from spinal segment L4 and sends its grey ramus (rami) to the spinal nerve L5, ganglion L7 sends its grey ramus (rami) to spinal nerve S1, etc. (Baron et al., 1985a). This kind of labelling is at variance with that of Langley (1903), who named the lumbar ganglia according to the spinal nerve to which they are connected by way of the grey rami.

Most sympathetic preganglionic neurones which are involved in regulation of distal colon, rectum, sphincter ani internus, internal generative organs and lower urinary tract are situated in the segments L3 and L4, some in L5 and very few in L2 (Langley and Anderson, 1895a–d). The observations made by the latter authors on the effector responses (pallor, contractions, inhibition of motility) in these organs (Fig. 3A, lower part) correspond quite well to the segmental distribution of preganglionic neurones which project in the lumbar splanchnic nerves

(Fig. 3B, open columns): more than 80% of the preganglionic neurones lie in the segments L3 and L4, the rest in L5 and L2 (Baron et al., 1985c). Preganglionic neurones which project through the hypogastric nerves to pelvic organs are concentrated in L4, those which only synapse in the inferior mesenteric ganglion, and are probably involved in the regulation of colonic motility and blood flow through the colon, are mostly located in segment L3 (Baron et al., 1985b,d).

On one side, about 4500 preganglionic neurones project in the distal lumbar sympathetic trunk and about 2300 in the lumbar splanchnic nerves (Baron et al., 1985c; Jänig and McLachlan, 1986a). For the lumbar segments to L5, the total numbers of preganglionic neurones can be estimated from the experimental work with horseradish peroxidase (Fig. 3C): the segment L3 contains about 2500, segment L4 about 2000 and segment L5 about 300 sympathetic preganglionic neurones on one side (Jänig and McLachlan, 1986b). These numbers correspond approximately to the total numbers of preganglionic neurones in the thoracic segments which project in the cervical sympathetic trunk and to the stellate ganglion (T2, about 2500; T3, about 2000 preganglionic neurones; Oldfield and McLachlan, 1981).

Most preganglionic neurones (> 90%) projecting in the distal lumbar sympathetic trunk beyond the most caudal lumbar splanchnic nerve lie in the pars funicularis (ILf) and pars principalis (ILp) of the nucleus intermediolateris (which ends in the upper part of L4; see Rexed, 1954) and at equivalent positions in the segments L4 and L5. They appear as a small band of densely packed, stained cells at the border between white and grey matter after horseradish peroxidase solution has been applied to the proximal end of the lumbar sympathetic trunk cut distally to ganglion L5. Very few cells are found medial to this part of the spinal cord in the nucleus intercalatus and in the nucleus central autonomicus. In contrast, preganglionic neurones which project in the lumbar splanchnic nerves (LSN) have a different location in the spinal cord. Most LSN cells lie just medial to the LST cells; no LSN cells are situated in the ILf but some are in the ILp. Variable proportions of LSN cells are located in the nucleus intercalatus and in the nucleus central autonomicus. Further differences probably exist, in these spinal locations, between preganglionic neurones projecting to pelvic organs through the hypogastric nerves and preganglionic neurones which project to the inferior mesenteric ganglion only (for details see Baron et al., 1985d; Jänig and McLachlan, 1986a,b). These results clearly indicate that preganglionic neurones with different functions have distinct topographical locations in the spinal cord. Future work will show whether this also applies to functionally different classes of preganglionic neurones (see Fig. 3A).

Neurones supplying target organs in skeletal muscle and skin

Animals with intact neuraxis

Six types of sympathetic neurones to skeletal muscle and skin have been functionally characterized (Fig. 2). Three types have ongoing activity in anaesthetized cats and in non-anaesthetized human beings and exhibit characteristic reflexes upon natural stimulation of deep and superficial sensory receptors (muscle vasoconstrictor neurones, MVC; cutaneous vasoconstrictor neurones, CVC; sudomotor neurones, SM). A simple reflex pattern in MVC and CVC neurones is illustrated in Fig. 4. Three types of sympathetic neurones exhibit no ongoing activity in anaesthetized cats and probably not in unanaesthetized humans (pilomotor neurones, PM; muscle vasodilator neurones, MVD; cutaneous vasodilator neurones, CVD); these neurones can only be activated by very specific stimuli and in very specific behavioural contexts. The functional properties of all six pre-/postganglionic channels have been extensively described (Jänig, 1985); furthermore, results obtained in anaesthetized cats have been compared with those obtained in human beings (Jänig et al., 1983b).

One of the most powerful afferent inputs to the

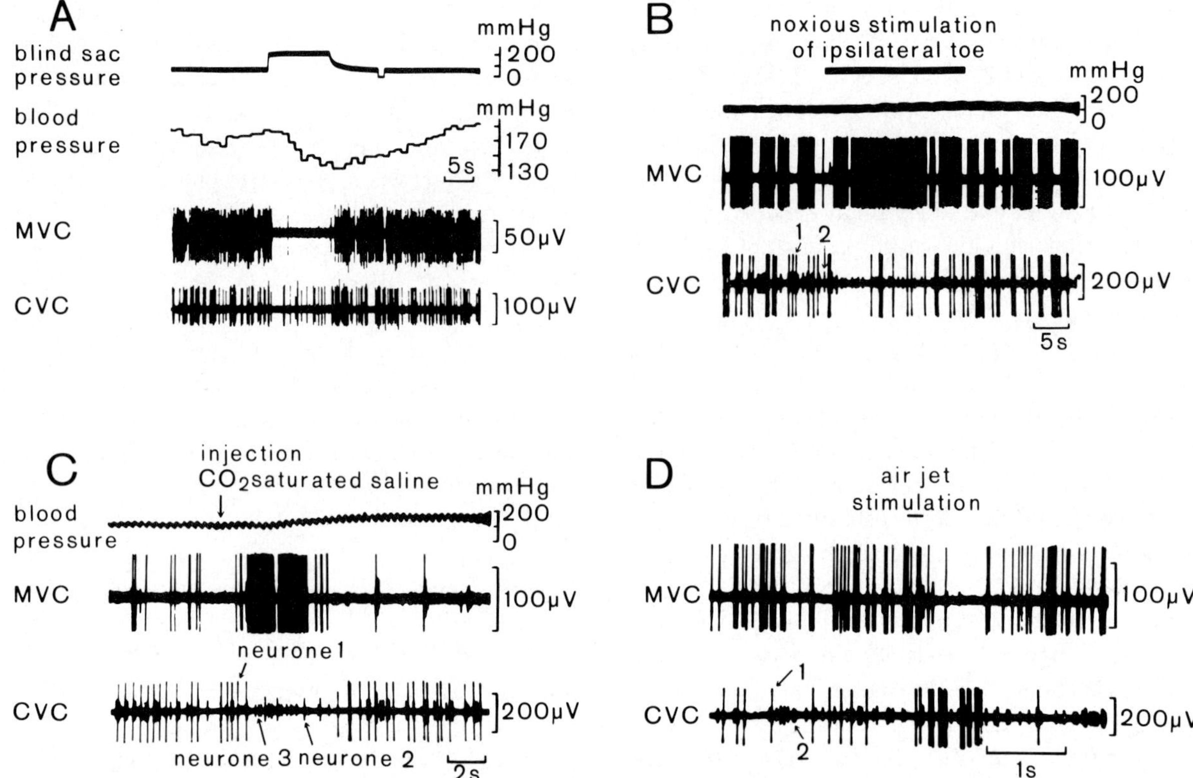

Fig. 4. Reflex patterns in postganglionic vasoconstrictor neurones supplying skeletal muscle (MVC; deep peroneal nerve) and postganglionic vasoconstrictor neurones supplying hairy skin (CVC; superficial peroneal nerve) of the cat hindlimb. A, pressure increase applied in a left isolated carotid blind sac. The carotid sinus nerve to the blind sac was left intact; right carotid sinus nerve and both cervical vagosympathetic trunks, including the aortic nerves, were cut. Both bundles from which the recordings were made contained several postganglionic axons. B–C, simultaneous recordings from a single MVC neurone and a bundle with three CVC neurones (1–3). B, mechanical stimulation of cutaneous nociceptors in a toe of the ipsilateral hindpaw. Upper record, blood pressure. Note that CVC neurones 1 and 2 were inhibited. C, stimulation of arterial chemoreceptors by a bolus injection of CO_2-enriched saline solution (0.8 ml) through a catheter in the left lingual artery close to the glomus caroticum. Note that the CVC neurones 1 and 2 were inhibited and CVC neurone 3 excited. D, short-lasting stimulation of hair follicle receptors on the trunk of the animal by air jets (ten trials superimposed). A and B, modified from Blumberg et al. (1980); C and D, from H. Blumberg and W. Jänig, unpublished observations.

MVC, CVC and SM neurones comes from the visceral organs. Contraction and distension of the urinary bladder and the colon, and even sometimes mechanical stimulation of the mucosal skin of the anus, excites MVC and SM neurones and leads to a decrease of activity in CVC neurones supplying the cat hindlimb (Fig. 5A). After cutting the hypogastric nerves, the reflexes remain virtually unchanged. Thus, the stimulation of pelvic nerve afferent fibres seems to have the major effect (see Jänig and Morrison, this volume). At present, we have no idea about the contribution of the lumbar visceral afferents which pass through the hypogastric nerves from pelvic organs and through the lumbar colonic nerves from the distal colon (Blumberg et al., 1983b). The reflexes elicited from visceral organs fit very well into the general reflex patterns of the sympathetic neurones elicited by stimulation of cutaneous receptors, arterial baro- and chemoreceptors and central (hypothalamic and spinal) heat-sensitive structures (Fig. 6A).

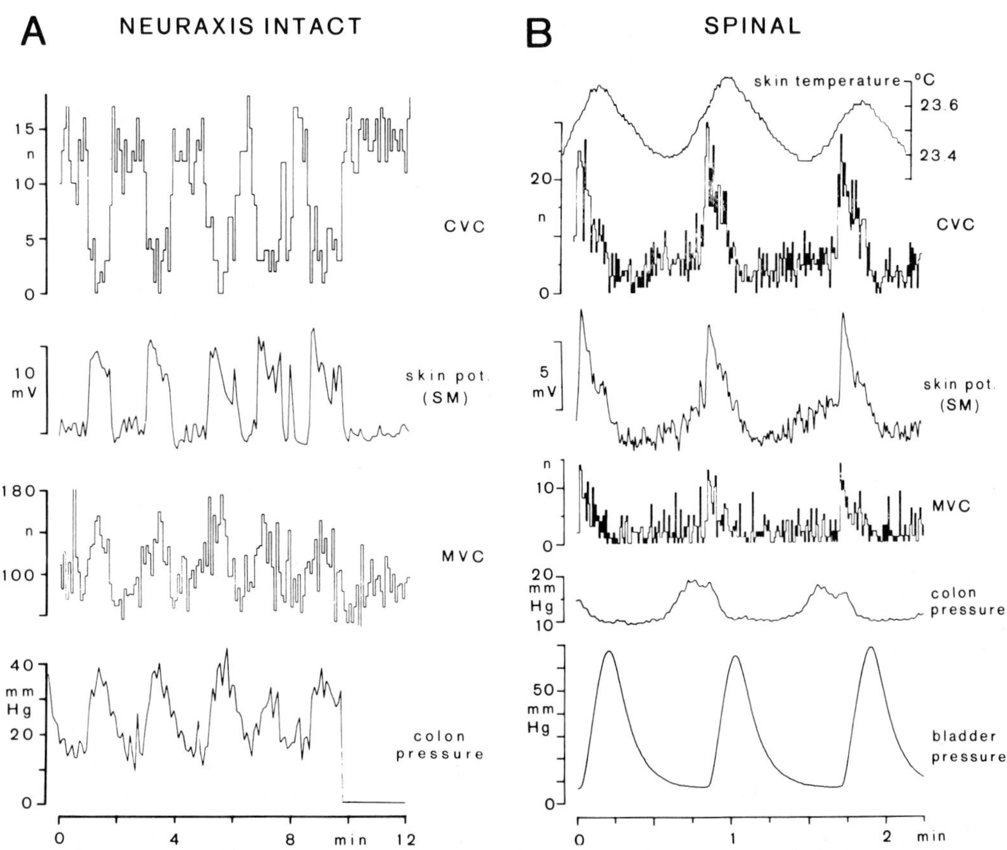

Fig. 5. Reactions of cutaneous vasoconstrictor (CVC), sudomotor (SM) and muscle vasoconstrictor neurones (MVC) during isovolumetric contractions of colon and urinary bladder in a cat with intact neuraxis (A) and in a chronic spinal cat (B); the cat in B was spinalized 135 days before the experiment at segment T_{10}. The postganglionic activities were recorded from multiunit bundles which were isolated from the superficial peroneal nerve (hairy skin) and from a muscle branch of the deep peroneal nerve. For the SM activity, the skin potential was recorded from the surface of the central pad of the ispilateral hindpaw (see Jänig and Kümmel, 1977). The skin temperature in B was recorded on the surface of the central pad of the left hindpaw. The colon was filled with about 30–60 ml fluid in a flexible balloon; the pressure in the balloon was measured by a transducer. The urinary bladder was filled with 20 ml saline and the intravesical pressure measured through the urethral catheter by a transducer. Note that the CVC activity is inhibited during the colon contractions in A and that CVC, SM and MVC neurones are synchronously excited in B. Note, furthermore, that the discharges in the CVC neurones are followed by a decrease in skin temperature, and that urinary bladder and colon contract alternately in B. *n*, number of impulses per 5 seconds in A and per 0.5 second in B. A, from H. Kümmel (unpublished observation); B, modified from Kümmel (1983).

Spinal cats

A question of general interest is: to what extent are the reflexes and reactions of the sympathetic neurones relayed by the spinal cord and dependent on integrating circuits in the spinal cord? At present, this question cannot easily be answered since we have a complete lack of knowledge about the synaptic connections between the spinal afferent inflows, interneurones and sympathetic preganglionic neurones in the spinal cord. Electrical stimulation of spinal nerves elicits short- and long-latency reflexes in preganglionic neurones. The short-latency reflexes probably have a spinal pathway, the long-latency reflexes supraspinal pathways. The spinal pathways are not monosynaptic (see Dembowsky

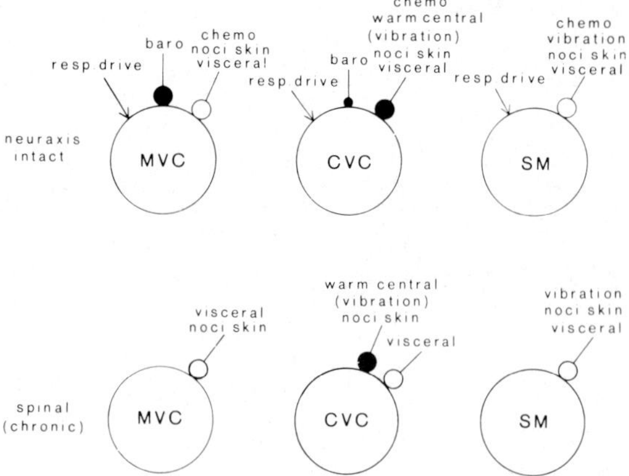

Fig. 6. Reaction patterns of muscle vasoconstrictor (MVC), cutaneous vasoconstrictor (CVC) and sudomotor (SM) neurones in animals with intact neuraxis and in chronic spinal animals. The open and closed small circles indicate excitatory and inhibitory actions, respectively, when the indicated afferent input systems are stimulated. Adequate stimulation of afferents: baro, arterial baroreceptors; chemo, arterial chemoreceptors; noci skin, cutaneous nociceptors of the ipsilateral hindpaw; visceral, visceral afferents from urinary bladder, colon and anus (distension, isovolumetric contraction, shearing stimulus); warm central, heat-sensitive neuronal structures in spinal canal and in hypothalamus; vibration, Pacinian corpuscles in hindpaw. Respiratory drive: grouping of discharges with respiration pronounced in MVC neurones. Note that the visceral spinal input produces inhibition in intact cats but excitation in spinal cats in CVC neurones. Some CVC neurones behave like MVC neurones (see neurone 3 in Fig. 4C).

et al., 1985a). Increasing the stimulus strengths to the C-fibre range also leads to long latency responses via the spinal pathways (Sato and Schmidt, 1973). These experiments show that spinal reflex pathways exist and, furthermore, that they not only have a segmental organization but also a strong intersegmental organization via polysynaptic spinal pathways, e.g., between afferent inflows from the cat hindlimb into the segments L6–S1 and the sympathetic outflow to the hindlimb from the segments L1–L4 (Sato and Schmidt, 1971, 1973). The latter is quite obvious in chronic spinal animals (see Horeyseck and Jänig, 1974b). Unfortunately, it is practically impossible to use electrical stimulation of afferent fibres in order to characterize pre- and postganglionic sympathetic neurones by way of their reflex patterns, neither in animals with intact neuraxis (see Jänig et al., 1972) nor in spinal animals (see Horeyseck and Jänig, 1974b). Furthermore, the existence of short-latency (spinal) and long-latency (probably supraspinal) reflexes elicited in sympathetic neurones by electrical stimulation of visceral and somatic nerves does not give information as to the type of sympathetic system in which the spinal pathway is functionally important, whether the spinal pathway functions under normal ongoing regulation of the sympathetic activity and whether these pathways relay not only excitation but also inhibition of preganglionic activity, etc. Answers to these and other questions can only be derived from experiments in which functionally identified sympathetic neurones are analyzed, since it is to be expected that the spinal pathways vary between different systems. From our analysis of sympathetic neurones supplying skeletal muscle and skin in intact cats, we already have, for example, an indication that the inhibitory reflex elicited by noxious cutaneous stimuli in cutaneous vasoconstrictor neurones is essentially a spinal reflex and unique for this system. This reflex has a spatial organization: it is strongest when the skin of the hindlimb (or tail), which is supplied by the cutaneous vasoconstrictor neurones, is stimulated and weaker or absent when other skin areas are stimulated (Horeyseck and Jänig, 1974a; Grosse and Jänig, 1976; for discussion, see Jänig, 1985).

In our first approach to the question of the spinal organization, we used chronic spinal cats in which the thoracic spinal cord had been cut 60–140 days before the experiments (Horeyseck and Jänig, 1974b; Jänig and Spilok, 1978; Jänig and Kümmel, 1981; Kümmel, 1983; Kümmel and Xu, 1983). Sympathetic systems to skeletal muscle and skin undergo severe "spinal shock" after transection of the spinal cord, and therefore cannot be analyzed in acutely spinalized animals. The duration of the "spinal shock" seems to vary between sympathetic systems (for discussion, see Jänig, 1985). One may argue that spinal circuits function entirely differently when isolated chronically from supraspinal influences since considerable changes may occur in the spinal cord and that, for this reason, studies of sympathetic systems under these conditions may render results which — though pathophysiologically interesting — are not relevant for the above questions. This point cannot be refuted at present. However, the analyses of our experiments on different sympathetic systems in chronic spinal cats have revealed the surprising fact that the sympathetic systems to skeletal muscle and skin do not lose most of their characteristic discharge patterns elicited by stimulation of spinal afferent systems from the skin and the viscera (compare Fig. 6A and 6B). This point should be stressed, since it shows — at least for the MVC, CVC and SM systems — that the spinal cord may contain the neuronal circuits which determine these patterns. Details of quantitative differences between spinal and intact animals have been discussed extensively in the literature (see Jänig, 1985).

The reflexes which changed completely after spinalization were those elicited by visceral stimuli (isovolumetric contraction of urinary bladder and colon, mechanical shearing stimuli applied to the anal canal) in cutaneous vasoconstrictor neurones. Before spinalization these neurones were inhibited (Fig. 5A); after spinalization they were excited and discharged synchronously with the muscle vasoconstrictor and sudomotor neurones (Fig. 5B). The discharges evoked in the cutaneous vasoconstrictor neurones were followed by decreases in skin temperature, indicating vasoconstriction (see upper record in Fig. 5B) (Kümmel, 1983; Kümmel and Xu, 1983).

Sympathetic neurones supplying colon and pelvic organs

The lumbar preganglionic sympathetic outflow, which projects in the lumbar splanchnic nerves, synapses with postganglionic neurones in the inferior mesenteric ganglion and in the pelvic ganglia. These neurones supply the middle and distal colon and pelvic organs. Experiments in which this sympathetic supply was electrically stimulated or abolished indicate that it may have the following functions: (1) Regulation of blood flow and resistance to blood flow in the colon (Langley and Anderson, 1895a; Hultén, 1969), in the urinary bladder (Langley and Anderson, 1895b) and in the internal and reproductive organs (Langley and Anderson, 1895c,d). (2) Regulation of contraction of internal and reproductive organs (Langley and Anderson, 1895c,d); the latter effect and some vascular effects in the pelvic organs may also be induced by stimulation of sympathetic fibres which pass through the sympathetic trunk and then through the pelvic and pudendal nerves (Langley and Anderson, 1895c; Kuo et al., 1984). (3) Regulation of motility of descending colon-rectum (inhibition) and internal anal sphincter (contraction) (Langley and Anderson, 1895a; Bayliss and Starling, 1900; Learmonth and Markowitz, 1929; Garry, 1933; Hultén, 1969; De Groat and Krier, 1976, 1979; Rostad, 1973). (4) Regulation of motility of the urinary bladder (contraction of the sphincter vesicae internus, inhibition of detrusor; inhibition of parasympathetic impulse transmission in pelvic ganglia) (Langley and Anderson, 1895b; De Groat and Saum, 1972; De Groat and Theobald, 1976; De Groat and Booth, 1980); this may lead to a decrease of rhythmic contractions, to an increase of the micturition threshold and to a prolongation of the collecting (continence) phase (Gjone, 1965, 1966a,b; Edvardson, 1968a,b). However, the latter is not well established (Langley and Whiteside, 1951; Klevmark, 1977).

Recording of effector responses in the visceral domain and correlating these effector responses with activity in sympathetic neurones is difficult. This is certainly due, firstly, to the fact that many visceral effector organs depend on several neuronal influences (enteric, sympathetic, parasympathetic) and on non-neural influences (see right side of Fig. 1), secondly, the sympathetic effect may require a parasympathetic or enteric neural background activity, and thirdly, the sympathetic activity might not influence the effector organs directly but inhibit the pre-/postganglionic parasympathetic transmission. This complex situation may be responsible for our poor understanding of the functional organization of the visceral sympathetic supply. Thus far, our knowledge of the above is based mainly on experiments in which gross effector responses or activity in whole sympathetic nerves were recorded, these nerves having been stimulated electrically, or visceral afferents were stimulated electrically or naturally (Hultén, 1969; De Groat and Lalley, 1972; De Groat and Saum, 1972; Rostad, 1973; Garrett et al., 1974; De Groat, 1975; De Groat and Theobald, 1976; De Groat and Krier, 1979; De Groat et al., 1979).

In order to obtain a general idea on the functional organization of the sympathetic outflow to viscera in comparison to that of the sympathetic systems supplying skeletal muscle and skin, we focussed on the discharge patterns of preganglionic neurones, which project in the lumbar splanchnic nerves, and of postganglionic neurones, which project in the hypogastric nerves, without concentrating on any particular organ function. The visceral sympathetic supply originates from the same spinal segments as the sympathetic supply to the hindlimb (see Fig. 2); its target organs are limited in number (though not easily accessible), when compared to other visceral sympathetic supplies; anatomically, it is relatively accessible (Baron et al., 1985a), and therefore experimentally not too difficult to handle, when the recordings are made from the pre- and postganglionic axons. The general idea with which we started was that there are two separate classes of sympathetic neurones, each having its characteristic reaction pattern: visceral vasoconstrictor and various types of motility-regulating neurones. The latter term is purely operational and means inhibitory or excitatory control of non-vascular smooth muscles.

Cats with intact neuraxis

Two classes of preganglionic neurones which project in the lumbar splanchnic nerves could be discriminated, by way of their discharge patterns, with relatively little overlap. The afferent input systems stimulated naturally were: arterial baro- and chemoreceptors, afferents from the urinary bladder and urethra, colon and anus and, occasionally, afferents from the perigenital hairy skin. Arterial baro- and chemoreceptors were stimulated as described by Blumberg et al. (1980) and visceral mechanoreceptors by distension and contraction of the organs (urinary bladder and colon), by tapping on or pulling of the urethral catheter (urethra) and by mechanical shearing (anus). The perigenital skin was stimulated mechanically (see Blumberg et al., 1983b; Bahns et al., 1985a,b, 1986; Jänig and Morrison, this volume).

Visceral vasoconstrictor neurones (VVC)

The first class of preganglionic neurones displayed a very homogeneous reaction pattern: they were strongly inhibited upon stimulation of arterial baroreceptors, exhibiting a pronounced "cardiac rhythmicity" of their activity (for definition, see Blumberg et al., 1980). Stimulation of the arterial chemoreceptors (either by injection of a small amount of CO_2-enriched saline solution through the lingual artery close to the arterial chemoreceptors in the left glomus caroticum, or by ventilating the animal with a hypoxic gas mixture of 8% O_2 in N_2) led to a weak excitation of the neurones. This excitation was much weaker than that of muscle vasoconstrictor neurones. Visceral stimuli had either no effect on most of these neurones, or a slight excitatory or inhibitory effect, when the visceral stimuli were very strong (e.g., contraction of the urinary bladder with intravesical pressures of more than 50 mmHg). These effects may be produced indirectly via the baroreceptor loop (inhibition) or directly via the spinal cord (excitation).

These preganglionic neurones, which we have called "visceral vasoconstrictor neurones" (VVC), behave like muscle vasoconstrictor neurones. Both classes of neurones also have a strong respiratory rhythmicity in their activity (for definition, see Jänig et al., 1980; Jänig, 1985). Because of the weak reaction of the VVC neurones to stimulation of chemoreceptors and of the visceral afferents from the urinary bladder and colon, as compared to the muscle vasocontrictor neurones (see Fig. 5), we believe that these VVC neurones are a third class of vasoconstrictor neurones (Jänig, 1984; Bahr et al., 1986b). The discharge pattern of these neurones is illustrated in Fig. 9.

An extensive analysis of the postganglionic neurones projecting in the hypogastric nerves, which was conducted recently in our laboratory, has revealed a class of neurones with a discharge pattern identical to that of the preganglionic VVC neurones (W. Jänig, M. Schmidt, A. Schnitzler and U. Wesselmann, unpublished observation). However, the percentage of neurones with the VVC pattern is considerably lower for the postganglionic neurones than for the preganglionic neurones (36% preganglionically versus 9% postganglionically). Therefore, it is likely that the VVC discharge pattern is transmitted without change from pre- to postganglionic neurones in the hypogastric nerve. A large part of the vasoconstrictor supply to the pelvic organs may pass through the distal sympathetic trunk and the pelvic nerve (Kuo et al., 1984). A small percentage of neurones was found, pre- as well as postganglionically, with the discharge pattern of both VVC and certain motility-regulating neurones (see Bahr et al., 1986b). We do not know yet whether or not this is a technical artefact.

Motility-regulating (MR) neurones

The second class of visceral preganglionic neurones was defined operationally as "motility-regulating neurones" (MR neurones) if the neurones were not inhibited upon stimulation of arterial baroreceptors and not excited or inhibited upon stimulation of arterial chemoreceptors, and if they reacted to at least one of the visceral stimuli used. Preganglionic neurones belonging to this class display a wealth of reactions to the visceral stimuli used. From experiments in which the hypogastric and lumbar colonic nerves were cut (thus abolishing the lumbar afferent input from pelvic organs and colon), we know that the sacral afferent inputs via the pelvic nerves and, possibly, via the pudendal nerves are important for these differentiated reactions (see Bahns et al., 1985a,b). The role of the lumbar visceral afferents is unclear; from experiments in which these afferents were stimulated electrically, we at least know that these have a weak effect on the MR neurones, as compared to the VVC neurones (see below, and Bahr et al., 1986c).

In principle, stimulation of the afferent inputs from the lower urinary tract (bladder and urethra), the colon, the anus and the perigenital skin can elicit excitation and inhibition in the preganglionic MR neurones. The most powerful inputs are from the anal skin and the urinary bladder. Stimulation of the anal skin elicits excitation in 78.5% of the MR neurones (Fig. 7A, B); the reflex is very often followed by an afterdischarge, which may last for several minutes (Fig. $7B_1$). Some MR neurones (8%) are inhibited by this stimulus. Mechanical stimulation of the perianal or perigenital hairy skin is mostly without effect. In some neurones, however, perigenital stimulation also elicits reflex excitation or inhibition; these reflexes may be opposite to those elicited from the anus (see Bahr et al., 1986a). About 67% of the MR neurones tested were excited during distension and contraction of the urinary bladder (Fig. $7A_1$, A_2, upper records) and 23% inhibited by these stimuli (Fig. $7A_1$, A_2, middle records). The excitatory reflexes were very often quite large, whereas the inhibitory ones were difficult to detect.

For technical reasons, it is difficult to elicit reflexes from the colon. This usually requires filling of the colon with up to 60–80 ml, and leads consequently to considerable displacement of the abdominal contents, and thus to an impairment of the recording conditions, if not to a loss of the fibre bundles which had been isolated from one of the lumbar splanchnic or hypogastric nerves. The reflexes, if successfully elicited from the colon, usually result in a decrease of ongoing activity in the MR neurones (Fig. $7B_2$) or, more rarely, an increase in activity. Many MR neurones do not react at all. These reactions are mostly discrete and not as pronounced at those produced by either anal stimulation or isovolumetric contraction of the urinary bladder (Fig. $7B_1$).

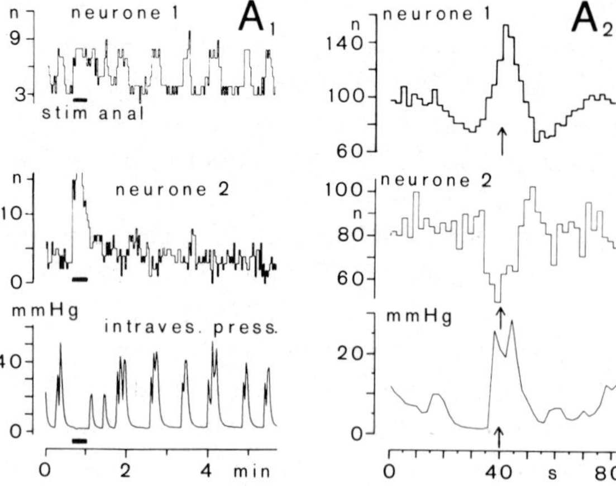

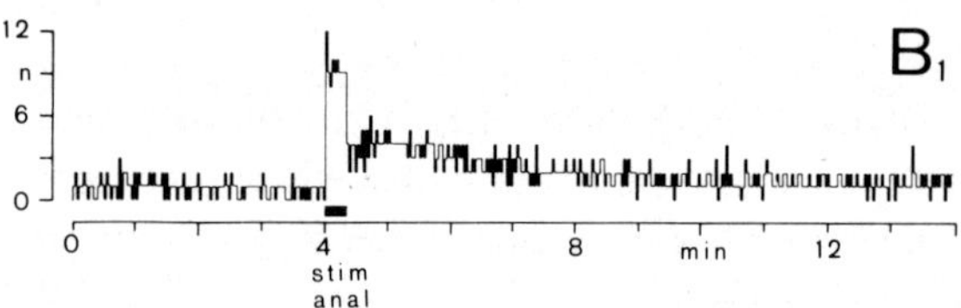

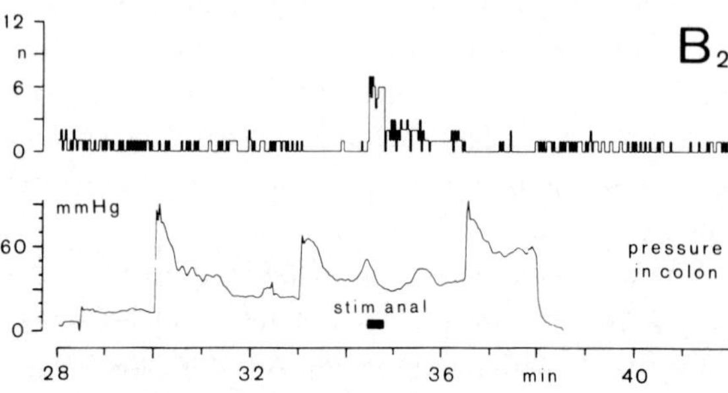

Fig. 7. Reactions of visceral preganglionic neurones projecting in the lumbar splanchnic nerves to the inferior mesenteric ganglion. A_1, A_2, simultaneous recording from two motility-regulating (MR) neurones during isovolumetric contractions of the urinary bladder (lower record). Neurone 1 (MR_1) was excited and 2 (MR_2) inhibited. In A the activities of the neurones were superimposed several times with respect to the bladder contractions. Both neurones were excited by mechanical stimulation of the mucosal skin of the anus (black bar). B_1, B_2, neurone being excited by anal stimulation (B_1) and inhibited by distension and contraction of the colon (B_2). Note that the anal reflex is followed by afterdischarges (B_1) and that the anal reflex is also depressed from the colon. *n*, number of impulses per 2 seconds. A, modified from Bahr et al. (1986a); B, unpublished observations.

If one tries to combine the different excitatory and inhibitory visceral reflexes in the MR neurones, at least two reflex patterns emerge (Fig. 9). Taking the reflexes elicited by contraction and distension of the urinary bladder as "leading" reflexes and the reflexes to distension and contraction of the colon as supplementary criteria, most neurones can be divided into two complementary classes: MR_1 neurones, which are excited from the urinary bladder and inhibited from the colon (or are excited from the urinary bladder but show no effect from the colon or, rarely, show no effect from the urinary bladder but are inhibited from the colon); MR_2 neurones, which are inhibited from the urinary bladder and excited from the colon (or are inhibited from the urinary bladder but show no effect from the colon, or show no effect from the urinary bladder but are excited from the colon). About 50% of the preganglionic MR neurones belong to the MR_1 class and about 25% to the MR_2 class. About 25% of the MR neurones were only excited from the anus or could not be further classified with the experimental protocol used. At present, we are not able to use the anal reflex for subclassifying the MR_1 and MR_2 neurones (see Bahr et al., 1986a).

An extensive analysis of the postganglionic neurones projecting in the hypogastric nerves which was conducted recently in our laboratory revealed, cum grano salis, besides the postganglionic visceral vasoconstrictor neurones (VVC in Fig. 9), the same two classes of postganglionic MR_1 and MR_2 neurones (W. Jänig, M. Schmidt, A. Schnitzler and U. Wesselmann, unpublished observations). About 51% of the postganglionic MR neurones belong to the MR_1 class, and about 16% to the MR_2 class; the remainder were only excited from the anus or could not be further classified with the experimental protocol used. This finding substantiates the idea that the discharge patterns of the MR neurones are transmitted in functionally separate pre-/postganglionic channels to the pelvic organs.

The experiments show that each set of pelvic visceral afferents (from the anus, colon, lower urinary tract; see Bahns et al., 1985a,b), and probably also afferents from the perigenital skin and the distal part of the urethra that pass through the pudendal nerve (Todd, 1964), can elicit qualitatively and quantitatively distinct reflexes in preganglionic sympathetic MR neurones. It also shows that this part of the sympathetic nervous system is probably highly differentiated. In this context, it is interesting to note that interneurones in the sacral spinal cord (with and without ascending axons), which respond to stimulation of the urinary bladder and the colon, exhibit discharge patterns very similar to those of the MR neurones. About 75–91% of the interneurones have either the pattern of the MR_1 neurones or that of the MR_2 neurones (De Groat et al., 1981; McMahon and Morrison, 1982a,b).

At present, we have no ideas as to the role of the lumbar visceral afferents from the colon (Blumberg et al., 1983a; Haupt et al., 1983) and from the pelvic organs (Bahns et al., 1986a; see Jänig and Morrison, this volume). Electrical stimulation of visceral afferents in the white rami L2–L5 elicit weak reflexes in MR neurones (Bahr et al., 1985c). Floyd et al. (1982) analyzed the discharge pattern of postganglionic sympathetic neurones projecting in the hypogastric nerves to distension of urinary bladder and colon, in cats which had been spinalized at the 6th lumbar segment. In this way, the effect of the lumbar visceral afferents from the organs on the visceral sympathetic neurones could be tested without interfering with the activity in the pelvic afferents. About 60% of the efferent postganglionic units which were tested in their reactions to distension were excited from both organs, and 20% were not affected from both. No reciprocal reflex patterns were found.

Spinal animals

After spinalization of the cat by cutting the spinal cord between T7 and T13, preganglionic visceral vasoconstrictor neurones can no longer be recognized by way of their discharge pattern. Analysis of two vasoconstrictor neurones, before and after spinalization, revealed that they lose their ongoing activity (Bartel et al., 1986). Thus, it might well be

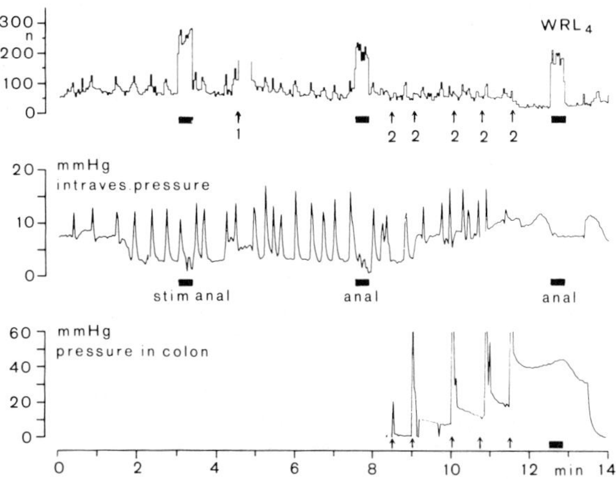

Fig. 8. Reaction of preganglionic neurones projecting in the white ramus L4 (WRL_4) to contraction of the urinary bladder, distension of the colon and mechanical stimulation of the anal mucosal skin in a spinal cat (spinalized 1 hour before at T10). The preganglionic activity increased upon the bladder contractions and anal stimulation and decreased upon distension of the colon. At the arrows labelled with "2" the balloon in the colon was filled with 10 ml saline each. The preganglionic activity started to decrease when the pressure in the colon reached values of 20–40 mmHg. Note that anal stimulation and colon distension inhibited the bladder contractions. At "1", the WRL_4 was cut distal to the recording electrode in order to exclude the possibility of afferent activity being recorded. *n*, number of impulses per 2 seconds. From Bartel et al. (1986).

that this system goes through a long phase of "spinal shock", as is the case with vasconstrictor neurones supplying skeletal muscle and skin (see Jänig, 1985), and that spinal reflexes in these neurones can only be tested in the chronic state after spinalization.

Motility-regulating (MR) neurones, however, behave differently; excitatory reflexes upon anal stimulation and contraction and distension of the urinary bladder are fully preserved and inhibitory reflexes upon colon distension and contraction may become very pronounced. Fig. 8 illustrates the records from an experiment in which, about 1 hour after spinalization, the activity was recorded from the white ramus L4; the urinary bladder exhibited weak contractions, the colon was distended. Mechanical stimulation of the anus excited the preganglionic neurones, the contractions of the urinary

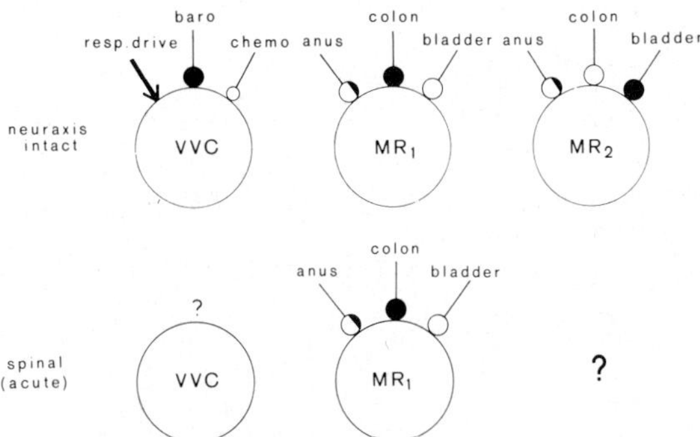

Fig. 9. Reaction patterns of lumbar visceral vasoconstrictor (VVC) and lumbar motility-regulating (MR) neurones in cats with intact neuraxis and in acutely spinalized cats. The open and closed small circles indicate excitatory and inhibitory effects, respectively, when the indicated afferent input systems are stimulated. Respiratory drive, baro and chemo, see legend of Fig. 6; anus, stimulation of the mucosal skin of the anus by mechanical shearing stimuli; colon, distension and isovolumetric contraction of the colon; bladder, distension and isovolumetric contraction of the urinary bladder. MR neurones were neither inhibited upon stimulation of arterial baroreceptors nor excited upon stimulation of arterial chemoreceptors. For details, see text and Bahr et al. (1986a,b) and Bartel et al. (1986).

bladder were accompanied by excitation of the neurones and, during distension of the colon with intraluminal pressures of 20–40 mmHg, the activity was decreased. This is the reflex pattern of MR_1 neurones; it was obtained in the same preganglionic neurones before and after spinalization, whereby the inhibitory effect from the colon became either stronger or appeared after spinalization. Thus, the pattern of the MR neurones is preserved after spinalization, and therefore is fully dependent on spinal neuronal mechanisms (Fig. 9). This does not mean that these spinal neuronal circuits are not under descending control from supraspinal brain structures. In some MR_1 neurones it was observed that the excitation upon contraction and distension of the urinary bladder became enhanced and that the depression of activity upon colon distension appeared enhanced following spinalization. Thus, it might be hypothesized that both spinal reflex pathways are normally under inhibitory descending control.

A second interesting observation was that the inhibitory reflexes elicited in MR neurones by mechanical stimulation of anal and perianal skin and by contraction of the urinary bladder disappeared or even changed to excitatory reflexes after spinalization (Bartel et al., 1986). This finding may mean that these inhibitory reflexes have a supraspinal pathway or that the spinal pathways which relay these reflexes require considerable facilitation from supraspinal brain structures (see also De Groat and Lalley, 1972). I favour the latter possibility, since we have found visceral preganglionic neurones in the spinal animal which were inhibited from the anal and perigenital skin and one neurone which was inhibited upon contraction of the urinary bladder. This latter neurone might well have been an MR_2 neurone (Bartel et al., 1986).

Functional considerations

The functional separation of the lumbar visceral preganglionic neurones into VVC and MR neurones is sound. This separation is strongly supported by the difference in other properties between both classes of neurones (Bahr et al., 1986c): (1) segmental distribution (VVC: L1–L4; MR: L3–L5); (2) conduction velocity of axons (VVC: 2.8 ± 2.5 m/second, n = 49 (mean ± S.D.); MR: 8.1 ± 4.7 m/second, n = 131); (3) rate of ongoing activity (VVC: 1.6 ± 0.9 imp/second, n = 46; MR: 0.8 ± 0.7 imp/second, n = 91, 16% silent); (4) reflexes to electrical stimulation of lumbar white rami and lumbar spinal nerves (VVC: segmental and suprasegmental in all neurones; MR: only about 50% of the neurones have weak reflexes, mainly segmental).

The population of MR neurones is functionally heterogeneous. Besides the MR_1 and MR_2 neurones, there probably are other types of MR neurones which were not recognized by our experimental protocol. Considering the possible types of target organs (urinary bladder and urethra, sphincter ani internus, rectum-colon, internal generative organs, pelvic ganglia), one could expect to find functionally different types of lumbar visceral sympathetic neurones. Theoretically, each type of target organ may receive its separate sympathetic supply.

According to De Groat and co-workers (De Groat and Lalley, 1972; De Groat, 1975; De Groat and Theobald, 1976; De Groat et al., 1979), stimulation of pelvic nerve afferents leads to excitatory spinal reflexes in postganglionic sympathetic neurones which project in the hypogastric nerve. It is hypothesized that this sympathetic excitation induces inhibition of the detrusor muscle, contraction of the trigone region and depression of transmission in vesical parasympathetic ganglia, and leads consequently to an increase in the micturition threshold and in the continence volume. When micturition is initiated this spinal vesico-sympathetic reflex is inhibited by the pontine "micturition centre", thus allowing micturition to proceed uninhibited. From this hypothesis it could be assumed that our MR_1 neurones are involved in regulation of micturition and continence of the urinary bladder. Two observations have been made which go against this assumption: first, MR_1 neurones are excited at low and high intravesical pressures during bladder contractions; secondly, distension of the colon depresses the activity in many MR_1 neurones.

An alternative hypothesis could be that MR_1 neurones supply the sphincter ani internus and rectum-colon, whereas MR_2 neurones supply detrusor muscle, the trigone region and visceral parasympathetic ganglia. This pattern of innervation would be consistent with the reciprocal reaction pattern of both types of neurones with respect to the afferent stimuli from both organs. It would also fit with the reciprocal contraction pattern of both organs when they are filled with fluid, which can be observed both in cats with intact neuraxis and in spinal cats (see Fig. 5B, lower two recordings).

Most MR_1 and MR_2 neurones are excited by anal stimulation. In spinal cats and in cats with an intact neuraxis, bladder and colon contractions can be inhibited by mechanical stimulation of the anus (Bahr et al., 1986a). Similar results have been obtained for the urinary bladder in humans (Kock and Pompeius, 1963; Sundin et al., 1974). We have no idea as to the function of the inhibition induced in some MR (particularly MR_1) neurones by anal stimulation or of the reflexes (excitation or inhibition) elicited by perigenital stimuli in some MR_1 and MR_2 neurones. We have no idea about the discharge pattern of the sympathetic neurones which supply the internal generative organs. These neurones, under our experimental conditions, are probably silent and can only be excited by very specific central and peripheral stimuli (which we did not use). Quantiative comparison of the HRP histology on the lumbar splanchnic nerves (Baron et al., 1985c,d) with the electrophysiological results leads to the following estimations: about 350 visceral preganglionic neurones have vasoconstrictor function and about 1000 motility-regulating function with properties as measured by Bahr et al. (1986c); about 1000 preganglionic neurones which project in the lumbar splanchnic nerves do not exhibit MR or VVC neurone reflexes. Many of the latter neurones may supply internal reproductive organs.

Organization of the sympathetic systems. The "spinal sympathetic functional units"

Fig. 10 provides a general idea as to how the lumbar sympathetic nervous systems might be organized at the spinal level and peripherally. This idea is, of course, largely speculative and based completely on the experimental results which have been obtained in our laboratory over the last 12 years.

(1) The sympathetic outflow of the spinal cord is organized in functionally separate pre-/postganglionic channels which we call — taking the above restrictions into consideration — "final common sympathetic motor paths". These peripheral paths are the links between the CNS and the sympathetic target organs. The activity in the preganglionic neurones is probably modified by integrative processes in the sympathetic para- and prevertebral ganglia. The nature of these peripheral processes during ongoing neuronal regulation of the target organs is largely unknown, but enough knowledge has been accumulated showing that there are several possible mechanisms by which this may occur. There may be differences in these inte-

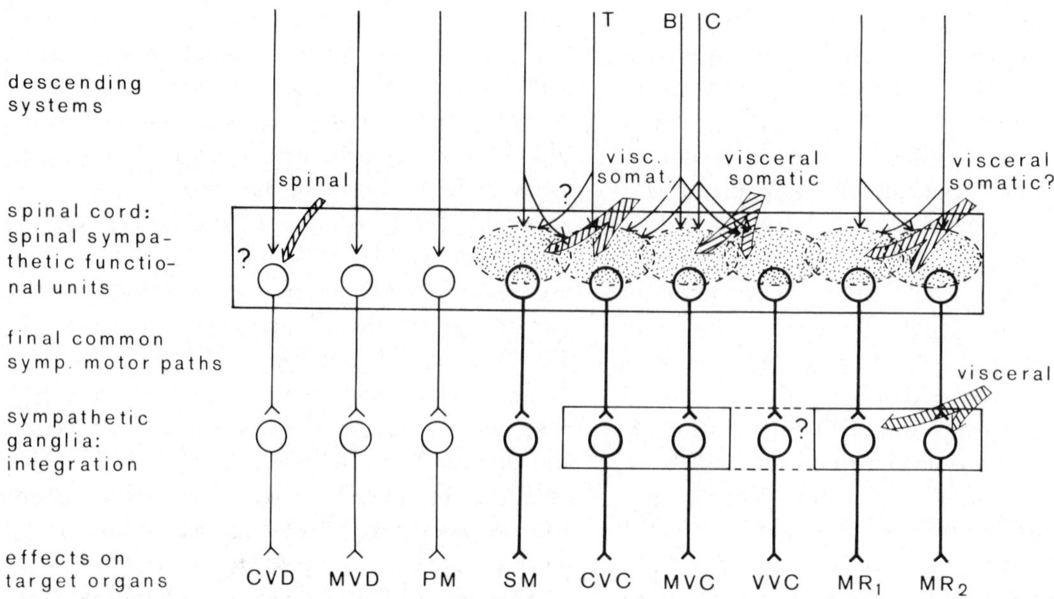

Fig. 10. Diagrammatic representation of the spinal organization of the lumbar sympathetic systems supplying skeletal muscle, skin, distal colon and pelvic organs (systems projecting in the distal lumbar sympathetic trunk, distal to ganglion L5, and in the lumbar splanchnic nerves). At the base of this organization are the sympathetic target organs which are supplied by the "final common sympathetic motor paths". The "target organs" of some MR neurones may be other neurones or the synaptic terminals on these neurones in the pelvic ganglia to the urinary bladder (De Groat and Saum, 1972; De Groat and Theobald, 1976; De Groat and Booth, 1980) and in the enteric nervous system of the colon. The transmission of information in the "final common sympathetic motor paths" from the pre- to the postganglionic neurones may be modified in the CVC and MVC systems in the ganglia of the sympathetic trunk (Hoffmeister et al., 1978; Jänig et al., 1982, 1983a, 1984a; Blumberg and Jänig, 1983) and in the inferior mesenteric ganglion (Simmons, 1985). The stippled areas symbolize "spinal sympathetic functional units" which consist of preganglionic neurones, interneurones and their synaptic connections with the spinal primary afferent inputs from the somatic and visceral domains (shaded arrows) and with the descending systems. These spinal units may determine the characteristic discharge patterns of the sympathetic neurones which are drawn in thick lines (these systems also have ongoing activity). The other three systems (right side) are probably largely dependent on the activity in the descending systems. The existence of the CVD system is not as well established as that of the other systems (see Jänig and Kümmel, 1981; Bell et al., 1985). The "spinal sympathetic functional units" are under control of various descending systems from brainstem and hypothalamus (T, thermo; B, baro; C, chemo). CVD, cutaneous vasodilator; MVD, muscle vasodilator; PM, pilomotor; SM, sudomotor; CVC, cutaneous vasoconstrictor; MVC, muscle vasoconstrictor; VVC, visceral vasoconstrictor; MR, motility-regulating. Modified from Jänig (1985).

grative processes between sympathetic systems: for example, in the systems on the left side in Fig. 10 (CVD, MVD, PM, SM), the impulses may be transmitted from the pre- to the postganglionic neurones in a "relay-like" fashion without any further modulating mechanisms; in the systems on the right side (CVC, MVC, VVC, MR), integration may occur; this certainly applies to the MR systems. The postganglionic neurones of the latter systems may get peripheral synaptic input from afferents which have their cell bodies in the periphery and also from collaterals of spinal visceral afferent neurones. The synaptic processes may also use peptidergic transmitters and induce long-term postganglionic processes (see Szurszewski, 1981; Simmons, 1985).

The postganglionic CVC and MVC neurones in the paravertebral ganglia probably do not receive peripheral synaptic inputs, but long-term synaptic (non-nicotinic, cholinergic and non-cholinergic) processes can also be shown to exist in these neurones (Hoffmeister et al., 1978; Jänig et al., 1982, 1983a, 1984; Blumberg and Jänig, 1983). Thus, there are first of all considerable differences between sympathetic systems in ganglionic transmission of impulses and, second, between para- and prevertebral ganglia.

(2) The analysis of the discharge patterns of the lumbar pre- and postganglionic neurones in cats with intact neuraxis and in spinal cats shows that the spinal cord plays an important role in the generation of the reflex patterns of several types of sympathetic neurones (see Figs. 6 and 9). This probably applies to the systems which have been drawn in thick lines in Fig. 10. Many, if not most, of the neurones of these systems have ongoing activity in anaesthetized cats (see Jänig, 1985) and, as far as the SM, CVC and MVC systems are concerned, also in awake humans (Jänig et al., 1983b). I have postulated for these systems, in analogy to the functional motor units in the spinal cord (Baldissera et al., 1981), "spinal sympathetic functional units" (stippled in Fig. 10; see Jänig, 1985). A "spinal sympathetic functional unit" may consist of the respective preganglionic neurones, interneurones and their synaptic connections with the spinal primary afferent inputs and with the descending spinal systems from the brainstem and hypothalamus. Related spinal sympathetic functional units may share common interneurone pools and common inputs from spinal primary afferents and descending spinal systems. In Fig. 10 functionally related spinal sympathetic functional units are shown close together, such as the CVC and SM system, the CVC and MVC system, the MVC and VVC system, and both MR systems. This functional relation is reflected in the similarity, but not identity, of the discharge patterns of the neurones with respect to the afferent inputs (for example, in MVC and VVC neurones; see Figs. 6 and 9), and in the reciprocity of the discharge patterns of different types of neurones with respect to the afferent inputs (for example, in CVC and SM neurones, in CVC and MVC neurones and in MR_1 and MR_2 neurones; see Figs. 6 and 9). Also, the VVC and MR systems may overlap: some visceral preganglionic neurones have been found which have both the VVC and the MR discharge patterns (see Bahr et al., 1986b).

It is unclear whether the MVD and the PM systems can be activated by spinal afferent inputs. The properties of the CVD system are not well established; these neurones can probably be activated by warm inputs in the spinal canal (see Jänig and Kümmel, 1981; Bell et al., 1985; Jänig, 1985).

(3) Spinal sympathetic functional units are under control of spinal descending systems from the brainstem and hypothalamus. From our work and the work of others, it follows that several functionally distinct descending systems must exist which are related to the sympathetic systems. For example, the information from the arterial baroreceptors is transmitted to the CVC, MVC and VVC systems but not to the other systems (B in Fig. 10), that from the arterial chemoreceptors preferentially to the CVC, MVC, VVC and SM systems (C in Fig. 10), and the information from the hypothalamic thermosensitive structures preferentially to the CVC but not to the MVC system (T in Fig. 10). Furthermore, the descending control of the MR systems is probably different from the descending control of most other systems, etc. There is ample morphological evidence showing a diversity of descending spinal systems, from lower and upper brainstem and hypothalamus, which may be functionally related to the sympathetic systems (Amendt et al., 1979; Loewy and McKellar, 1980; Loewy and Neil, 1981; Loewy, 1982), and also some neurophysiological evidence about different types of descending systems (Illert and Seller, 1969; Illert and Gabriel, 1972; Foreman and Wurster, 1973; Coote and MacLeod, 1974a,b, 1975; Jänig and Szulczyk, 1979; Dampney et al., 1982; Caverson et al., 1983; for discussion, see Dampney, 1981; Dembowsky et al., 1985a). The conduction velocities of the descending axons range from about 2 m/second or less to 25 m/second (see Dembowsky et al., 1985a). No clear-cut information is available about the functional properties of any descending spinal system and its relation to the sympathetic systems.

The organization of the sympathetic systems may be expressed metaphorically in a picture: the final common sympathetic motor paths plus the respective spinal sympathetic functional units are the keyboard on which brainstem, hypothalamus and higher brain structures play by way of the descending spinal systems; the effector responses are the sounds, the combinations of the effector responses are the chords, and the temporal courses of the different combinations of effector responses are the melodies, according to the functional conditions. The afferent inputs from the somatic and visceral domains modify these sounds, chords and melodies, and are the registers. The integration in the ganglia, including the non-nicotinic and peptidergic synaptic long-term mechanisms, may correspond to the forte and piano pedals or similar mechanisms.

Comparison of extracellularly and intracellularly obtained data on sympathetic preganglionic neurones

No systematic attempt has been made to analyze intracellular events in sympathetic preganglionic neurones with respect to the different types of adequate stimuli applied to the body surface and visceral domain. The reason for this deficit is obvious: (1) it is difficult to obtain acceptable intracellular records from sympathetic preganglionic neurones over longer periods of time, probably because of the small size, spindle shape and rostrocaudal orientation of most of these neurones (Oldfield and McLachlan, 1981; Baron et al., 1985b,c; Dembowsky et al., 1985b); (2) natural stimuli, whether applied to the skin, viscera, arterial baro- and chemoreceptors or elsewhere, may produce mechanical irritation of the preparation and may lead to a change in the arterial blood pressure, venous pressure and heart rate, influencing in this way the recording conditions; (3) conceptually, the differentiation in the sympathetic nervous system is not well established. The first studies were restricted to the description of the features of the action potentials (Fernandez de Molina et al., 1965; Coote and Westbury, 1979) and of the naturally occurring ongoing synaptic activity (McLachlan and Hirst, 1980). The latter study is the only one in which synaptic activity in thoracic preganglionic vasoconstrictor neurones in response to stimulation of arterial baroreceptors was studied, showing that the excitation of the neurones decreased due to inhibitory synaptic potentials or to disfacilitation of synaptic activity.

An extensive intracellular study of ongoing synaptic activity and synaptic activity, evoked by electrical stimulation of white rami, intercostal nerves, cervical dorsolateral funiculus and cervical dorsal root entry zone, in preganglionic neurones of the thoracic segment T3, has been conducted by Dembowsky et al. (1985a,c). This segment contains about 2500 preganglionic neurones (Oldfield and McLachlan, 1981) which are involved in the regulation of various target organs (head, upper extremity, heart, inner eye muscles, erector pili muscles, blood vessels of skeletal muscle and skin, sweat glands, heart muscle, etc.); practically all of these neurones are situated in the nucleus intermediolateralis, about 80–90% lying in the pars principalis and the rest in the pars funicularis (Oldfield and McLachlan, 1981; Wesselmann and McLachlan, 1984). The dendritic fields of these neurones are confined to the intermediolateral nucleus, extending about 1.5–2.50 mm in the rostro-caudal, about 150–400 μm in the medio-lateral and about 5.0–200 μm in the dorso-ventral direction (Réthelyi, 1972; Dembowsky et al., 1985b). Based on the passive and active electrophysiological properties, the preganglionic neurones can be divided into three types (Dembowsky et al., 1985c). About 50% of these neurones showed pronounced and 50% very slight excitatory synaptic ongoing activity; inhibitory potentials rarely occurred. Electrical stimulation of visceral (white ramus) and somatic (intercostal nerve) afferents elicits early and late excitatory postsynaptic potentials (EPSPs) in nearly all preganglionic neurones; electrical stimulation of descending pathways in the dorso-lateral funiculus also elicits responses in all of these neurones, inhibitory postsynaptic potentials being very rare. Taking the possible target organs of sympathetic preganglionic neurones in the thoracic segment T3 into consideration, it is surprising that Dembowsky et al. (1985a,c) could not make any functional classification of their neurones by way of the spinal and supraspinal synaptic inputs. Their population of preganglionic neurones appeared to be quite homogeneous. In my opinion, this conclusion, derived from the work of Dembowsky's group, is an enigma; it shows that the only way to approach questions as to the central organization of the sympathetic systems is to use natural afferent stimuli as has been done by McLachlan and Hirst (1980).

Summary

The lumbar sympathetic outflow supplying skeletal muscle, skin, distal colon and pelvic viscera is composed of several subsystems with different functions: muscle vasoconstrictor (MVC), cutaneous vasoconstrictor (CVC), sudomotor (SM), pilomotor (PM), muscle vasodilator (MVD), cutaneous vasodilator (CVD), visceral vasoconstrictor (VVC) and different types of motility-regulating (MR) neurones. (1) Each subsystem is functionally characterized by the discharge pattern of its pre- and postganglionic neurones. Six systems (MVC, CVC, SM, VVC, MR_1, MR_2) have ongoing activity and exhibit distinct reflexes upon stimuli applied to skin, viscera, arterial chemo- and baroreceptors and upon central stimuli (warming, coupling to respiratory neurones). Spinal afferent inputs from the viscera have pronounced effects on MVC, CVC and SM neurones and determine almost fully the discharge patterns of the MR neurones. Three systems (PM, MVD, CVD) are silent and probably only excited by very specific central stimuli. (2) It is probable that in all systems the pattern of activity in the preganglionic neurones is selectively transmitted to the respective type of postganglionic neurone. In this sense, the pre-/postganglionic neurone chains can be considered as being the "final common sympathetic motor paths", i.e., the liaison between spinal cord and target tissues. (3) The idea of the "final common sympathetic motor path" does not preclude integrative processes in the sympathetic ganglia. Integration may occur in particular in prevertebral ganglia in which the postganglionic neurones receive inputs, other than the preganglionic synaptic inputs, from the viscera; but in some systems (MVC, CVC) synaptic mechanisms other than the nicotinic cholinergic one can also be shown to exist. The physiological role of these integrative synaptic mechanisms is a matter of speculation. (4) Investigations of the reflex patterns of the sympathetic neurones in spinal animals have revealed that the spinal cord contains important neuronal circuits which determine the characteristic discharge patterns of the sympathetic systems. This is very obvious for the MR, SM and CVC systems but probably also applies to the MVC and VVC systems. (5) The interneurones, preganglionic neurones and their synaptic connections with the spinal somatic and visceral afferent input systems, and with the systems descending from brainstem and hypothalamus, have tentatively been called "spinal sympathetic functional units"; such a functional unit may exist for each sympathetic system (SM, CVC, MVC, VVC, MR_1, MR_2). Functionally related spinal units share interneurones, afferent input systems and descending systems.

Acknowledgement

This work was supported by the Deutsche Forschungsgemeinschaft.

References

Amendt, K., Czachurski, J., Dembowsky, K. and Seller, H. (1979) Bulbospinal projections to the intermediolateral cell column; a neuroanatomical study. J. Auton. Nerv. Systems, 1: 103–117.

Bahns, E., Ernsberger, U., Jänig, W. and Nelke, A. (1986) Functional characteristics of lumbar visceral afferent fibres from the urinary bladder and the urethra in the cat. Pflügers Arch., in press.

Bahns, E., Halsband, U. and Jänig, W. (1985a) Reaction of visceral afferents in the pelvic nerve to distension and contraction of the urinary bladder in the cat. Neurosci. Lett., Suppl., 22: S86.

Bahns, E., Halsband, U. and Jänig, W. (1985b) Functional characteristics of sacral afferent fibres from the urinary bladder, urethra, colon and the anus. Pflügers Arch., 405, Suppl., 2: R51.

Bahr, R., Bartel, B., Blumberg, H. and Jänig, W. (1986a) Functional characterization of preganglionic neurons projecting in the lumbar splanchnic nerves: neurons regulating motility. J. Auton. Nerv. Systems, in press.

Bahr, R., Bartel, B., Blumberg, H. and Jänig, W. (1986b) Functional characterization of preganglionic neurons projecting in the lumbar splanchnic nerves: vasoconstrictor neurons. J. Auton. Nerv. Systems, 15: 131–140.

Bahr, R., Bartel, B., Blumberg, H. and Jänig, W. (1986c) Secondary functional properties of lumbar visceral preganglionic neurons. J. Auton. Nerv. Systems, 15: 141–152.

Baldissera, F., Hultborn, H. and Illert, M. (1981) Integration in spinal neuronal systems. In J. M. Brookhart, V. B. Mountcastle, V. B. Brooks and S. R. Geiger (Eds.), Handbook of Physiology, Section 1, The Nervous System, Vol. II, Motor Control, Part I, American Physiological Society, Bethesda, MD, pp. 509–595.

Baron, R., Jänig, W. and McLachlan, E. M. (1985a) On the anatomical organization of the lumbosacral sympathetic chain and the lumbar splanchnic nerves of the cat — Langley revisited. J. Auton. Nerv. Systems, 12: 289–300.

Baron, R., Jänig, W. and McLachlan, E. M. (1985b) The afferent and sympathetic components of the lumbar spinal outflow to the colon and pelvic organs in the cat. I. The hypogastric nerve. J. Comp. Neurol., 236, 238: 135–146.

Baron, R., Jänig, W. and McLachlan, E. M. (1985c) The afferent and sympathetic components of the lumbar spinal outflow to the colon and pelvic organs in the cat. II. The lumbar splanchnic nerves. J. Comp. Neurol, 238: 147–157.

Baron, R., Jänig, W. and McLachlan, E. M. (1985d) The afferent and sympathetic components of the lumbar spinal outflow to the colon and pelvic organs in the cat. III. The colonic nerves, incorporating an analysis of all components of the lumbar prevertebral outflow. J. Comp. Neurol., 238: 158–168.

Bartel, B., Blumberg, H. and Jänig, W. (1986) Discharge patterns of motility-regulating neurons projecting in the lumbar splanchnic nerves to visceral stimuli in spinal cats. J. Auton. Nerv. Systems, 15: 153–163.

Bayliss, W. M. and Starling, E. H. (1900) The movements and the innervation of the large intestine. J. Physiol. (Lond.), 26: 107–118.

Bell, C., Jänig, W., Kümmel, H. and Xu, H. (1985) Differentiation of vasodilator and sudomotor responses in the cat paw pad to preganglionic sympathetic stimulation. J. Physiol (Lond.), 364: 93–104.

Blumberg, H. and Jänig, W. (1983) Enhancement of resting activity in postganglionic vasoconstrictor neurones following short-lasting repetitive activation of preganglionic axons. Pflügers Arch., 396: 89–94.

Blumberg, H., Jänig, W., Rieckmann, C. and Szulczyk, P. (1980) Baroreceptor and chemoreceptor reflexes in postganglionic neurones supplying skeletal muscle and hairy skin. J. Auton. Nerv. Systems, 2: 223–240.

Blumberg, H., Haupt, P., Jänig, W. and Kohler, W. (1983a) Encoding of visceral noxious stimuli in the discharge patterns of visceral afferent fibres from the colon. Pflügers Arch., 398: 33–40.

Blumberg, H., Hilbers, K. and Jänig, W. (1983b) Viscero-sympathetic reflexes in postganglionic neurones supplying skin and skeletal muscle in brain-intact cats. Naunyn-Schmiedeberg's Arch. Pharmacol., 322: Suppl., R69.

Caverson, M. M., Ciriello, J. and Calaresu, F. R. (1983) Direct pathway from cardiovascular neurons in the ventrolateral medulla to the region of the intermediolateral nucleus of the upper thoracic cord: an anatomical and electrophysiological investigation in the cat. J. Auton. Nerv. Systems, 9: 451–475.

Coote, J. H. and MacLeod, V. H. (1974a) The influence of bulbospinal monoaminergic pathways on sympathetic nerve activity. J. Physiol. (Lond.), 241: 453–475.

Coote, J. H. and MacLeod, V. H. (1974b) Evidence for the involvement in the baroreceptor reflex of a descending inhibitory pathway. J. Physiol. (Lond.), 241: 477–496.

Coote, J. H. and MacLeod, V. H. (1975) The spinal root of sympatho-inhibitory pathways descending from the medulla oblongata. Pflügers Arch., 359: 335–347.

Coote, J. H. and Westbury, D. R. (1979) Intracellular recordings from sympathetic preganglionic neurones. Neurosci. Lett., 15: 171–175.

Dampney, R. A. L. (1981) Functional organization of central cardiovascular pathways. Clin. Exp. Pharmacol. Physiol., 8: 241–259.

Dampney, R. A. L., Goodchild, A. K., Robertson, L. G. and Montgomery, W. (1982) Role of ventrolateral medulla in vasomotor regulation: a correlative anatomical and physiological study. Brain Res., 249: 223–235.

De Groat, W. C. (1975) Nervous control of the urinary bladder of the cat. Brain Res., 87: 201–211.

De Groat, W. C. and Booth, A. M. (1980) Inhibition and facilitation in parasympathetic ganglia of the urinary bladder. Fed. Proc., 39: 2990–2996.

De Groat, W. C. and Krier, J. (1976) An electrophysiological study of the sacral parasympathetic pathway to the colon in the cat. J. Physiol. (Lond.), 260: 425–445.

De Groat, W. C. and Krier, J. (1979) The central control of the lumbar sympathetic pathway to the large intestine of the cat. J. Physiol. (Lond.), 289: 449–468.

De Groat, W. C. and Lalley, P. M. (1972) Reflex firing in the lumbar sympathetic outflow to activation of vesical afferent fibres. J. Physiol. (Lond.), 226: 289–309.

De Groat, W. C. and Saum, W. R. (1972) Sympathetic inhibition of the urinary bladder and of pelvic ganglionic transmission in the cat. J. Physiol. (Lond.), 220: 297–314.

De Groat, W. C. and Theobald, R. J. (1976) Reflex activation of sympathetic pathways to vesical smooth muscle and parasympathetic ganglia by electrical stimulation of vesical afferents. J. Physiol. (Lond.), 259: 223–237.

De Groat, W. C., Booth, A. M., Krier, J., Milne, R. J., Morgan, C. and Nadelhaft, I. (1979) Neural control of the urinary bladder and large intestine. In C. McC. Brooks, K. Koizumi and A. Sato (Eds.), Integrative Functions of the Autonomic Nervous System, Elsevier/North-Holland Biomedical Press, Amsterdam, pp. 50–67.

De Groat, W. C., Nadelhaft, I., Milne, R. J., Booth, A. M., Morgan, C. and Thor, K. (1981) Organization of the sacral parasympathetic reflex pathways to the urinary bladder and large intestine. J. Auton. Nerv. Systems, 3: 135–160.

Dembowsky, K., Czachurski, J., Amendt, K. and Seller, H. (1980) Tonic descending inhibition of the spinal somatosympathetic reflex from the lower brainstem. J. Auton. Nerv. Systems, 2: 157–182.

Dembowsky, K., Czachurski, J. and Seller, H. (1985a) An intracellular study of the synaptic input to sympathetic preganglionic neurones in the third thoracic segment of the cat. J. Auton. Nerv. Systems, 13: 201–244.

Dembowsky, K., Czachurski, J. and Seller, H. (1985b) Morphology of sympathetic preganglionic neurons in the thoracic spinal cord of the cat: an intracellular horseradish peroxidase study. J. Comp. Neurol., 238: 453–465.

Dembowsky, K., Czachurski, J. and Seller, H. (1985c) Three types of sympathetic preganglionic neurones with different electrophysiological properties are identified by intracellular recordings in the cat. Pflügers Arch., 406: 112–120.

Edvardsen, P. (1968a) Nervous control of urinary bladder in cats. I. The collecting phase. Acta Physiol. Scand., 72: 157–171.

Edvardsen, P. (1968b) Nervous control of urinary bladder in cats. II. The expulsion phase. Acta Physiol. Scand., 72: 172–182.

Fernandez de Molina, A., Kuno, M. and Perl, E. R. (1965) Antidromically evoked responses from sympathetic preganglionic neurones. J. Physiol. (Lond.), 180: 321–335.

Floyd, K., Hick, V. E. and Morrison, J. F. B. (1982) The influence of visceral mechanoreceptors on sympathetic efferent discharge in the cat. J. Physiol. (Lond.), 323: 65–75.

Foreman, R. D. and Wurster, R. D. (1973) Localization and functional characteristics of descending sympathetic pathways. Am. J. Physiol., 225: 212–217.

Garrett, J. R., Howard, E. R. and Jones, W. (1974) The internal anal sphincter in the cat: a study of nervous mechanisms affecting tone and reflex activity. J. Physiol. (Lond.), 243: 153–166.

Garry, R. C. (1933) The nervous control of the caudal region of the large bowel. J. Physiol. (Lond.), 77: 422–431.

Gjone, R. (1965) Peripheral autonomic influence on the motility of the urinary bladder in the cat. I. Rhythmic contractions. Acta Physiol. Scand., 65: 370–377.

Gjone, R. (1966a) Peripheral autonomic influence on the motility of the urinary bladder in the cat. II. Tone. Acta Physiol. Scand., 66: 72–80.

Gjone, R. (1966b) Peripheral autonomic influence on the motility of the urinary bladder in the cat. III. Micturition. Acta Physiol. Scand., 66: 81–90.

Grosse, M. and Jänig, W. (1976) Vasoconstrictor and pilomotor fibres in skin nerves to the cat's tail. Pflügers Arch., 361: 221–229.

Haupt, P., Jänig, W. and Kohler, W. (1983) Response pattern of visceral afferent fibres, supplying the colon, upon chemical and mechanical stimuli. Pflügers Arch., 398: 41–47.

Hoffmeister, B., Hussels, W. and Jänig, W. (1978) Long-lasting discharge of postganglionic neurones to skin and muscle of the cat's hindlimb after repetitive activation of preganglionic axons in the lumbar sympathetic trunk. Pflügers Arch., 376: 15–20.

Horeyseck, G. and Jänig, W. (1974a) Reflexes in postganglionic fibres within skin and muscle nerves after noxious stimulation of skin. Exp. Brain Res., 20: 125–134.

Horeyseck, G. and Jänig, W. (1974b) Reflex activity in postganglionic fibres within skin and muscle nerves elicited by somatic stimuli in chronic spinal cats. Exp. Brain Res., 21: 155–168.

Hultén, L. (1969) Extrinsic nervous control of colonic motility and blood flow. Acta Physiol. Scand., Suppl., 335: 1–116.

Illert, M. and Gabriel, M. (1972) Descending pathways in the cervical cord of cats affecting blood pressure and sympathetic activity. Pflügers Arch., 335: 109–124.

Illert, M. and Seller, H. (1969) A descending sympathoinhibitory tract in the ventrolateral column of the cat. Pflügers Arch., 313: 343–360.

Jänig, W. (1984) Vasoconstrictor systems supplying skeletal muscle, skin, and viscera. Clin. Exp. Hypertension, A6: 329–346.

Jänig, W. (1985) Organization of the lumbar sympathetic outflow to skeletal muscle and skin of the cat hindlimb and tail. Rev. Physiol. Biochem. Pharmacol., 102: 119–213.

Jänig, W. and Kümmel, H. (1977) Functional discrimination of postganglionic neurones to the cat's hindpaw with respect to the skin potentials recorded from the hairless skin. Pflügers Arch., 371: 217–225.

Jänig, W. and Kümmel, H. (1981) Organization of the sympathetic innervation supplying the hairless skin of the cat's paw. J. Auton. Nerv. Systems, 3: 215–230.

Jänig, W. and McLachlan, E. M. (1986a) The sympathetic and sensory components of the caudal lumbar sympathetic trunk in the cat. J. Comp. Neurol., 245: 62–73.

Jänig, W. and McLachlan, E. M. (1986b) Identification of distinct topographical distributions of lumbar sympathetic and sensory neurons projecting to end organs with different functions in the cat. J. Comp. Neurol., 246: 104–112.

Jänig, W. and Spilok, N. (1978) Functional organization of the sympathetic innervation supplying the hairless skin of the hindpaws in chronic spinal cats. Pflügers Arch., 377: 25–31.

Jänig, W. and Szulczyk, P. (1979) Conduction velocity in spinal descending pathways of baro- and chemoreceptor reflex. J. Auton. Nerv. Systems, 1: 149–160.

Jänig, W., Sato, A. and Schmidt, R. F. (1972) Reflexes in postganglionic cutaneous fibres by stimulation of group I to group IV somatic afferents. Pflügers Arch., 331: 244–256.

Jänig, W., Kümmel, H. and Wiprich, L. (1980) Respiratory rhythmicities in vasoconstrictor and sudomotor neurones supplying the cat's hindlimb. In H. P. Koepchen, S. M. Hilton and A. Trebski (Eds.), Central Interaction Between Respiratory and Cardiovascular Control Systems, Springer-Verlag, Berlin, pp. 128–135.

Jänig, W., Krauspe, R. and Wiedersatz, G. (1982) Transmission of impulses from pre- to postganglionic vasoconstrictor and sudomotor neurons. J. Auton. Nerv. Systems, 6: 95–106.

Jänig, W., Krauspe, R. and Wiedersatz, G. (1983a) Reflex activation of postganglionic vasoconstrictor neurones supplying skeletal muscle by stimulation of arterial chemoreceptors via non-nicotinic synaptic mechanisms in sympathetic ganglia. Pflügers Arch., 396: 95–100.

Jänig, W., Sundlöf, G. and Wallin, B. G. (1983b) Discharge patterns of sympathetic neurons supplying skeletal muscle and skin in man and cat. J. Auton. Nerv. Systems, 7: 239–256.

Jänig, W., Krauspe, R. and Wiedersatz, G. (1984) Activation of postganglionic neurones via non-nicotinic synaptic mechanisms by stimulation of thin preganglionic axons. Pflügers Arch., 401: 318–320.

Klevmark, B. (1977) Motility of the urinary bladder in cats during filling at physiological rates. II. Effects of extrinsic bladder denervation on intraluminal tension and intravesical pressure patterns. Acta Physiol. Scand., 101: 176–184.

Kock, N. G. and Pompeius, R. (1963) Inhibition of the vesical motor activity induced by anal stimulation. Acta Chir. Scand., 126: 244–250.

Kümmel, H. (1983) Activity in sympathetic neurons supplying skin and skeletal muscle in spinal cats. J. Auton. Nerv. Systems, 7: 319–327.

Kümmel, H. and Xu, H. (1983) Viscero-sympathetic reflexes in postganglionic neurones supplying the hindlimb of chronic spinal cats. Naunyn-Schmiedeberg's Arch. Pharmacol., 322: Suppl., R69.

Kuo, D. C., Hisamitsu, T. and De Groat, W. C. (1984) A sympathetic projection from sacral paravertebral ganglia to the pelvic nerve and to postganglionic nerves on the surface of the urinary bladder and large intestine of the cat. J. Comp. Neurol., 226: 76–86.

Langley, J. N. (1891a) On the course and connections of the secretory fibres supplying the sweat glands of the feet of the cat. J. Physiol. (Lond.), 12: 347–374.

Langley, J. N. (1891b) Note on the connection with nerve cells of the vaso-motor nerves for the feet. J. Physiol. (Lond.), 12: 375–377.

Langley, J. N. (1894) The arrangement of the sympathetic nervous system based chiefly on observations upon pilo-motor nerves. J. Physiol. (Lond.), 15: 176–244.

Langley, J. N. (1894/5) Further observations on the secretory and vaso-motor fibres of the foot of the cat, with notes on other sympathetic nerve fibres. J. Physiol. (Lond.), 17: 296–314.

Langley, J. N. (1903) Das sympathische und verwandte nervöse Systeme der Wirbeltiere (autonomes nervöses System). Ergebn. Physiol., 2/II: 818–872.

Langley, J. N. and Anderson, H. K. (1895a) On the innervation of the pelvic and adjoining viscera. Part I. The lower portion of the intestine. J. Physiol. (Lond.), 18: 67–105.

Langley, J. N. and Anderson, H. K. (1895b) The innervation of the pelvic and adjoining viscera. Part. II. The bladder. J. Physiol. (Lond.), 19: 71–84.

Langley, J. N. and Anderson, H. K. (1895c) The innervation of the pelvic and adjoining viscera. Part III. The external generative organs. J. Physiol. (Lond.), 19: 85–121.

Langley, J. N. and Anderson, H. K. (1895d) The innervation of the pelvic and adjoining viscera. Part IV. The internal generative organs. J. Physiol. (Lond.), 19: 122–130.

Langley, J. N. and Sherrington, C. S. (1891) On pilo-motor nerves. J. Physiol. (Lond.), 12: 278–291.

Langley, L. L. and Whiteside, J. A. (1951) Mechanisms of accommodation and tone of urinary bladder. J. Neurophysiol., 14: 147–152.

Learmonth, J. R. and Markowitz, J. (1929) Studies of the function of the lumbar sympathetic outflow. I. The relation of the lumbar sympathetic outflow to the sphincter ani internus. Am. J. Physiol., 89: 686–691.

Lloyd, D. P. C. (1960) Spinal mechanisms involved in somatic activities. In J. Field, H. W. Magoun and V. E. Hall (Eds.), Handbook of Physiology, Section 1, Neurophysiology, Vol. II, American Physiological Society, Washington, DC, pp. 929–949.

Loewy, A. D. (1982) Descending pathways to the sympathetic preganglionic neurons. In H. G. J. M. Kuypers and G. F. Martin (Eds.), Anatomy of Descending Pathways to the Spinal Cord, Progress in Brain Research, Vol. 57, Elsevier Science Publishers, Amsterdam, pp. 267–277.

Loewy, A. D. and McKellar, S. (1980) The neuroanatomical basis of central cardiovascular control. Fed. Proc., 39: 2495–2503.

Loewy, A. D. and Neil, J. J. (1981) The role of descending monoaminergic systems in central control of blood pressure. Fed. Proc., 40: 2778–2785.

McLachlan, E. M. and Hirst, G. D. S. (1980) Some properties of preganglionic neurons in upper thoracic spinal cord of the cat. J. Neurophysiol., 43: 1251–1265.

McLachlan, E. M. and Jänig, W. (1983) The cell bodies of origin of sympathetic and sensory axons in some skin and muscle nerves of the cat hindlimb. J. Comp. Neurol., 214: 115–130.

McLachlan, E. M., Clark, E. L. and Cassell, J. F. (1984) Electrophysiologic characteristics of two classes of sympathetic ganglion cells in the guinea-pig. Proc. Austr. Physiol. Pharmacol. Soc., 15: 140.

McMahon, S. B. and Morrison, J. F. B. (1982a) Spinal neurones with long projections activated from the abdominal viscera of the cat. J. Physiol. (Lond.), 322: 1–20.

McMahon, S. B. and Morrison, J. F. B. (1982b) Two groups of spinal interneurones that respond to stimulation of the abdominal viscera of the cat. J. Physiol. (Lond.), 322: 21–34.

Oldfield, B. J. and McLachlan, E. M. (1981) An analysis of the sympathetic preganglionic neurons projecting from the upper thoracic spinal roots of the cat. J. Comp. Neurol., 196: 329–345.

Réthelyi, M. (1972) Cell and neuropil architecture of the intermedio-lateral (sympathetic) nucleus of cat spinal cord. Brain Res., 46: 203–213.

Rexed, B. (1954) A cytoarchitectonic atlas of the spinal cord in the cat. J. Comp. Neurol., 100: 297–379.

Rostad, H. (1973) Colonic motility in the cat. II. Extrinsic nervous control. Acta Physiol. Scand., 89: 91–103.

Sato, A. and Schmidt, R. F. (1971) Spinal and supraspinal components of the reflex discharges into lumbar and thoracic white rami. J. Physiol. (Lond.), 212: 839–850.

Sato, A. and Schmidt, R. F. (1973) Somatosympathetic reflexes: afferent fibers, central pathways, discharge characteristics. Physiol. Rev., 53: 916–947.

Simmons, M. (1985) The complexity and diversity of synaptic transmission in the prevertebral sympathetic ganglia. Prog. Neurobiol., 24: 43–93.

Skok, V. I. and Ivanov, A. Y. (1983) What is the ongoing activity of sympathetic neurons? J. Auton. Nerv. Systems, 7: 263–270.

Sonnenschein, R. R. and Weissman, M. L. (1978) Sympathetic vasomotor outflows to hindlimb muscles of the cat. Am. J. Physiol., 235: H482–H487.

Sundin, T., Carlson, C. and Kock, N. (1974) Detrusor inhibition induced from mechanical stimulation of the anal region and from electrical stimulation of the pudendal nerve afferents. Invest. Urol., 5: 374–378.

Szurszewski, J. H. (1981) Physiology of mammalian prevertebral ganglia. Annu. Rev. Physiol., 43: 53–68.

Todd, J. K. (1964) Afferent impulses in the pudental nerves of the cat. Q. J. Exp. Physiol., 49: 258–267.

Wesselmann, U. and McLachlan, E. M. (1984) The effect of previous transection on quantitative estimates of the preganglionic neurones projecting in the cervical sympathetic trunk of the guinea pig and the cat made by retrograde labelling of damaged axons by horseradish peroxidase. Neuroscience, 13: 1299–1309.

F. Cervero and J. F.B. Morrison
Progress in Brain Research, Vol. 67

CHAPTER 17

Brainstem control of visceral afferent pathways in the spinal cord

B. M. Lumb

Department of Physiology, University of Leeds Medical School, LS2 9TJ, U.K.

Introduction

A role for centrifugal control of sensory transmission in the determination of sensory experience has been recognised since early this century (see, e.g., Head and Holmes, 1911). The dorsal horns of the spinal cord and medulla are considered to be important sites of centrifugal control since there is considerable potential at this early level in sensory pathways to filter out unwanted information and, in so doing, to modulate the transmission of afferent information to higher levels of the neuroaxis. It is probable that all afferent pathways in the dorsal horn are subject to some form of centrifugal control originating from supraspinal structures. There is considerable evidence to suggest that this is the case for somatic information (see Willis, 1982); however, little is known of the supraspinal control of visceral pathways.

Although non-painful sensations are evoked from certain viscera (e.g., bladder fullness and a desire to void), it is generally reported that the only sensations arising from most viscera are discomfort and pain. Our understanding of the centrifugal control of the spinal transmission of nociceptive information has increased greatly in recent years. Most studies, however, have been concerned with the processing of information from somatic structures. The aim of this chapter is to discuss to what extent the spinal transmission of information from the viscera is subject to supraspinal control and to consider the functional significance of such control in relation to visceral sensation.

Brain stem control of nociceptive transmission in the spinal cord

In recent years a great deal of attention has focussed on the supraspinal control of nociceptive transmission in the spinal cord. Impetus for these studies came largely from initial reports of the antinociceptive effects of electrical stimulation within the periaqueductal grey (PAG) region of the midbrain in awake rats (Reynolds, 1969; Mayer et al., 1971). This phenomenon was later termed stimulation-produced analgesia (SPA). Subsequent investigations confirmed the importance of the PAG in SPA and revealed that similar effects could be produced by stimulation at more rostral sites in the periventricular grey (PVG) in cats (Liebeskind et al., 1973; Melzack and Melinkoff, 1974; Oliveras et al., 1974a, b; Gebhart and Toleikis, 1978), rats (Balagura and Ralph, 1973; Mayer and Liebeskind, 1974; Soper, 1976; Yeung et al., 1977; Rhodes and Liebeskind, 1978; Fardin et al., 1984) and primates, including humans (Goodman and Holcombe, 1976; Richardson and Akil, 1977a, b; Oleson et al., 1980). Other studies demonstrated that stimulation at more caudal sites in the medulla, in particular in nucleus raphe magnus (NRM) and the immediately adjacent reticular formation (nucleus magnocellularis or nucleus paragigantocellularis), could result in potent "analgesia" (Oliveras et al., 1975, 1977, 1978, 1979; Proudfit and Anderson, 1975; Oleson et al., 1980; Satoh et al., 1980; Zorman et al., 1981).

All these studies used electrical stimulation of brainstem sites, which has the disadvantage that not only cell bodies located in these regions, but also fibres of passage from other structures would be activated. In other studies the importance of NRM neurones themselves has been confirmed, since the selective stimulation of their cell bodies and dendrites by direct microinjection of L-glutamate has been shown to suppress nociceptive responses in awake rats (Satoh et al., 1983).

It is generally believed that the antinociceptive effects of stimulation at sites in the brainstem are mediated, at least partly, by descending inhibitory pathways that modulate the nociceptor-evoked responses of spinal cord neurones, some of which transmit information rostrally towards the brain. Stimulation in the PAG (Liebeskind et al., 1973; Oliveras et al., 1974a; Carstens et al., 1979, 1980, 1981; Duggan and Griersmith, 1979; Hayes et al., 1979) and in NRM (Fields et al., 1977; Guilbaud et al., 1977; Willis et al., 1977; Duggan and Griersmith, 1979; Rivot et al., 1980; Iggo et al., 1981; Blum, 1981; Edeson and Ryall, 1983) can depress the activities of dorsal horn neurones, including some which project to the thalamus (Beall et al., 1976; Willis et al., 1977; Hayes et al., 1979; McCreery et al., 1979; Gerhart et al., 1981; Giesler et al., 1981a; Yezierski et al., 1982). The fact that stimulation at these brainstem sites can modulate the activities of spinothalamic neurones is of considerable importance since such neurones are thought to be concerned with the transmission of nociceptive information, especially in primates (see Willis and Coggeshall, 1978).

In terms of the functional classification of dorsal horn neurones, stimulation in the PAG and in NRM can depress the activities of "convergent" (wide dynamic range) neurones (i.e., those receiving both high- and low-threshold inputs) and "noxious-specific" neurones (i.e., those receiving only high-threshold inputs). With regard to convergent neurones, many studies have suggested that the PAG preferentially inhibits their high-threshold inputs (presumably by presynaptic mechanisms), without having any clear effect on their low-threshold inputs (however, see Duggan and Griersmith, 1979). This might account for the observation that responses to tactile stimuli are unaffected during stimulation of the PAG in awake animals (see Mayer and Price, 1976). As for NRM, its inhibitory effects on dorsal horn neurones appear to be complex and to involve postsynaptic as well as presynaptic mechanisms (see Willis, 1982).

There is a large body of evidence to suggest that the inhibitory effects of stimulation in NRM are due to the activation of direct projections to the spinal cord, many of which travel in the dorsolateral funiculus (DLF) (Brodal et al., 1960; West and Wolstencroft, 1977; Basbaum et al., 1978; Leichnetz et al., 1978; Martin et al., 1978; Basbaum and Fields, 1979; Tohyama et al., 1979; Watkins et al., 1980). In support of this, section of the DLF has been shown to reduce NRM-mediated inhibitions of dorsal horn neuronal activity (Fields et al., 1977; Willis et al., 1977). A proportion of spinally-projecting raphe neurones are serotonergic (Dahlstrom and Fuxe, 1965; Wessendorf et al., 1981; Bowker et al., 1981, 1982, 1983) and the inhibitory effects of NRM stimulation are thought to be due, to some extent, to the release of 5-hydroxytryptamine (5-HT) in the dorsal horn (see references in Miletic et al., 1984).

The PAG has few direct projections to the spinal cord and is thought to exert its inhibitory effects on dorsal horn neurones after a relay in NRM or the adjacent reticular formation (Fields and Anderson, 1978; Lovick et al., 1978; Behbehani and Fields, 1979; Pomeroy and Behbehani, 1979; Shah and Dostrovsky, 1980; Sandkuhler and Gebhart, 1984; Vanegas et al., 1984).

This account has concentrated on the mechanisms responsible for the antinociceptive effects of stimulation in the PAG and NRM; however, similar inhibitory effects on the activities of dorsal horn neurones have been reported following stimulation at sites in the PVG (Carstens, 1982; Carstens et al.,

1982). The similarity between the inhibitions produced by PAG and PVG stimulation plus the recent demonstration of excitatory inputs from the PVG on to antidromically identified raphe-spinal neurones (Lumb and Morrison, 1985) suggests that the antinociceptive effects of PVG stimulation may also depend, to some extent, on the integrity of descending projections from the medulla.

In summary, there is general agreement that the activation of spinal projections (some of which are serotonergic) from NRM and the adjacent reticular formation can modulate the responses of dorsal horn neurones to high-threshold somatic inputs and that this may be responsible, at least in part, for the antinociceptive effects of brainstem stimulation.

Brainstem control of visceral afferent pathways in the spinal cord

The analgesic effects of central stimulation are thought to extend to visceral structures since electrical stimulation at sites within the PAG and PVG has been shown to relieve pain associated with visceral carcinomas in man (Hosobuchi et al., 1977; Richardson and Akil, 1977a, b) and to attenuate behavioural responses to intraperitoneal injections of hypertonic saline in rats (Giesler and Liebeskind, 1976). However, despite these observations and the enormous interest in brainstem control of spinal mechanisms, the control of visceral afferent pathways in the spinal cord has largely been neglected.

There is no evidence for the existence of spinal cord neurones receiving exclusively visceral information since those spinal cord neurones which are driven by visceral afferents also receive excitatory inputs from somatic structures, including muscle (viscero-somatic neurones) (see Cervero and Tattersall, this volume). A considerable proportion of these cells receive noxious (high-threshold) somatic inputs and can be classified, by their responses to somatic stimulation, as noxious-specific or convergent (see above). With regard to their somatic inputs, noxious-specific and convergent neurones have been shown to be under descending controls from the brainstem. It might be expected that the visceral inputs to these cells would be under similar descending controls, especially as a component of the inhibition appears to be non-selective and possibly mediated by postsynaptic mechanisms (Giesler et al., 1981a). This view is supported by several recent studies, as described below.

A population of viscero-somatic neurones in the thoracic spinal cord has been shown to be under tonic and phasic descending inhibition (Cervero, 1983; Cervero et al., 1985a). These cells were driven by electrical stimulation of a visceral nerve (the splanchnic nerve) and by transcutaneous electrical stimulation within their somatic receptive fields. The existence of tonic supraspinal inhibition of these neurones was indicated by their increased responses to stimulation of visceral and somatic afferents after interruption of descending pathways in the spinal cord during functional "spinalisation" (produced by cold block of the thoracic or cervical spinal cord). The increased response of a lamina V viscero-somatic neurone to stimulation of the splanchnic nerve during reversible spinalisation is illustrated in Fig. 1B. Powerful tonic descending inhibition of the responses of dorsal horn neurones to noxious cutaneous stimuli has been reported previously (see, e.g., Wall, 1967; Handwerker et al., 1975; Duggan et al., 1977, 1981). A feature of these studies and those of Cervero (1983) is that tonic descending inhibition was often reported to be selective and to affect differentially the responses of convergent neurones to high-threshold inputs.

Phasic inhibitions which, like tonic inhibition, affected both the visceral and the somatic inputs to neurones in the thoracic cord have been observed following stimulation of the ipsilateral DLF (Cervero, 1983). Unlike the tonic inhibition (which appeared to be selective), phasic inhibitions were reported to be non-selective, as both high- and low-threshold somatic inputs to convergent neurones were supressed. Phasic inhibitions of neuronal responses to electrical stimulation of the splanchnic nerve (Fig. 1D; Cervero et al., 1985a) and/or distension of the biliary system (Cervero et al., 1986)

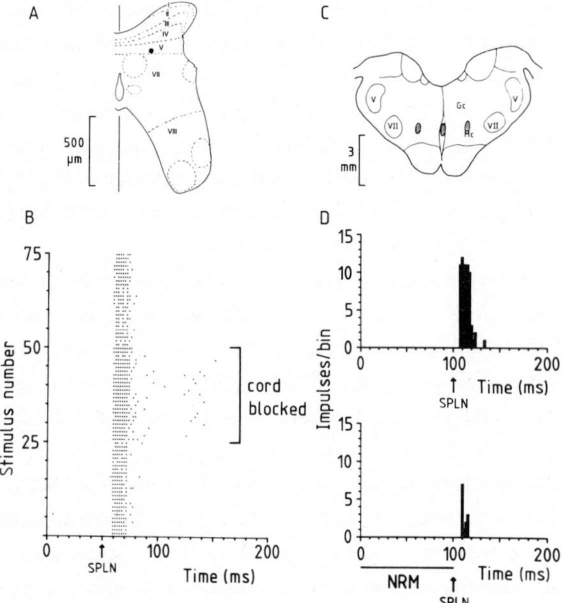

Fig. 1. Viscero-somatic neurone of the thoracic spinal cord showing tonic descending inhibition and phasic inhibition from NRM. A, location of the recording site of the neurone in lamina V of the dorsal horn. B, dot-raster display of the responses of the neurone to supramaximal electrical stimulation of the splanchnic nerve (SPLN) before, during and after reversible spinalisation by cold block. (Note that in this example both the A- and C-fibre responses to stimulation of SPLN are increased during reversible spinalisation.) C, locations of stimulating electrodes in the brain stem as reconstructed from electrolytic lesions (cross-hatched areas). D, peri-stimulus time histograms (10 sweeps) of the responses of the neurone to supramaximal electrical stimulation of the splanchnic nerve (SPLN) before (top histogram) and during (bottom histogram) electrical stimulation of the NRM (continuous train at 333 Hz and 200 μA). Results obtained from experiment on chloralose-anaesthetised cat. From Cervero et al. (1985a).

were also seen following stimulation in NRM and the adjacent reticular formation. These observations suggest that the inhibitory influences reported by Cervero (1983) might have originated from midline medullary structures that contribute axons to the DLF.

A large proportion of the cells which were reported by Cervero and his colleagues to be under tonic and/or phasic inhibition were recorded in the dorsal horn, particularly in lamina V. These authors noted that other cells, located mainly in the ventral horn, were excited from midline medullary structures, and in fact received their visceral input after a supraspinal relay. Neurones of this type, and the functional significance of their supraspinal connections, are considered in a later section of this chapter.

In the case of pelvic viscera, it is of considerable interest that areas of the brainstem that are known to be concerned with regulating sensory transmission have also been shown to influence urinary bladder motility. Stimulation in midline medullary regions (including NRM) can inhibit urinary bladder motility and reflexly evoked activity in pelvic nerve efferents (McMahon and Spillane, 1982). Such inhibitions of visceral motility could represent an important means of centrifugal control of visceral sensation since physiological contractions are an adequate stimulus to the afferent fibres, and are often present in the rectum and bladder when patients report sensation. Furthermore, patients with hyperexcitable bladder reflexes experience urgency, or pain, during contractions at low bladder volumes (see Jänig and Morrison, this volume).

Subsequent investigations have revealed that, in addition to influencing efferent pathways to the bladder, NRM can exert inhibitory influences on spinal cord neurones that receive afferent information from this viscus (J. F. B. Morrison and K. Spillane, unpublished observations). In agreement with previous reports from this laboratory (McMahon and Morrison, 1982a, b), Morrison and Spillane found that neurones in the sacral spinal cord which were driven by electrical stimulation of the pelvic nerves always showed inputs from somatic nerves. Stimulation in NRM was found to inhibit both the visceral and the somatic inputs to these cells. In these experiments, the background activity of spontaneously active neurones was often suppressed during NRM conditioning stimulation. However, in some instances the inhibition was preceded by a short burst of activity and neurones without ongoing activity were either unaffected or excited by stimulation in the medulla.

The experiments described above suggest that

activity evoked in thoracic and sacral spinal cord neurones, by stimulation of visceral afferents, is under similar supraspinal controls as activity evoked by somatic inputs. Furthermore, several observations suggest that a component of this inhibition is non-specific and might involve postsynaptic mechanisms: (i) stimulation of the DLF can inhibit the responses of viscero-somatic neurones in the thoracic spinal cord to visceral and to both high- and low-threshold somatic inputs, (ii) stimulation in NRM can inhibit the background activity of many viscero-somatic neurones, (iii) although stimulation in NRM can inhibit pelvic nerve-evoked responses of neurones in the sacral cord, it apparently does not increase pelvic nerve afferent terminal excitability (J. F. B. Morrison and K. Spillane, unpublished observations), which suggests that the inhibitory mechanisms are not presynaptic.

With regard to the supraspinal control of visceral sensory pathways, it is of particular interest that not only unidentified viscero-somatic neurones but also spinothalamic viscero-somatic neurones are under descending control from brain stem structures (Ammons et al., 1984). Viscero-somatic spinothalamic neurones in the thoracic spinal cord that receive inputs from cardiopulmonary afferents and are excited by noxious cardiac stimuli (such as intracardiac injection of bradykinin and coronary artery occlusion) are believed to be important mediators of cardiac pain (Blair et al., 1981, 1982, 1984). Ammons and his colleagues (1984) have recently reported that stimulation in NRM inhibited the Aδ- and C-fibre responses to stimulation of cardiopulmonary nerves of all the thoracic viscero-somatic spinothalamic neurones which they studied. The responses of these cells to intracardiac injections of bradykinin were similarly affected. Furthermore, as reported by other authors and described above, medullary raphe stimulation inhibited the background activities of these cells and the responses to both high- and low-threshold somatic inputs to convergent spinothalamic neurones.

Functions of descending inhibition in sensory control

As discussed above, there is a wealth of experimental and clinical evidence to suggest that stimulation of certain supraspinal structures can result in antinociception in animals and the relief of pain in man and that these effects are mediated, at least partly, by the activation of descending inhibitory pathways from NRM and the adjacent reticular formation. Most investigations of the supraspinal control of visceral and somatic afferent information have used chemical or electrical stimulation to activate these descending pathways from the brainstem. However, a further understanding of these controls and their possible physiological roles has resulted from investigations of their activation by "natural" stimuli. One means of triggering supraspinal controls by natural stimulation has been provided in the concept of "diffuse noxious inhibitory controls" (Le Bars et al., 1979a, b; and see below).

In the anaesthetised rat with an intact CNS, the activities of certain neurones in the spinal dorsal horn can be depressed by noxious stimulation of remote areas of the body, including the viscera (Le Bars et al., 1979a, b). These inhibitory effects, termed "diffuse noxious inhibitory controls" (DNIC), can only be produced by noxious stimuli and only affect the activities of "convergent" neurones (i.e., those receiving both high- and low-threshold afferents). Nearly all convergent neurones tested have been shown to be influenced by DNIC, including some which project to the thalamus (Dickenson and Le Bars, 1983). It is probable, therefore, that DNIC can modulate the transmission of sensory information to higher centres of the CNS and, by so doing, produce a "contrast signal" whereby the activity evoked by the strongest stimulus to the body is "seen" against a background of silence or inactivity in other pathways. It has been proposed that DNIC may provide the neural basis for certain counter-irritation procedures and, more importantly, that they may play a role in the signalling of pain (Le Bars et al., 1979b).

It should be noted that although propriospinal mechanisms undoubtably contribute to these inhibitory effects, DNIC are also thought to involve supraspinal structures since the effects of remote noxious stimuli are weaker, of shorter duration and affect a smaller proportion of convergent neurones in spinal animals (Cadden et al., 1983). Thus, DNIC appear to involve a supraspinal loop, and the following evidence suggests that the descending limb of this loop is the same pathway as that activated by chemical or electrical stimulation of NRM. (1) DNIC are greatly reduced following electrolytic lesions of NRM (Dickenson et al., 1980). (2) A proportion of spinally-projecting neurones in NRM contain 5-HT (see a previous section of this chapter) and depletion of 5-HT (Dickenson et al., 1981) or blockade of 5-HT receptors (Chitour et al., 1982) strongly reduces DNIC. (3) Administration of a 5-HT precursor (5-hydroxytryptophan) potentiates DNIC (Chitour et al., 1982). (4) Stimuli known to produce DNIC evoke 5-HT synthesis and release in the spinal cord and brainstem (Yaksh and Tyce, 1981; Weil-Fugazza et al., 1984).

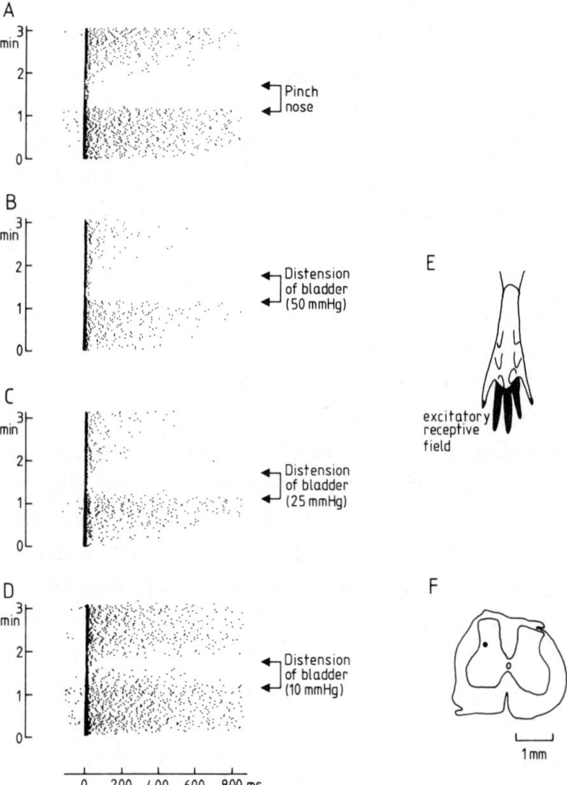

Fig. 2. Results from experiment on urethane-anaesthetised rat. A–D, dot display analyses showing succesive responses (bottom to top) of a lumbar dorsal horn convergent neurone to repeated electrical stimulation of its receptive field (1.8 mA, 2 mseconds; 1/1.5 seconds). Note that although the presence of both short- and long-latency responses is typical for this neuronal type, the asynchronous nature of the long-latency responses shown here is less commonly found. Arrows illustrate the periods of application of noxious somatic (A) and of visceral (B–D) conditioning stimuli. E, excitatory receptive field on ipsilateral hind paw. F, recording site in dorsal horn. From S. W. Cadden and J. F. B. Morrison (unpublished results).

Role of visceral afferents in diffuse noxious inhibitory controls

The fact that visceral afferents can trigger DNIC was shown by the original report of Le Bars and his colleagues (Le Bars et al., 1979a) in which intraperitoneal injections of bradykinin produced profound inhibitions of the activities of rat dorsal horn convergent neurones. Subsequent experiments have demonstrated that intraperitoneal injections of acetic acid can also depress the activities of convergent neurones and can produce behavioural antinociception (Calvino et al., 1984). Furthermore, recent experiments indicate that distensions of the urinary bladder or the colon can produce DNIC-like effects on rat lumbar dorsal horn neurones (Cadden, 1985; Cadden and Morrison, 1984).

The effects of DNIC on the activity of a "convergent" neurone in the rat lumbar dorsal horn are illustrated in Fig. 2. This figure shows the effects of either noxious somatic (pinch of the nose) or visceral (distension of the urinary bladder) conditioning stimuli on both the short-latency (A-fibre) and long-latency (C-fibre) responses of a "convergent" neurone to transcutaneous electrical stimulation within its excitatory receptive field. Fig. 2A, where the conditioning stimulus is a noxious pinch of the nose, demonstrates some of the features of DNIC described by Le Bars and his colleagues. First, both the A- and C-fibre-evoked activities are depressed by the conditioning stimulus, with the effect more marked for the C-fibre activity; secondly, the inhibition clearly outlasts the period of stimulation. The effects of urinary bladder distension (Fig. 2B–D) are qualitatively similar to those of noxious somatic stimulation (Fig. 2A).

Since the effects of spinalisation, medullary lesions and pharmacological manipulations were not determined in these recent experiments, it is not possible to be certain that the effects were mediated by DNIC and, as such, involved raphe-spinal neurones. However, a role for DNIC seems most likely since there were several similarities between the present results and those previously reported for DNIC; the inhibitory effects were qualitatively similar (see above), they were found for almost all convergent neurones but rarely for any other type of dorsal horn neurone which received a cutaneous input (S. W. Cadden, personal communication; cf. Le Bars et al., 1979a, b) and were proportional to the intensity of the conditioning stimulus (see Fig. 1B–D; cf. Le Bars et al., 1981).

If DNIC are mediated after a relay in NRM it might be expected that neurones in this region of the medulla would be driven by the same stimuli which inhibit the activities of "convergent" neurones (i.e., noxious stimulation of widespread areas of the body). Many studies indicate that this is indeed the case. Although a brisk tap is often an adequate stimulus to activate neurones in NRM, many neurones in this region respond exclusively or maximally to noxious somatic stimuli in rats (Guilbaud et al., 1980) and cats (Moolenaar et al., 1976; Anderson et al., 1977; Eisenhart et al., 1983). Typically, these cells have very large receptive fields. Neurones in NRM can also be driven by visceral stimuli such as intraperitoneal injections of bradykinin (Guilbaud et al., 1980) or distensions of the urinary bladder (Lumb and Spillane, 1984) and, as discussed above, these stimuli also appear to trigger DNIC. It is of particular interest that some cells in NRM which are driven by noxious somatic (Lumb and Morrison, 1984; Maciewicz et al., 1984; Yen and Blum, 1984) or visceral stimuli (Lumb and Morrison, 1984) send descending axons to the spinal cord.

The hypothesis that neurones in NRM, including those with visceral inputs, might form the descending limb of a spino-bulbo-spinal pathway which is triggered by widespread noxious stimuli and thought to mediate DNIC is further supported by the following observations:

(1) Although it has been reported that NRM contains neurones whose activities are depressed by visceral distension as well as neurones which are excited by such stimuli, it has also been found that threshold pressures that cause excitations (mean, 22 mmHg) are generally higher than those that cause depressions of activity (mean, 9 mmHg) (Lumb and Spillane, 1984). In subsequent studies of the receptive field properties of raphe-spinal neurones, only neurones whose activities were increased at higher bladder pressures were found to project to the spinal cord (Lumb and Morrison, 1984). Furthermore, the majority of these neurones exhibited a convergence of visceral and somatic input. Generally, the somatic receptive fields covered large areas of the body surface and neurones were driven by noxious mechanical (pinch or deep pressure) and thermal (52°C water) stimuli but not by innocuous stimuli (brush, stroke, 37°C water). An example of the convergence of visceral and high-threshold somatic input on to a raphe-spinal neurone is shown in Fig. 3.

Threshold intravesical pressures which caused excitations in raphe-spinal neurones ranged from 10 to 44 mmHg (Lumb and Morrison, 1984), and in the example in Fig. 3 was between 30 and 40 mmHg. However, threshold pressures which evoke activity in pelvic and hypgastric afferents, which convey sensory information from the bladder, range from 4 to 30 mmHg (see Jänig and Morrison, this volume). One mechanism which could account for the higher threshold values observed in some medullary neurones is that their threshold for excitation might depend on a balance between inhibitory and excitatory influences of bladder distension. Inhibitory effects of bladder distensions have been described for neurones in the sacral spinal

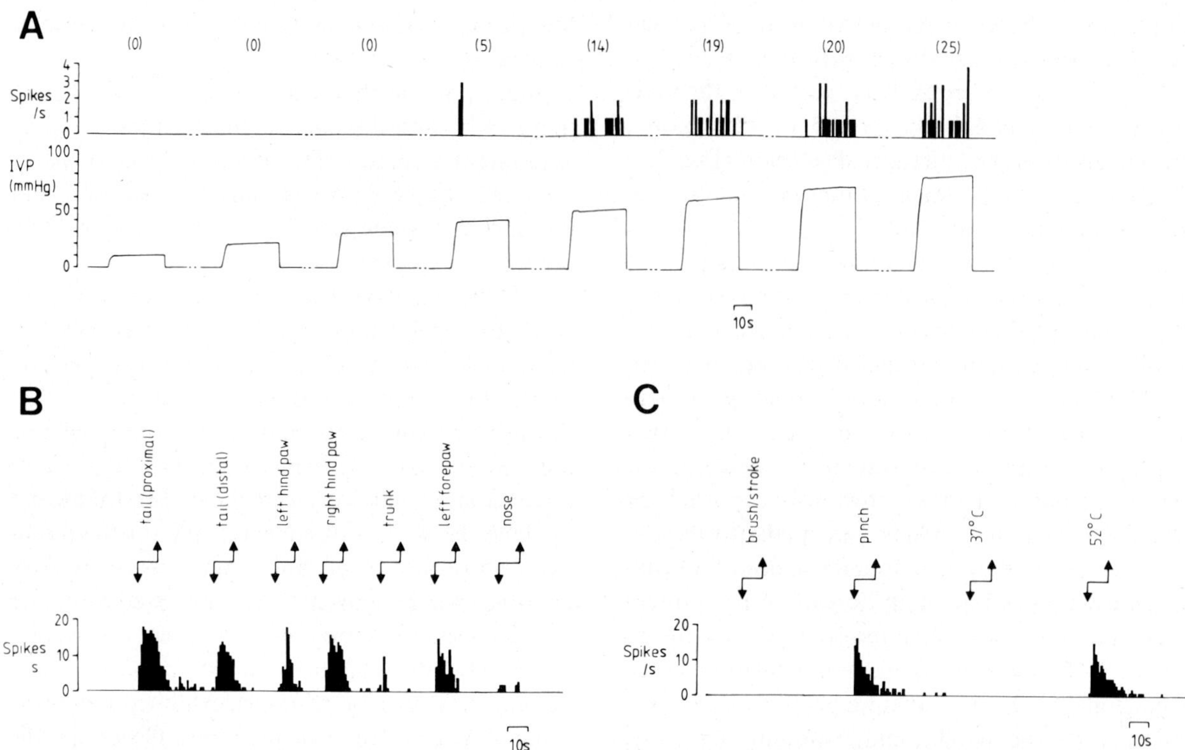

Fig. 3. Results obtained from a recording made in NRM in a urethane-anaesthetised rat. A–C, ratemeter records showing the excitatory responses of an antidromically identified raphe-spinal neurone to visceral and noxious somatic stimuli. Stimuli applied; urinary bladder distensions of 10–80 mmHg (A), sustained pinches at the times indicated by the arrows (B), noxious and non-noxious mechanical and thermal stimuli applied to the tail (C). Broken lines indicated 30-second breaks in the record. Numbers in parentheses are total spike counts. IVP, intravesical pressure. From B. M. Lumb and J. F. B. Morrison (unpublished results).

cord, some of which contribute axons to ascending fibre tracts (Milne et al., 1981; McMahon and Morrison, 1982a) and, indeed, inhibitory influences of bladder distension were observed in some neurones in NRM (see above).

(2) As mentioned above, the degree of DNIC is proportional to the intensity of the conditioning stimulus applied (Le Bars et al., 1981). It might be expected, therefore, that increasing the intensity of the conditioning stimulus would result in either excitation of a larger pool of neurones in NRM, or increases in the magnitude of responses of single raphe neurones. The available evidence suggests that with regard to visceral conditioning stimuli both of these mechanisms might operate. First, the threshold intravesical pressures that cause excitation of raphe-spinal neurones range from 10 to 44 mmHg and, as most neurones respond tonically during suprathreshold bladder distensions (see Fig. 3), an increase in bladder pressure would result in a greater number of neurones responding to the stimulus. Secondly, many neurones respond in a graded manner to increases in bladder distension, i.e., an increase in bladder pressure causes an increase in the magnitude of the responses of individual neurones (Fig. 3).

(3) With regard to the degree of DNIC being proportional to the intensity of the conditioning stimulus applied, it is interesting to note that thermal cutaneous stimuli of 52°C appear to be approximately 1.5–2.0 times as "effective" as bladder distensions of 50 mmHg in depressing the C-fibre-evoked responses of dorsal horn convergent neurones (see Cadden, 1985; S. W. Cadden, personal communi-

cation) and that 52°C cutaneous stimuli produce mean increases in the firing rate of raphe neurones which are approximately double that produced by bladder distensions of 50 mmHg (B. M. Lumb and J. F. B. Morrison, unpublished observations).

Visceral afferents other than those activated by distensions of the urinary bladder or colon or by intraperitoneal injections of bradykinin or acetic acid may also trigger descending inhibition. For example, effects similar to those manifested by DNIC have been reported following genital stimulation. Distension of the vaginal canal, produced by applying a 200 g force to the cervix with a blunt rod, has been shown to be antinociceptive in rats (Komisaruk and Wallman, 1977). It is not known whether vaginal stimulation can depress the activities of dorsal horn convergent neurones. However, several observations suggest that distension of the vaginal canal and subsequent activation of pelvic visceral afferents may trigger DNIC:

(1) An involvement of supraspinal structures in the antinociceptive effects of vaginal stimulation (measured in the tail-flick test) is indicated by the observation that these effects are reduced in rats with thoracic cord transections (Watkins et al., 1984). The supraspinal structures involved appear to be located in the caudal brainstem since mid-collicular decerebration has no significant effect on vaginal stimulation-produced antinociception. Furthermore, a role for raphe-spinal neurones is suggested by the attenuation of antinociception following DLF lesions (Watkins et al., 1984).

(2) Further support for the involvement of NRM is provided by reports that midline medullary neurones, including neurones in NRM, can be driven by probing of the cervix in rats (Hornby and Rose, 1976) and cats (Rose, 1975). It is not known whether any of these cells project to the spinal cord, but it is interesting to note that many of them show sustained responses to cervical probing which sometimes outlast the period of stimulation (cf. the time course of DNIC-mediated inhibitions).

(3) As with DNIC, the antinociceptive effects of vaginal stimulation are attenuated by administration of 5-HT antagonists (Steinman et al., 1983) and vaginal stimulation evokes the release of 5-HT in the spinal cord (Steinman et al., 1983).

(4) Just as the degree of DNIC-mediated inhibitions is proportional to the intensity of the noxious conditioning stimuli, the magnitude of the antinociceptive effects of vaginal stimulation is proportional to the intensity of the pressure applied to the cervix (Crowley et al., 1976).

To summarise, the antinociceptive effects of vaginal stimulation, together with the effects of distensions of abdominal viscera and of intraperitoneal injections of bradykinin and acetic acid on the activities of neurones in the caudal medulla and the dorsal horn, strongly suggest that afferent inputs from visceral structures may trigger descending inhibition from the brainstem. These afferents may therefore play an important role in the processing of sensory information in the dorsal horn of the spinal cord.

Possible mechanisms underlying the time course of DNIC: involvement of visceral afferents

One feature of DNIC in intact anaesthetised rats is that the inhibitory effects on dorsal horn convergent neurones generally outlast the period of conditioning stimulation (see Fig. 1). It has been suggested (Cervero and Wolstencroft, 1984) that the long time-course of DNIC may be due to activation of a positive feedback loop between neurones in the ventral horn of the spinal cord and neurones in the midline of the medulla. These authors described a population of neurones in laminae VII and VIII of the ventral horn that were driven antidromically from sites in NRM and the adjacent reticular formation and could also be activated orthodromically by stimulation of midline medullary sites, thus creating a positive feedback loop. They proposed that ascending activity from neurones in laminae VII and VIII of the ventral horn may also trigger descending inhibition from neurones in NRM and the adjacent reticular formation on to neurones in the dorsal horn and, because of the positive feedback nature of the loop from the ventral horn, the inhibitory effects would be maintained beyond the period of stimulation.

The somatic receptive fields of these ventral horn neurones were complex, but all could be driven by deep pressure of the limbs, which is consistent with the view that such cells are involved in control mechanisms activated by noxious stimuli. In many respects these neurones are similar to a subpopulation of spinothalamic tract neurones described by Giesler et al. (1981b). These cells, located in or around laminae VII and VIII, send collaterals to the reticular formation and can be driven orthodromically by electrical stimulation within the reticular formation and by noxious peripheral stimuli.

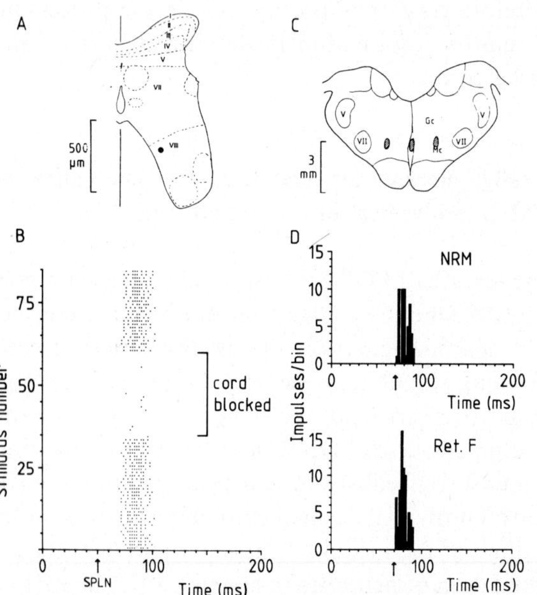

Fig. 4. Viscero-somatic neurone of the thoracic spinal cord with a suprasegmental visceral input and phasic excitation from the brain stem. A, location of the recording site of the neurone in lamina VIII of the ventral horn. B, dot-raster display of the responses of the neurone to supramaximal electrical stimulation of the splanchnic nerve (SPLN) before, during and after reversible spinalisation by cold block. C, locations of stimulating electrodes in the brain stem as reconstructed from electrolytic lesions (cross-hatched areas). D, peri-stimulus time histograms (10 sweeps) of the responses of the neurone to electrical stimulation of the NRM (200 μA, bottom histogram). Results obtained from experiment in chloralose-anaesthetised cat. From Cervero et al. (1985a).

Further support for the existence of positive feedback loops between the spinal cord and medulla is provided by the description of a group of spinothalamic tract neurones which increase their excitatory responses to stimulation in the reticular formation on repetitive stimulation (Haber et al., 1980).

Some viscero-somatic neurones in the thoracic spinal cord are thought to receive their visceral inputs after a supraspinal relay (Cervero, 1983). Recent studies have indicated that the visceral inputs to these cells might contribute to positive feedback loops between the spinal cord and medulla and, as such, might participate in the maintenance of the supraspinal control of dorsal horn neurones (Cervero et al., 1985a). These authors identified cells in the thoracic cord whose excitatory visceral (splanchnic) input was attenuated or abolished during functional "spinalisation" by cold block (Fig. 4B), which indicated that they received their visceral inputs after a supraspinal relay. Cells which responded in this manner were located predominantly in laminae VII and VIII of the ventral horn (Fig. 4A) and could be driven orthodromically from sites in NRM and the adjacent reticular formation (Fig. 4D). The anatomical location of these cells, their excitatory responses to stimulation of medullary structures, plus the observation that some had long axons projecting to the brainstem suggest that they might participate in the positive feedback system described by Cervero and Wolstencroft (1984). Further support for a positive feedback loop activated by stimulation of visceral afferents is provided by the observation that the responses to stimulation of pelvic nerve afferents of some neurones in and adjacent to NRM often outlast the period of stimulation by many seconds (Hornby and Rose, 1976).

Concluding remarks

The evidence presented in this chapter indicates that the spinal transmission of visceral information can be modulated by supraspinal structures. Stimulation at sites in NRM and the adjacent reticular formation can result in inhibitory or facilitatory effects on the visceral-evoked responses of spinal cord neurones.

Cells whose responses to visceral stimulation were depressed following activation of descending pathways from the medulla were located predominantly in the dorsal horn. In addition to phasic inhibition, some of these cells were considered to be under tonic descending inhibitory control from supraspinal structures.

The phasic modulation of visceral afferent transmission in the spinal cord is similar in many respects to that reported for the transmission of noxious somatic information and may account for the "analgesic" effects of central stimulation which extend to visceral structures. This view is supported by the report that descending inhibitory influences affect the visceral-evoked responses of some dorsal horn neurones that project to the thalamus (Ammons et al., 1984). Inhibition of transmission in this particular ascending pathway might well account for the antinociceptive effects of central stimulation. Indeed, Ammons and his colleagues proposed that activation of descending inhibitory pathways from NRM on to spinothalamic tract cells in the upper thoracic cord may modulate ascending information related to cardiac pain and may provide an explanation for painless episodes of myocardial ischaemia (Foreman et al., this volume).

As well as data suggesting that visceral afferent pathways are under supraspinal controls, evidence described earlier suggests that activity in these pathways may trigger DNIC. In such a way visceral afferent input may participate in the signalling of pain by "convergent" neurones (see Le Bars et al., 1979b). Other evidence presented above suggests that visceral afferents may not only trigger DNIC but may also contribute to mechanisms thought to be responsible for the long time-course of inhibitory influences on convergent neurones.

Although visceral afferent fibres may trigger descending inhibitory controls from the medulla, it is not known whether the responses of dorsal horn neurones to stimulation of viscera are themselves subject to DNIC. This is likely to be the case, however, as there is evidence that DNIC are finally mediated by post-synaptic inhibition of convergent neurones (Villanueva et al., 1984).

Acknowledgements

I thank Drs. S. W. Cadden and J. F. B. Morrison for permission to use Fig. 2 and for their discussion of the manuscript.

References

Ammons, W. S., Blair, R. W. and Foreman, R. D. (1984) Raphe magnus inhibition of primate T_1–T_4 spinothalamic cells with cardiopulmonary visceral input. Pain, 20: 247–260.

Anderson, S. D., Basbaum, A. I. and Fields, H. L. (1977) Responses of medullary raphe neurons to peripheral stimulation and to systemic opiates. Brain Res., 123: 363–368.

Balagura, S. and Ralph, T. (1973) The analgesic effect of electrical stimulation of the diencephalon and mesencephalon. Brain Res., 60: 369–379.

Basbaum, A. I. and Fields, H. L. (1979) The origin of descending pathways in the dorsolateral funiculus of the spinal cord of the cat and rat: further studies on the anatomy of pain modulation. J. Comp. Neurol., 187: 513–532.

Basbaum, A. I., Clanton, C. H. and Fields, H. L. (1978) Three bulbospinal pathways from the rostral medulla of the cat: an autoradiographic study of pain modulating systems. J. Comp. Neurol., 178: 209–224.

Beall, J. E., Martin, R. F., Applebaum, A. E. and Willis, W. D. (1976) Inhibition of primate spinothalamic tract neurons by stimulation in the region of the nucleus raphe magnus. Brain Res., 114: 328–333.

Behbehani, M. M. and Fields, H. L. (1979) Evidence that an excitatory connection between the periaqueductal gray and nucleus raphe magnus mediates stimulation produced analgesia. Brain Res., 170: 85–93.

Blair, R. W., Weber, R. N. and Foreman, R. D. (1981) Characteristics of primate spinothalamic neurons receiving viscerosomatic convergent inputs in T_3–T_5 segments. J. Neurophysiol., 46: 797–811.

Blair, R. W., Weber, R. N. and Foreman, R. D. (1982) Responses of thoracic spinothalamic neurons to intracardiac injections of bradykinin in the monkey. Circ. Res., 51: 83–94.

Blair, R. W., Ammons, W. S. and Foreman, R. D. (1984) Responses of thoracic spinothalamic and spinoreticular cells to coronary artery occlusion. J. Neurophysiol., 51: 636–648.

Blum, P. S. (1981) Control of sensory transmission by electrical stimulation within the caudal raphe nuclei of the cat. Exp. Neurol., 72: 570–581.

Bowker, R. M., Steinbusch, H. W. M. and Coulter, J. D. (1981) Serotonergic and peptidergic projections to the spinal cord demonstrated by a combined retrograde HRP histochemical and immunocytochemical staining method. Brain Res., 211: 412–417.

Bowker, R. M., Westlund, K. N., Sullivan, M. C. and Coulter, J. D. (1982) Organisation of descending serotonergic projections to the spinal cord. In H. G. J. M. Kuypers and G. F. Martin (Eds.), Descending Pathways to the Spinal Cord, Progress in Brain Research, Vol. 57, Elsevier, Amsterdam, pp. 239–265.

Bowker, R. M., Westlund, K. N., Sullivan, M. C., Wilber, J. F. and Coulter, J. D. (1983) Descending serotonergic, peptidergic and cholinergic pathways from the raphe nuclei: a multiple transmitter complex. Brain Res., 288: 33–48.

Brodal, A., Taber, E. and Walberg, F. (1960) The raphe nuclei of the brain stem in the cat. II. Efferent connections. J. Comp. Neurol., 114: 239–260.

Cadden, S. W. (1985) A comparison of visceral and noxious somatic influences on neurons in the rat lumbar dorsal horn. Phil. Trans. Roy. Soc. B, 308: 414.

Cadden, S. W. and Morrison, J. F. B. (1984) The effects of visceral distension on the activities of lumbar dorsal horn neurones in the rat. J. Physiol. (Lond.), 350: 71P.

Cadden, S. W., Villanueva, L., Chitour, D. and Le Bars, D. (1983) Depression of activities of dorsal horn convergent neurones by propriospinal mechanisms triggered by noxious inputs; comparison with diffuse noxious inhibitory controls (DNIC). Brain Res., 275: 1–11.

Calvino, B., Villanueva, L. and Le Bars, D. (1984) The heterotopic effects of visceral pain; behavioural and electrophysiological approaches in the rat. Pain, 20: 261–271.

Carstens, E. (1982) Inhibition of spinal dorsal horn neuronal responses to noxious skin heating by medial hypothalamic stimulation in the cat. J. Neurophysiol., 48: 809–823.

Carstens, E., Yokota, T. and Zimmermann, M. (1979) Inhibition of spinal neuronal responses to noxious skin heating by stimulation of mesencephalic periaqueductal gray in the cat. J. Neurophysiol., 42: 558–568.

Carstens, E., Klumpp, D. and Zimmermann, M. (1980) Time course and effective sites for inhibition from midbrain periaqueductal gray of spinal dorsal horn neuronal responses to cutaneous stimuli in the cat. Exp. Brain Res., 38: 425–430.

Carstens, E., Bihl, H., Irvine, D. R. F. and Zimmermann, M. (1981) Descending inhibition from medial and lateral midbrain of spinal dorsal horn neuronal responses to noxious and nonnoxious cutaneous stimuli in the cat. J. Neurophysiol., 45: 1029–1042.

Carstens, E., MacKinnon, J. D. and Guinan, M. J. (1982) Inhibition of spinal dorsal horn neuronal responses to noxious skin heating by medial preoptic and septal stimulation in the cat. J. Neurophysiol., 48: 981–991.

Cervero, F. (1983) Supraspinal connections of neurones in the thoracic spinal cord of the cat: ascending projections and effects of descending impulses. Brain Res., 275: 251–261.

Cervero, F. and Wolstencroft, J. H. (1984) A positive feedback loop between spinal cord nociceptive pathways and antinociceptive areas of the cat's brain stem. Pain, 20: 125–138.

Cervero, F., Lumb., B. M. and Tattersall, J. E. H. (1985) Supraspinal loops that mediate visceral inputs to thoracic spinal cord neurones: involvement of descending pathways from raphe and reticular formation. Neurosci. Lett., in press.

Cervero, F., Lumb, B. M. and Tattersall, J. E. H. (1986) Supraspinal excitation and inhibition of viscero-somatic neurones in the thoracic spinal cord of the cat. J. Physiol. (Lond.), in press.

Chitour, D., Dickenson, A. H. and Le Bars, D. (1982) Pharmacological evidence for the involvement of serotonergic mechanisms in diffuse noxious inhibitory controls (DNIC). Brain Res., 236: 329–337.

Crowley, W. R., Jacobs, R., Volpe, J., Rodriguez-Sierra, J. F. and Komisaruk, B. R. (1976) Analgesic effects of vaginal stimulation in rats: modulation by graded stimulus intensity and hormones. Physiol. Behav., 16: 483–488.

Dahlström, A. and Fuxe, K. (1965) Evidence for the existence of monoamine neurons in the central nervous system. II. Experimentally induced changes in the intraneuronal amine levels of bulbospinal neuron systems. Acta Physiol. Scand. (Suppl. 247), 64: 1–36.

Dickenson, A. H. and Le Bars, D. (1983) Diffuse noxious inhibitory controls (DNIC) involve trigeminothalamic and spinothalamic neurones in the rat. Exp. Brain Res., 49: 174–180.

Dickenson, A. H., Le Bars, D. and Besson, J. M. (1980) An involvement of nucleus raphe magnus in diffuse noxious inhibitory controls (DNIC) in the rat. Neurosci. Lett. Suppl., 5: S375.

Dickenson, A. H., Rivot, J. P., Chaouch, A., Besson, J. M. and Le Bars, D. (1981) Diffuse noxious inhibitory controls (DNIC) in the rat with or without pCPA pretreatment. Brain Res., 216: 313–321.

Duggan, A. W. and Griersmith, B. T. (1979) Inhibition of the spinal transmission of nociceptive information by supraspinal stimulation in the cat. Pain, 6: 149–161.

Duggan, A. W., Hall, J. G., Headley, P. M. and Griersmith, B. T. (1977) The effect of naloxone on the excitation of dorsal horn neurons of the cat by noxious and non-noxious cutaneous stimuli. Brain Res., 138: 185–189.

Duggan, A. W., Griersmith, B. T. and Johnson, S. M. (1981) Supraspinal inhibiton of the excitation of dorsal horn neurons by impulses in unmeylinated primary afferents: lack of effect by strychnine and bicuculline. Brain Res., 210: 231–241.

Edeson, R. O. and Ryall, R. W. (1983) Systematic mapping of descending inhibitory control by the medulla of nociceptive spinal neurones in cats. Brain Res., 271: 251–262.

Eisenhart, S. F., Morrow, T. J. and Casey, K. L. (1983) Sensory and motor properties of bulboreticular and raphe neurons in awake and anaesthetised cats. In J. J. Bonica, U. Lindblom and A. Iggo (Eds.), Advances in Pain Research and Therapy, Vol. 5, Raven Press, New York, pp. 161–168.

Fardin, V., Oliveras, J. L. and Besson, J. M. (1984) A reinvestigation of the analgesic effects induced by stimulation of the periaqueductal gray matter in the rat. II. Differential characteristics of the analgesia induced by ventral and dorsal PAG stimulation. Brain Res., 306: 125–139.

Fields, H. L. and Anderson, S. D. (1978) Evidence that raphe-spinal neurons mediate opiate and midbrain stimulation-produced analgesias. Pain, 5: 333–349.

Fields, H. L., Basbaum, A. I., Clanton, C. H. and Anderson, S. D. (1977) Nucleus raphe magnus inhibition of spinal cord dorsal horn neurons. Brain Res., 126: 441–453.

Gebhart, G. F. and Toleikis, J. R. (1978) An evaluation of stimulation-produced analgesia in the cat. Exp. Neurol., 62: 570–579.

Gerhart, K. D., Wilcox, T. K., Chung, J. M. and Willis, W. D. (1981) Inhibition of nociceptive and nonnociceptive responses of primate spinothalamic cells by stimulation in medial brain stem. J. Neurophysiol., 45: 121–136.

Giesler, G. J. and Liebeskind, J. C. (1976) Inhibition of visceral pain by electrical stimulation of the periaqueductal gray matter. Pain, 2: 43–48.

Giesler, G. J., Gerhart, K. D., Yezierski, R. P., Wilcox, T. K. and Willis, W. D. (1981a) Postsynaptic inhibition of primate spinothalamic neurons by stimulation of nucleus raphe magnus. Brain Res., 204: 184–188.

Giesler, G. J., Yezierski, R. P., Gerhart, K. D. and Willis, W. D. (1981b) Spinothalamic tract neurons that project to medial and/or lateral thalamic nuclei: evidence for a physiologically novel population of spinal cord neurons. J. Neurophysiol., 46: 1285–1308.

Goodman, S. J. and Holcombe, V. (1976) Selective and prolonged analgesia in the monkey resulting from brain stimulation. In J. J. Bonica and D. Albe-Fessard (Eds.), Advances in Pain Research and Therapy, Vol. 1, Raven Press, New York, pp. 495–502.

Guilbaud, G., Oliveras, J. L., Giesler, G. and Besson, J. M. (1977) Effects induced by stimulation of the centralis inferior nucleus of the raphe on dorsal horn interneurons in cat's spinal cord. Brain Res., 126: 355–360.

Guilbaud, G., Peschanski, M., Gautron, M. and Binder, D. (1980) Responses of neurons of the nucleus raphe magnus to noxious stimuli. Neurosci. Lett., 17: 149–154.

Haber, L. H., Martin, R. F., Chung, J. M. and Willis, W. D. (1980) Inhibition and excitation of primate spinothalamic tract neurons by stimulation in region of nucleus reticularis gigantocellularis. J. Neurophysiol., 43: 1578–1593.

Handwerker, H. O., Iggo, A. and Zimmermann, M. (1975) Segmental and supraspinal actions on dorsal horn neurons responding to noxious and non-noxious skin stimuli. Pain, 1: 147–165.

Hayes, R. L., Price, D. D., Ruda, M. and Dubner, R. (1979) Suppression of nociceptive responses in the primate by electrical stimulation of the brain or morphine administration: behavioural and electrophysiological comparisons. Brain Res., 167: 417–421.

Head, H. and Holmes, G. (1911) Sensory disturbances from cerebral lesions. Brain, 34: 102–254.

Hornby, J. B. and Rose, J. D. (1976) Responses of caudal brainstem neurons to vaginal and somatosensory stimulation in the rat and evidence of genital-nociceptive interactions. Exp. Neurol., 51: 363–376.

Hosobuchi, Y., Adams, J. E. and Linchitz, R. (1977) Pain relief by electrical stimulation of the central gray matter in humans and its reversal by naloxone. Science, 197: 183–186.

Iggo, A., McMillan, J. A. and Mokha, S. S. (1981) Modulation of spinal cord multireceptive neurones from locus coeruleus and nucleus raphe magnus in the cat. J. Physiol. (Lond.), 319: 107–108P.

Komisaruk, B. R. and Wallman, J. (1977) Antinociceptive effects of vaginal stimulation in rats: neurophysiological and behavioural studies. Brain Res., 137: 85–107.

Le Bars, D., Dickenson, A. H. and Besson, J. M. (1979a) Diffuse noxious inhibitory controls (DNIC). I. Effects on dorsal horn covergent neurones in the rat. Pain, 6: 283–304.

Le Bars, D., Dickenson, A. H. and Besson, J. M. (1979b) Diffuse noxious inhibitory controls (DNIC). II. Lack of effect on non-convergent neurones, supraspinal involvement and theoretical implications. Pain, 6: 305–327.

Le Bars, D., Chitour, D. and Clot, A. M. (1981) The encoding of thermal stimuli by diffuse noxious inhibitory controls (DNIC). Brain Res., 230: 394–399.

Leichnetz, G. L., Watkins, L., Griffin, G., Murfin, R. and Mayer, D. J. (1978) The projection from the nucelus raphe magnus and other brainstem nuclei to the spinal cord in the rat: a study using the HRP blue-reaction. Neurosci. Lett., 8: 119–124.

Liebeskind, J. C., Guilbaud, G., Besson, J. M. and Oliveras, J. L. (1973) Analgesia from electrical stimulation of the periaqueductal gray matter in the cat: behavioural observations and inhibitory effects on spinal cord interneurones. Brain Res., 50: 441–446.

Lovick, T. A., West, D. C. and Wolstencroft, J. H. (1978) Responses of raphespinal and other bulbar raphe neurones to stimulation of the periaqueductal gray in the cat. Neurosci. Lett., 8: 45–49.

Lumb, B. M. and Morrison, J. F. B. (1984) Convergence of visceral and somatic information on to identified reticulo- and raphe-spinal neurones in the rat. J. Physiol. (Lond.), 357: 33P.

Lumb, B. M. and Morrison, J. F. B. (1985) Effects of ventromedial forebrain stimulation on the activities of raphe- and reticulo-spinal neurones in the rat. J. Physiol. (Lond.), 365: 28P.

Lumb, B. M. and Spillane, K. (1984) Visceral inputs to brainstem neurones in the rat. J. Physiol. (Lond.), 346: 46P.

Maciewicz, R., Sandrew, B. B., Phipps, B. S., Poletti, C. E. and Foote, W. E. (1984) Pontomedullary raphe neurons: intracellular responses to central and peripheral electrical stimulation. Brain Res., 293: 17–33.

Martin, R. F., Jordan, L. M. and Willis, W. D. (1978) Differential projections of cat medullary raphe neurons demonstrated by retrograde labelling following spinal cord lesions. J. Comp. Neurol., 182: 77–88.

Mayer, D. J. and Liebeskind, J. C. (1974) Pain reduction by focal electrical stimulation of the brain: an anatomical and behavioral analysis. Brain Res., 68: 73–93.

Mayer, D. J. and Price, D. D. (1976) Central nervous system mechanisms of analgesia. Pain, 2: 379–404.

Mayer, D. J., Wolfle, T. L., Akil, H., Carder, B. and Liebeskind, J. C. (1971) Analgesia from electrical stimulation in the brainstem of the rat. Science, 174: 1351–1354.

McMahon, S. B. and Morrison, J. F. B. (1982a) Spinal neurones with long projections activated from the abdominal viscera of the cat. J. Physiol. (Lond.), 322: 1–20.

McMahon, S. B. and Morrison, J. F. B. (1982b) Two groups of spinal interneurones that respond to stimulation of the abdominal viscera in the cat. J. Physiol. (Lond.), 322: 21–34.

McMahon, S. B. and Spillane, K. (1982) Brain stem influences on the parasympathetic supply to the urinary bladder of the cat. Brain Res., 234: 237–249.

McCreery, D. B., Bloedal, J. R. and Hames, E. G. (1979) Effects of stimulating in raphe nuclei and in reticular formation on response of spinothalamic neurons to mechanical stimuli. J. Neurophysiol., 42: 166–182.

Melzack, R. and Melinkoff, D. F. (1974) Aanlgesia produced by brain stimulation: evidence of a prolonged onset period. Exp. Neurol., 43: 369–374.

Miletic, V., Hoffert, M. J., Ruda, M. A., Dubner, R. and Shigenaga, Y. (1984) Serotonergic axonal contacts on identified cat spinal dorsal horn neurons and their correlation with nucleus raphe magnus stimulation. J. Comp. Neurol., 228: 129–141.

Milne, R. J., Foreman, R. D., Giesler, G. J. and Willis, W. D. (1981) Convergence of cutaneous and pelvic visceral nociceptive inputs on to primate spinothalamic neurons. Pain, 11: 163–183.

Moolenaar, G. M., Holloway, J. A. and Trouth, C. O. (1976) Responses of caudal raphe neurons to peripheral somatic stimulation. Exp. Neurol., 53: 304–313.

Oleson, T. D., Kirkpatrick, D. B. and Goodman, S. J. (1980) Elevation of pain threshold to tooth shock by brain stimulation in primates. Brain Res., 194: 79–95.

Oliveras, J. L., Besson, J. M., Guibaud, G. and Liebeskind, J. C. (1974a) Behavioral and electrophysiological evidence of pain inhibition from midbrain stimulation in the cat. Exp. Brain Res., 20: 32–44.

Oliveras, J. L., Woda, A., Guilbaud, G. and Besson, J. M. (1974b) Inhibition of the jaw opening reflex by electrical stimulation of the periaqueductal gray matter in the awake, unrestrained cat. Brain Res., 72: 328–331.

Oliveras, J. L., Redjemi, F., Guilbaud, G. and Besson, J. M. (1975) Analgesia induced by electrical stimulation of the inferior centralis nucleus of the raphe in the cat. Pain, 1: 139–145.

Oliveras, J. L., Hosobuchi, Y., Redjemi, F., Guilbaud, G. and Besson, J. M. (1977) Opiate antagonist naloxone, strongly reduces analgesia induced by stimulation of a raphe nucleus (centralis inferior). Brain Res., 120: 221–229.

Oliveras, J. L., Hosobuchi, Y., Guilbaud, G. and Besson, J. M. (1978) Analgesic electrical stimulation of the feline nucleus raphe magnus: development of tolerance and its reversal by 5-HTP. Brain Res., 146: 404–409.

Oliveras, J. L., Guilbaud, G. and Besson, J. M. (1979) A map of serotonergic structures involved in stimulation producing analgesia in unrestrained freely moving cats. Brain Res., 164: 317–322.

Pomeroy, S. L. and Behbehani, M. M. (1979) Physiological evidence for a projection from the periaqueductal gray to nucleus raphe magnus in the rat. Brain Res., 176: 143–147.

Proudfit, H. K. and Anderson, E. G. (1975) Morphine analgesia: blockade by raphe magnus lesions. Brain Res., 98: 612–618.

Reynolds, D. V. (1969) Surgery in the rat during electrical analgesia induced by focal brain stimulation. Science, 164: 444–445.

Rhodes, D. L. and Liebeskind, J. C. (1978) Analgesia from rostral brain stem stimulation in the rat. Brain Res., 143: 521–532.

Richardson, D. E. and Akil, H. (1977a) Pain reduction by electrical brain stimulation in man: Part 1: acute administration in periaqueductal and periventricular sites. J. Neurosurg., 47: 178–183.

Richardson, D. E. and Akil, H. (1977b) Pain reduction by electrical brain stimulation in man: Part 2: chronic self-administration in the periventricular gray matter. J. Neurosurg., 47: 184–194.

Rivot, J. P., Chaouch, A. and Besson, J. M. (1980) Nucleus raphe magnus modulation of response of rat dorsal horn neurons to unmyelinated fiber inputs: partial involvement of serotonergic pathways. J. Neurophysiol., 44: 1039–1057.

Rose, J. D. (1975) Response properties and anatomical organisation of pontine and medullary units responsive to vaginal stimulation in the cat. Brain Res., 97: 79–93.

Sandkuhler, J. and Gebhart, G. F. (1984) Relative contributions of the nucleus raphe magnus and adjacent medullary reticular formation to the inhibition by stimulation in the periaqueductal gray of a spinal nociceptive reflex in the pentobarbital-anaesthetised rat. Brain Res., 305: 77–87.

Satoh, M., Akaike, A., Nakazawa, T. and Takagi, H. (1980) Evidence for the involvement of separate mechanisms in the production of analgesia by electrical stimulation of the nucleus reticularis paragigantocellularis and nucleus raphe magnus in the rat. Brain Res., 194: 525–529.

Satoh, M., Oku, R. and Akaike, A. (1983) Analgesia produced by microinjection of L-glutamate into the rostral ventromedial bulbar nuclei of the rat and its inhibition by intrathecal alpha-adrenergic blocking agents. Brain Res., 261: 361–364.

Shah, Y. and Dostrovsky, J. O. (1980) Electrophysiological evidence for a projection of the periaqueductal gray matter to nucleus raphe magnus in cat and rat. Brain Res., 193: 534–538.

Soper, W. Y. (1976) Effects of analgesic midbrain stimulation on reflex withdrawal and thermal escape in the rat. J. Comp. Physiol. Psychol., 90: 91–101.

Steinman, J. L., Komisaruk, B. R., Yaksh, T. L. and Tyce, G. M. (1983) Spinal cord monoamines modulate the antinociceptive effects of vaginal stimulation in rats. Pain, 16: 155–166.

Tohyama, M., Sakai, K., Touret, M., Salvert, D. and Jouvet, M. (1979) Spinal projections from the lower brain stem in the cat as demonstrated by the horseradish peroxidase technique. II. Projections from the dorsolateral pontine tegmentum and raphe nuclei. Brain Res., 176: 215–231.

Vanegas, H., Barbaro, N. M. and Fields, H. L. (1984) Midbrain stimulation inhibits tail-flick only at currents sufficient to excite rostral medullary neurons. Brain Res., 321: 127–133.

Villanueva, L., Cadden, S. W. and Le Bars, D. (1984) Diffuse noxious inhibitory controls (DNIC): evidence for post-synaptic inhibition of trigeminal nucleus caudalis convergent neurones. Brain Res., 321: 165–168.

Wall, P. D. (1967) The laminar organisation of the dorsal horn and effects of descending impulses. J. Physiol. (Lond.), 188: 403–423.

Watkins, L. R., Griffin, G., Leichnetz, G. R. and Mayer, D. J. (1980) The somatotopic organisation of the nucleus raphe magnus and surrounding brain stem structures as revealed by HRP slow-release gels. Brain Res., 181: 1–15.

Watkins, L. R., Faris, P. L., Komisaruk, B. R. and Mayer, D. J. (1984) Dorsolateral funiculus and intraspinal pathways mediate vaginal stimulation-induced suppression of nociceptive responding in rats. Brain Res., 294: 59–65.

Weil-Fugazza, J., Godefroy, F. and Le Bars, D. (1984) Increase in 5-HT synthesis in the dorsal part of the spinal cord, induced by a nociceptive stimulus: blockade by morphine. Brain Res., 297: 247–264.

Wessendorf, M. W., Proudfit, H. K. and Anderson, E. G. (1981) The identification of serotonergic neurons in the nucleus raphe magnus by conduction velocity. Brain Res., 214: 168–173.

West, D. C. and Wolstencroft, J. H. (1977) Location and conduction velocity of raphe-spinal neurones in nucleus raphe magnus and raphe pallidus in the cat. Neurosci. Lett., 5: 147–151.

Willis, W. D. (1982) Control of nociceptive transmission in the spinal cord. In D. Ottoson (Ed.), Progress in Sensory Physiology, Vol. 3, Springer-Verlag, Berlin, pp. 1–159.

Willis, W. D. and Coggeshall, R. E. (1978) Sensory mechanisms of the spinal cord, Plenum Press, New York, pp. 1–485.

Willis, W. D., Haber, L. H. and Martin, R. F. (1977) Inhibition of spinothalamic tract cells and interneurons by brain stem stimulation in the monkey. J. Neurophysiol., 40: 969–981.

Yaksh, T. L. and Tyce, G. M. (1981) Release of norepinephrine and serotonin in cat spinal cord: direct in vivo evidence for the activation of descending monoamine pathways by somatic stimulation. J. Physiol. (Paris), 77: 483–487.

Yen, C. T. and Blum, P. S. (1984) Response properties and functional organisation of neurones in midline region of medullary reticular formation in cats. J. Neurophysiol., 52: 961–979.

Yeung, J. C., Yaksh, T. L. and Rudy, T. A. (1977) Concurrent mapping of brain sites for sensitivity to the direct application of morphine and focal electrical stimulation in the production of antinociception in the rat. Pain, 4: 23–40.

Yezierski, R. P., Wilcox, T. K. and Willis, W. D. (1982) The effects of serotonin antagonists on the inhibition of primate spinothalamic tract cells produced by stimulation in nucleus raphe magnus or the periaqueductal gray. J. Pharmacol. Exp. Ther., 220: 266–277.

Zorman, G., Hentall, I. D., Adams, J. E. and Fields, H. L. (1981) Naloxone-reversible analgesia produced by microstimulation in the rat medulla. Brain Res., 219: 137–148.

F. Cervero and J. F.B. Morrison
Progress in Brain Research, Vol. 67

CHAPTER 18

Brainstem integration of cardiovascular and pulmonary afferent activity

D. Jordan and K. M. Spyer

Department of Physiology, Royal Free Hospital School of Medicine, Rowland Hill Street, London NW3 2PF, U.K.

The central projection of cardiovascular and respiratory afferents

The central terminations of afferents from the heart and cardiovascular system have been studied for many years by a variety of methods. It is only in the last few years, however, that definitive results have been forthcoming. This has been due to the development of more sensitive and precise histological and physiological techniques. Since the earlier work has been reviewed previously (Spyer, 1981), only a brief summary will be given of this; a more detailed account is given of the numerous studies undertaken over the last 10 years.

Histological studies

Early histological studies using degeneration techniques investigated the termination of glossopharyngeal (IXth) and vagal (Xth) nerve afferents after intracranial rootlet section. These studies agreed that, in the cat, the majority of myelinated Xth and IXth afferents entered the tractus solitarius (TS) and descended in the tractus, sending off collaterals to the main nuclear regions of the solitary tract (NTS), where they terminated. Some Xth afferents, however, entered the spinal trigeminal tract and others decussated at the level of the obex and terminated in the contralateral commissural nucleus (Foley and Dubois, 1934; Ingram and Dawkins, 1945).

With the advent of the Nauta technique, which also visualises degenerating unmyelinated fibres, these studies were extended. The most complete report is that of Cottle (1964), in which she selectively cut individual IXth and Xth nerve rootlets. Degenerating fibres were followed across the descending trigeminal tract and most became incorporated into the TS, only a few remaining within the trigeminal tract. From this level the fibres in the TS coursed caudally, sending off small bundles of fibres medially and dorsomedially, where they terminated. Further caudally, some fibres entered the lateral (Slt) and ventrolateral (Svl) regions of the NTS, and yet others crossed via the commissural nucleus (Com) to terminate in the contralateral dorsomedial NTS (Sdm). The pattern of degeneration indicated that the fibres terminating in the rostral third of the NTS were exclusively from IXth nerve afferents whereas those in the caudal third were of Xth origin. The maximal density of degeneration, however, was found in an area extending rostrally 2.5 mm from the obex, the intermediate third of the nucleus. The fibres in this region originated in both IXth and Xth rootlets. Since the Xth fibres terminating in this region came from rootlets which had previously been shown to contain cardiovascular afferents (Von Baumgarten and Aranda Coddou, 1959), Cottle (1964) suggested that this was the most likely area to be important in cardiovascular control.

Other histological studies have shown that the

projection of IXth and Xth nerve afferents to this intermediate region of the NTS is similar in the rat (Torvik, 1956), cat (Kerr, 1962), guinea-pig (Kimmel and Kimmel, 1964), monkey (Rhoton et al., 1966), opossum (Culberson and Kimmel, 1972) and mallard duck (Dubbeldam et al., 1979). Most recently, the degeneration studies of Gwyn and Leslie (1979) have, in addition, identified a previously unreported heavy vagal projection to the dorsal and dorsomedial parts of the cat NTS, a region termed the area subpostrema or subnucleus gelatinosus (SNG), and their electron microscopical investigation (Leslie et al., 1982) provided evidence that these degenerating Xth terminals did indeed make synaptic contact with neurones in this region.

These anterograde degeneration studies have indicated the major areas to which the IXth and Xth nerves project, although little specific information is provided from this type of study since there is only partial transganglionic degeneration after cutting individual nerve branches distal to the sensory ganglion. The elucidation of the central projection of sensory fibres from particular nerve branches or individual organs awaited a methodological breakthrough, which came with the use of neural tracer substances which are transported transganglionically, and therefore can be employed to label selectively the afferent nerves from particular organs. Various tracer substances have been employed in these studies, and all rely on uptake of the substance by neurones and its subsequent anterograde transport by axoplasmic transport mechanisms.

Autoradiographic localization of transported radioactively labelled amino acids such as proline and leucine was the first of this type of study to be reported on the IXth and Xth nerves. After injection of these labelled amino acids into the petrosal ganglia of monkeys, Beckstead and Norgren (1979) localized afferent fibres entering the medulla ventrolaterally at the level of the rostral pole of the inferior olivary nucleus. Groups of fibres then coursed dorsomedially as fascicles through, and above, the spinal tract of the trigeminal nucleus. On reaching the NTS the fibres dispersed mainly into the lateral part of the nucleus, both rostral and caudal to the site of entry, only sparse labelling being noted in the medial parts of the nucleus. Labelled fibres were restricted to the region of the NTS rostral to the obex and ipsilateral to the site of injection. An unexpected finding was the lack of rostrocaudally running labelled fibres in the TS. Following amino acid injections into the nodose ganglion, labelled fibres were seen entering the medulla in a similar fashion to glossopharyngeal afferents and at a level immediately caudal to them. These fibres solidly filled the TS throughout its rostro-caudal extent. Both Slt and Sm were labelled in these animals; most concentrated in the lateral region at the level of the Xth nerve entry but most dense in the medial region, including the Com more caudally. The contralateral Sm and Com were also labelled. Outside the NTS, dense bilateral labelling of fibres was noted in the area postrema and sparse labelling was noted in the dorsomedial portion of the spinal V nucleus.

Similar injections of labelled amino acids into cat nodose ganglia (Gwyn et al., 1979; Kalia and Mesulam, 1980a) showed a pattern of labelling similar to that described in the monkey. Whilst most subnuclei of the NTS and the area postrema were labelled bilaterally, all ipsilateral areas were more heavily labelled than were contralateral regions. The most heavily labelled area was the Sm, including the SNG (parvocellular nucleus), which in the cat stains heavily for cholinesterases (Gwyn and Wolstencroft, 1968).

In the rat (Contreras et al., 1982) a very similar distribution of IXth and Xth afferents has been described to that seen in the monkey; however, in the rat no terminals were labelled rostral to the level of nerve entry and in this species some IXth afferents terminated as far caudal as the ipsilateral Com. In addition, Sumal et al. (1983) have recently provided evidence that Xth afferent terminals overlie catecholamine-containing neurones in the Sm. Synaptic contacts between labelled Xth axons and dendrites, some of which contained catecholamine, were also visualised.

More specific information regarding the central projections of visceral sensory afferents has been produced using the transganglionic anterograde transport of the enzyme horseradish peroxidase (HRP), alone or in conjugation with a variety of larger molecules such as the lectins and albumins. HRP is taken up by cut nerves or after injection into sensory ganglia, whole nerves or organs of innervation. Over the last few years a wealth of data has accumulated from using this technique on both the IXth and Xth nerves or their various branches and organs of innervation. Whilst these show that the NTS is the prime site of termination of these afferents, there does appear to be a differential termination for afferents from different organs (Kalia and Mesulam, 1980b; Katz and Karten, 1983).

The anterograde transport of HRP following its application to the central cut ends of the IXth and Xth nerves (Ciriello et al., 1981b) or injection into the nodose ganglion (Gwyn et al., 1979; Kalia and Mesulam, 1980a; Chernicky et al., 1984) has confirmed the earlier degeneration studies showing that sensory afferents of the IXth and Xth cranial nerves project primarily to the ipsilateral NTS. Although most sub-nuclei received some input, the relative density varied (Table I). On the contralateral side of the brain the Sm and Com were the most consistently labelled. Most workers have noted a bilateral innervation of the area postrema whilst there are various reports of an innervation of the dorsal motor nucleus of the vagus and external cuneate nucleus.

In respect of sensory afferents from specific visceral sites, those of the arterial baroreceptors especially have received most interest. Table II summarizes the results of a variety of authors, mainly working in the cat, after application of HRP to the carotid sinus nerve (CSN). There is agreement that the Sdm, Sm, Slt and Com are the most likely to receive a CSN input, whilst the extent of any input to the area postrema and contralateral brainstem remains controversial. Outside this immediate area there are also claims of a direct CSN input to the medial reticular formation, external cuneate nucleus, spinal nucleus V (Ciriello et al., 1981a), the nucleus ambiguus and dorsal reticular formation (Davies and Kalia, 1981).

The central projections of the aortic depressor nerve (ADN), containing afferents from the aortic baroreceptors, have been studied in a wider variety

TABLE I

A comparison of the central distribution of vagal nerve terminals after injection of HRP into nodose ganglia or applications to the central end of the cut cervical vagus

Animal (Reference)		Sm	Sdm	Spc	Svl	Is	Slt	Int	Com	AP	Extent	Other areas
Cat (Kalia and Mesulam, 1980a)	i	+++	++	+++	++	+	++	++	+++	++	+2.8 → −4.4	DVN
	c	+	○	○	○	○	○	○	+	+		
Cat (Ciriello et al., 1981b)	i	+++	+++	+++	+++	++	+++	○	+++	+	+4.0 → −2.0	ECN
	c	+	+	+	○	○	+	○	+	+	+2.0 → −2.0	
Cat (Gwyn et al., 1979)	i	++	++	+++	−	−	++	−	+++	++		
	c	○	○	○	○	○	○	○	○	○		
Dog (Chernicky et al., 1984)	i	++	++	++	+	+++	+++	−	++	++	+4.5 → −3.5	DVN
	c	+	+	○	○	○	○	○	○	+	+2.5 → −3.5	

In all cases HRP was visualised by the tetramethylbenzidine (TMB) technique (Mesulam, 1978). The nuclear groups are an extended version of those described by Loewy and Burton (1978). AP, area postrema; c, contralateral; Com, commissural nucleus; DVN, dorsal vagal nucleus; ECN, external cuneate nucleus; i, ipsilateral; Int, intermediate nucleus; Is, interstitial nucleus; nA, nucleus ambiguus; Sdm, dorsomedial solitary nucleus; Slt, lateral solitary nucleus; Sm, medial solitary nucleus; Spc, parvocellular solitary nucleus; Svl, ventrolateral solitary nucleus; +, positive representation, density indicated by number of (+); ○, absence of representation; −, no information relating to involvement.

TABLE II

A comparison of the central distribution of carotid sinus nerve terminals after application of horseradish peroxidase to the central end of the cut CSN or injection of HRP into the intact CSN (Davies and Kalia, 1981)

Animal studied (Reference)		Sm	Sdm	Spc	Svl	Is	Slt	Int	Com	AP	Extent	Other areas
Cat (Berger, 1979)	i	+ +	+ + +	+	+	+ +	+ +	+	+ +	○	+2.5 → −2.5	
	c	+	+	○	○	+	○	○	+	○	+0.5 → −3.0	
Cat (Panneton and Loewy, 1980)	i	+ +	+ + +	○	+	+	+	○	+ +	+	+2.4 → −2.0	
	c	+	+	○	○	○	○	○	+	○	+1.5 → −2.0	
Cat (Cieriello et al., 1981a)	i	+ +	+ + +	+	+	+	+ + +	+	+ +	○	+5.0 → −2.0	mRF
											most	ECN
											+2.0 → −1.0	spV
	c	+	+ +	+	○	○	+	+	+ +	○	+1.0 → −2.0	
Cat (Davies and Kalia, 1981)	i	+ +	+ + +	+	+ +	○	+ +	+	+ + +	+ +	−4.0	nA
	c	+	+ +	○	+	○	+	○	+ +	+	+2.4 → −4.0	dRF
Cat (Nomura and Mizuno, 1982)	i	+ +	+ + +	○	○	+ +	+ +	○	+ +	○	+2.5 → −1.0	
	c	○	○	○	○	–	○	○	+	○		
Rat (Seiders and Stuesse, 1984)	i	+	+ +	–	+	○	–	–	+	+	+2.0 → −1.0	
	c	○	○	○	○	○	○	○	+	○		

In all cases HRP was visualised by the tetramethyl benzidine (TMB) technique (Mesulam, 1978). The nuclear groups are an extended version of those described by Loewy and Burton (1978).

TABLE III

A comparison of the central distribution of aortic depressor nerve terminals after application of HRP to the central end of the cut ADN

Animal studied (Reference)		Sm	Sdm	Spc	Svl	Is	Slt	Int	Com	AP	Extent	Other areas
Cat (Kalia and Welles, 1980)	i	+ +	+ + +	–	○	–	+ +	○	+ +	+ +	+3.0 → −1.0	DVN
	c	+	+	–	○	–	○	○	+	+	+2.0 → −1.0	
Cat (Ciriello et al., 1981a)	i	+ +	+ + +	+	○	+	+ +	○	+ +	○	+4.0 → −1.0	not DVN
	c	+	+	+	○	–	+	○	+	○	+2.0 → −1.0	
Rabbit (Wallach and Loewy, 1980)	i	+ +	+ + +	○	○	○	○	○	+ +	○	+1.6 → −1.5	not DVN
	c	+	+	○	○	○	○	○	+	○	+1.0 → −1.0	
Rabbit (Higgins and Schwaber, 1981)	i	–	+ + +	–	–	–	–	–	–	–	–	
	c	–	–	–	–	–	–	–	–	–	–	
Rat (Ciriello, 1983)	i	+ +	+ + +	–	+	+ + +	+ + +	–	+ +	○	+2.0 → −1.5	not DVN
	c	+	+	–	○	○	○	–	+	○	0 → −1.5	
Rat (Higgins et al., 1984)	i	+ +	+ + +	–	○	–	+	○	+ + +	○	–	DVN
	c	○	○	○	○	○	○	○	+	○	–	
Pigeon (Kats and Karten, 1979)	i		+ + +								+1.7 → +1.1	
	c		+									

In all cases the TMB technique was used to visualise the HRP reaction product. The nuclear groups are an extended version of those described by Loewy and Burton (1978).

of species (Table III). As with the CSN, the Sdm, Slt, Sm and Com appear to be the most likely sites of termination of these fibres. In general, the extent of the ADN input appears more restricted than the CSN input. This may reflect claims that in the rabbit and rat the ADN is solely barosensory (Heymans and Neil, 1958; Sapru and Krieger, 1977; Sapru et al., 1981) whereas the CSN also contains afferents from the carotid body chemoreceptors.

The brainstem projections from other visceral afferents in the airways and thoracic cavity are detailed most thoroughly in the report by Kalia and Mesulam (1980b), who injected HRP into various sites in the larynx, trachea, bronchi, lungs and heart. The NTS received sensory projections from all these sites, with the Sm, Sdm, dorsolateral (Sdl), Svl and Com all receiving varying degrees of input from all these viscera, the remaining subnuclei only being connected to some of them.

It is clear from these data that there is no distinct specific region of the NTS dedicated to receiving afferent information from any particular visceral organ. Indeed, many subnuclei of the NTS appear to be the site of termination of a variety of afferent nerves. Differences, however, in the central representation of viscera have been documented in terms of the relative importance of the different subnuclei of the NTS. A similar conclusion has been reported in a recent study in the pigeon (Katz and Karten, 1983).

The techniques described have clearly delineated the areas of termination of sensory afferents from a variety of visceral organs. However, the function of these labelled afferents can only be surmised. Until recently, electrophysiological techniques have been required to study this problem (see below). However, a new autoradiographic technique has now been developed using a marker substance, 2-[^{3}H]deoxyglucose. This technique, developed by Sokoloff et al. (1977), uses 2-deoxyglucose as a marker for the increased glucose utilization which occurs when neural activity occurs. During prolonged physiological activation of a group of sensory afferents increased uptake of 2-deoxyglucose would be expected and this could be visualized autoradiographically. Of course, not only the primary afferent terminals but all areas of increased activity will be visualized by this technique. So far, the input to the NTS from stimulation of the Xth, CSN (Kostreva, 1983), aortic baroreceptors (Ciriello et al., 1983) and carotid body chemoreceptors (Harris and Banks, 1985) has been reported. Unfortunately, the resolution of this technique does not, as yet, approach that of the other tracer techniques, but no doubt this will soon be improved.

Finally, the terminal branching of physiologically identified, slowly adapting lung stretch afferents (SARs) has been visualised after intracellular injections of HRP-wheatgerm agglutinin (WGA) into their axons within the brainstem (Kalia and Richter, 1985a,b). Single SARs had terminal branches which arborized over a considerable rostro-caudal extent within the ipsilateral Sv, Svl and intermediate nucleus (Int).

Antidromic mapping studies

The histological studies summarised in the previous section have provided evidence that the NTS, and its immediate vicinity, is the sole site of termination in the medulla of the afferents contained in the IXth and Xth cranial nerves and their various peripheral branches. Traditional neurophysiological recording studies have lent support to this contention (see Spyer, 1981, for review), although these failed to reveal the specific patterns of projection of the individual classes of afferent contained within these nerves. Antidromic excitation of CSN, ADN and a variety of vagal branches on microstimulation within the NTS has added further confirmation (Spyer, 1981, 1982), but an adaptation of this approach involving recordings from the cell bodies of individual afferent neurones in the nodose (Xth) and petrosal (IXth) ganglia has provided the opportunity to define the projections of specific afferents.

Baroreceptor afferents

Studies in both rabbits and cats indicate that baroreceptor afferents project to distinct, and lo-

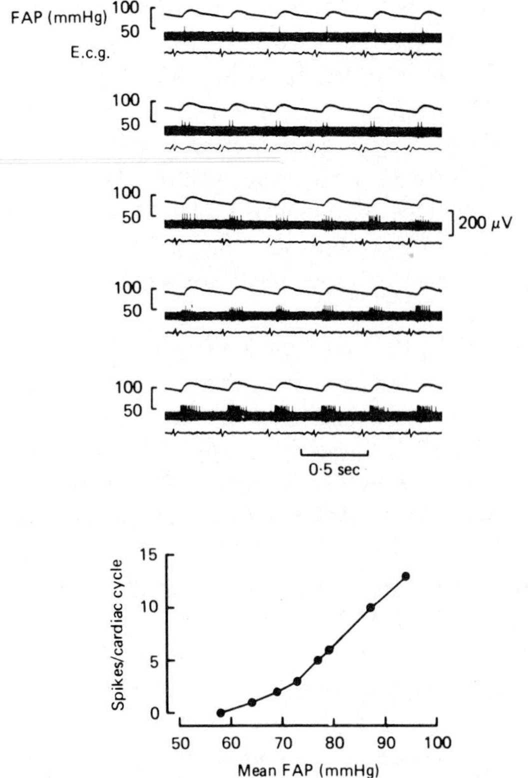

Fig. 1. Nodose ganglion of cat: A, original records of femoral arterial blood pressure (FAP), electrocardiogram (e.c.g.) and spontaneous activity of an aortic baroreceptor afferent, showing the relationship between FAP and afferent activity. B, a graph of the number of spikes/cardiac cycle (average of ten cycles) against mean FAP. Reproduced, with permission, from Donoghue et al. (1982a).

calised, regions of the NTS. Considering aortic arch baroreceptors, evidence has been obtained that the receptors with myelinated axons (conduction velocity 12.5–22.0 m/second in cat; 14–23 m/second in rabbit) innervate almost exclusively the ipsilateral NTS at levels rostral to the obex (Donoghue et al., 1982a). Using the example of such an afferent recorded in the nodose ganglion of the cat (Fig. 1), the discharge was seen to be related to the level of arterial blood pressure. Furthermore, the afferent was antidromically activated on stimulating within restricted regions of the NTS, the pattern of projection being assessed by noting the threshold current for activation at 100-μm steps through serial

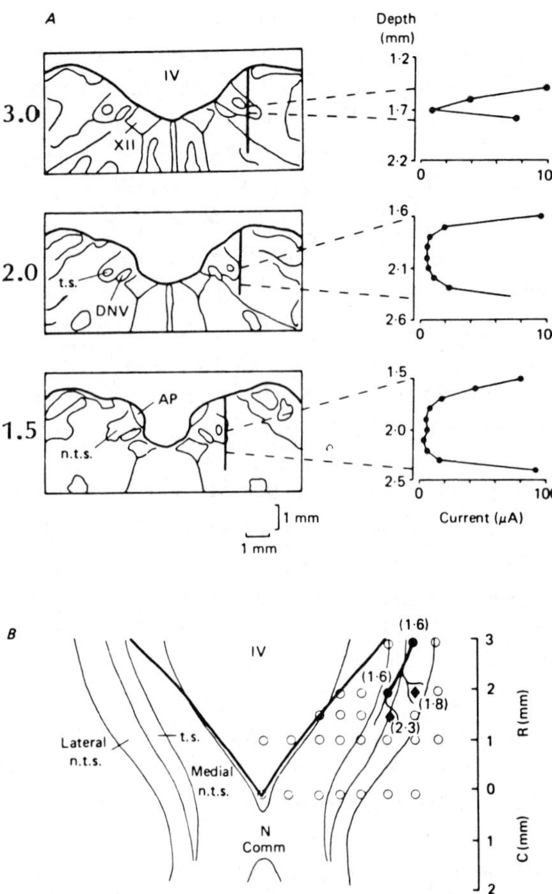

Fig. 2. Myelinated aortic baroreceptor afferent (cat). A, cross-sections of the dorsomedial region of the medulla oblongata at intervals rostral to the obex. The thick vertical lines each represent a stimulating electrode track. On the right are shown depth-threshold curves corresponding to the penetrations. That at the top is of the "point" type, the lower two of the "field" type. B, a schematic view of the dorsal surface of the medulla oblongata showing the fourth ventricle. Superimposed on this is the medial and lateral extent of the tractus solitarius and its nucleus. Scales indicate distances (in mm) rostral (R), caudal (C) and lateral to the obex. Sites of stimulating electrode penetration are indicated, classed according to the type of depth-threshold contour obtained from the penetration, i.e., point (●), field (◆) or no response (○). The main axon is shown by the thick line connecting point types, and regions of branching by thin lines. AP, area postrema; DNV, dorsal motor nucleus of vagus; NComm, nucleus commissuralis; nts, nucleus tractus solitarius; ts, tractus solitarius; XII, hypoglossal nucleus; IV, fourth ventricle. Reproduced, with permission, from Donoghue et al. (1982a).

penetrations within the dorsomedial medulla. On the basis of the latency for activation and the family of depth-threshold contours, a reasonable picture of the distribution of each fibre was inferred (Fig. 2). In the cat, five of six afferents projected to the Slt, and in three of these there was also an input to the Sm. In a single case this continued into the Com and crossed the midline to the contralateral side, to innervate the Sm on that side. In the rabbit seven out of eight afferents similarly innervated the Slt rostral to the obex whilst in a single afferent there was an innervation of the Sm. Only ipsilateral projections were observed.

In the cat the central projections of both myelinated and unmyelinated baroreceptors with endings in the carotid sinus have been assessed using equivalent techniques (Donoghue et al., 1984). No marked differences were apparent in the patterns of projection and termination of these two classes of baroreceptor afferent, although as yet no afferent with conduction velocity of >10 m/second has been studied. All gave only ipsilateral projections, which always involved the Slt at levels rostral to the obex, usually with additional innervations of the Sm, and in some cases there was also an innervation of the Svl. The dorsal regions of both Slt and Sm were particular sites of termination. In seven of the 12 afferents investigated some innervation of the Com was identified.

In summary, baroreceptors, whether with endings in the aorta or carotid sinus, project to essentially similar areas of the NTS. The dorsolateral and dorsomedial regions at levels rostral to the obex appear to receive the densest innervations, although lateral, and to a lesser extent ventrolateral, subdivisions receive a significant input.

Chemoreceptor afferents

In the cat both the CSN and ADN contain chemoreceptor afferents as well as baroreceptor afferents. The central projections of the carotid body chemoreceptor afferents have also been studied using antidromic mapping. 13 afferents, all with unmyelinated axons and discharging under eupnoiec conditions, have been shown to have projections that differ considerably from those of the arterial baroreceptors. All were activated on stimulation within the ipsilateral Sm, particularly its dorsomedial aspect, and in 12 of these there was an additional projection into the Com. In 25% of cases this continued into the Com on the contralateral side. There was also evidence of an ipsilateral projection in four afferents to the Slt at levels rostral to the obex.

Slowly adapting lung stretch afferents (SARs)

Xth afferents with endings in the airways are known to exert influences over both respiration and the cardiovascular system (Widdicombe, 1982). Myelinated Xth afferents with a discharge that adapts slowly to maintained lung inflation play an important role in the "off-switch" that terminates inspiration and exert that role through an action on one group of neurone within the Svl (Von Baumgarten and Kanzow, 1958). The central projection of these afferents has been detailed using antidromic mapping (Donoghue et al., 1982b). In the cat six of seven SARs projected to the ipsilateral Sm, with two of these also innervating the Slt and Svl at levels rostral to the obex. The other afferent had exclusive projections to Slt and Svl. In the rabbit the pattern of projection was largely the same (nine of 11 afferents projected to the Sm, one of which also projected to Svl and Slt; two afferents gave only inputs to the Slt and Svl).

These observations have been confirmed using the alternative technique of spike-triggered averaging of extracellular activity in the brainstem using the spike activity of SARs recorded in the nodose ganglion as the trigger (Berger and Averill, 1983). Potentials reflecting terminal activity were recorded maximally in a region 1 mm rostral to the obex within the Sm (in six cases) and in the Sdl in two cases. Maximal synaptic potentials were also restricted to these areas. In conjunction with the data of Donoghue et al. (1982b), this emphasises the importance of the Sm in the mediation of the reflex effects of SARs.

The limited input of SARs to the Svl and Sv is, however, of considerable importance in respiratory control since a monosynaptic input to the Rβ inspiratory neurones of the Svl has been demonstrated by the spike-triggered averaging of the membrane potential of Rβ neurones using the spikes of SARs as the trigger (Backman et al., 1984; Berger et al., 1985) or by cross-correlating the activity of SARs and extracellularly recorded Rβ neuronal activity (Averill et al., 1984). Neither group could show a monosynaptic activation of the Rα group of respiratory neurones, but Averill et al. (1984) could show such a monosynaptic excitatory input to "P" cells, which have no central respiratory rhythm but fire in phase with lung inflation (Berger, 1977). The monosynaptic excitatory postsynaptic potentials (EPSPs) in Rβ cells had amplitudes of 30–265 μV and latencies between 1.6 and 3.1 mseconds (Backman et al., 1984). Even with the inherent problem of averaging over the whole respiratory cycle, there was a suggestion, on the basis of the shape of the averaged EPSP, either that the monosynaptic input was distributed to several regions of the Rβ neurone or that there was an additional polysynaptic input.

Rapidly adapting lung stretch afferents (RARs)

In addition to the detailed information on the projection and synaptic connections of SARs, there are some limited data available on the projections of RARs. These airway mechanoreceptors, which also relay via the Xth, respond to rapid lung inflations or deflations with an irregular discharge which rapidly adapts to a maintained lung volume. In the cat, antidromic mapping has shown these fibres to project to the NTS, but to a region further caudal to the region of termination of SARs (Kubin and Davies, 1985). In the majority of cases the ventral parts of the Sm received an innervation, which in most continued into the contralateral Sm. The Slt received only a few branches and in only two of the 11 RARs studied did these branches reach the Svl, where inspiratory neuronal activity could be recorded.

The major projections of these cardiovascular and pulmonary sensory afferents as determined by the antidromic mapping technique are summarised in Fig. 3.

Afferent interactions with the NTS

From the above review it is clear that whilst individual classes of IXth and Xth nerve afferents have distinctive patterns of projection to the NTS, specific regions of the nucleus receive inputs from several different afferents. In particular, the Sm at levels rostral to the obex represents an area with a variety of inputs and an extensive innervation. However, there is as yet little information available on the synaptic role of this apparent convergence (see Donoghue et al., 1985, for review) and only a limited appraisal of the role of presynaptic interactions has been made (Rudomin, 1967, 1968; Barillot, 1970; Jordan and Spyer, 1979; Ballantyne et al., 1985). Both levels of interaction have considerable potential physiological inportance since there is a large literature describing the interaction of respiratory and cardiovascular reflexes (Daly, 1984). Also, respiratory activity itself alters the effectiveness of these reflexes and this involves the action of both the neuronal substrate responsible for the generation of respiratory activity and inputs related to lung inflation (see Spyer, 1981, 1982). These effects may be so powerful as to prevent the arterial che-

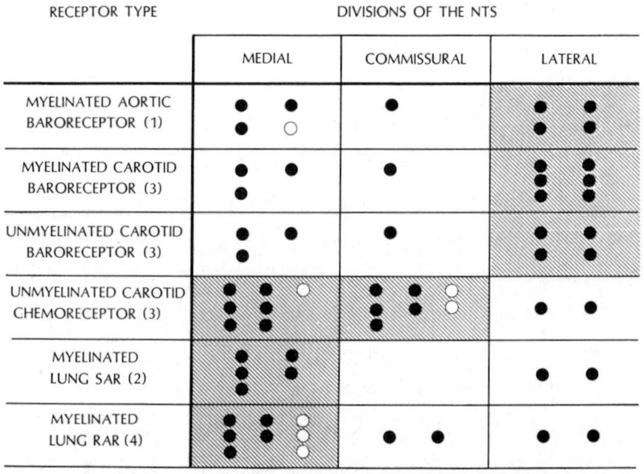

RECEPTOR TYPE	DIVISIONS OF THE NTS		
	MEDIAL	COMMISSURAL	LATERAL
MYELINATED AORTIC BARORECEPTOR (1)	● ● ● ○	●	● ● ● ●
MYELINATED CAROTID BARORECEPTOR (3)	● ● ●	●	● ● ● ● ● ●
UNMYELINATED CAROTID BARORECEPTOR (3)	● ● ●	●	● ● ● ●
UNMYELINATED CAROTID CHEMORECEPTOR (3)	● ● ● ● ● ● ○	● ● ● ● ● ○ ○	● ●
MYELINATED LUNG SAR (2)	● ● ● ● ●		● ●
MYELINATED LUNG RAR (4)	● ● ● ● ● ○ ○ ○	● ●	● ●

Fig. 3. Terminations within the cat NTS of cardiovascular and pulmonary afferents. A summary of the relative density of ipsilateral (●) and contralateral (○) regions of termination based on antidromic mapping studies. 1, Donoghue et al. (1982a); 2, Donoghue et al. (1982b); 3, Donoghue et al. (1984); 4, Kubin and Davies (1985). Shading represents the major projection for each afferent.

moreceptors from exciting NTS inspiratory neurones during expiration (Lipski et al., 1977), and brief stimuli, applied to both the arterial chemoreceptors and carotid sinus baroreceptors, will only excite vagal cardio-inhibitory neurones if timed to occur during expiration (Spyer, 1981). Lung inflation is also able to block effectively these reflex inputs to these neurones (Potter, 1981). Whilst, in the case of vagal cardio-inhibitory neurones, much of this respiratory "gating" is a consequence of a respiratory control of the activity of these neurones themselves (Gilbey et al., 1984), at least a portion of these variations in reflex sensitivity may occur through pre- and postsynaptic processes within the NTS.

Presynaptic interactions

Present evidence suggests that interactions between afferents at a presynaptic level may result in modifications in synaptic transmission in the CNS. In this respect there is a limited literature indicating that such interactions may occur between vagal afferent fibres (Rudomin, 1967, 1968). These interactions have been inferred from measurements of the terminal excitability of vagal afferents to conditioning stimuli delivered to other Xth branches or to stimuli delivered within the NTS (Rudomin, 1967, 1968; Barillot, 1970; Jordan and Spyer, 1979). This has been clearly illustrated for superior laryngeal nerve (SLN) afferents antidromically activated by stimulation within the NTS (Rudomin, 1967), an influence that has been shown to be mediated by SARs (Barillot, 1970). Furthermore, SARs themselves are also affected by conditioning stimuli delivered to the SLN and the NTS (Barillot, 1970). These inferences have received direct support from the observations of Ballantyne et al. (1985), who have recorded the membrane potentials of SAR fibres in close proximity to their points of termination within the NTS. In these recordings two waves of depolarisation were observed in response to SLN stimulation. These had latencies of 3–8 and 27–35 mseconds, respectively, the long-latency response showing considerable sensitivity to the period of the respiratory cycle in which the stimulus was delivered. Effects were maximal in phase with each burst of phrenic nerve activity (i.e., inspiration). This also indicated that a depolarisation of SAR terminals must occur in phase with inspiration. Indeed, in a proportion of SARs such waves of depolarisation were recorded. Additional effects of lung inflation were seen superimposed on the inspiratory waves of depolarisation, indicating an additional interaction at presynaptic level between SARs (Ballantyne et al., 1986). Such influences were also evident in the case of SARs whose activity was recorded in the nodose ganglion and which were antidromically activated on stimulation within the NTS (Ballantyne et al., 1986).

On the basis of such observations it is clear that these changes in terminal excitability may allow a degree of control of afferent transmission through presynaptic inhibition. This process can be evoked by peripheral inputs and also by central inputs related to inspiratory activity and presumably involving the dorsal group of respiratory neurones (Von Baumgarten and Kanzow, 1958). Is there a physiological role for this control of afferent transmission? In the case of SLN-evoked effects on SARs there is at least some suggestive evidence of a genuine role. Activation of laryngeal receptors is known to suppress inspiration in order to prevent the aspiration of materials into the airways. This input actively inhibits Rα and Rβ inspiratory neurones, but the action of SLN activation on SARs would lead in addition to a depolarisation of their terminals, and hence a reduction of transmitter release. This would effectively disfacilitate Rβ neurones, which depend, at least in part, on SAR input for their discharge. In addition, the interaction between SARs described above may well act to produce synchronisation of discharge in Rβ neurones similar to the effects reported previously for Ia afferent inputs in regulating a motoneuronal discharge (Rudomin et al., 1975). In a rhythmically active system such as the medullary respiratory network this may have particular importance.

Whilst we have presented convincing evidence from several different laboratories that afferents with endings in the lungs and airways are amenable to presynaptic influences, the same does not seem to hold for CSN and ADN afferents (Rudomin, 1967, 1968; Barillot, 1970; Jordan and Spyer, 1979; Ballantyne et al., 1986). Stimulating the ADN can certainly evoke presynaptic excitability changes in SLN afferents (Rudomin, 1967) but conditioning stimuli within the NTS do not affect the threshold for the antidromic response in the ADN to a test stimulus within the NTS (Rudomin, 1967; Jordan and Spyer, 1979). Nor does the threshold for the activation of ADN baroreceptor afferents recorded in the nodose ganglion show systematic variations in phase with either phrenic nerve activity or lung inflation (Ballantyne et al., 1986). This difference between baroreceptor afferents and SARs may reflect the marked differences between their patterns of termination within the NTS (Ballantyne et al., 1986). As was described earlier, whilst both groups of afferents terminate within the Sm, SARs make monosynaptic connections with Rβ neurones whose cell bodies are located in the Svl. Conversely, baroreceptors appear to provide their densest innervation of the NTS to dorsomedial and dorsolateral divisions of the Slt and Sm. The K^+ activity in the vicinity of the dorsal group of respiratory neurones has been shown to change dramatically during the respiratory cycle, with a periodic increase of 0.05–0.20 mM in the Svl during inspiration and of 0.3–0.5 mM on repetitive vagal stimulation (Richter et al., 1978). Such changes could account for the waves of depolarisation observed in recordings from SARs. However, during the respiratory cycle there are no measurable changes in K^+ activity in the dorsal regions of the NTS described above.

Whilst the ionic mechanism described above may account for some of the presynaptic interactions within the NTS, anatomical data are available which support the possibility of interactions occurring independent of such ionic changes. Electron-microscopic studies have identified axo-axonal synapses within the Com (Chiba and Doba, 1976) but not the intermediate (Chiba and Doba, 1975) regions of the NTS, and in a recent study Kalia and Richter (1985b) described SAR terminals, labelled with HRP, which form the postsynaptic element of axo-axonal synapses within the Sv and Svl.

Postsynaptic interactions

Whilst it is clear that presynaptic influences may modulate the reflex effectiveness of some afferent inputs, others, such as arterial baroreceptors, appear to be devoid of such control. However, it is known that many of these afferents can interact substantially when producing their reflex effects (see Heymans and Neil, 1958; Korner, 1979; Daly, 1984). However, the postsynaptic sites at which such interactions may occur are still a matter of speculation. Both sympathetic and vagal preganglionic neurones are known to have the ability to behave in an integrative manner (see Spyer (1981) for discussion). Hence, the question which needs to be addressed is whether the NTS is simply a relay station for its wide range of afferent input or whether it too can contribute to their postsynaptic integration into appropriate physiological patterns of response dependent upon the prevailing spectrum of afferent input.

The majority of studies to approach this problem have used the technique of extracellular recording from brainstem neurones whilst electrically stimulating the afferent nerves or physiologically activating the specific receptors in the periphery. Clearly, the majority of NTS neurones receive an input from peripheral receptors of one sort or another, e.g., baroreceptor, chemoreceptor, receptors in the thorax or respiratory tract (see above), However, there is no consensus in the literature as to whether neurones in this area can receive inputs from more than one type of receptor. An expansive study by Biscoe and Sampson (1970) described a wealth of convergence of afferents in the IXth, CSN, ADN and SLN onto medullary neurones. Few, however, were shown to be within the NTS. A more detailed study of the convergence between ADN and CSN afferents was made by Gabriel and Seller (1970), who detailed the time course of the occlusive interactions which occur between the field potentials evoked by stimulation of the two sets of baroreceptor nerves. This would clearly indicate a level of postsynaptic interaction between these afferents but, in his thesis, McAllen (1973) failed to observe neurones in the NTS which received a convergent input from any combination of the CSN, ADN or the cardiac branches of the Xth. In contrast to this Hildebrandt (1974) provided evidence of a limited convergence of inputs from CSN, ADN and Xth onto single neurones, though again most of the responsive neurones lay outside the NTS. Most recently, Ciriello and Calaresu (1980, 1981) have shown a significant population of NTS neurones (27 of 122) which could be activated from both CSN and ADN, these being located primarily in the Sm, Svl and INT. In areas outside the NTS, a higher percentage of cells received convergent input (26 of 55).

The most extensive studies of convergence between afferent fibres travelling in the Xth nerve came from the work of Kidd and his colleagues (Donoghue et al., 1981a,b; Kidd, 1979). On the basis of their pattern of activity, response to carotid occlusion and electrical stimulation of the CSN and Xth, only a very few neurones in the NTS of their dogs could be shown to receive an input from both CSN and Xth afferents (Fussey et al., 1967; Kidd, 1979), a result Kidd (1979) admits was surprising. A later series of studies in cats (Donoghue et al., 1981a; Bennett et al., 1981) described the convergence in the NTS from afferents in the thoracic branches of the Xth, both cardiac and pulmonary. Between 20 and 40% of neurones showed such convergence, but it was noticeable that neurones receiving an unmyelinated input from one branch would receive only an unmyelinated input from the other branch(es) and, similarly, neurones receiving a myelinated input from one set of afferents would receive only a myelinated input from the others. Only a single neurone was reported to receive both a myelinated and unmyelinated input. Whilst no neurones receiving an input from the cardiac branches of the Xth could be shown to receive an input from the ADN (Donoghue et al., 1981a), a limited convergence of myelinated and unmyelinated ADN afferents to the same NTS neurone was demonstrated (Donoghue et al., 1981b). Since these neurones were intermingled within the NTS, many within the Sm, it would appear that myelinated and non-myelinated afferent fibres from the heart and lungs terminate within the same anatomical region but, functionally, inputs appear to take distinctly separate pathways.

A bilateral convergence between myelinated Xth afferents onto neurones in the caudal part of the NTS and Com has been described by Porter (1963) in the cat and Nosaka et al. (1978) in rats. However, in this same region Nosaka et al. (1978) also describe clear convergence between both myelinated and unmyelinated Xth afferents. Whether this reflects a true species difference or the result of activation of afferents of non-thoracic origin remains to be determined.

The central interactions of another group of Xth afferents — those innervating the larynx and travelling in the SLN — have also come under scrutiny. There is now overwhelming evidence that the terminals of these afferents within the NTS are subject to presynaptic control (see above). There appears, however, to be only a limited degree of postsynaptic interaction described for these afferents. Whilst Porter (1963) could show no convergence of input from the afferents in the cervical vagus or recurrent laryngeal nerve onto neurones receiving an SLN input, Sessle (1973) describes only six neurones from a population of 84 receiving a SLN input could also be activated by stimulating the IXth nerve. Using long-term recording and correlation techniques in cats and dogs, Stroh-Werz et al. (1977a,b) have shown peaks of activity in the discharge of NTS neurones which were correlated with the arterial pulse and respiratory rhythm. These responses were mediated by both Xth and non-Xth inputs and lead to the conclusion that different cardiovascular afferents converge onto single neurones.

The lack of convergent sensory input in many of these studies may well indicate a limited degree of interaction between these inputs at this level of their reflex pathway. However, it could also be due to the fact that all studies used only extracellular re-

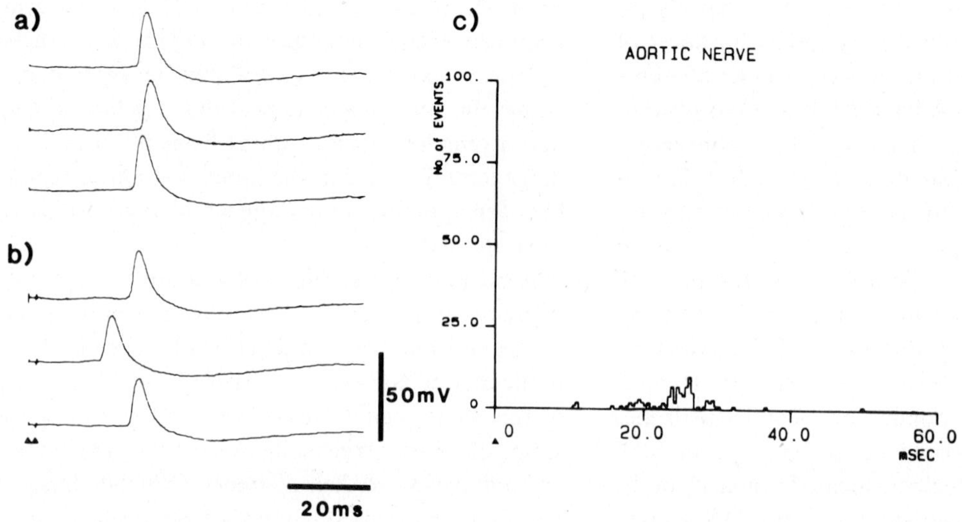

Fig. 4. Intracellular recording from a neurone exclusively excited by stimulation of the aortic nerve. Three successive oscilloscope traces of intracellular recordings (membrane potential, −63 mV) show the response of the neurone to (a) single and (b) pairs of stimuli to the aortic nerve given at ▲. c, the effect of a single stimulus is shown in the form of a post-stimulus time histogram (100 sweeps, 128 bins, 0.8 mseconds). Reproduced, with permission, from Donoghue et al. (1985).

cording techniques which would show only interactions which were suprathreshold, stringent condition-test procedures being required to uncover more subtle subliminal effects. In a recent study from our own laboratory (Donoghue et al., 1985), we have tried to overcome this problem by using both extracellular and intracellular techniques to record the activity of neurones in the immediate vicinity of the NTS during activation of afferent fibres in the CSN, ADN and Xth. We confirmed the previous studies showing that the predominant effect of stimulating these nerves was an excitatory input which in the majority of cases was exclusively from one set of afferents. These responses showed the expected postsynaptic characteristics, including temporal summation, and in intracellular records, a summation of evoked EPSPs and an afterhyperpolarization showing these recordings were not made from the afferent fibres themselves (Fig. 4). A significant population of neurones had a convergent input from more than one nerve and in nearly 25% (10 of 43) this could be identified in intracellular records such as Fig. 5, where stimulation of neither Xth nor CSN alone was sufficient to activate the neurone.

In our study a specific baroreceptor input to several neurones was inferred on the basis of ECG-related spike activity or discharge of EPSPs. The majority of visceral sensory nerves, however, are heterogeneous in terms of both the size of afferent fibre and the function served. Therefore, little can be said with certainty about functional considerations in any of the studies previously detailed. Only a handful of studies have investigated convergence between afferents of known function. In the first of these reports, Miura and Reis (1972) could find no evidence that neurones in the cat NTS which they considered to have a carotid sinus baroreceptor input (i.e., having a pulse-related discharge which could be abolished by carotid occlusion) also responded to carotid body chemoreceptor stimulation. A later report (Lipski et al., 1976) studied neurones excited by electrical stimulation of the CSN. Ten of these could be shown to be activated by inflation of a perfused carotid sinus. Eight of these neurones also received an input from carotid body

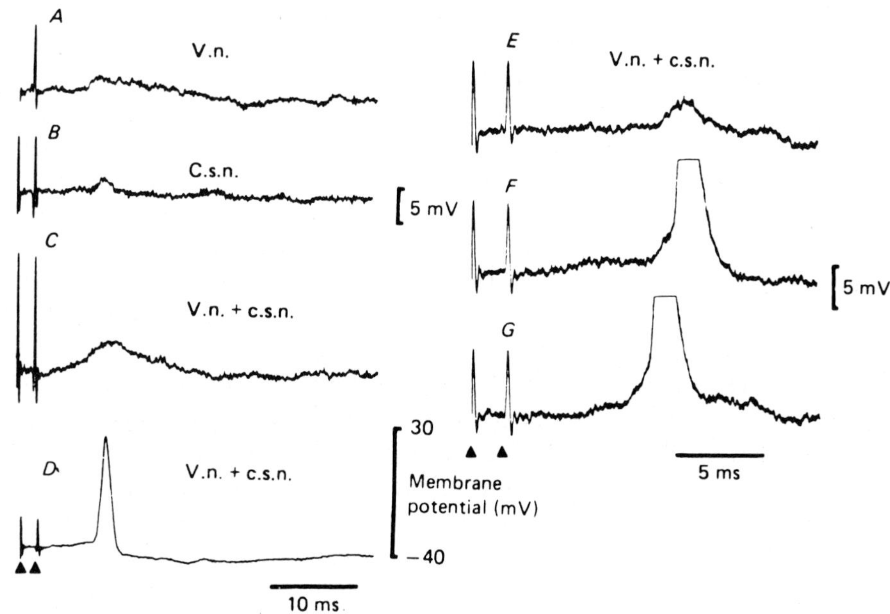

Fig. 5. Intracellular recordings from a neurone responsive to stimulation of carotid sinus nerve (CSN) and vagus nerve (VN). Single oscilloscope traces show the intracellular recorded response of the neurone to stimulation of the VN with one pulse (A), a pair of stimuli to the CSN (B) and the effect of these two stimulations combined (C). Increasing the stimulus voltage evoked a larger response and eventually spike initiation (E, F and G), which can also be seen at a lower gain in D. Reproduced, with permission, from Donoghue et al. (1985).

chemoreceptors, only two receiving an exclusive baroreceptor input. Few of these neurones, however, were actually located in the NTS. In view of the marked antagonistic patterns of cardiovascular and respiratory responses which can be evoked by stimulation of baroreceptors and chemoreceptors, such a marked convergence could appear surprising. Indeed, in rats, Nosaka (1976) could find < 10% of neurones which could be inferred as receiving both baroreceptor and chemoreceptor inputs on the basis of the neurones response to carotid occlusion. Finally, McCall et al. (1977) described NTS neurones responsive to both baroreceptor inputs and activation of afferents in the inferior cardiac nerve, whilst Schwaber and Schneiderman (1975) showed in rabbits that stimulation of the ADN, which in this animal is totally barosensory, activated NTS neurones receiving an input from sensory fibres in the Xth.

Whilst by far the majority of afferent input is of an excitatory nature, there are several reports in the literature that activation of sensory fibres can evoke inhibitory responses within the NTS. In his detailed electrophysiological study of the medullary projections of the CSN, Humphrey (1967) described some neurones in the ventromedial NTS (an area from which he recorded a positive-going wave evoked by CSN stimulation) whose spontaneous discharge was reduced by repetitive CSN stimulation. A similar inhibitory action on NTS neurones mediated by carotid sinus baroreceptors was later confirmed by Lipski and Trzebski (1975). A brief report (Bennett et al., 1982) shows that NTS neurones can also receive long-lasting inhibitory inputs from myelinated and unmyelinated afferents from the heart and lungs and Sessle (1973) noted that NTS neurones with SLN or IXth nerve inputs could show depressed responses if conditioning stimuli were applied to either nerve. These reports of inhibitory effects are rare. However, extracellular recordings can only demonstrate inhibition in spontaneously active neurones or by inhibition of other evoked responses and cannot distinguish between effects mediated pre- and postsynaptically. In the few studies where intracellular recordings have been made, reports of inhibitory postsynaptic responses are more common. Hildebrandt (1974) noted three cells in which CSN stimulation evoked inhibitory postsynaptic potentials (IPSPs), though all were within the medial reticular formation. Within the NTS, Miura (1975) described IPSPs evoked in neurones by activation of A-fibres in the CSN, and in our own laboratory (Donoghue et al., 1985) we have extended this to include slower-conducting CSN, ADN and Xth afferents. Finally, using an in vitro rat medullary slice preparation, Champagnat et al. (1985) provided a variety of evidence for synaptic inhibition in NTS neurones. This included (i) a reduction in the amplitude of test EPSP by a subthreshold conditioning stimulus to the TS, (ii) hyperpolarizing postsynaptic potentials with characteristics similar to IPSPs could be recorded in some neurones using potassium acetate-filled electrodes and (iii) groups of spontaneous postsynaptic potentials likely to be reversed IPSPs were recorded only after injection of Cl^- into these cells.

At this point it might be appropriate to consider one widely discussed contradiction: whilst baroreceptor afferents with an obvious pulsatile discharge have been shown to terminate within a wide area of the NTS where they activate neurones through both mono- and polysynaptic pathways, despite repeated attempts by various groups, surprisingly few neurones (mainly restricted to the dorsomedial NTS) have also been shown to have such a pulse-related discharge (see Spyer, 1981, for review). Several possibilities may contribute to such findings. Firstly, Seller and Illert (1969) described a marked attentuation in the amplitude of the evoked potential recorded in the NTS with repetitive stimulation of the CSN, and concluded that frequency transmission across the first synapse was the limiting step in the frequency response of the baroreceptor reflex as a whole. Secondly, the convergent, occlusive nature of the interaction between the various baroreceptor afferents (Gabriel and Seller, 1970) could confuse the pulsatile input from one nerve, since aortic and carotid sinus afferent impulses will reach the NTS at different times relative to one another, and therefore act as a conditioning stimulus. Even this condition-test regime will vary since the delay between the activation of the different baroreceptors will be dependent on the velocity of the pulse wave in the ascending aorta and common carotid arteries. Thirdly, it is clear from intracellular records in cat (Donoghue et al., 1985) and rat (Champagnat et al., 1985) that orthodromic action potentials in many NTS neurones exhibit large and prolonged afterhyperpolarizaitons which would contribute to the frequency limiting seen in the studies of Seller and Illert (1969). Whether all, or any, of these effects contribute to the scarcity of "pulse-modulated neurones" in the NTS is a matter for debate; however, it is interesting that clear cardiac rhythm becomes obvious once again at the level of the autonomic preganglionic neurones — both vagal and sympathetic (see Spyer, 1981).

Suprabulbar control of visceral inputs

The results of a variety of different studies have provided a substantial body of evidence implicating suprabulbar areas in the organisation of visceral responses, much of it acting at the level of the brainstem. Since the bulk of this evidence has been thoroughly reviewed in a series of articles (Calaresu et al., 1975; Korner, 1979; Spyer, 1981, 1984; Stock et al., 1983), only a brief summary of the important conclusions will be given here.

Suprabulbar areas are involved in producing patterns of autonomic and behavioural responses related to certain "species-characteristic" behaviours, and in this respect the "defence" or "arousal" reaction has been particularly well investigated. In anaesthetised cats stimulation of the perifornical region of the hypothalamus, termed the "hypothalamic defence area" (HDA), evokes pupillary dilatation, piloerection, a maintained tachycardia and pressor response. These cardiovascular responses are due to a widespread sympathetic activation leading to vasoconstriction in most vascular beds but a characteristic cholinergic vasodilatation in the supply to hindlimb skeletal muscle (Abrahams et al., 1960). The maintained tachycardia and pressor responses during such activation would suggest a modification of the baroreceptor reflex and it has been claimed that this reflex is either totally (Coote et al., 1979) or partially (Djojosugito et al., 1970) suppressed during HDA stimulation (see Spyer, 1981, for review). In contrast, stimulation of a region of the anterior hypothalamus evoked changes in blood pressure, heart rate and respiration qualitatively identical to the baroreceptor reflex (Hilton and Spyer, 1971). A qualitatively similar response can be elicited by stimulation of the central nucleus of the amygdala (ACE), which in the awake cat elicits a variety of behavioural responses ranging from alerting to full-blown defensive behaviour (Hilton and Zbrozyna, 1963; Stock et al., 1978).

A wealth of anatomical data is available showing reciprocal connections between the ACE, the hypothalamus and the NTS (Saper et al., 1976; Hopkins and Holstege, 1978; Ricardo and Koh, 1978; Ross et al., 1981; Van der Kooy et al., 1984). In addition, evidence is accumulating for connections between these regions and the insular cortex — a region which may well be important in visceral control (Saper, 1982; Van der Kooy et al., 1984).

Little electrophysiological data are available in this field, but what is available complements well the anatomical evidence. Neurones in both the hypothalamus (see Calaresu and Ciriello, 1980; Spyer, 1981, for review) and ACE (Cechetto and Calaresu, 1984, 1985) respond to activation of arterial baroreceptors and chemoreceptors, and these same amygdaloid cells would also appear to receive inputs from other sources, such as the locus coeruleus, acoustic, optic and tactile stimuli (Schutze et al., 1982).

Conversely, stimulation of the hypothalamus in the region of the HDA has been reported to inhibit the response of NTS neurones to CSN stimulation (Adair and Manning, 1975) and baroreceptor stimuli (McAllen, 1976). Weiss and Crill (1969) proposed that such descending inputs could modify presynaptically the transmission of baroreceptor information through the NTS. However, this was not supported by more recent studies in this laboratory (Jordan and Spyer, 1979); we could find no influence of stimulating the HDA on the terminal excitability of CSN afferents, though the stimulus evoked a central suppression of the baroreceptor reflex (Coote et al., 1979). This same stimulus, however, did influence the excitability of other IXth nerve afferents, indicating that such descending inputs can modulate sensory transmission in the NTS, but as this does not include baroreceptor afferents any descending influence on these reflexes must involve synaptic actions at a later stage in the reflex pathway. In an ongoing study in our laboratory (Jordan et al., 1985), we have indeed shown in extracellular recordings that NTS neurones receiving a CSN or Xth input, or both, could be either excited or inhibited by HDA stimulation. Similarly, in these same experiments stimulation of the ACE could have both excitatory or inhibitory effects on such NTS neurones. Interestingly, a single NTS neurone could have either similar or opposing effects from the ACE and HDA. Intracellular recordings are now being carried out to identify more fully the postsynaptic mechanisms producing such effects.

A similar series of studies is being undertaken in the rabbit (Moruzzi et al., 1984), where it has been shown that NTS neurones receiving either an ADN or Xth input can be excited at short latency by stimulation of the ACE, which in this species evoked a bradycardia and hypotension. In recent studies in rats, however, Nosaka (1984) has shown that some NTS neurones activated by both hypothalamic and vagal afferent stimulation also had axons projecting to this same hypothalamic area, whilst Kannan and Yamashita (1985) have shown that NTS neurones projecting to the paraventricular nucleus (PVN) can receive afferent inputs from both the PVN itself and the carotid baroreceptors.

Therefore, it is apparent that reciprocal connections can occur between both the hypothalamus-NTS and the amygdala-NTS and these may have particular importance in the behavioural integration of visceral responses.

Concluding remarks

The present report has summarised the current literature relating to the afferent innervation of the NTS from cardiopulmonary receptors and the arterial baroreceptors and chemoreceptors. The processing of these inputs has been described and the influence of descending inputs from the diencephalon on these mechanisms has been indicated. Whilst these afferent inputs exert powerful reflex influences and modify the state of arousal (see Spyer, 1981), their role in conscious perception and in the control of visceral sensation remains to be documented.

Acknowledgements

The original studies reported were supported by grants from the M.R.C. and the British Heart Foundation. Thanks are extended to Marion Roper for assistance in the preparation of the manuscript.

References

Abrahams, V. C., Hilton, S. M. and Zbrozyna, A. (1960) Active muscle vasodilatation produced by stimulation of the brain stem: Its significance in the defence reaction. J. Physiol., 154: 491–513.

Adair, J. R. and Manning, J. W. (1975) Hypothalamic modulation of baroreceptor afferent unit activity. Am. J. Physiol., 229: 1357–1364.

Averill, D. B., Cameron, W. E. and Berger, A. J. (1984) Monosynaptic excitation of dorsal medullary respiratory neurons by slowly adapting pulmonary stretch receptors. J. Neurophysiol., 52: 771–785.

Backman, S. B., Anders, C., Ballantyne, D., Röhrig, N., Camerer, H., Mifflin, S., Jordan, D., Dickhaus, H., Spyer, K. M. and Richter, D. W. (1984) Evidence for a monosynaptic connection between slowly adapting pulmonary stretch receptor afferents and inspiratory beta neurones. Pflügers Arch., 402: 129–136.

Ballantyne, D., Jordan, D., Meesmann, M., Richter, D. W. and Spyer, K. M. (1986) Presynaptic depolarization in myelinated vagal afferent fibres terminating in the nucleus of the tractus solitarius in the cat. Pflügers Arch., 406: 12–19.

Barillot, J.-C. (1970) Dépolarisation présynaptique des fibres sensitives vagales et laryngées. J. Physiol. (Paris), 62: 273–294.

Beckstead, R. M. and Norgren, R. (1979) An autoradiographic examination of the central distribution of the trigeminal, facial, glossopharyngeal and vagal nerves in the monkey, J. Comp. Neurol., 184: 455–472.

Bennett, J. A., Goodchild, C. S., Kidd, C. and McWilliam, P. N. (1981) Neurones in the brain stem of the cat activated by myelinated and non-myelinated fibres in the cardiac and pulmonary branches of the vagus. J. Physiol., 310: 64P.

Bennett, J. A., Goodchild, C. S., Kidd, C. and McWilliam, P. N. (1982) Inhibition of evoked and spontaneous activity of neurones in the nucleus of the tractus solitarius and dorsal motor vagal nucleus by cardiac and pulmonary vagal afferent fibres in the cat. J. Physiol., 332: 77P.

Berger, A. J. (1977) Dorsal respiratory group neurons in the medulla of cat: Spinal projections, responses to lung inflation and superior laryngeal nerve stimulation. Brain Res., 135: 231–254.

Berger, A. J. (1979) Distribution of carotid sinus nerve afferent fibers to solitary tract nuclei of the cat using transganglionic transport of horseradish peroxidase. Neurosci. Lett., 14: 153–158.

Berger, A. J. and Averill, D. B. (1983) Projection of single pulmonary stretch receptors to solitary tract region. J. Neurophysiol., 49: 819–830.

Berger, A. J., Averill, D. B., Cameron, W. E. and Dick, T. E. (1985) Anatomical and functional correlates of dorsal respiratory group neurones. In A. L. Bianchi and M. Denavit-Saubié (Eds.), Neurogenesis of Central Respiratory Rhythm, MTP Press Limited, Lancaster, pp. 130–137.

Biscoe, T. J. and Sampson, S. R. (1970) Responses of cells in the brainstem of the cat to stimulation of the sinus, glossopharyngeal, aortic and superior laryngeal nerves. J. Physiol., 209: 359–373.

Calaresu, F. R. and Ciriello, J. (1980) Projections to the hypothalamus from buffer nerves and nucleus tractus solitarius in the cat. Am. J. Physiol., 239: R130–R136.

Calaresu, F. R., Faiers, A. A. and Mogenson, G. J. (1975) Central neural regulation of heart and blood vessels in mammals. Prog. Neurobiol., 5: 1–35.

Cechetto, D. F. and Calaresu, F. R. (1984) Units in the amygdala responding to activation of carotid baro- and chemoreceptors. Am. J. Physiol., 246: R832–R836.

Cechetto, D. F. and Calaresu, F. R. (1985) Central pathways relaying cardiovascular afferent information to amygdala. Am. J. Physiol., 248: R38–R45.

Champagnat, J., Siggins, G. R., Koda, L. Y. and Denavit-Saubié, M. (1985) Synaptic responses of neurons of the nucleus tractus solitarius in vitro. Brain Res., 325: 49–56.

Chernicky, C. L., Barnes, K. L., Ferrario, C. M. and Conomy,

J. P. (1984) Afferent projections of the cervical vagus and nodose ganglion in the dog. Brain Res. Bull., 13: 401–411.

Chiba, T. and Doba, N. (1975) The synaptic structure of catecholaminergic axon varicosities in the dorso-medial portion of the nucleus of the tractus solitarius of the cat: possible roles in the regulation of cardiovascular reflexes. Brain Res., 84: 31–46.

Chiba, T. and Doba, N. (1976) Catecholaminergic axo-axonic synapses in the nucleus of the tractus solitarius (Pars commissuralis) of the cat: possible relation to presynaptic regulation of baroreceptor reflexes. Brain Res., 102: 255–265.

Ciriello, J. (1983) Brainstem projections of aortic baroreceptor afferent fibres in the rat. Neurosci. Lett., 36: 37–42.

Ciriello, J. and Calaresu, F. R. (1980) Monosynaptic pathway from cardiovascular neurons in the nucleus tractus solitarii to the paraventricular nucleus in the cat. Brain Res., 193: 529–533.

Ciriello, J. and Calaresu, F. R. (1981) Projections from buffer nerves to the nucleus of the solitary tract: an anatomical and electrophysiological study in the cat. J. Auton. Nerv. Systems, 3: 299–310.

Ciriello, J., Hrycyshyn, A. W. and Calaresu, F. R. (1981a) Horseradish peroxidase study of brainstem projections of carotid sinus and aortic depressor nerves in the cat. J. Auton. Nerv. Systems, 4: 43–61.

Ciriello, J., Hrycyshyn, A. W. and Calaresu, F. R. (1981b) Glossopharyngeal and vagal afferent projections to the brainstem of the cat: a horseradish peroxidase study. J. Auton. Nerv. Systems, 4: 63–79.

Ciriello, J., Rohlicek, C. V. and Polosa, C. (1983) Aortic baroreceptor reflex pathway: a functional mapping using [^{3}H]2-deoxyglucose autoradiography in the rat. J. Auton. Nerv. Systems, 8: 111–128.

Contreras, R. J., Beckstead, R. M. and Norgren, R. (1982) The central projections of the trigeminal, facial, glossopharyngeal and vagus nerves: an autoradiographic study in the rat. J. Auton. Nerv. Systems, 6: 303–322.

Coote, J. H., Hilton, S. M. and Perez-Gonzalez, J. F. (1979) Inhibition of the baroreceptor reflex on stimulation in the brainstem defence centre. J. Physiol., 288: 549–560.

Cottle, M. K. (1964) Degeneration studies of primary afferents of IXth and Xth cranial nerves in the cat. J. Comp. Neurol., 122: 329–343.

Culberson, J. L. and Kimmel, D. L. (1972) Central distribution of primary afferent fibres of the glossopharyngeal and vagal nerves in the opossum *Didelphis virginiana*. Brain Res., 44: 325–335.

Daly, M. De B. (1984) Breath-hold diving: Mechanisms of cardiovascular adjustments in the mammal. In P. F. Baker (Ed.), Recent Advances in Physiology, Vol. 10, Churchill Livingstone, Edinburgh, pp. 201–245.

Davies, R. O. and Kalia, M. (1981) Carotid sinus nerve projections to the brain stem in the cat. Brain Res. Bull., 6: 531–541.

Djojosugito, A. M., Folkow, B., Kylstra, P. H., Lisander, B. and Tuttle, R. S. (1970) Differentiated interaction between hypothalamic defence reaction and baroreceptor reflexes. Acta Physiol. Scand., 78: 376–385.

Donoghue, S., Fox, R. E., Kidd, C. and Koley, B. N. (1981a) The distribution in the cat brain stem of neurones activated by vagal non-myelinated fibres from the heart and lungs. Q. J. Exp. Physiol., 66: 391–404.

Donoghue, S., Fox, R. E., Kidd, C. and McWilliam, P. N. (1981b) The terminations and secondary projections of myelinated and non-myelinated fibres of the aortic nerve in the cat. J. Exp. Physiol., 66: 405–422.

Donoghue, S., Garcia, M., Jordan, D. and Spyer, K. M. (1982a) Identification and brain-stem projections of aortic baroreceptor afferent neurones in nodose ganglia of cats and rabbits, Q. J. Physiol., 322: 337–352.

Donoghue, S., Garcia, M., Jordan, D. and Spyer, K. M. (1982b) The brain-stem projections of pulmonary stretch afferent neurones in cats and rabbits. J. Physiol., 322: 353–363.

Donoghue, S., Felder, R. B., Jordan, D. and Spyer, K. M. (1984) The central projections of carotid baroreceptors and chemoreceptors in the cat: a neurophysiological study. J. Physiol., 347: 397–409.

Donoghue, S., Felder, R. B., Gilbey, M. P., Jordan, D. and Spyer, K. M. (1985) Post-synaptic activity evoked in the nucleus tractus solitarius by carotid sinus and aortic nerve afferents in the cat. J. Physiol., 360: 261–273.

Dubbeldam, J. L., Brus, E. R., Menken, S. B. J. and Zeilstra, S. (1979) The central projections of the glossopharyngeal and vagus ganglia in the Mallard (*Anas platyrhynchos* l.). J. Comp. Neurol., 183: 149–168.

Foley, J. O. and Dubois, F. S. (1934) An experimental study of the rootlets of the vagus nerve in the cat. J. Comp. Neurol., 60: 137–159.

Fussey, I. F., Kidd, C. and Whitwam, J. C. (1967) Single unit activity associated with cardiovascular events in the brainstem of the dog. J. Physiol., 191: 57P–58P.

Gabriel, M. and Seller, H. (1970) Interaction of baroreceptor afferents from carotid sinus and aorta at the nucleus tractus solitarii. Pflügers Arch., 318: 7–20.

Gilbey, M. P., Jordan, D., Richter, D. W. and Spyer, K. M. (1984) Synaptic mechanisms involved in the inspiratory modulation of vagal cardio-inhibitory neurones in the cat. J. Physiol., 356: 65–78.

Gwyn, D. G. and Leslie, R. A. (1979) A projection of vagus nerve to the area subpostrema in the cat. Brain Res., 161: 335–341.

Gwyn, D. G. and Wolstencroft, J. H. (1968) Cholinesterases in the area subpostrema. J. Comp. Neurol., 133: 289–308.

Gwyn, D. G., Leslie, R. A. and Hopkins, D. A. (1979) Gastric afferents to the nucleus of the solitary tract in the cat. Neurosci. Lett., 14: 13–17.

Harris, M. C. and Banks, D. (1985) Midbrain and hindbrain structures activated by carotid body chemoreceptor stimulation: a 14C-2-deoxyglucose study in the rat. Neurosci. Lett. Suppl., 21: S59.

Heymans, C. and Neil, E. (1958) Reflexogenic Areas of the Cardiovascular System, Churchill, London.

Higgins, G. A. and Schwaber, J. S. (1981) Afferent organization of the nucleus tractus solitarius of the rabbit: evidence for overlap of forebrain and primary afferent inputs. Anat. Rec., 199: 114A.

Higgins, G. A., Hoffman, G. E., Wray, S. and Schwaber, J. S. (1984) Distribution of neurotensin immunoreactivity within baroreceptive portions of the nucleus tractus solitarius and dorsal vagal nucleus of the rat. J. Comp. Neurol., 226: 155–164.

Hildebrandt, J. R. (1974) Central connections of aortic depressor and carotid sinus nerves. Exp. Neurol., 45: 590–605.

Hilton, S. M. and Spyer, K. M. (1971) Participation of the anterior hypothalamus in the baroreceptor reflex. J. Physiol., 218: 271–293.

Hilton, S. M. and Zbrozyna, A. W. (1963) Amygdaloid region for defence reactions and its efferent pathway to the brain stem. J. Physiol., 165: 160–173.

Hopkins, D. A. and Holstege, G. (1978) Amygdaloid projections to the mesencephalon, pons and medulla oblongata in the cat. Exp. Brain Res., 32: 529–547.

Humphrey, D. R. (1967) Neuronal activity in the medulla oblongata of cat evoked by stimulation of the carotid sinus nerve. In P. Kezdi (Ed.), Baroreceptors and Hypertension, Pergamon Press, Oxford, pp. 131–168.

Ingram, W. R. and Dawkins, E. A. (1945) The intramedullary course of afferent fibres of the vagus in the cat. J. Comp. Neurol., 82: 157–168.

Jordan, D. and Spyer, K. M. (1979) Studies on the excitability of sinus nerve afferent terminals. J. Physiol., 297: 123–134.

Jordan, D., Spyer, K. M. and Wood, L. M. (1985) Forebrain influences on brainstem neurones receving inputs from cardiovascular afferents. In R. Hainsworth (Ed.), International Symposium on Cardiogenic Reflexes, Leeds, September 1985, Oxford University Press, Oxford.

Kalia, M. and Mesulam, M. M. (1980a) Brain stem projections of sensory and motor components of the vagus complex in the cat: I. The cervical vagus and nodose ganglion. J. Comp. Neurol., 193, 435–465.

Kalia, M. and Mesulam, M. M. (1980b) Brain stem projections of sensory and motor components of the vagus complex in the cat: II. Laryngeal, tracheobronchial, pulmonary, cardiac and gastrointestinal branches. J. Comp. Neurol., 193: 467–508.

Kalia, M. and Richter, D. W. (1985a) Morphology of physiologically identified slowly adapting lung stretch receptor afferents stained with intra-axonal horseradish peroxidase in the nucleus of the tractus solitarius of the cat. I. A light microscopic analysis. J. Comp. Neurol., 241: 503–520.

Kalia, M. and Richter, D. W. (1985b) Morphology of physiologically identified slowly adapting lung stretch receptor afferents stained with intra-axonal horseradish peroxidase in the nucleus of the tractus solitarius of the cat. II. An ultrastructural analysis. J. Comp. Neurol., 241: 521–535.

Kalia, M. and Welles, R. V. (1980) Brain stem projections of the aortic nerve in the cat: A study using tetramethylbenzidine as the substrate for horseradish peroxidase. Brain Res., 188: 23–32.

Kannan, H. and Yamashita, H. (1985) Connections of neurons in the region of the nucleus tractus solitarius with the hypothalamic paraventricular nucleus: their possible involvement in neural control of the cardiovascular system in rats. Brain Res., 329: 205–212.

Katz, D. M. and Karten, H. J. (1979) The discrete anatomical localization of vagal aortic afferents within a catecholamine-containing cell group in the nucleus solitarius. Brain Res., 171: 187–195.

Katz, D. M. and Karten, H. J. (1983) Visceral representation within the nucleus of the tractus solitarius in the pigeon (*Columba livia*). J. Comp. Neurol., 218: 42–73.

Kerr, F. W. L. (1962) Facial, vagal and glossopharyngeal nerves in the cat. Arch. Neurol., 6: 264–281.

Kidd, C. (1979) Central neurons activated by cardiac receptors. In R. Hainsworth, C. Kidd and R. J. Linden (Eds.), Cardiac Receptors, Cambridge University Press, Cambridge, pp. 377–403.

Kimmel, D. L. and Kimmel, C. B. (1964) Spinal distribution of glossopharyngeal and vagal afferent fibres in the cat, rat and guinea pig. Anat. Rec., 148: 299–300.

Korner, P. I. (1979) Central nervous control of autonomic cardiovascular function. In R. M. Berne, N. Sperelakis and S. R. Geiger (Eds.), Handbook of Physiology: The Cardiovascular System, Vol. 1, American Physiological Society, Washington, DC, pp. 691–739.

Kostreva, D. R. (1983) Functional mapping of cardiovascular reflexes and the heart using 2-[^{14}C]deoxyglucose. The Physiologist, 26: 333–350.

Kubin, L. and Davies, R. O. (1985) Antidromic mapping of the brainstem projection of pulmonary rapidly adapting receptor neurons in the cat. In A. L. Bianchi and M. Denavit-Saubié (Eds.), Neurogenesis of Central Respiratory Rhythm, MTP Press Ltd., Lancaster, pp. 262–265.

Leslie, R. A., Gwyn, D. G. and Hopkins, D. A. (1982) The ultrastructure of the subnucleus gelatinosus of the nucleus of the tractus solitarius in the cat. J. Comp. Neurol., 206: 109–118.

Lipski, J. and Trzebski, A. (1975) Bulbospinal neurones activated by baroreceptor afferents and their possible role in inhibition of preganglionic sympathetic neurons. Pflügers Arch., 356: 181–192.

Lipski, J., McAllen, R. M. and Trzebski, A. (1976) Carotid baroreceptor and chemoreceptor inputs onto single medullary neurones. Brain Res., 107: 132–136.

Lipski, J., McAllen, R. M. and Spyer, K. M. (1977) The carotid chemoreceptor input to the respiratory neurones of the nucleus of tractus solitarius. J. Physiol., 269: 797–810.

Loewy, A. D. and Burton, H. (1978) Nuclei of the solitary tract: efferent projections to the lower brain stem and spinal cord of the cat. J. Comp. Neurol., 181: 421–450.

McAllen, R. M. (1973) Projections of the Carotid Sinus Baroreceptors to the Medulla of the Cat, Ph.D. Thesis, University of Birmingham.

McAllen, R. M. (1976) Inhibition of the baroreceptor input to the medulla by stimulation of the hypothalamic defence area. J. Physiol., 257: 45–46P.

McCall, R. S., Gebber, G. L. and Barman, S. M. (1977) Spinal interneurones in the baroreceptor reflex arc. Am. J. Physiol., 232: H657–H665.

Mesulam, M. M. (1978) Tetramethyl benzidine for horseradish peroxidase neurohistochemistry: A non-carcinogenic blue reaction product with superior sensitivity for visualizing neural afferents and efferents. J. Histochem. Cytochem., 26: 106–117.

Miura, M. (1975) Postsynaptic potentials recorded from the nucleus of the solitary tract and its subadjacent reticular formation elicited by stimulation of the carotid sinus nerve. Brain Res., 100: 437–440.

Miura, M. and Reis, D. J. (1972) The role of the solitary and paramedian reticular nuclei in mediating cardiovascular reflex responses from carotid baro- and chemoreceptors. J. Physiol., 223: 525–548.

Moruzzi, P., Schwaber, J. S., Spyer, K. M. and Turner, S. A. (1984) Amygdaloid influences on brainstem neurones in the rabbit. J. Physiol., 353, 43P.

Nomura, S. and Mizuno, N. (1982) Central distribution of afferent and efferent components of the glossopharyngeal nerve. An HRP study in the cat. Brain Res., 236: 1–13.

Nosaka, S. (1976) Responses of rat brainstem neurons to carotid occlusion. Am. J. Physiol., 231: 20–27.

Nosaka, S. (1984) Solitary nucleus neurons transmitting vagal visceral input to the forebrain via a direct pathway in rats. Exp. Neurol., 85: 493–505.

Nosaka, S., Kamaike, T. and Yasunaga, K. (1978) Central vagal organization in rats: An electrophysiological study. Exp. Neurol., 60: 405–419.

Panneton, W. M. and Loewy, A. D. (1980) Projections of the carotid sinus nerve to the nucleus of the solitary tract in the cat. Brain Res., 191: 239–244.

Porter, R. (1963) Unit responses evoked in the medulla oblongata by vagus nerve stimulation. J. Physiol., 168: 717–735.

Potter, E. K. (1981) Inspiratory inhibition of vagal responses to baroreceptor and chemoreceptor stimuli in the dog. J. Physiol., 316: 177–190.

Rhoton, A. L., O'Leary, J. L. and Ferguson, J. P. (1966) The trigeminal, facial, vagal and glossopharyngeal nerves in the monkey. Arch Neurol., 14: 530–540.

Ricardo, J. A. and Koh, E. T. (1978) Anatomical evidence of direct projections from the nucleus of the solitary tract to the hypothalamus, amygdala, and other forebrain structures in the rat. Brain Res., 153: 1–26.

Richter, D. W., Camerer, H. and Sonnhof, U. (1978) Changes in extracellular potassium during the spontaneous activity of medullary respiratory neurones. Pflügers Arch., 376: 139–149.

Ross, C. A., Ruggiero, D. A. and Reis, D. J. (1981) Afferent projections to cardiovascular portions of the nucleus of the tractus solitarius in the rat., Brain Res., 223: 402–408.

Rudomin, P. (1967) Presynaptic inhibition induced by vagal afferent volleys. J. Neurophysiol., 30: 964–981.

Rudomin, P. (1968) Excitability changes of superior laryngeal, vagal and depressor afferent terminals produced by stimulation of the solitary tract nucleus. Exp. Brain Res., 6: 156–170.

Rudomin, P., Burke, R. E., Nuñez, R., Madrid, J. and Dutton, H. (1975) Control by presynaptic correlation: a mechanism affecting information transmission from la fibers to motoneurones. J. Neurophysiol., 38: 267–284.

Saper, C. B. (1982) Convergence of autonomic and limbic connections in the insular cortex of the rat. J. Comp. Neurol., 210: 163–173.

Saper, C. B., Loewy, A. D., Swanson, L. W. and Cowan, W. N. (1976) Direct hypothalmo-autonomic connections. Brain Res., 117: 305–312.

Sapru, H. N. and Krieger, A. J. (1977) Carotid and aortic chemoreceptor function in the rat. J. Appl. Physiol., 42: 344–348.

Sapru, H. N., Gonzalez, E. and Krieger, A. J. (1981) Aortic nerve stimulation in the rat: cardiovascular and respiratory responses. Brain Res. Bull., 6: 393–398.

Schutze, I., Knuepfer, M. M. and Stock, G. (1982) Afferent input to the amygdaloid complex in the cat. Pflügers Arch., 394: R54.

Schwaber, J. and Schneiderman, N. (1975) Aortic nerve-activated cardioinhibitory neurons and interneurons. Am. J. Physiol., 229: 783–789.

Seiders, E. P. and Stuesse, S. L. (1984) A horseradish peroxidase investigation of carotid sinus nerve components in the rat. Neurosci. Lett., 46: 13–18.

Seller, H. and Illert, M. (1969) The localisation of the first synapse in the carotid sinus baroreceptor reflex pathway and its alteration of the afferent input. Pflügers Arch., 306: 1–19.

Sessle, B. J. (1973) Excitatory and inhibitory inputs to single neurones in the solitary tract nucleus and adjacent reticular formation. Brain Res., 53: 319–331.

Sokoloff, L., Reivich, M., Kennedy, C., Des Rosiers, M. H., Patlak, C. S., Pettigrew, K. D., Sakurada, O. and Shinohara, M. (1977) The [C^{14}]deoxyglucose method for the measurement of local cerebral glucose utilization; theory, procedure, and normal values in conscious and anesthetized albino rat. J. Neurochem., 28: 897–916.

Spyer, K. M. (1981) Neural organisation and control of the baroreceptor reflex. Rev. Physiol. Biochem. Pharmacol., 88: 23–124.

Spyer, K. M. (1982) Central nervous integration of cardiovascular control. J. Exp. Biol., 100: 109–128.

Spyer, K. M. (1984) Central control of the cardiovascular system. In P. F. Baker (Ed.), Recent Advances in Physiology, Vol. 10, Churchill Livingstone, Edinburgh, pp. 163–200.

Stock, G., Schlör, K. H., Heidt, H. and Buss, J. (1978) Psychomotor behaviour and cardiovascular patterns during stimulation of the amygdala. Pflügers Arch., 376: 177–184.

Stock, G., Schmelz, M., Knuepfer, M. M. and Forssmann, W. G. (1983) Functional and anatomic aspects of central nervous cardiovascular regulation. In D. Ganten and D. Pfaff (Eds.), Current Topics in Neuroendocrinology, Vol. 3, Central Cardiovascular Control, Springer Verlag, Berlin, pp. 1–30.

Stroh-Werz, M., Langhorst, P. and Camerer, H. (1977a) Neuronal activity with cardiac rhythm in the nucleus of the solitary tract in cats and dogs. I. Different discharge patterns related to the cardiac cycle. Brain Res., 133: 65–80.

Stroh-Werz, M., Langhorst, P. and Camerer, H. (1977b) Neuronal activity with cardiac rhythm in the nucleus of the solitary tract in cats and dogs. II. Activity modulation in relationship to the respiratory cycle. Brain Res., 133: 81–93.

Sumal, K. K., Blessing, W. W., Joh, T. H., Reis, D. J. and Pickel, V. M. (1983) Synaptic interaction of vagal afferents and catecholaminergic neurons in the rat nucleus tractus solitarius. Brain Res., 277: 31–40.

Torvik, A. (1956) Afferent connections to the sensory trigeminal nuclei, the nucleus of the solitary tract and adjacent structures. J. Comp. Neurol., 106: 51–141.

Van der Kooy, D., Koda, L. Y., McGinty, J. F., Gerfen, C. R. and Bloom, F. E. (1984) The organisation of projections from the cortex, amygdala and hypothalamus to the nucleus of the solitary tract in rat. J. Comp. Neurol., 224: 1–24.

Von Baumgarten, R. and Aranda Coddou, L. (1959) Distribucion de las aferencias cardiovasculares y respiratorias en las raices bulbares del nervio vago. Acta Neurol. Lat. Am., 5: 267–278.

Von Baumgarten, R. and Kanzow, E. (1958) The interaction of two types of inspiratory neurones in the region of the tractus solitarius of the cat. Arch. Ital. Biol., 96: 361–373.

Wallach, J. H. and Loewy, A. D. (1980) Projections of the aortic nerve to the nucleus tractus solitarius in the rabbit. Brain Res., 188: 247–251.

Weiss, G. K. and Crill, W. E. (1969) Carotid sinus nerve: primary afferent depolarisation evoked by hypothalamic stimulation. Brain Res., 16: 269–272.

Widdicombe, J. G. (1982) Pulmonary and respiratory tract receptors. J. Exp. Biol., 100: 41–57.

Subject Index